Health and Fitness for Life

Raschel Larsen

Health and Fitness for Life

ISBN: 978-1-943536-34-4

Beta Edition 1.0 Winter 2018

Chemeketa Press

Chemeketa Press is a nonprofit publishing endeavor at Chemeketa Community College that works with faculty, staff, and students to create affordable and effective alternatives to commercial textbooks. All proceeds from the sales of this textbook go toward the development of new textbooks. To learn more, visit www.chemeketapress.org.

Publisher: Tim Rogers

Managing Editor: Steve Richardson

Production Editor: Brian Mosher

Instructional Editor: Stephanie Lenox

Manuscript Editors: Catherine Shride and Chris Cottrell

Design Editor: Ronald Cox IV

Cover Design: Ronald Cox IV

Interior Design: Faith Martinmaas, Michael Ovens, Noah Barerra, Keyiah McClain, Shaun Jaquez

Cover photo by Holly Mandarich is in the public domain (https://unsplash.com/photos/c2aLW24QqGc).

Printed in the United States of America.

Contents

Chapter 1: **Introduction to Health and Wellness**................1

Chapter 2: **Fitness and Exercise**................27

Chapter 3: **Cardiorespiratory Fitness**................ 55

Chapter 4: **Muscular Strength and Endurance**................79

Chapter 5: **Flexibility**................103

Chapter 6: **Body Composition Basics**................121

Chapter 7: **Nutrition**................153

Chapter 8: **Stress Management**................195

Chapter 9: **Chronic Disease** 243

Chapter 10: **Infectious Disease** 267

Chapter 11: **Substances** 303

Chapter 12: **Environmental Health** 345

Acknowledgments................385

Chapter 1
Introduction to Health and Wellness

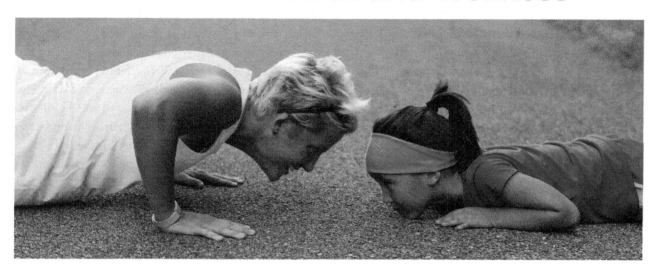

Have you ever thought about what it means to be healthy? We hear a lot about exercise, diet, weight, and illnesses when we talk about health, but the word "healthy" often makes us think about being "unhealthy." The same is true about being "well." When a friend asks you "How are you?" and you respond with "I'm well, thank you," what are you really saying? Does it just mean not sick? Are you envisioning someone with constant physical and emotional struggles because of their lifestyle choices as someone who is *not* well? Or does it mean that you personally feel great and highly functional in your daily routine? Sure, in comparison to your friend Chuck who eats fast food from the comfort of his recliner all day, you *do* seem healthy, but are you being honest with yourself about your own functionality? Are you doing enough to maintain or improve your quality of life?

We've all heard the phrases "life is short" and "live life to the fullest." Chuck may be enjoying those onion rings and his recliner, but you'd hardly consider his life full and are likely concerned about his longevity. When you ask him to hike up to the top of Multnomah Falls with you to see the view, will he go? Can *you* make it to the top (Figure 1)?

It's easy to say that you don't want to, that it's not important. Who really wants to witness the sunrise peeking through white, fluffy clouds above the Columbia River while listening to the water plunge down the side of a mountain as birds sing in your ear? It may suggest that witnessing something majestic really isn't interesting to you, or it may suggest that your health is impacting your quality of life. Can you get through your work or school day giving everything your best effort? If the answer is no, your life may not be as meaningful as you would like it to be.

The little choices and small decisions you make each day add up over the course of your lifetime — good or bad. They can make the difference not only in how long you live but also what you are able to do with that time. Your decision to exercise this morning before work gave you the energy to get through your shift and smile at customers. The salad you chose at lunch gave you the nutrients you needed to fight off that flu bug that has been going around.

Your friend Chuck in the recliner probably made a series of choices that have now impacted his quality of life. Imagine if that had been a series of different choices,

Figure 1. Multnomah Falls.

even small choices, over the course of a year. He may have been hiking the Pacific Crest Trail with his friends or getting a promotion due to his efforts at work. He may have been helping in his local community or building orphanages in developing countries. There are short- and long-term payoffs when we make decisions that impact our health and wellness.

Health is a person's physical and mental state. Public health refers to the health condition in a group of people, and is linked to life expectancy, disease, and wellness. Wellness is a set of multidimensional factors of individuals' health that can be improved through changes in behavior. In order to improve public health, individuals must make choices that improve their individual health and wellness. That's all you have control over. You may not be able to get Chuck to put down the junk food and take a walk, but you can make sure that you don't end up trapped in your own recliner.

The more individuals who take charge of their health or wellness, the happier and healthier we are as a society. We are able to respond in times of need. We spend less money on illness and more on prevention. You can use the terms "health" and "wellness" to refer to big picture and individual statuses. This book will encourage you to be healthy yourself and to focus on your personal wellness.

This chapter will define and explain health and wellness, show why wellness is so important, and describe a basic goal-setting method for improving individual behaviors associated with wellness.

What Are Health and Wellness?

Health and wellness are linked in definition and so are often used interchangeably. While **health** refers to the general condition of our bodies and minds, **wellness** can be considered a deliberate effort to actually be healthy.

The term "health" has evolved since Hippocrates, one of the most noted medical practitioners in ancient Greece, began teaching people ways to fight diseases and to look at the body as a whole unit. In 1948, the **World Health Organization (WHO)**, a division of the United Nations, defined health as "a state of complete physical, mental, and social well-being, and not merely the absence of disease or infirmity," a definition they still utilize today. What both have in common is the idea that health is not just about being free of sickness, but also about the holistic nature of the body and its capability to keep us thriving in life.

Wellness is a work in progress in the US, and its importance comes down to keeping people alive longer and maintaining or improving quality of life. As a nation, our population's average life expectancy, its likelihood of developing disease and disability, and the average amounts of physical activity we perform are all used to measure health status and determine longevity and quality of life. That status helps determine public policy about individuals' well-being, leading to a healthier population. Our collective health only improves if lots of individuals make improvements to these areas.

Wellness is an active process. It is the individual pursuit of improvements to all the different dimensions of personal success. Each dimension of wellness factors into individual wellness, and each well person contributes to the health status of their community. All people

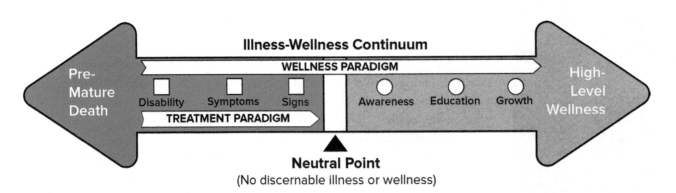

Figure 2. Illness-wellness continuum.

are somewhere on a continuum, with wellness at one end and illness at the other, and every action they take causes them to shift their position on that continuum, either toward illness or wellness (Figure 2).

The US still struggles with certain health-related issues, but it has come a long way compared to the time of Hippocrates (around 460 BC) and the foundation of the WHO in 1948. Much of this is due not only to advances in medical care but also to programs that bring awareness to individuals — to you, for example — about the importance of health and wellness. You can make changes to your lifestyle to help you live a longer, happier life and avoid disease. Those changes happen in the dimensions of wellness. If enough people pursue wellness, the health status of the population can improve.

Dimensions of Wellness

Wellness includes seven dimensions of an individual's well-being. These dimensions should be thought of as an interactive web where each dimension overlaps and intersects with others in different ways. The whole group of seven dimensions makes up overall wellness, and each dimension has important qualities. The dimensions all have this in common: they are equal parts recognition of the dimension's qualities and acting on that knowledge.

Physical wellness is the complete physical conditioning and functioning of the body. It includes physical fitness, eating habits, sleeping habits, and choices that affect your risk of illness or injury, such as substance use/abuse, sexual habits, safe-driving habits, and other self-care practices like getting regular check-ups and

Factors	Percentage of Students Affected
Stress	32.2%
Anxiety	24.9%
Sleep Difficulties	20.6%
Depression	15.4%
Work	14.2%
Cold/Flu/Sore Throat	13.0%
Concern for Troubled Friend or Family Member	10.1%
Extracurricular Activities	9.4%
Internet/Computer Games	9.0%
Relationship Difficulties	8.5%

Figure 3. Top 10 reported impediments to academic performance — past 12 months.

recognizing symptoms of disease. Physically well individuals recognize the differences between healthy habits that increase their physical well-being and destructive habits that decrease their well-being, and then make choices that help them rather than hurt them. Knowing which habits lead to physical wellness is part of this dimension and actions make up the rest.

Emotional wellness describes the ability to cope with the inevitable challenges of daily life. An emotionally well person acknowledges that difficulties are normal, and embraces and shares equally the ups of joy, hope, and happiness and the downs of anger, fear, and sadness. They handle their emotions with a generally positive outlook and control their behavioral response to strong feelings. They may experience stress but learn to manage and cope

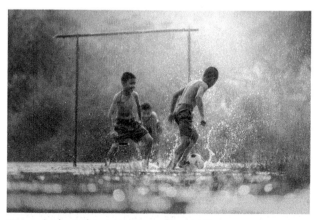

Figure 4. Physical activity is important at all ages.

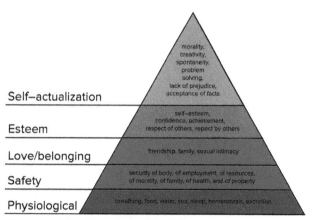

Figure 5. Maslow's hierarchy of needs.

Social Wellness	is the ability to relate to and connect with other people in our world. Our ability to establish and maintain positive relationships with family, friends and co-workers contributes to our Social Wellness.
Emotional Wellness	is the ability to understand ourselves and cope with the challenges life can bring. The ability to acknowledge and share feelings of anger, fear, sadness or stress; hope, love, joy and happiness in a productive manner contributes to our Emotional Wellness.
Spiritual Wellness	is the ability to establish peace and harmony in our lives. The ability to develop congruency between values and actions and to realize a common purpose that binds creation together contributes to our Spiritual Wellness.
Environmental Wellness	is the ability to recognize our own responsibility for the quality of the air, the water and the land that surrounds us. The ability to make a positive impact on the quality of our environment, be it our homes, our communities or our planet contributes to our Environmental Wellness.
Occupational Wellness	is the ability to get personal fulfillment from our jobs or our chosen career fields while still maintaining balance in our lives. Our desire to contribute in our careers to make a positive impact on the organizations we work in and to society as a whole leads to Occupational Wellness.
Intellectual Wellness	is the ability to open our minds to new ideas and experiences that can be applied to personal decisions, group interaction and community betterment. The desire to learn new concepts, improve skills and seek challenges in pursuit of lifelong learning contributes to our Intellectual Wellness.
Physical Wellness	is the ability to maintain a healthy quality of life that allows us to get through our daily activities without undue fatigue or physical stress. The ability to recognize that our behaviors have a significant impact on our wellness and adopting healthful habits (routine check ups, a balanced diet, exercise, etc.) while avoiding destructive habits (tobacco, drugs, alcohol, etc.) will lead to optimal Physical Wellness.

Figure 6. The dimensions of wellness.

with it as it occurs . People with emotional wellness often share certain qualities, such as optimism, trust, enthusiasm, self-confidence, self-acceptance, resiliency, and self-esteem.

Intellectual wellness describes the ability to use logic and problem-solving to respond to experiences and continue to learn throughout life. An intellectually well person applies this open-mindedness to their own decisions, their interactions with others, and the improvement of their community as a whole. They want to learn about new things. They want to improve their sense of self, build upon their skills, and challenge themselves to see life in new ways.

Social wellness describes the ability to interact and connect with others in your family, your community, and the world around you. A socially well person develops and nurtures positive relationships with acquaintances, co-workers and colleagues, friends, and family. Social wellness is about more than just spending time with others. It's about taking an active role in establishing and fostering positive contact with the people in your life. Socially well people confide in and communicate with others respectfully, nurture and support others in different social interactions, and receive love openly and willingly.

Spiritual wellness may be less concrete than the other dimensions but is just as important. A spiritually well person has a sense of meaning and purpose in their life. They can identify their important values, such as compassion, forgiveness, altruism, tolerance, and capacity for love. They can then connect their values with their actions. There are many ways a person can experience spiritual wellness. Some find it through religion. Others practice it through volunteering, spending time in nature, being creative, meditating, or contributing to a greater cause (Figure 9).

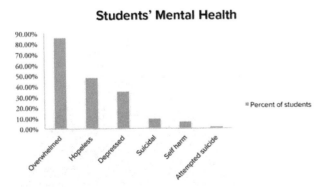

Figure 7. Mental health concerns of American college students — past 12 months.

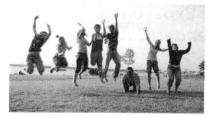

Figure 8. Social wellness.

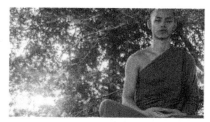

Figure 9. Spiritual wellness.

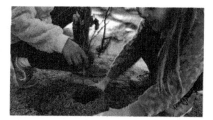

Figure 10. Envionmental wellness.

Environmental wellness describes the ability to take responsibility for the quality of our surroundings. An environmentally well person understands that their actions and decisions have an impact on the safety of the air, water, and land around them and beyond. They finds ways to have a net positive impact on that safety. This dimension of wellness can be experienced at a local level and more broadly at a global level. Positive global impact is possible through participating with others in networks of environmental wellness (Figure 10).

Occupational wellness describes the ability to take pride in the jobs and career fields that we pursue while balancing the demands of our work and home life. A person who is occupationally well contributes to their career with the desire to have a positive impact on the organization or people they work with. They also maintain a healthy balance between that contribution and not working too much or too little. Being able to recognize what this balance looks like for you is critical to your occupational wellness. This enables you to grow at work and still feel satisfied.

Each dimension of wellness needs attention, and many dimensions overlap with one another and can be improved with a single action. For example, some types of exercise, like biking instead of driving to work, can positively impact your physical, emotional, social, and environmental wellness. Each dimension works together to impact your life, and when proper attention is paid to each, your life can be more fulfilling and even be extended by the habits that you've built through your focus on wellness.

Health Challenges in the United States

Medical and technological advancements have improved life expectancy in the US, but we still have areas where we need to improve. Let's look at how some of the measurable factors of health — including causes of death, life expectancy, and health care costs — have changed over the last 100 years.

Causes of Death

The leading causes of death have shifted over the years with advances in science, medical technology, and public health initiatives. In 1900, the leading causes of death were infectious diseases, including pneumonia, influenza, and tuberculosis. We have much lower rates of infectious disease today than we did 100 years ago. The development of vaccines and antibiotics, and improvements in food safety and environmental conditions, are some of the major factors that have reduced the death rate in the US (Figure 11).

Infectious diseases and injuries are still a public health concern, and you can find more information about infectious diseases in Chapter 10.

In 2010, the leading causes of death are chronic

Leading Causes of Death	Number	Percent Of Total Death
All causes	2,626,418	100
Disease of heart	614,348	23.4
Malignant neoplasms	591,700	22.5
Chronic lower respiratory disease	147,101	5.6
Accidents (unintentional injuries)	135,928	5.2
Cerebrovascular disease	133,103	5.1

Figure 11. Leading causes of death in the US.

Top 10 Leading Causes of Death by Gender 2015

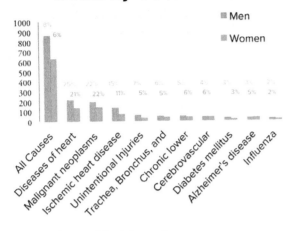

Figure 12. Causes of death by gender.

Life Expectancy by Gender/Country

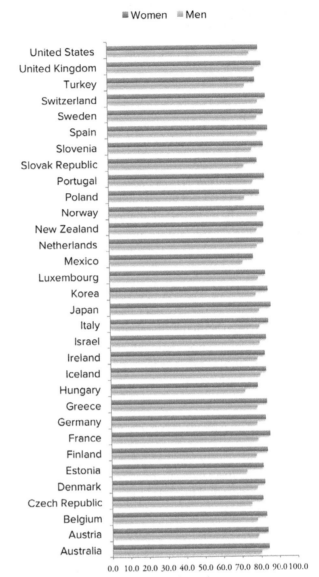

Figure 13. Life expectancy by gender and country.

diseases such as heart disease, cancer, chronic lower respiratory diseases, and cerebrovascular disease (stroke). In fact, nearly half of Americans have at least one chronic disease. Approximately 70% of all deaths in the US are caused by chronic diseases. Other common serious health concerns among Americans today include obesity, unintentional injuries (drug overdose, motor vehicle accidents, unintentional falls), suicide, Alzheimer's disease, depression, anxiety, and other mental health issues.

You can learn more about the causes and treatment of chronic diseases in Chapter 9, but stopping or slowing their development is often related to lifestyle behaviors, such as our level of physical activity, nutrition, and tobacco and alcohol use. Preventing obesity, injuries, and infections is also possible. All of these topics are addressed in later chapters in this book.

The leading causes of death vary by age and gender. Adults in the US age 15–24 are more likely to die from unintentional injuries, homicide and suicide, and adults in the US age 24–44 have higher death rates from unintentional injuries, cancer, and heart disease. Heart disease is the leading cause of death for both men and women in the United States. Cancer is the second leading cause of death for both men and women, with lung cancer

Life Expectancy

Life expectancy is the number of years the average American is predicted to live. This number has risen significantly during the last century. In 1901, the average American could expect to live 49.3 years. In other

having the highest mortality rate. Men, however, are often affected by prostate cancer, while women have higher rates of breast cancer. Men experience higher rates of death from unintentional injury, suicide, and chronic liver disease. Women experience higher death rates from stroke, Alzheimer's disease, and septicemia.

words, most Americans died before their 50th birthday. In 2010, the average life expectancy in the US was 78.8 years, an increase of almost 30 years.

When considering life expectancy, it isn't just about how long we live but how many of those years are lived in good health. This is our **healthy life expectancy**. Your friend Chuck, for example, may live to be 70. Let's face it — he isn't likely to experience an accident if he rarely leaves his recliner. But he could spend the last 20 of those 70 years with a chronic illness like heart disease, cancer, or diabetes related to his physical activity and nutrition. The WHO indicated in 2015 that the healthy life expectancy for an average person in the US was 69.1 years of age, just behind the United Kingdom at 71.4 years.

Average life expectancy in the US varies based on gender, ethnicity, and geography. For example, women have a life expectancy of 81.2 years, and men have a life expectancy of 76.3 years according to the Centers for Disease Control (CDC). The average life expectancy for white Americans is 79 years, while the average life expectancy of African Americans is 75.6 years and Hispanic Americans is 81 years.

The dramatic increase from 1901 to today can be attributed to changes in public policy, such as community education, immunization programs, and the availability of health care, as well as advances in science and technology. Basically, the new ideas in the late 1800s and early 1900s about germ theory and disease led to better health infrastructure and personal behavior. This led to major life-saving scientific innovations like vaccines and medical procedures like surgery and transplants. All of these factors have contributed to the rising life expectancy not just in the US but in developed countries around the world (Figure 13).

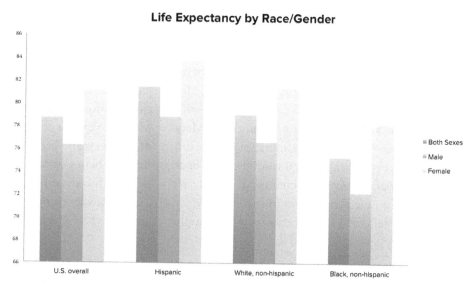

Figure 14. Life expectancy by race and gender.

Health Care Costs

Public health experts also use the cost of health care to measure health in a given population. The dollar amounts spent on treating health problems indicates two things: the frequency and seriousness of health conditions in that population and the relative cost of treatment in their area. This isn't the best way to determine health because it doesn't adjust well for that cost. If the cost of health care in one population is high and the number of health problems are low, the amount spent on health care might still be the same as a population where costs are lower but problems are higher. This doesn't give us a complete picture of health because the cost impacts the amount spent so directly.

However, as a tool for measuring health, cost is an example of how health and wellness intersect. Take the example above. If costs are high and health problems are low, the relative burden on an individual's expenses for

health care causes greater stress in other areas of their lives. They may even have to choose between paying for health care and, say, paying their college tuition. In this scenario, the population's health status (ill or healthy) is relatively positive, but the cost of care negatively impacts the population's wellness.

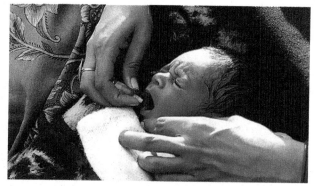

Figure 15. Infant receiving oral vaccine.

Health Disparities and Inequalities

Life expectancy may have increased over time, but there are still too many people who experience younger than average deaths because of factors in their life that are beyond their control. An important thing to consider when describing public health challenges is the unequal way those challenges affect different groups of people. This is called **health disparity** (Figure 17).

Health disparities and inequalities are avoidable, unfair differences in health status that occur within and between populations. For example, differences in chronic disease rates by age, receipt of preventative vaccinations by socioeconomic status, or risky behaviors by race are all examples of health disparities. According to the World Health Organization, the social determinants of health — the conditions in which persons are born, grow, live, work, and age — are mostly responsible for health inequalities.

Let's say, for example, that you and your cousin Mary both have asthma. You have health insurance and live in a quiet, suburban neighborhood. You visit the doctor once each year and your asthma is well controlled. You haven't had a trip to the emergency room in five years. Mary lives in a congested, urban neighborhood of Pittsburgh,

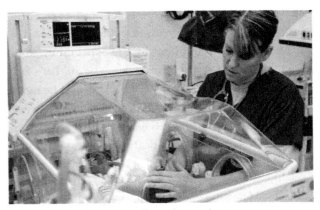

Figure 16. Healthcare provider with a newborn.

Pennsylvania. Her apartment is in a smoggy area on a busy street not far from an industrial plant. She has been forced to make eight trips to the emergency room in the past year. Her asthma is not well-controlled, but she cannot afford to move to an area with better air quality. Mary also cannot afford health insurance that may cover medications and better preventative care. If the air quality were better (something Mary has no control over), her health care costs and need for care would decrease.

Let's look at some examples of health disparities from a Centers for Disease Control report published in 2013.

Mortality

Mortality rate is the statistical odds for when a person will die. When a person dies, basic identifying information about them — age, ethnicity, sex, geographic location, cause of death — is collected in a database.

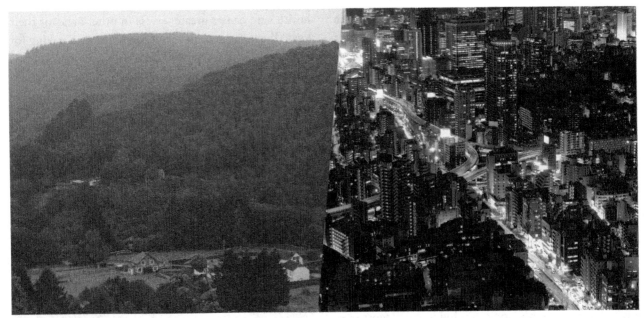

Figure 17. Health outcomes and health care options often differ by geographic location.

The total numbers of death, sorted into these categories, form mortality rates for those segments of a population. For example:

- The rates of premature death (death before age 75 years) from stroke and coronary heart disease were higher among non-Hispanic blacks than among whites.

- The infant mortality rate (death before age one year) for non-Hispanic black women was more than double that for non-Hispanic white women in both 2005 and 2008.

- In 2009, homicide rates were 263% higher among males than females and 665% higher among non-Hispanic blacks compared with non-Hispanic whites. Homicide rates for American Indian/Alaska Natives and Hispanics also far exceeded those of non-Hispanic whites.

- The motor vehicle-related death rate for men is approximately 2.5 times that for women. The motor vehicle-related death rate for American Indian/Alaska Natives is two to five times those for other races/ethnicities.

- Suicide rates were higher for non-Hispanic whites and American Indian/Alaska Natives compared with non-Hispanic blacks, Asian/Pacific Islanders, and persons of Hispanic ethnicity.

Morbidity

Morbidity is the rate people contract infectious or chronic diseases. Morbidity is measured like mortality, by tracking categories of information when people are sick. The information can be used to determine an individual's statistical odds of contracting a disease if they are a member of a given population. For example:

- During 1999–2008, both life expectancy and expected years of life free of activity limitations caused by chronic conditions were significantly greater for females than for males and for whites than for blacks.

- Among persons with asthma, attacks were reported more frequently for children than adults, adults with incomes under 250% of the federal poverty level (FPL) than adults with incomes over 450% of the federal poverty level, and those living in the

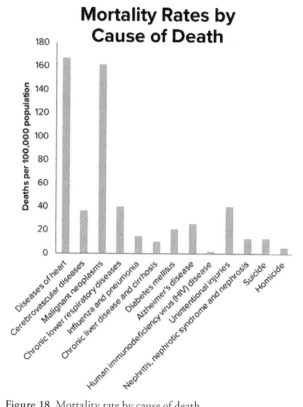

Figure 18. Mortality rate by cause of death.

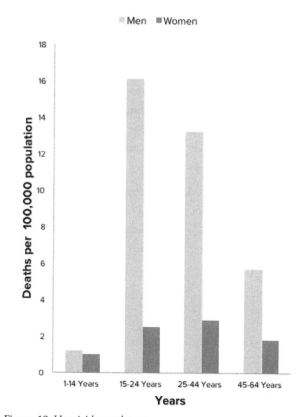

Figure 19. Homicide rate by age.

South and West than the Northeast and Midwest. When discussing the poverty level specifically, the FPL in 2017 was $12,060 for individuals. So, for example, someone with an annual income of less than $30,150 would be more likely to have an asthma attack than someone making $54,270 or more.

- Approximately 50% of people under 30 years had some form of periodontitis (gum disease) during 2009–2010. Prevalence was highest among older adults, non-Hispanic blacks and Mexican Americans, those with lower household income, those with less than a high school education, and current smokers.

- During 1999–2002 and 2007–2010, the prevalence of obesity increased significantly among boys and men but did not increase significantly among girls and women. Disparities persisted in the prevalence of obesity by race/ethnicity, sex, and education.

- Diabetes prevalence was highest among males, people 65 years and older, non-Hispanic blacks and those of mixed race, Hispanics, people with less than a high school education, people who were poor, and people with a disability.

Health Care Access and Preventive Health Services

Health care access and access to preventive health services is a disparity because it may be linked to morbidity. When people don't have easy access to health care, they're less likely to seek care when they need it or advice to avoid illnesses.

- During 2010, 64.5% of the US population aged 50–75 years met the US Preventive Services Task Force's criteria for up-to-date colorectal (colon) cancer screening. Screening increased with age,

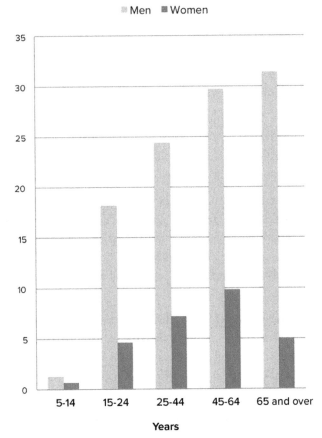

Deaths per 100,00

Figure 20. Suicide rate by age.

education level, and household income. Screening varied by insurance status and race/ethnicity.

- Influenza (flu) vaccination coverage for children increased from the 2009–10 to the 2010–11 season. Among adults aged 65 years and older, coverage increased among Hispanics but decreased among non-Hispanic whites.

Behavioral Risk Factors

Some behaviors put you at greater risk for morbidity and mortality. The statistical likelihood of this can be tracked as well. If more people in a given population engage in risky behaviors, that population is said to be at risk for those behaviors and the consequences that potentially accompany them.

- Binge drinking is more common among persons aged 18–34 years, men, non-Hispanic whites, and people with higher household incomes. Binge drinkers aged 65 years and older report the highest binge drinking frequency, and those 18–24 years and American Indian/Alaska Natives report the highest binge drinking intensity.

- Adolescent birth rates (delivering a child before age 18 years) for non-Hispanic black and Hispanic teenagers remain approximately double those for non-Hispanic whites and Asian/Pacific Islanders. This is despite an 18% decrease in these rates overall during 2007–2010.

- Little progress has been made in reducing cigarette smoking among persons of low socioeconomic status despite improvements in racial/ethnic groups in recent years (Figure 21).

Smoking Status	Total (285)	White (82)	Black/African American (119)	Hispanic (84)
Current Cigarette Smoker	77% (219)	72% (59)	86% (102)	69% (58)
Former Cigarette Smoker	23% (66)	28% (23)	14% (17)	31% (26)

Figure 21. Comparison of current and past smokers (who have quit smoking) by race.

Environmental Hazards

Risks associated with hazardous living, working, and air quality conditions can be tracked using the number of deaths and injuries resulting from those conditions, and comparing that to the categories of people in those environments.

- Racial/ethnic minorities, foreign-born people, and people who speak Spanish or another non-English language at home were more likely to be living near major highways in 2010, suggesting increased exposure to traffic-related air pollution and an elevated risk for adverse health outcomes.

- The likelihood of working in a high risk occupation — an occupation with an elevated injury and illness rate — is greatest for those who are Hispanic, are low wage earners, were born outside of the US, have no education beyond high school, or are male (Figure 22).

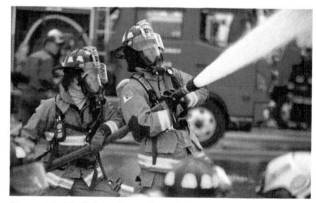

Figure 22. Firefighters have a hazardous job.

- Work-related death rates are highest for those who are Hispanic, are born outside of the United States, or are male. Work-related homicide rates were highest for non-Hispanic blacks, American Indian/Alaska Natives, and Asian/Pacific Islanders.

Social Determinants of Health

Some disparities result from social factors, such as unemployment, poor or incomplete education, and living area. These factors increase morbidity and mortality based on the social impact they have on individual health.

- The prevalence of unemployment was much higher among blacks, Hispanics, and American Indian/Alaska Natives than among whites in 2006 and 2010. In 2010, unemployed adults were much less likely than employed adults to report their health as excellent or very good.

- The highest percentage of adults not completing high school were Hispanic, people with income less than 1.9% of the federal poverty level, those with a disability, or foreign born. The highest percentage of adults living below the federal poverty level were non-Hispanic black or Hispanic, those with less than a high school education, those with a disability, or foreign born.

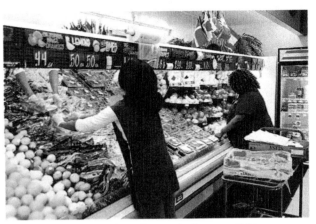

Figure 23. Healthy food retailers aren't always available.

- Persons living in rural census tracts, or living in areas with a higher percentage of senior citizens, or with a higher percentage of non-Hispanic whites, more often lacked at least one healthy food retailer nearby (within ½-mile of the tract boundary) compared with persons living in other census tracts (Figure 23).

What Can Be Done about Health Disparities?

The goal of these public health initiatives, and of looking at health disparities in general, is to achieve health equity, eliminate health disparities, and improve the health of all Americans. The future health of the nation will be determined, to a large extent, by how effectively government and private agencies and organizations work to eliminate disparities that cause disease, disability, and death. The CDC and its partners can use the information they collect to stimulate action on disparities in the US (Figure 24).

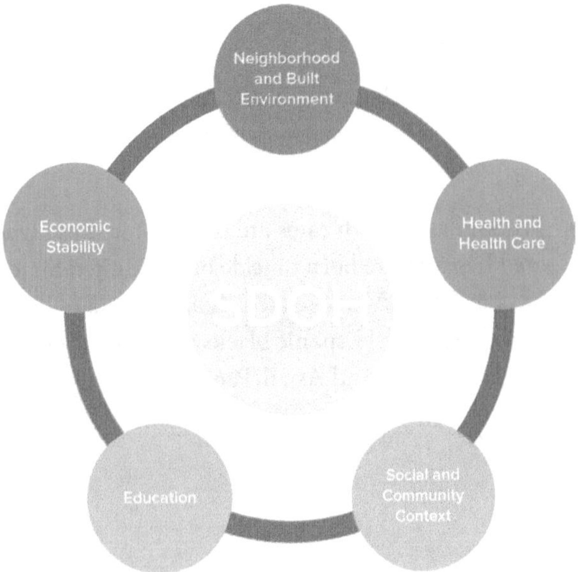

The multiple, complex causes of health disparities can be fully addressed only with the involvement of many people and organizations in fields that influence health such as housing, transportation, education, and business.

Other Determinants

Some barriers to healthy behaviors that come from social disparities can also occur among any group of people, even those without the socioeconomic risk factors listed above. We are all products of our environment, to some extent. Chuck may have been raised by parents who valued the relative safety of their recliner, just as he does. Junk food may have been a main staple of his diet as a child. If we have unhealthy behaviors keeping us from pursuing wellness, the behavioral change we need might take some hard work.

Figure 24. Social determinants of health.

Issues with a lack of motivation, knowledge, resources, willpower, energy, and support can frequently arise from inside the home and from the examples surrounding us in our families and neighborhoods. A tendency to procrastinate or have a negative attitude toward change can be hard-wired into us from an early age. Experiences with public health programs like the ones in public schools can give us knowledge and a desire to improve wellness, but without support at home or in your community, relapsing into poor behaviors after a positive change is common. We have to consider how our behaviors are reinforced and enabled by people around us, and use that knowledge to break the cycle of bad behavior.

Reinforcing

If you've ever spent time with a toddler or trained a pet, then you know what it means to reinforce actions. A toddler might throw herself, kicking and screaming, on the grocery store floor store because she wants a candy bar. If you panic and give her the treat, you are reinforcing her negative behavior. The next time she wants a candy bar at the store, the tantrum might be her first approach. It worked as a strategy to get what she wanted before, so why not try it again?

When a puppy learns to sit on command, you give him a dog treat or say "good boy" in your best puppy voice, motivating him to repeat his behavior. The treat reinforces his positive behavior.

Adults are more complex, of course, and our behaviors can be harder to reinforce. Why? First, our experience with toddlers and puppies makes so we know when reinforcing is happening. We are not so easy to please. Second, we have more control over our situation. If we don't perform to get our "treat," we can often get it ourselves, even if we didn't earn it. Third, our learned behaviors may have become habits after years of bad choices. It may take a lot of the right kind of reinforcement to change them. That doesn't mean we can't do it. It just means that we need to remind ourselves who is in control and choose reinforcements that makes sense for us.

Chuck once spent three months trying to lose weight. He got up from his recliner, took walks, and ate a fairly healthy diet. Each time he lost a few pounds he treated himself to a night of binge-eating. It took him a few days to get back on track after these episodes and he never really lost weight. Instead, he reinforced the same behavior that caused him to gain weight in the first place.

For Chuck, a reward like a new pair of jeans might have done more to reinforce his positive changes in a healthy way. Chuck could have called some friends to take walks with him, giving him a chance to tell them about his progress. They would probably praise his efforts. Both the time spent with friends and their encouraging words would have reinforced his positive behavior change.

Enabling

Certain factors in our environment enable us to slip backward into old habits. Say, for example, that your partner has been instructed by their physician to cut sugar out of their diet. It has been your habit to offer them a homemade cookie each night after dinner. It's really hard for you to give that up, so you continue to do so (you're proud of your baking skills). You tell them that one little cookie won't hurt them. As if on cue, they can't seem to turn down such an amazing cookie. This makes you an enabler of the negative behavior they need to change.

Enabling can be positive, too. Maybe you and a friend have both decided to hit the gym together, but you're really struggling to get motivated. Each time you make an excuse not to go to the gym, your friend shows up in your driveway. They are enabling your success. When we surround ourselves with positive enablers, we set ourselves up for success. Avoiding negative enabling doesn't have to mean you have to stop baking for your spouse. How about finding a sugar-free cookie recipe?

You may not always be in a supportive environment that offers positive reinforcement or enables your success, but that kind of environment can help you make healthier choices more often. You can't always just remove certain people or temptations from your life. We love our families and friends, and we need their support, but forming new support systems to offset unhelpful environments can make a huge difference.

Improving Wellness and Health in the United States

Part of the reason textbooks like this one exist is to help solve challenges to public health. If public health is seen as a problem worth solving, then working toward better public health is everyone's responsibility. The rest of this chapter looks first at how communities are taking action, then provides guidance for how individuals can assess their health status, create a plan for improvements, and effectively take action to improve.

Public Health Initiatives and Programs

The Centers for Disease Control are leading multiple initiatives that address each of the challenges to public health listed above and more. These initiatives range from "action plans" to "strategies," and offer road maps to elimination of the targeted problem within a certain number of years. These initiatives represent the majority of public health programming at the federal governmental level.

One major initiative is the program Healthy People 2020. This is a nationwide set of goals and objectives bringing together many individuals' and organizations' efforts. It is a 10-year program — begun in 2010 and updated in 2012 and 2014 — with objectives that align with measurable improvements to health across the country. These objectives strive to:

- Attain high-quality, longer lives free of preventable disease, disability, injury, and premature death

- Achieve health equity, eliminate disparities, and improve the health of all groups

- Create social and physical environments that promote good health for all

- Promote quality of life, healthy development, and healthy behaviors across all life stages

The initiative began when CDC data revealed that chronic diseases such as heart disease, cancer, and diabetes are responsible for seven out of every ten deaths in the US each year, and that their treatment accounts for 75% of the nation's health spending. Preventing these diseases from occurring in the first place is the primary challenge facing the Department of Health and Human Services, according to a Healthy People 2020 press release.

Healthy People 2020 published a list of objectives that target specific areas of public health in 2010. Each area below has its own set of goals that must be met in order for the initiative to claim improvements in that area:

- Access to Health Services

- Adolescent Health

- Arthritis, Osteoporosis, and Chronic Back Conditions

- Blood Disorders and Blood Safety

- Cancer

- Chronic Kidney Diseases

- Diabetes

- Disability and Secondary Conditions

- Early and Middle Childhood

- Educational and Community-Based Programs

- Environmental Health

- Family Planning

- Food Safety

- Genomics

- Global Health

- Health Communication and Health Information Technology

- Healthcare-Associated Infections

- Hearing and Other Sensory or Communication Disorders (Ear, Nose, Throat — Voice, Speech, and Language)

- Heart Disease and Stroke

- HIV

- Immunization and Infectious Diseases

- Injury and Violence Prevention

- Maternal, Infant, and Child Health

- Medical Product Safety

- Mental Health and Mental Disorders

- Nutrition and Weight Status
- Occupational Safety and Health
- Older Adults
- Oral Health
- Physical Activity and Fitness
- Public Health Infrastructure
- Quality of Life and Well-being
- Respiratory Diseases
- Sexually Transmitted Diseases

- Social Determinants of Health
- Substance Abuse
- Tobacco Use
- Vision

As progress is made in each objective area, the Healthy People 2020 initiative has adjusted their targets based on continuous tracking of the health indicators. Changes were proposed in 2012 and 2014 to adapt to improvements to most objectives and to worsening trends in a few categories.

Assessments of Health and Determinants of Wellness

There are many factors that contribute to public health and individual wellness. You can assess your own health and wellness by investigating the aspects of your life that impact health. The following influences on health and wellness can help you see things you can do every day and long-term habits that can help you maintain a healthy lifestyle.

Be Physically Active

The amount and intensity of recommended physical activity varies for adults and children based on a variety of factors, but the basic guidelines from the US Department of Health and Human Services recommend aerobic activity and strength training for all individuals. At least 150 minutes of moderate activity or 75 minutes of vigorous activity per week is recommended for adults, spread out over several days during a given week. Additional benefits occur with higher levels of activity. Adults should also perform strengthening exercises of moderate or high-intensity at least twice a week with all major muscle groups (Figure 25).

You can find more information on physical activity in chapters 2, 3, 4, and 5.

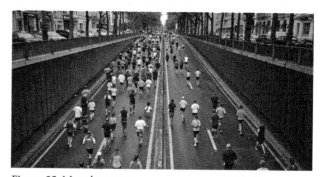

Figure 25. Marathon runners.

Choose a Healthy Diet to Maintain a Healthy Body Weight

A healthy diet gives you the energy and nutrients you need and can help prevent future health problems. Several of the leading causes of disease are connected to nutrition, and choosing healthful foods can help improve your quality of life and overall wellness. According to the *Dietary Guidelines for Americans 2015–2020*, a healthy eating plan:

- Emphasizes fruits, vegetables, whole grains, and fat-free or low-fat milk and milk products (Figure 26)

- Includes lean meats, poultry, fish, beans, eggs, and nuts

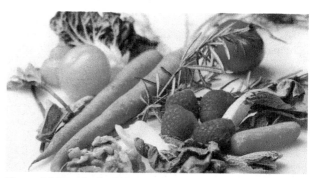

Figure 26. Healthy food choices include vegetables.

- Is low in saturated fats, trans fats, cholesterol, salt (sodium), and added sugars

- Stays within your daily calorie needs

You can find more information on body composition and nutrition in chapters 6 and 7.

Manage Stress

Stress is a normal psychological and physical reaction to the ever-increasing demands of life. Some days by the time we make it to work or school we've already argued with our roommate, spilled coffee on our shirt, been stuck in traffic, and arrived 20 minutes late with the phrase "I'm so stressed" on the tip of our tongue. And those are only the small stressors, the insignificant ones that only matter because they accumulate. Larger stressors, like job loss, illness, or financial worries can pose an even stronger reaction. None of us are immune to it. Surveys show that many Americans experience challenges with stress at some point during the year.

In looking at the causes of stress, remember that your brain comes hard-wired with an alarm system for your protection. When it perceives a threat, it signals your body to release a burst of hormones to fuel your capacity for a response. This has been labeled the "fight-or-flight" response. Once the threat is gone, your body is meant to return to a normal relaxed state. Unfortunately, the nonstop stress of modern life means that your alarm system rarely shuts off.

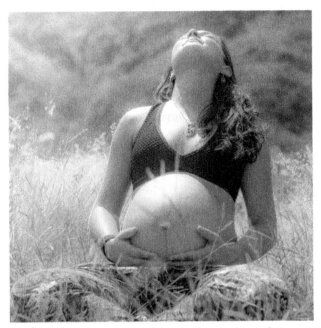

Figure 27. Meditation is just one stress management tool.

That's why learning how to handle it is so important. Stress management gives you a range of tools to reset your alarm system (Figure 27). Without stress management, all too often your body is always on high alert. Over time, high levels of stress can lead to serious health problems. Don't wait until stress has a negative impact on your health, relationships, or quality of life. Start practicing a range of stress management techniques today.

You can find more information about stress management techniques in Chapter 8.

Stressor	Examples
Environmental Stressors	Hypo or hyper-thermic temperatures, elevated sound levels, over-illumination, overcrowding
Daily Stress Events	Traffic, lost keys, quality and quantity of physical activity
Life Changes	Divorce, bereavement
Workplace Stressors	High job demand vs. low job control, repeated or sustained exertions, forceful exertions, extreme postures
Chemical Stressors	Tobacco, alcohol, drugs
Social Stressors	Societal and family demands

Figure 28. Examples of common stressors.

Avoid Tobacco

Tobacco use leads to disease and disability and harms nearly every organ of the body. More than 16 million Americans are living with a disease caused by smoking. For every person who dies because of smoking, at least 30 people live with a serious smoking-related illness. Smoking contributes to cancer, heart disease, stroke, lung diseases, diabetes, and chronic obstructive pulmonary diseases, including emphysema and chronic bronchitis. It also increases risks for tuberculosis, certain eye diseases, and problems of the immune system, including rheumatoid arthritis.

Being around someone who smokes for an extended period of time (such as living with a smoker) or working in a smoke-laden environment can also present risk. Secondhand smoke exposure contributes to approximately 41,000 deaths among nonsmoking adults and 400 deaths in infants each year (Figure 29). It increases the risk of stroke, lung cancer, and coronary heart disease in adults. Children who are exposed to secondhand smoke are at increased risk for sudden infant death syndrome, acute respiratory infections, middle ear disease, more severe asthma, respiratory symptoms, and slowed lung growth.

Second hand smoke impairs a child's ability to learn, and high levels of exposure are associated with deficits in reading, math, and spatial reasoning.

Children who breathe second hand smoke are at an increased risk for ear infections.

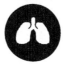
Children who breathe second hand smoke are more likely to suffer from pneumonia, bronchitis, asthma, and other lung diseases.

Pets in smoking households have a 60% higher risk of developing lung cancer.

Figure 29. Second hand smoke affects those around you, even animals.

The good news is that people who use tobacco can quit and the body is able to recover from much of the damage, especially if a person stops using tobacco while a young adult (Figure 30).

You can find more information about the dangers of tobacco and strategies for quitting in Chapter 11.

After Quitting for	Results
20 Minutes	Circulation improves in the hands and feet.
2 Hours	Pulse, heartbeat, and blood pressure normalize.
8 Hours	Carbon monoxide is reduced and no longer stops oxygen from reaching the blood cells.
24 Hours	Your risk of heart attack drops.
48 Hours	Nicotine is completely eliminated from your body.
1 Week	Blood pressure falls.
3 Months	On average lung capacity rises by 39 percent.
3 to 9 Months	Smokers cough and susceptibility to infections are reduced.
12 Months	The risk of cardiovascular disease is halved.
5 Years	The risk of stomach, mouth, throat, esophageal, and lung cancer is halved.
10 Years	Cell and tissue that were precancerous have largely been replaced.
15 Years	Your risk of cancer is the same amount as that of a nonsmoker.

Figure 30. The benefits of quitting smoking begin almost immediately and continue for several years.

Get Adequate Sleep

Insufficient sleep is associated with a number of chronic diseases and conditions — such as diabetes, cardiovascular disease, obesity, and depression — which threaten our nation's health. Inadequate sleep is also responsible for motor vehicle and machinery-related crashes, causing substantial injury and disability each year (Figure 31). In testing done on sleep-deprived individuals using a driving simulator, the participants often performed the same or worse than a person who was intoxicated. Some Americans have become so accustomed to functioning while sleep deprived that they don't even realize the toll it takes on their minds and bodies — it just becomes a new, riskier version of normal.

Often, this lack of sleep is self-inflicted and well within our control. How many times have you stayed up late bingeing a television series, playing a game on your laptop, or checking social media? How often have you put off writing an essay for a class until 2:00am the day it is due? You knew you would be tired the next day, but you may not have known how dangerous it might be to you or those around you. That is because many of us have allowed ourselves to accept being tired as a part of life.

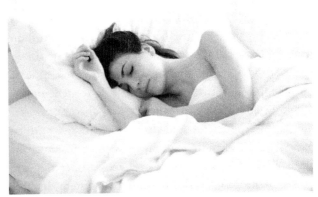

Figure 31. Not getting enough sleep can affect your health.

Over 25% of the US population report occasionally not getting enough sleep, while nearly 10% experience chronic insomnia. However, new methods for assessing and treating sleep disorders bring hope to the millions suffering from insufficient sleep. For those of us who miss out on adequate sleep due to poor planning or poor choices, it's time for a "wake up call." Getting sufficient sleep is not a luxury — it is a necessity — and should be thought of as a "vital sign" of good health.

Limit Alcohol Consumption

Excessive alcohol use, including underage drinking and binge drinking (drinking 5 or more drinks on an occasion for men or 4 or more drinks on an occasion for women), can lead to an increased risk of health problems such as injuries, violence, liver disease, and cancer. Excessive alcohol use was responsible for approximately 88,000 deaths and 2.5 million years of potential life lost (the amount of expected life left after early deaths) each year in the United States from 2006–2010, shortening the lives of those who died by an average of 30 years. In addition, excessive drinking was responsible for one in every ten deaths among working-age adults aged 20–64 years.

Excessive alcohol use has immediate effects that increase your risk for many harmful health conditions. People who have been binge drinking have increased risk of:

- Injuries, such as motor vehicle crashes, falls, drownings, and burns

- Violence, including homicide, suicide, sexual assault, and intimate partner violence

- Alcohol poisoning, a potentially fatal medical emergency that results from high blood alcohol concentration

- Risky sexual behaviors including unprotected sex or sex with multiple partners, potentially resulting in unintended pregnancy or sexually transmitted diseases (including HIV)

- Non-consensual sexual activity

- Miscarriage and stillbirth or fetal alcohol spectrum disorders among pregnant women

Over time, excessive alcohol use can lead to the development of chronic diseases and other serious problems including:

- High blood pressure, heart disease, stroke, liver disease, and digestive problems

- Cancer of the breast, mouth, throat, esophagus, liver, and colon

- Learning and memory problems, including dementia and poor school performance

- Mental health problems, including depression and anxiety

- Social problems, including lost productivity, family problems, and unemployment

- Alcohol dependence or alcoholism

By limiting alcohol consumption, you can reduce the risk of these short and long-term health risks. You can find more information about alcohol abuse and treatment in Chapter 11.

Protect Yourself from Infectious Diseases

Everyone is exposed to germs on a regular basis. You can't help it. Some can live on surfaces like door handles and ATM buttons for up to 24 hours, making it easy for them to spread from person to person. Some may be the common cold virus, while others, like bacterial meningitis, can be dangerous and cost you a stay in the hospital or even your life.

While you may have heard that it is good to challenge your immune system on occasion, there are steps you can take to avoid being constantly bombarded by infectious agents. Stopping the spread of disease can be as simple as regular, effective hand washing. To wash your hands adequately, follow these steps:

- Wet your hands with running water — either warm or cold

- Apply liquid, bar, or powder soap

- Lather well

- Rub your hands vigorously for at least 20 seconds

- Remember to scrub all surfaces, including the backs of your hands, wrists, between your fingers and under your fingernails

- Rinse well

- Dry your hands with a clean or disposable towel or air dryer

- If possible, use a towel or your elbow to turn off the faucet

In addition to frequent, thorough hand washing, you can often prevent illness or lessen its effects by taking good care of yourself in general. A healthy diet and adequate sleep can keep your body ready to fight what comes its way. When you're fatigued or malnourished, your body doesn't have what it takes to do the job.

Protect Yourself from Injuries

Like avoiding infections, there are simple steps you can take to avoid injuries at home and at play. Whether you're climbing one step too high on a ladder or going swimming in a river with no lifeguard, most of us look at caution or warning signs and think, "It won't happen to me." Instead of considering why certain guidelines exist and being respectful of them, we take that extra step up the ladder, or stupidly jump off the high rock.

Some injuries are more avoidable than others, of course. Be especially careful concerning poisonous household products, playing in or around water, prescription and over-the-counter drug storage, fire safety, motor vehicle and bicycle safety, pedestrian safety, and caring for older adults and children. If the dosage instructions are to take two tablets of acetaminophen every 4 to 6 hours, do that rather than assuming more is better because you're 6 feet tall. Don't play doctor. If the box says to "Keep away from small children," you should probably do that — every time.

Practice Good Self-Care and Seek Appropriate Medical Care

Many people avoid a trip to the doctor like it's a luxury rather than a necessity, but getting regular preventative care and prompt emergency care should be part of your lifestyle. It is important to know your body's limits and understand when you need to seek professional medical help. This is an essential part of maintaining personal health and striving toward wellness. This means being aware of your personal health, identifying the possibility of problems, and not waiting too long to see a doctor, of course, but it also means scheduling regular checkups to find hidden problems before they begin to affect your life.

Apply Critical Thinking Skills as a Health Consumer

In the 21st century, most people who recognize a problem with their health — maybe an unexpected pain or discomfort — visit one of the many health websites on the Internet to seek advice. These websites are a great place to learn introductory information about different verifiable conditions. But they can be alarming to naïve users who go looking for the cause of the pain in their foot, and come away thinking it "could be cancer!" This jump to an extreme conclusion seems to happen all the time, and there's no wonder, since most health information seems so foreign to most readers. It's is an easy trap to fall into, so thinking critically about health advice from a website should be your first line of defense against alarmist cancer fears.

You should always apply your critical thinking skills when researching health information on your own, but this same attitude is helpful when you see advertisements

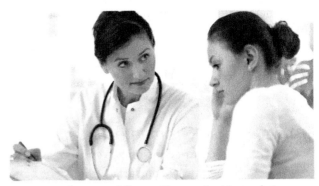

Figure 32. Always carefully consider your healthcare choices..

for prescription medication, pick up a health-related brochure, or even when speaking with a healthcare professional (Figure 32). You don't always need a "second opinion," but being equipped with the knowledge that other opinions are out there can be really useful when a serious situation — like high treatment costs or dangers in a procedure — comes up. Some level of critical thinking is essential in all interactions regarding our health.

Cultivate Relationships and Social Support

Social interactions are some of the most impactful life experiences you will have. Without overstating it, your relationships help define who you are, what your interests are, how you spend your time, and how much enjoyment you get out of life. Nourishing these relationships is a key ingredient to wellness, and represents a significant investment in your health.

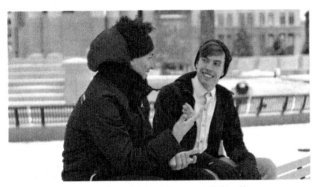

Figure 33. Fostering friendships is key to social wellness.

Don't overlook or take for granted the people in your life who encourage you to improve and grow (Figure 33). The people who rely on you for the same should be met with honesty and loyalty so that you can mutually benefit from your relationships. Responsibility to others is a mark of good citizenship, and becoming a thoughtful and involved member of your community — whatever its size — creates meaningful bonds. Those bonds may come and go, but the experience of growing together and apart is essential to being supported by and supportive of others.

Nourish Your Spiritual Side

Spirituality takes many forms, not just religion and belief in a "higher power." The simplest way to describe spiritual wellness is an alignment between personal values and the purpose of one's life (Figure 34). The idea of spirituality is not that different today than what some in the 19th century called "transcendentalism," or the belief that all of humanity and nature held a divine connection. Today, we might see this universal energy as a god or deity, or we may see it as a deep understanding of our self, our connection to the world and everything in it, or the belief that we have a higher purpose. The things and ideas each person holds up as their values can be totally different, so take time to investigate what your values are. As you do that, think about why you value each of those things. Identifying your values and then pursuing them is a key step to becoming spiritually well.

Isolation and Social Withdrawal	Defining spirituality as a connection to the sacred, and encouraging trauma survivors to seek supportive, healthy communities can directly address these symptoms.
Guilt and Shame	Though not part of the diagnostic criteria for PTSD, guilt and shame are recognized as important clinical issues. Spirituality may lead to self-forgiveness and an emphasis on compassion toward self.
Anger and Irritability	Beliefs and practices related to forgiveness can address anger and chronic hostile attitudes that lead to social isolation and poor relationships with others.
Hypervigilance, Anxiety, and Physiological Arousal	Inwardly-directed spiritual practices such as mindfulness, meditation, and prayer may help reduce hyperarousal.
Foreshortened Future and Loss of Interest in Activities	Rediscovery of meaning and purpose in one's life may potentially have enormous impact on these symptoms.

Figure 34. Focusing on spiritual wellness can have physical effects.

Setting Goals and Understanding How Changes Happen

If you need to change your behavior to better strive toward wellness, there are strategies you can use to increase your chances of success. Two of those strategies are goal-setting and becoming aware of the stages of behavior change that you will likely go through.

Your goals should be short- and long-term. Don't be tempted to have just one humongous goal, like "lose weight," for example. Having a long-term goal is okay, but you should fill the space between the present and your long-term goal with many more short-term goals that you can celebrate meeting along the way. Behavior change is not always an easy process and can be a bit like learning to ride a bike. In case you don't remember, you probably fell a lot when you first got on a bike. To avoid as many of those falls as possible, you should be SMART about the goals you set.

SMART Goals

For your goals to be effective, they should represent SMART thinking. SMART goals are:

- **S — Specific.** Choose goals that target particular actions or behavior. For example, if you want to eat healthier, select a specific nutritional issue. Saying you're going to eat healthier is too general and vague. Instead, say that you will eat more vegetables or prepare more meals at home would be more specific.

- **M — Measurable.** Be sure you can measure your completion and your progress along the way. Creating a nutrition goal to eat more vegetables is specific but not measurable. Include a way to measure the amount of vegetables you eat, such as aiming for three servings per day. If planning to cook more dinners at home, establish a number, such as five per week. If you can't tell whether you've completed your goals or not, chances are you won't be certain if you're meeting them and may be disappointed.

- **A — Achievable.** Set goals that you can actually complete. You may want to lose 20 pounds by next month, but you can't do it safely, if at all, and will be setting yourself up for disappointment. To make goals achievable, it's important to set meaningful goals and goals that are within your limits. Becoming a vegetarian may not be an achievable goal, but eating more vegetables throughout the day and one meatless meal a week may.

- **R — Relevant.** For the same reasons, set goals that are relevant to your life. If you are making a change, make sure that the goals you set put you on a path to that change, and that meeting your goal will let you see progress. Realistic goals are all about meaning. You need to believe they are important and will have a positive impact.

- **T — Time-based.** Your goals should have a limit and be based on some kind of deadline system. Without deadlines attached to your goals, they can go on forever. You may never reach them (Figure 35).

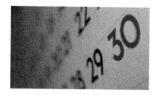

Figure 35. Set deadlines.

We often need to make adjustments to our goals and change the plan over time. It could be that your goals need to be more challenging or more reasonable. Some goals require more lifestyle changes than others and might require more adjustments. When this occurs, it can help to focus on process goals (what you are doing) rather than outcome goals (where you want to be).

For example, you may initially have been trying to lose 15 pounds over a 4-month period but it was more difficult than expected. Try focusing on process, the behaviors you need to change in order to lose the weight. Maybe one goal is to always pack your lunch for school or work so that you don't eat fast food. This process goal can help you adjust your behavior over time and reach your goal.

It's also important to keep your approach flexible. Sometimes things happen beyond our control that can force us to modify our goals. Adjust them to better suit your situation. This is fine as long as you are still progressing toward your goals. No matter what changes you may need to make along the way, making SMART, short- and long-term goals can help you find encouragement in your ability to complete steps toward improving your wellness.

Stages of Change Model

One model for how behavior change happens is the Stages of Change, or Transtheoretical model. It includes six different stages of change individuals must go through on their way to changing their behavior: pre-contemplation, contemplation, preparation, action, maintenance, and termination. The model suggests that each of us is in one of the different stages for any given behavior. Because it can be hard to identify whether you've actually changed your behavior or not, this model can be helpful as you see your progress from one stage to the next. It is also helpful to identify the current stage you are in so that you can develop strategies to help you move to the next stage.

The main idea behind the Stages of Change model is that all the stages are normal parts of changing your behavior. Lapses and relapses are common. Most of the time, people don't fall all the way back to pre-contemplation. People can learn through their mistakes, and moving through the stages can help a person learn what success feels like. With progress comes improved self-efficacy and motivation, so we shouldn't feel too discouraged with some amount of backwards movement (Figure 36).

During the **pre-contemplation** stage, you haven't thought about any changes to your behavior, but you might be noticing unpleasant feelings or conditions that could be connected to the behavior you end up changing. At this stage, you do not intend to start the healthy behavior in the near future (within 6 months), and may be unaware of the need to change. You may also have tried to change in the past but were unsuccessful and now feel frustrated or discouraged. You may be more focused on the reasons not to change than the reasons to change. You may be like Chuck who is still parked in

his recliner, but is noticing that his energy level is deteriorating. He's starting to wonder if he'll ever get to go windsurfing in Hawaii. You haven't yet connected your

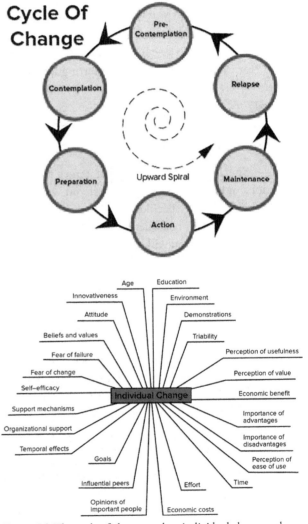

Figure 36. The cycle of change and an individual change web.

feelings to a behavior you have, but something is starting to simmer in the back of your mind about yourself.

During the **contemplation** stage, you start to think that your behavior is problematic and that you might want to make a change in your life (within the next 6 months). You might fantasize about what that change would take or the pros and cons of making the change. You might even start researching ways of taking action. No actions have happened yet, but the wheels are turning. People in this stage learn about the kind of person they could be if they changed their behavior and learn more from people who behave in healthy ways. Others can influence and help you at this stage by encouraging you to reduce the cons of changing your behavior. Chuck wants to exercise more, but he worries that it will make him even more tired. His friend, Roy encourages him by saying that exercising actually gave him more energy, not less.

During the **preparation** stage, you're ready to start taking action within the next 30 days. You take small steps that you believe can help make healthier behavior a part of your life. Chuck might tell his friends and family that he wants to be more active and has started doing a bit of research on diet and exercise. People in this stage should be encouraged to seek support from friends they trust, tell people about their plan to change the way they act, and think about how they would feel if they behaved in a healthier way. Their number one concern is: when they act, will they fail? They learn that the better prepared they are, the more likely they are to keep progressing.

During the **action** stage, you have changed your behavior within the last 6 months and need to work hard to keep moving ahead. Above all, you need to learn how to strengthen your commitments to change and to fight urges to slip back. People in this stage progress by learning techniques for keeping up their commitments (Figure 37), such as replacing activities related to the unhealthy behavior with more positive ones, rewarding themselves for taking steps toward changing, and avoiding people and situations that tempt them to behave in unhealthy ways. In other words, Chuck has been taking brisk walks each day and has been letting his dog take naps in his recliner, making it more difficult for Chuck to get comfortable in it. He has bought a Hawaiian shirt and is saving his money for a vacation to Maui.

During the **maintenance** stage, you changed your behavior at least 6 months ago. It is important to be aware of situations that may tempt you to slip back into doing the unhealthy behavior — particularly stressful situations. The maintenance stage may never end. It is a continual choice to engage in behaviors that are healthy. People in this stage benefit when they seek support from friends and talk with people they trust, spend time with people who behave in healthy ways, and engage in healthy activities to cope with stress instead of relying on unhealthy behavior. Chuck walks his dog with a neighbor every day, practices surfing balance techniques when he watches TV, and is watching airline prices every week for a cheap ticket to Maui.

Termination is the sixth stage that may be reached. This is where people have exited the cycle of change and are no longer tempted to fall into their old behavior. They have developed ways of coping with behaviors and mastered those mechanisms. This may or may not be

Self-Management	Employment of behavior analytic interventions to the behavior of oneself; requires the desired change in the behavior
Self-Monitoring	Procedure in which a person observes his/her own behavior systematically and records occurrence or nonoccurrence of behavior
Self-Instruction	Self generated verbal responses, covert or overt, that function as response prompts for desired behavior; often used to guide a person through a behavior change
Massed Practice	Forcing oneself to perform an undesired behavior repeatedly; occasionally this strategy may decrease behavior
Habit Reversal	A multi-component treatment package for reducing unwanted habits that involves identifying events that precede a target behavior and engaging in competing responses
Token Economy	A contingency package that includes a specified list of responses to reinforce, tokens for exhibiting the specified responses, back-up reinforcers that can be purchased with the token; effectiveness of tokens as reinforcers depends upon the power of back-up reinforcers; response cost is used with most; tokens are generalized conditioned reinforcers for target responses

Figure 37. Behavior change systems.

possible with certain behaviors. Chuck knows his weaknesses. He has replaced his favorite recliner with a chair that is comfortable enough to watch a bit of television from but not comfy enough for meals and naps. Now instead of burrowing into his recliner with a large bag of candy when he's stressed, he goes for a run with his dog, watches just one old episode of *The Three Stooges*, or calls up a friend to go have coffee. The trip to Maui last fall was a blast, and he has the photos to prove it. He now tries to plan at least one surfing trip closer to home every year.

Decisional Balance

When deciding to make a behavioral change, individuals go through a process known as decisional balance, where they weigh the pros and cons of the change (Figure 38). The balance factor of this process is how the number or importance of pros and cons must shift over time as a person gets closer to changing their behavior. The cons of changing outweigh the pros in the pre-contemplation stage. The pros surpass the cons in the middle stages. The pros outweigh the cons in the action stage. Think about how Chuck adjusted his pros and cons above.

Self-Efficacy

Your self-efficacy is your belief in your own ability to succeed in certain situations or under certain influences that may or may not be within your control. This can impact how we approach behavior change and the goals we've set for ourselves. We measure our self-efficacy by how confident we are in high-risk situations that may trigger relapse or present temptation to veer away from our goals.

Let's say, for example, that you are trying to lose weight. Your sister Karen is coming to visit. The two of you typically spend your time trying out new bars and restaurants in Portland and making late-night runs to Voodoo Doughnut. This presents some serious temptation. Your level of confidence that you can keep your calorie intake reasonable is your degree of self-efficacy.

Relapse is not necessarily a stage in itself, but is a return from the action or maintenance stages to an earlier stage. The word "relapse" is most often associated with addictive behaviors, but is very common in other unhealthy behaviors, as well. Achieving a long-term behavior change often requires ongoing support from family members, a health coach, a physician, or another motivational source. Supportive literature and other resources can also be helpful to avoid a relapse.

Cons	Pros
Withdrawal Symptoms including sweating, nausea, headaches, coughing, sore throat, insomnia, and difficulty concentrating	Sharper Hearing
	Better Vision
	Clean Mouth
Cravings	Clear Skin
Difficulty Changing Habits	Decreased Heart Risks
Increased Stress	Lower Cholesterol
Changes In Relationships	Stop Lung Damage
	Money no longer being spent on cigarettes

Figure 38. Sample pros and cons list for quitting smoking.

During the first two stages of change, pre-contemplation and contemplation, the temptation to relapse may be stronger than our ability to refrain from the negative behavior. While we are in the preparation stage and moving to the action stage, the gap between temptation and feelings of self-efficacy closes, and we make a behavior change. Relapse occurs when your self-efficacy to maintain the change is not as great as the temptation in front of you.

Motivation

People who decide to make a behavioral change must be motivated to do so by something in their life. That motivation to change can come from yourself or from others. The source of your motivation can impact your decision making. Internal motivation can be more personally fulfilling, but it lacks the accountability that an external motivation source can provide (e.g., the doctor asking if you've been eating better or your trainer measuring your percentage of body fat).

Your motivation is often impacted by whether you believe you have control over your behavior or not. If you believe you have control over your personal outcomes, it is known as an **internal locus of control** (control is located inside you). If you believe control is internal, changes occur as a result of effort on your part, and your commitment to change will result in positive changes.

If you believe your ability to change is out of your control, it is known as an **external locus of control** (control is outside of you). If you believe control is external, any behavioral change can only result from luck or chance. People who believe they control changes to their behavior are more likely to pursue those changes than people who think they have no control over their behavior.

Being honest with yourself can often help you find an internal locus of control. People are great at making excuses for why they can't make a change or find reasons why their problem is caused by someone or something else. Let's face it — it's easier that way. It's much harder to admit the reality that you haven't yet chosen your health as a priority over the gratification you gain from a particular behavior.

For example, it's easy to say that you can't lose weight because the people around you aren't helping. But maybe if you tracked what you ate during the day you would find that you consumed way more than what is recommended for healthy weight loss. Yes, it's often true that weight loss is more difficult for some people than others due to their gender, a genetic predisposition, or environmental factors. People in those situations can still set realistic goals that they can achieve.

For most people, it comes down to honesty and acceptance of their unique reality. Be honest with yourself about your limitations and strengths and what that means for you as you are setting goals.

Consider all the things you could gain by achieving your goals compared to the things you are giving up by never trying to change. Is the candy you snacked on last night or the pack of cigarettes you smoked yesterday worth the potentially lost years with your family? Do you want to look back on your life and wonder if you could have controlled your behavior, or do you want to do something about it now? If the answer is yes, then you believe you have the power to make positive changes, an internal locus, that can help you as you work toward your goals.

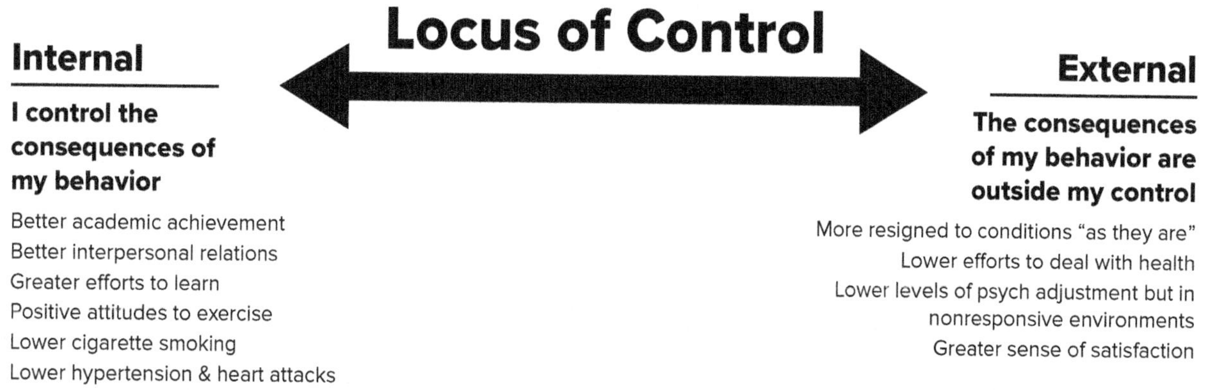

Locus of Control

Internal

I control the consequences of my behavior

Better academic achievement
Better interpersonal relations
Greater efforts to learn
Positive attitudes to exercise
Lower cigarette smoking
Lower hypertension & heart attacks

External

The consequences of my behavior are outside my control

More resigned to conditions "as they are"
Lower efforts to deal with health
Lower levels of psych adjustment but in nonresponsive environments
Greater sense of satisfaction

Figure 39. Internal and external locus of control.

Conclusion

This introductory chapter gives you some critical tools and techniques to learn about public and personal health. We described:

- Definitions of health and wellness dimensions that prepare you to discuss health topics with a community and individual scope

- Challenges to public and personal health as defined by health agency guidelines

- Objectives of several public health initiatives to improve public health and quality of life

- Basic frameworks for assessing your fitness and health status

- SMART goals to help you improve your health status

- Stages of Change model of behavior modification

As you can see from this chapter, learning about health and fitness is not just about defining the terms health scientists use to talk about their field, but applying those terms to your own life to improve your own health. The best thing about studying health and wellness is that it can make an actual difference in people's lives. The following chapters each focus on particular improvement areas, encourage assessment along with SMART goal setting and planning, and recommend training for each area.

Chapter 2
Fitness and Exercise

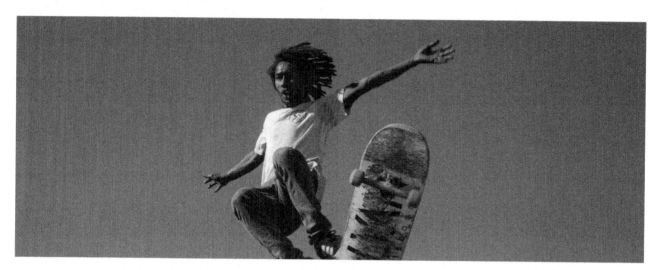

One of the most important aspects of health and wellness is fitness. Fitness is one of the components of the physical dimension of wellness, and several chapters in this book address how fitness plays a role in other dimensions of wellness. Most Americans today begin learning the importance of physical fitness as early as elementary school, yet many of us are not fit and not doing enough to meet the recommended levels of physical activity established by the US Department of Health and Human Services.

In the past, physical fitness was frequently part of the work that people did for their jobs. Today, fitness is something we need to make time for. Technological advancements have erased the physical aspect of work for many people, as productivity, communication, and many other areas of work become digitized or automated. If you think about it, most Americans cruise through life from behind a computer screen or from a smartphone in the palm of their hand.

This chapter will define and explain the differences between fitness, physical activity, and exercise and show why it is important to implement a fitness plan. You will also learn how to create a safe, effective exercise plan. A lifestyle that includes physical activity can have a positive impact on social, intellectual, emotional, and physical wellness that can improve your overall quality of life.

What Does It Mean to Be Fit?

Fitness is the ability to conduct one's daily life without undue fatigue. When we are young and naturally more active, we rarely think about our energy after tying our shoes or walking up a flight of stairs. Things like that never made us tired. But as we get older or we become less physically active, the fatigue that can come from these simple tasks might surprise us (Figure 1). Climbing stairs, doing laundry, shopping, or playing with our children and pets should be easy, but for many Americans with a sedentary lifestyle, routine physical activity can become a struggle, even something to dread.

Being fit is really as simple as being able to just do the things you want to do without worrying about being too tired. It sounds easy, but consider an example where what you want to do and what you're able to do don't quite align. Imagine that you've finally saved enough to take the vacation of your dreams to Brazil. The first day, your family decides to go on a walking tour of Rio de Janeiro, but you know you won't be able to keep up with the kids. You decide to skip it. You spend your afternoon playing Sudoku on your phone in the hotel lobby. The next day, they book a bus tour to an exotic waterfall. You ride along with them, but when it's time to hike to the top of waterfall, you stay on the bus and resume your Sudoku. At the end of the trip, you're late for your flight, and everyone must run to get to the gate in time. Can you make it?

True fitness is really a type of freedom. When we maintain our fitness, we have more energy and agility and fewer physical limitations (Figure 2).

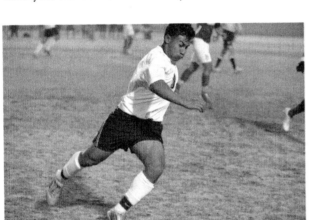

Figure 1. Staying fit means regular activity.

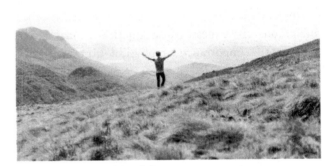

Figure 2. Freedom through fitness.

Defining Fitness

We commonly use the terms, "physical activity," "exercise," and "physical fitness," as if they are the same, but the terms are not interchangeable. Students of health need to know the difference.

Physical activity is any body movement that expends energy. Just getting through your day requires physical activity. This could be as gentle as walking to class, pulling weeds in your garden, or brushing your teeth. It could be as intense as running a half-marathon, biking five miles to work, or swimming laps in the pool at your gym. Different activities have different levels, defined by the amount of energy the activity requires. For example, you will expend more energy swimming laps than while planting flowers. The energy is measured by calories, which are units of heat that are burned during our movements. The amount of calories burned varies based on the intensity of the activity and on each person's physical makeup. For example, swimming at high intensity for ten minutes would result in more energy spent than if you tread water for the same amount of time. Additionally, someone with greater muscle mass may burn more calories during the same swim.

We often think that if we are busy during the day then we are "getting exercise," particularly if the activity makes us tired. Most of our routine physical activities, however, are considered "baseline" rather than "health-enhancing." As we move around doing dishes, folding clothes, or walking the occasional flight of stairs, we are participating in baseline activities that will burn fewer calories than the health-enhancing ones we perform when we exercise.

Exercise is sustained and planned physical activity that results in improvements to your fitness. You may engage in a great deal of physical activity in your day-to-day life. This is great and certainly much better than nothing, but it may not have the same impact on your health as an exercise routine. A routine might include walking, running, swimming, aerobics, or weight training. As long as it's sustained, it's exercise. These activities have regular sessions, adjustable goals, and intervals, all of which are the result of a plan. A pizza delivery job may keep you moving from place to place rather than sitting, but your day-to-day physical activity is probably not intense enough to count as real exercise, so it doesn't contribute significantly to your physical fitness.

Physical fitness is the result of planned exercise. It is a set of attributes related to health, many of which can be measured. Our cardiorespiratory (heart and lung) and muscular endurance, muscle strength, flexibility, and the composition of our bodies, such as our weight and body fat percentage, can all be assessed and evaluated to determine just how fit we are and what we need to do to improve our overall health (Figure 3). Each of

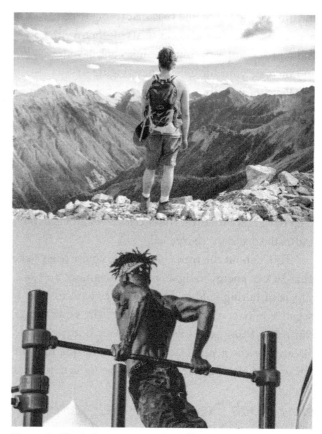

Figure 3. Physical activity can take different forms.

these areas of fitness are covered in much more detail in chapters 3, 4, 5, and 6.

Benefits

In general, people have praised the numerous benefits that consistent exercise has on our health. This can be seen throughout western history, but it wasn't until the 1950s that we had the scientific data to prove what we seem to have known for so long — that maintaining a healthy fitness level helps us physically and psychologically.

According to the Centers for Disease Control, one of the largest physical benefits of exercise is lowering your risk of developing chronic diseases. You can find more information in Chapter 1 and Chapter 9. About half of all Americans are living with at least one chronic disease, such as Type 2 diabetes, heart disease, stroke, high blood pressure, and osteoporosis. These issues can often be lessened or avoided if a person is physically fit. Fitness reduces our risk of developing Alzheimer's disease, reduces symptoms of premenstrual syndrome, and helps

women manage menopausal symptoms. Even the risk of developing some forms of cancer, such as colon, breast, and endometrial, can be reduced. The bike ride you take in the morning, the run with your dog after dinner, and

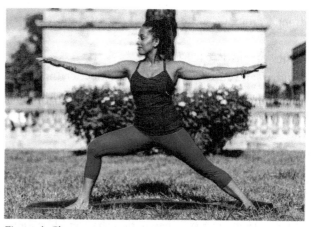

Figure 4. Choose activities you enjoy.

the time you spend on the yoga mat trying to achieve the perfect warrior pose all help to strengthen your bones and muscles, improve your stamina, control your weight, and increase your life expectancy (Figure 4).

Psychologically, regular exercise helps your mental health as well. We tend to sleep better after regular exercise, and improvements to mood and self-confidence lower the risk of depression and anxiety. Even in people who suffer from these mental health issues, exercise can help make their symptoms more manageable. Exercise can even help our cognition, or thinking. This helps us keep our ability to learn, think critically and creatively, and make decisions sharpened.

Think about the times in your life you've been sick. That lack of energy, fatigue, mental fogginess, and side effects of taking cold or flu medicines tend to have a negative impact on your mood, right? The same things can result from excess weight on your body, chronic diseases, or the general lack of stamina related to poor physical fitness. It can feel similar to being sick, or even

worse. It's no wonder that we are happier when we are fit, when you think about it in this way.

Scientific research is continuing on the nature and significance of the benefits of physical activity and exercise. We're still learning about the full impact on different health concerns, both physical and mental. It's a safe bet at this point in time, with the information currently available, that future studies are likely to show even more benefits to fitness.

Mental	Physical
Fights depression	Lowers cholesterol levels
Relieves stress	Builds stronger bones, joints, and ligaments
Boosts confidence	Boost in energy level
Improves memory	Improves sleeping habits
Lengthens attention span	Postpones fatigue

Figure 5. Benefits of exercise.

How Much Exercise Do We Need?

According to the US Department of Health and Human Services in their 2008 Physical Activity Guidelines, adults should complete a minimum of 150 minutes of moderate-intensity physical activity or 75 minutes of vigorous-intensity physical activity each week for health benefits. Studies suggest that the benefits increase as the minutes increase. The greatest possible improvements are seen when a person goes from sedentary to active.

Individuals focused on weight loss or wanting additional fitness in general should increase to 300 minutes of moderate intensity activity or 150 minutes of vigorous-intensity (or a combination of both). The DHHS strongly promotes adding muscle-strengthening activities

of moderate or high intensity at least two days per week to improve results even more. More information on muscular endurance is available in Chapter 4.

Activity Levels Based on Steps Per Day	
Steps Per Day	**Lifestyle Activity Level**
Under 5000	Sedentary
5000 to 7499	Low Active
7500 to 9999	Somewhat Active
10000 to 12499	Active
More than 12500	Highly Active

Figure 6. Activity levels based on steps per day.

Children and Adolescents

Children and adolescents today have it better and worse than past generations. The increase in technology-based forms of play and social communication has enabled and encouraged many young people to maintain a more sedentary lifestyle. They don't have to leave the house, or even their bedroom, to spend time with their friends. When we combine this with public schools moving to shorter recesses and less physical education in some states, we have a generation that could be more

at risk for chronic diseases, and at younger ages than ever before.

The good news is that young people today are still being encouraged to join sports, dance, gymnastics, and many other competitive programs. This, too, is happening at younger ages and with greater variety and better access to these programs across the country.

The DHHS Physical Activity Guidelines recommend at least 60 minutes of physical activity each day for people under 18 years. This should include aerobic activity of moderate or vigorous intensity at least 3 days per week, muscle-strengthening at least 3 days per week, and bone-strengthening at least 3 days each week. Muscle-strengthening activities can be unstructured, like climbing on playground equipment or playing tug-of-war, or they can be structured, like weight lifting or resistance training. Bone-strengthening activities put force on the bones to encourage growth and strength. Running, jumping, and sports like tennis, football, and basketball all meet this standard. Any activities of this nature during the day count toward the minimum 60 minutes.

Older Adults

Medical improvements have led to people living longer than previous generations. This is great, of course, but those later years can be especially difficult for older adults to stay healthy and maintain a good quality of life. Physical activity plays a large role in this. Inactivity at this age can begin a downward slide in abilities that can be difficult to reverse. Older adults vary widely in the level of deterioration of their bodies, affecting what they are capable of doing. Most people over 65 years have at least one chronic condition, making regular exercise even harder.

The DHHS Physical Activity Guidelines for adults over 65 years are the same as for other adults as far as aerobic and muscle-strengthening exercises, with the added category of balance training activities. Adults over 65 years are more at risk for falls than any other population. Their bones are more brittle than younger people, so unexpected impacts can result in serious injury (e.g. hip fractures) that could potentially have irreversible effects.

Balance exercises include walking on their toes and heels, walking backwards and side-to-side, and standing from a sitting position. To most of us, this sounds pretty easy, but seniors may need to begin doing these activities with support and progress to doing them unsupported.

	Key Guidelines for Health	Additional Benefits	Additional Exercise
Children and Adolescents	Most of the 60 or more minutes a day should be either moderate or vigorous-intensity aerobic physical activity, and should include vigorous-intensity physical activity at least 3 days a week.	It is important to encourage young people to participate in physical activities that are appropriate for their age, that are enjoyable, and that offer variety.	As part of their 60 or more minutes of daily physical activity, children and adolescents should include muscle-strengthening physical activity on at least 3 days of the week.
Adults	For substantial health benefits, adults should do at least 150 minutes (2 hours and 30 minutes) a week of moderate-intensity, or 75 minutes (1 hour and 15 minutes) a week of vigorous-intensity aerobic physical activity, or an equivalent combination of moderate- and vigorous intensity aerobic activity.	For additional and more extensive health benefits, adults should increase their aerobic physical activity to 300 minutes (5 hours) a week of moderate intensity, or 150 minutes a week of vigorous intensity aerobic physical activity, or an equivalent combination of moderate- and vigorous-intensity activity.	Adults should also do muscle-strengthening activities that are moderate or high intensity and involve all major muscle groups on 2 or more days a week.
Older Adults	When older adults cannot do 150 minutes of moderate-intensity aerobic activity a week because of chronic conditions, they should be as physically active as their abilities and conditions allow.	Older adults should do exercises that maintain or improve balance if they are at risk of falling.	Older adults with chronic conditions should understand whether and how their conditions affect their ability to do regular physical activity safely.

Figure 7. Health guidelines by age.

General Guidelines

While it is true that some exercise is always better than none, the DHHS Physical Activity Guidelines suggest that we don't see and feel significant results until we are consistently meeting or surpassing the recommended minutes for physical activity (Figure 7).

There is recent emphasis on the importance of moving throughout the day, not just during an exercise session.

You may have noticed that many of our "smart" devices — our phones, watches, and even special gadgets we wear like bracelets — now also function as pedometers that track how many steps we take, miles we walk, or flights of stairs we climb during the day. These can be used to track activity both when we are exercising and as we are moving during our daily activities, helping us avoid being sedentary for too long. Healthy adults can reasonably target 8,000–10,000 steps each day.

Tracking your activity with steps can be especially helpful if you are time-constrained and are trying to build more physical activity into your lifestyle. Once you determine how many steps you normally take, you might try increasing your daily step count by about 500 to 1000 a few weeks at a time to progress safely.

The Health-Related Components of Exercise

There are many types of exercises, each with distinct benefits and guidelines. The types you choose to do should be enjoyable to you, but they should also push you to improve. In different types, this progressive thinking appears differently, so look at later chapters for more detailed information on each type.

Cardiorespiratory exercise, moves our large muscles for a sustained period and gets our heart pumping at a faster rate. This strengthens our cardiorespiratory system, which is really a couple of systems that work together — the cardiovascular and respiratory systems, which include the heart, lungs, and blood vessels. Over time the heart is able to pump more blood with each beat and our resting heart rate often lowers. The lungs become more efficient, take in more oxygen with each breath and increase their ability to deliver oxygen and remove carbon dioxide in the blood.

Your heart rate should be elevated for at least ten minutes during this type of exercise to be most effective. Ideally your 150 minutes of cardiorespiratory exercise will be 20–60 minutes per day, three to five days per week, depending upon intensity. Exercises that tend to be aerobic are shown below (Figure 8).

Any combination of moderate and vigorous-intensity exercise is helpful. You may choose to bike for 40 minutes one day and swim laps for 20 the next. Maybe your dog looks forward to his 30-minute run every morning and his brisk, 20-minute walk after dinner. No matter the exercise, a good rule of thumb is to consider two minutes of moderate activity as the equivalent of one minute of vigorous activity. If you are short on time, increasing the intensity is a good way to compensate depending on fitness level and ability.

So how do we determine if an activity is light, moderate, or vigorous? We measure it. **Absolute intensity** refers to the amount of energy expended per minute during

Moderate Intensity		Vigorous Intensity	
Walking briskly (3 mph or faster but not race-walking)	200 cal/hr	Running	600–1000 cal/hr
Water aerobics	250–300 cal/hr	Swimming laps	400–700 cal/hr
Tennis (doubles)	280 cal/hr	Aerobics	350–500 cal/hr
Bicycling (10 mph or less)	400 cal/hr	Tennis (singles)	500–600 cal/hr
Ballroom dancing	200–400 cal/hr	Bicycling (over 10 mph)	500–800 cal/hr
General gardening	200–400 cal/hr	Heavy gardening (continuous digging/hoeing with elevated heart rate)	400–600 cal/hr
Race-walking, jogging, or running	300 cal/hr	Hiking (uphill or with heavy backpack)	500–cal/hr

Figure 8. Physical activity guidelines from the US Department of Health and Human Services.

the activity. Vigorous activity uses six times the amount of energy that we expend when we are at rest, moderate 3.0–5.9 times, and light 1.1–2.9 times.

A simpler way to determine intensity is by measuring **relative intensity**. What is moderate to a fit person may be vigorous for someone who is not regularly active. We can estimate relative intensity using a scale of 0–10. 0 is at rest and 10 is the maximum level of effort we are capable of. Moderate intensity would be approximately a 5 or 6 on this scale, and vigorous intensity would be a 7 or 8.

Your track star friend Kendall may run a mile in six minutes without breaking a heavy sweat. It is moderate to her. She might rate her relative intensity as a 5. You, on the other hand, find that running a mile in just six minutes requires vigorous activity. It causes you to exert much more effort than you are used to. By the end, you are breathing heavy, your heart rate is racing, and your legs feel like rubber. You might rate your relative intensity as an 8 or 9.

More information on cardiorespiratory fitness is available in Chapter 3.

Muscle strengthening and endurance activities that are moderate or high intensity should be done two or more days each week. **Muscular strength** refers to the muscle's ability to exert force against resistance — how much weight a person can lift, for example. **Muscular endurance** refers to the length of time the muscle can sustain or repeat the action (Figure 9).

The goal in muscle strengthening and endurance is to challenge your muscles, particularly the major muscle groups (chest, arms, legs, abdomen, shoulders, back, and hips), and at times push them beyond what they are used to. To do this, you should repeat the muscle movement until you reach a point where you think you can't do another repetition. Good examples of activities that strengthen muscles include working with weights or resistance bands, doing calisthenics, or using your body for resistance (e.g. push-ups and pull-ups). More information about muscle strength and endurance is available in Chapter 4.

Flexibility is the capacity of a joint or muscle to reach the full extent of its range of motion. These types of activities are an important piece of any exercise program. Certain physical activities require a person to be more flexible and have a greater range of motion than others. This can be very helpful in certain professions and hobbies where your ability to bend and move is important to your performance. Athletes and dancers will, of course, need to be flexible, but so do fire fighters and house painters when they stretch their limbs. Many jobs call for more flexibility than one would even imagine. Ask your Aunt Marge, the pre-school teacher, how many times she gets up and down off the floor, or bends over to tie a tiny shoe during the day. Your job and hobbies may not be physically demanding, but the ability to reach that upper cabinet in your kitchen, touch your toes, or get up off the ground without hanging on to a chair can contribute to your overall quality of life, particularly as you age. To do this, the American College of Sports Medicine recommends doing flexibility exercises (e.g. stretching or lunges) two or more days each week. For variety, consider activities such as yoga or Pilates, which also work your muscles and improve your balance (Figure 10). More information on flexibility is available in Chapter 5.

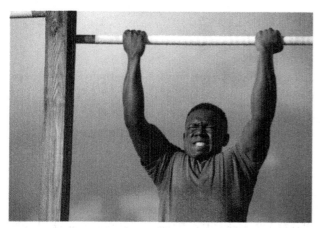

Figure 9. Pull ups test muscular endurance.

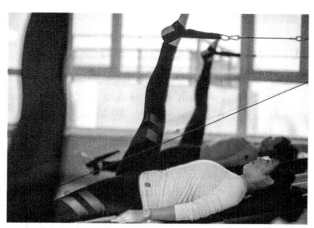

Figure 10. Some exercises require good flexibility.

Body composition, the relative amounts of muscle, fat, bone and other vital body tissues, plays an important role in our exercise goals. Body composition is one of the indicators that is used to assess fitness level and health risk. As you will read in Chapter 6, the amount of fat on our body impacts how our body functions and our life expectancy.

The next three chapters focus on how well we can move our body and how well our internal organs and bodily systems function, but they all relate in some way to body composition. The frequency, intensity, time, and type of your exercises — the FITT formula, featured in each chapter on fitness — may change based on your body composition. Each fitness component is measurable and can be targeted different ways, depending on your goals, interests, and abilities.

Your Aunt Marge, for example, has recently had her percentage of body fat measured and learned that it is too high for good health. She knew this, however, even before the trainer measured it. She had been having trouble keeping up with her preschoolers and was getting fatigued much easier than she used to. She knew she had gained some weight, but it wasn't until one of the adorable little cherubs asked her if she was having a baby (she isn't) that she realized things had gotten a bit out of hand (they had). Don't you love the honesty of children? Marge has decided to add more aerobic exercise — and a bit of yoga for strength, balance, and flexibility — to her daily activities to lower her body composition. She will also assess her nutrition to identify possible areas of improvement.

Are We Fit Enough?

Aunt Marge makes it sound easy, but the hard reality is that this kind of change is tough to do for most people. Unfortunately, most people in the US do not meet the recommended amounts of activity or exercise. According to the Centers for Disease Control, only one in five adults meet the federal recommendations for both aerobic and muscle strengthening activity, though nearly

.half met the guidelines for aerobic alone. This number is slightly higher among people aged 18–24 at close to 60 percent meeting aerobic guidelines but declines gradually with the age of the population. Among college students, approximately 46 percent meet the aerobic guidelines. Women are even less likely to meet the guidelines than men in the same age group.

In Oregon, approximately 60 percent of adults in 2015 met the guidelines for aerobic activity, almost 40 percent were exceeding the aerobic guidelines, and 22.6 percent met the guidelines for both aerobic and muscle-strengthening.

Though some of the statistics seem a bit bleak, the CDC's data shows that the numbers have risen since the federal guidelines were updated, indicating that we are doing better. Over the last few years, however, the numbers have been fairly stagnant, suggesting our progress as a nation has begun to slow.

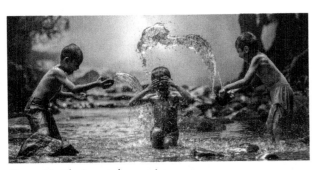

Figure 11. Playing can be exercise.

Improving Your Fitness

So what can we do to avoid being part of the population that isn't physically fit? The data is clear and the information is at our fingertips. We know that fitness can help us avoid chronic diseases and improve our

quality of life. We just need to take the necessary steps to be on the positive side of the statistics. To do this, it is important to assess our current level of fitness, plan our improvements, and follow a training program.

Assessing Your Current Activity Level

You must first assess your current activity level and set goals for improvements. There are a few common methods for assessing your cardiorespiratory fitness lev-

el and establishing a baseline from which to plan, such as the Physical Activity Readiness Questionnaire. The Physical Activity Readiness Questionnaire (PAR-Q) helps you determine any risk factors that may need to be discussed with your physician prior to beginning an exercise program or physical assessment. It presents a series of questions related to how you feel when you exercise, your medical history, medications, and general questions about your lifestyle. This should be done first to rule out any issues that could arise during physical

activity. Individuals with chronic pain or injuries (such as back or knee problems), illness or diseases (such as heart disease or high blood pressure), who are pregnant, or who experience pain or dizziness during exercise are examples of those who may need medical clearance before beginning an exercise program. A sample PAR-Q form can be found on pages 36–37.

Goals

Setting goals is an important step when establishing a fitness plan. These goals can involve improvement to health or skill. The Surgeon General states that while many Americans often begin an exercise program with excitement and good intentions, they frequently abandon their efforts. How many times have you decided to get up early to exercise before work and found yourself hitting the snooze button on your alarm? Or maybe you set a goal of completing a two-mile run each day

only to realize that you didn't have the stamina (you hadn't even walked briskly in several months) and ended up consoling yourself with a cold bowl of ice cream and a warm bath. Setting SMART goals (specific, measurable, achievable, relevant, and time bound) that fit with your lifestyle and current fitness level can help you avoid this pitfall, helping you stay encouraged and keeping you focused.

Goals for Improved Health

Health-related goals can be measured in five areas — improvements in cardiorespiratory health, muscular endurance, muscular strength, flexibility, and body composition. As pointed out earlier in this chapter, the benefits to improving your cardiorespiratory health, such as a reduced risk of heart disease and stroke, are significant. By measuring our cardiorespiratory capacity (such as with the Rockport Walking Test), we can set a goal that directly affects our health (see Chapter 3). Each time we are able to perform at a more intense level, such as running farther or faster, we see the benefits and can adjust our goals. The same applies to our muscular endurance and strength. We can assess these ini-

tially, for example, how much weight we can lift, how many repetitions we can complete, or how long we can run (see Chapter 4). Then we can set SMART goals and reassess. The same is true with body composition, the amount of fat we have in comparison to the amount of muscle and bone (see Chapter 6), and the flexibility of our muscles and joints (see Chapter 5). For many of us, our health-related goals are even more specific. We may want to lower our blood pressure, improve our cholesterol levels, or get high blood-sugar under control, all things that can be measured with goals adapted to suit our current needs.

Goals for Improved Skills

In addition to the more obvious health benefits, improvements to our skill levels can be valuable in our day-to-day lives and setting goals in this area could lead to a real difference in how we function. They might include improvements in:

- **Agility** — our ability to change positions quickly

- **Balance** — our ability to maintain equilibrium

- **Coordination** — our ability to conduct physical tasks smoothly

- **Power** — our ability to use force based on strength and speed

- **Reaction time** — our ability to respond quickly to a given situation

- **Speed** — our ability to move within a certain period of time

Most skill improvements can be measured, particularly if part of a sport. However, a person will most likely notice the change in how they are able to move and respond when presented with daily tasks. Remember the

ARE YOU READY FOR EXERCISE?

Physical activity and exercise have several benefits to individuals' health and wellness. Some of those benefits include improved cardiorespiratory function, decreased risk for chronic diseases, effective weight management, and improved body strength and capabilities.

If you are healthy, there is no reason to consider physical activity and exercise to be negative for your health because most exercise activities are safe and effective. However, before you start a physical activity and exercise program, you should evaluate your medical history. If any health problems or concerns are identified, it is advised that you consult with your doctor before participating in any type of exercise.

Read each statement and select the appropriate answer.

	Yes	No
I have been diagnosed with a heart disease.		
I have experienced chest pain during times of rest.		
I have experienced pain in my chest, neck, jaw, or arms during physical activity.		
I have high blood pressure.		
I have experienced dizziness or loss of consciousness.		
I have asthma.		
I have diabetes.		
I have arthritis.		
I have experienced shortness of breath with mild exertion, when resting, or when lying down.		
I have lower back pain.		
I have a bone, joint, or muscle injury.		
I experience lower leg pain when I walk.		
I am taking prescriptions drugs that may limit my activity.		
I have a medical reason not to exercise.		

If you selected yes for any of the statements, you should talk with your doctor before you engage in a physical activity or exercise program. If you selected no for each of the statements, you can start participating in a physical activity or exercise program. Remember to start slowly and increase the time and intensity gradually, as needed, or as recommended by your doctor or fitness trainer.

HPE295 – Health and Fitness for Life
Eric Colon-Cortes, MS

Most health experts suggest that you consult with your doctor before participating in a physical activity or exercise program if any of the following apply

- You have a heart condition
- You have asthma
- You have diabetes
- You have arthritis
- You are obese
- You have any signs or symptoms of heart or other condition that might be serious, including
  - Pain in your chest, neck, jaw, or arms when exercising
  - You have experienced fainting or dizziness when exercising
  - You experience shortness of breath when resting, lying down, or with mild exertion
  - You have an irregular heartbeat
  - You have high blood pressure or high cholesterol

vacation we imagined earlier in the chapter? A stronger cardiorespiratory system certainly helps you catch that flight you were about to miss, but so does your speed and response time. That hike your family wanted to take? Your agility, balance, and coordination skills help you navigate that uneven terrain.

With improvements in these areas, your life starts to become more manageable and enjoyable. Which goals you set will depend on your lifestyle, your age, your current fitness level, and how you need or want to use your body. Keeping them SMART will keep them reasonable and you'll be more likely to achieve them.

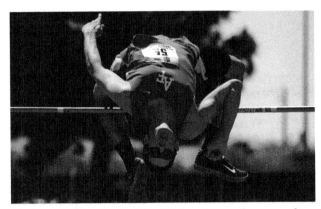

Figure 12. Athletes build their skills based on performance of a particular task.

Creating a Fitness Plan

Your fitness plan should be concerned with helping you meet your goals. One prominent type of fitness plan is the FITT Principle. FITT stands for Frequency, Intensity, Time, and Type, which focus on exercise strategies (Figure 13).

- **Frequency** refers to how often a particular physical activity is completed. Completing a cardiorespiratory activity at least three times each week can condition your body and reduce the risk of injury and excess fatigue from exercise. For strengthening and flexibility exercises, such as weight lifting, two to three days per week is a good guideline.

- **Intensity**, as mentioned earlier in the chapter, refers to how much energy a person exerts during the exercise — how hard he or she works (e.g. moderate or vigorous). Each different fitness component measures intensity differently, which will be discussed in future chapters.

- **Time** refers to the duration of the exercise. This varies depending upon the activity, the intensity, and/or part of the body being targeted. This is generally measured in minutes for cardiorespiratory exercise, repetitions and sets for muscular strength and endurance, and seconds and repetitions for flexibility.

- **Type**, or specificity, refers to the particular activity a person chooses to complete. For example, a person wanting to target their cardiovascular system and burn calories might choose to run or bike. Someone wanting to tone or gain strength in their arms may use weights (or body weight training if they have no access to equipment) to target their biceps and triceps.

	Cardiorespiratory	Flexibility	Muscular Endurance	Muscular Strength
Frequency	3–5 days per week	2–3 days per week	2–3 days per week (wait 48 hours between resistance training sessions)	2–3 days per week (wait 48 hours between resistance training sessions)
Intensity	55/65%–90% of max heart rate (21–31 B/10 sec for age 14)	To the point of slight discomfort	<50% Max weight Body weight 8–12 exercises	70–90% of max lift 8–12 Exercises
Time	20–60 min of continuous activity Progressive	2–4 reps Hold 10–30 seconds	15–20 reps 1–3 sets	8–12 reps 1–3 sets
Type	Large muscle groups Continual rhythmic	Static stretch Controlled dynamic stretching	Resistance training (Free weights/machines) Body weight Circuit training	Resistance training (Free weights/machines)

Figure 13. Applying the FITT Formula.

Training

Training involves the actual activities you perform to improve your fitness. There are many considerations that must be taken into account when developing a training plan, some general and some personal.

General Considerations in Your Fitness Plan

General considerations include overload, progression, specificity, reversibility, and recovery.

Overload is when we place a more intense level of stress on the body than it is used to, causing it to adapt and improve. When we do aerobic activities, our heart, lungs, and muscles are stressed and must work harder to do their job, increasing their overall efficiency. The same is true for exercises that impact muscle or bone strength. The effort taxes them and makes them stronger.

The amount of overload depends upon the person. Someone with very strong legs, for example, will not see much progression if they add just 5 squats to their training. Someone new to a fitness program or that particular type of training may find adding 5 squats to be helpful. It is important to increase based on your own needs. If your goal was to do 30 squats, you've reached it, and are happy with the results, continuing to do 30 squats will enable you to maintain that level.

Progression goes along with overload (often called progressive overload). Once our body is accustomed to the added intensity (the overload), we gradually increase it to cause the body to adapt again, gaining more benefits from the exercise. For example, you may find your brisk, one-mile walk tiring initially, but after a week or two you will notice that your breathing is easier and your leg muscles are not as tired. This is when progressive overload comes into play (Figure 14). You may choose to turn your walk into a jog or increase the distance.

It is important for the progression to be applied gradually. For example, if you want to add progress to your cardio program with time, you may want to add only 1–3% onto your timeyou're your body adapts to the overload, you can increase the progression. You will want to make sure to progress gradually to avoid injury. The amount of overload required varies from person to person. Make sure to check in with your body periodically to determine how much overload you should use.

Specificity means that we choose particular activities to work particular parts of the body and challenge particular systems. With specificity, we want to train in the way that we want our bodies to change or improve.

The gains that we make are directly tied to the type of workout that we do and exercises that are done. For example, if you found out with a sit-and-reach test that your flexibility is "poor," then you will want to include more stretches for the hamstrings and lower back as part of your workout. If you are not happy with your push-up score after completing a push-up assessment, then you will want to include push-ups and other upper body strength movements in your fitness program.

There is even specificity within types of fitness. A person who focuses on sprints for cardiorespiratory exercises is mostly training their anaerobic pathways and preparing their heart mostly for anaerobic movement. They are not focused on cardiorespiratory endurance. A body builder has to lift weights a certain way to get his body to look a certain way. A power lifter also lifts weights, but does it in a very different way in terms of intensity and the number of repetitions and sets.

Reversibility is essentially the "use it or lose it" principle and the opposite of progressive overload. Any improvements in fitness are reversible if the individual does not maintain his or her exercise program. To maintain the benefits of fitness, a person needs to continue to be active across his or her lifespan. If you have had to take time off from your workout due to an injury, health issue, or major life event, make sure that you progress gradually with your workout. If you have an injury

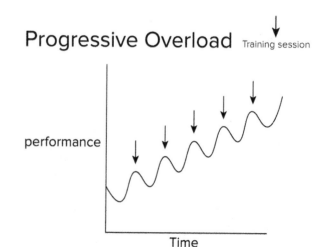

Figure 14. How progressive overload works.

that prevents you from continuing your normal fitness program, try to look for other ways that you can maintain your fitness level. For example, if knee pain is keeping you away from your running plan, look for ways to exercise that don't bother your knee while it's healing. You might try using an elliptical machine, cycling, or swimming (Figure 15).

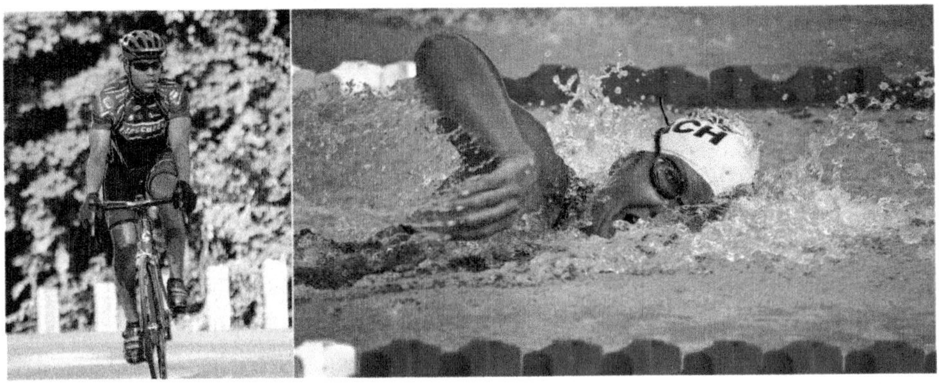

Figure 15. Different exercises can reduce painful impact on muscles or joints.

Recovery is the amount of time needed to rest and recover between exercises or workouts. Tissues experience slight damage when a body part is overloaded. It needs to rebuild — this is how muscles strengthen. Recovery is important to this rebuilding process and will be discussed in later chapters. It's important not to confuse recovery with inactivity. Unless you've sustained an injury, resting 1–2 days between the training of specific body parts

(such as when lifting weights) usually gives ample time for recovery. This doesn't mean that you will cease exercising entirely for several days. That could lead to reversibility and force you to start over again at a lower intensity.

The FITT Principle helps us safely implement overload, progression, and specificity. Determining the type of exercise we perform, how often, how intense we perform it, and for how long is important in order to see results in an effective and safe manner.

Personal Considerations in Your Fitness Plan

There is always a risk of injury or accident in any form of physical activity, though most often exercise is beneficial and safe for most people. With any fitness program, there are personal considerations that play a role in how we structure our plan. These include injury prevention

and safety (such as warm-up and cool-down times or previous injuries), adequate preparation for your environment and activity (such as clothing, weather, and air quality), as well as any previous medical conditions (e.g. high blood pressure or pregnancy).

Injury Prevention and Safety

In general, adapting to your age, personal limitations, surroundings, and previous experience with an activity can help prevent injury and keep you safe during physical activities.

Know your limits — If you are just getting started, begin slowly and remember to keep your FITT Principle SMART. Assess your fitness level first and make decisions based on your capabilities. Don't be fooled by weight loss and fitness programs that you see on television or online that show out of shape people suddenly working out at high levels and dropping lots of weight. It isn't reasonable to expect to be able to run three miles if you haven't run even one in several years. Listen to your body and what it is telling you about your intensity level.

Choose the appropriate type of activity — If you have a previous injury or a physical limitation, choose activities

that are safe for you. For example, if you have a chronic knee injury, then you will want to choose a form of exercise that doesn't aggravate your knee and cause pain.

Cost might also be a factor for you but it shouldn't be a deterrent. There are many ways to exercise that don't cost a dime in membership fees, training sessions, or classes. Famous NFL running back Herschel Walker built his healthy physique using only his surroundings and his own body weight for resistance. He performed push-ups, sit-ups, ran sprints and made use of what he had available and what he could afford, which when he first started exercising was nothing. Remember, it is the FITT principle — pick a type of exercise that you can do and that will help you progress (Figure 17).

Warm up and cool down — The primary purpose of warming up and cooling down the body is to prevent

Lack of Time	Identify available time slots. Monitor your daily activities for one week. Identify at least three 30-minute time slots you could use for physical activity.
	Add physical activity to your daily routine. For example, walk or ride your bike to work or shopping, organize school activities around physical activity, walk the dog, exercise while you watch TV, park farther away from your destination, etc.
	Select activities requiring minimal time, such as walking, jogging, or stairclimbing.
Social Influence	Explain your interest in physical activity to friends and family. Ask them to support your efforts.
	Invite friends and family members to exercise with you. Plan social activities involving exercise.
	Develop new friendships with physically active people. Join a group, such as the YMCA or a hiking club.
Lack of Energy	Schedule physical activity for times in the day or week when you feel energetic.
	Convince yourself that if you give it a chance, physical activity will increase your energy level; then, try it.
Lack of Motivation	Plan ahead. Make physical activity a regular part of your daily or weekly schedule and write it on your calendar.
	Invite a friend to exercise with you on a regular basis and write it on both your calendars.
	Join an exercise group or class.
Lack of Resources	Select activities that require minimal facilities or equipment, such as walking, jogging, jumping rope, or calisthenics.
	Identify inexpensive, convenient resources available in your community (community education programs, park and recreation programs, worksite programs, etc.).

Figure 16. Common excuses for sedentary behavior and possible solutions.

injury. Warm-ups are important for gradually increasing blood flow and building connections with the neuromuscular system. They allow the heart to prepare for increased activity and help you avoid a sudden increase in blood pressure. Exercising cold muscles and stiff connective tissues (e.g. ligaments, tendons) can not only limit range of motion and overall performance, but also result in sprains, strains, tears, and pulled muscles.

Begin your exercise at a lower speed or lower intensity initially, starting with light work to the cardiovascular system (e.g. walking or jogging), until the body has had a chance to warm up. Once your body has begun to warm, the particular body part you are working should be warmed too. For example, if you are lifting weights, start with a smaller weight initially, giving the muscle time to warm before moving to your target weight.

When you've finished your workout, slowly and progressively lower your intensity. Cool-downs help the body gradually return to its resting state. A warm-up and cool-down should each be about 5–10 minutes.

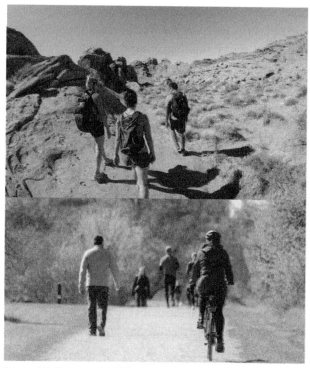

Figure 17. Pick an enjoyable exercise that you want to do.

If you integrate stretching into your warm-up be sure that it is done after the body is warm and that the stretching is dynamic (controlled, repetitive stretches). Static stretching (long holds in stretched positions) should only be done when the body is warm and is most effective and safe at the end of your workout. More information on stretching appears in Chapter 5.

Planning and Preparation

You should always consider your surroundings and other environmental concerns before exercising, such as what clothing or equipment you need or the weather you will be facing when you venture out your door. Preparing for your surroundings can help you stay safe, comfortable, and successful.

Wear the recommended protective gear for the sport or activity you've chosen. Riding a bicycle, for example, requires a helmet and reflectors. Playing soccer requires shin guards for protection. Manny contact sports, like basketball and wrestling, recommend mouth guards. Regardless of the activity, consider what you need to keep you safe, comfortable, and provide the protection you need (Figure 18). When active outdoors at night, for example, reflective gear and head lamps can alert your presence to passing vehicles. Wear layers when temperatures or conditions are variable. For those of us in the Pacific Northwest, for example, water repellant outer layers can help improve our comfort level in the rainy season. Adapting our clothing for heat and cold can have a big impact on how well you perform and your safety (see section on weather).

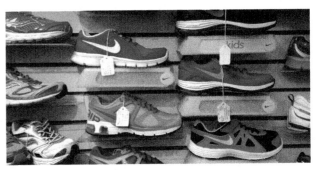

Figure 18. The right equipment can prevent injuries.

Shoes

For nearly every sport, a comfortable pair of shoes can make a difference in how successful we are with our exercise routine. Some shoes are specialized for the activity. Even traditional running/tennis shoes can be broken into categories based on the type of training you do (e.g. walking, distance running, crossfit). If you do a particular activity 3 or more days each week, it can be worth the investment to by a specialized shoe. It's not just a matter of picking a nice-looking shoe in your normal size with a sign that says "cross-training" underneath it. Try using the STRETCH test when selecting a pair of shoes:

- **S** — Wear the same **socks** you would use for your activities.
- **T** — **Try** them out. Run or walk around a bit, simulating the movements you will use during exercise.
- **R** — **Re-lace** the shoes. New shoes right out of the box are often not laced as they would be during exercise. Start at the toe and ensure that you lace the in the traditional, crisscross manner with enough pressure to make them secure and comfortable.

- **E** — Try them on at the **end** of the day when your feet are their largest.
- **T** — **Test** your toes. You should have three-eighths to one-half of an inch from your longest toe to the end of the shoe while standing and be able to wiggle your toes.
- **C** — **Comfort** should be instant. Your shoes should not need to be broken in.
- **H** — Your **heels** should be hugged by the shoe and not slipping as you move.

When your shoes start to show signs of wear and tear, replace them. A good pair of shoes can go a long way toward helping prevent discomfort and even injury during your workout. How often they last varies depending on how often they're used and the pattern with which your feet strike the surface, usually about 3–6 months.

Sports Bras and Athletic Supporters

Ladies, your daily bra is not designed for impact, heavy movement, or significant sweat. Sports bras offer additional support and come in many styles. The larger your breasts, the more support you may need to prevent strain on your neck and back and enable you to move freely and quickly.

Guys, protect yourself. A lack of support can be just as uncomfortable for you as for women, but impact to the area can be more damaging and incredibly painful. Wear an athletic strap (or similar undergarment) for support during exercise and add an athletic cup for protection when playing sports, particularly those with moving objects or potential contact with other players. It only takes one unprotected blow to teach you the importance of these barriers. It's best to learn it without having to first experience it.

Weather

When we make physical activity a part of our routine and start seeing and feeling the benefits of an active lifestyle, the last thing many of us want to do is interrupt our exercise plan. The can-do attitude is admirable and something to celebrate. However, it's important not to put yourself, and your fitness goals, at risk by subjecting yourself to an unsafe environment. Keep the elements of nature in mind when exercising, particularly outdoors. Extreme temperatures, snow, wind, rain, and humidity can present problems if you don't plan ahead.

Cold

Cold is relative to what we are used to. When Grandpa Fred comes to visit you from Minnesota in January, he wears his short-sleeved shirts and shorts for his power-walk in 32 degree temperatures (he's a pretty active senior). To him Salem, Oregon feels quite comfortable, even warm. He also lives in an area with adequate snow plows and city personnel who are experienced and knowledgeable at managing winter precipitation. He is accustomed to clear, salted or cindered sidewalks and roads. Were he to venture out for a walk while its "warm" in Northwestern Oregon and wander into an untended, shady or hilly area (and there are many of those), he would likely find himself lying on the ice. This is why the feeling of being cold is not always the best barometer for risk. Good measurements are *temperatures* and *wind chill factors*.

On most cold days the best approach is to dress in layers:

- *A bottom layer* made from a synthetic material, such as polypropylene, will draw sweat away from the body unlike cotton, which tends to keep the moisture next to your skin.

- Add *a middle layer* of fleece or wool for warmth and a top layer of something breathable and, if you're a Pacific Northwesterner, waterproof. Be prepared to remove these layers and replace them as needed.

If it's windy as well, adding:

- *Gloves*

- *A scarf*

- *Head protection* can shield your skin and those delicate digits from wind chafing and numbness (lets face it — it hurts like crazy when you bump numb fingers against something).

No matter how prepared you are some days are just too cold for outdoor exercise. Temperature and wind go together in the winter. The thermometer might read 30 degrees, but with the wind chill it may feel like 20 degrees. It's important to know the wind chill index (the temperature you feel) when exercising outdoors in the winter because frostbite and hypothermia can be dangerous. Your local weather channel provides this information routinely as do many online sources.

Frostbite occurs when the skin and underlying tissues begin to freeze. It primarily affects exposed areas of the skin, such as your ears, nose, and cheeks, along with your fingers and toes. Warning signs are numbness, loss of feeling, and stinging. Rubbing the affected area can irritate the problem even more by damaging the skin. If it's numb, you may not realize how hard you are rubbing. It's a bit like receiving a numbing injection at the dentist. While your mouth is numb, you're most at risk of biting your cheek or lip and not feel it.

Your best approach is to go inside and warm slowly. However, if the frostbite is severe, it's possible to have irreversible damage that can lead to amputation of the affected area. The following chart from the National Weather Service gives you an idea of how quickly frostbite can occur (Figure 19).

Hypothermia can also be quite dangerous. When your body's temperature (98.6) drops well below normal (approximately 95 or lower), it begins to lose heat faster than it produces it and responds with severe shivering, slurring speech, fatigue, poor coordination, and confusion. The confusion in particular can be very dangerous. It's not uncommon for individuals with hypothermia to make poor choices, such as removing garments and exposing themselves to greater risk. Get indoors or to shelter quickly and warm slowly. This is the key with both frostbite and hypothermia. Seek medical help if you suspect hypothermia or experience pain that doesn't resolve.

Exercising outdoors in the winter takes a bit of preparation. Look at the temperature and wind chill index (both available through your local weather channel or online), and for icy conditions that may create slipping hazards.

There may be times when it's too cold or risky to exercise outdoors. It doesn't mean that your routine has to freeze as well. It just means that you need to hit the treadmill or dust off one of those aerobics DVDs your mother gave you for your birthday. Doing calisthenics, lifting weights, jumping rope — the options are endless and present ample opportunity to keep you on track and maybe even work some muscles you haven't challenged in a while.

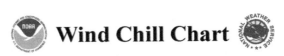

Wind Chill Chart

	Temperature (°F)																	
Calm	40	35	30	25	20	15	10	5	0	-5	-10	-15	-20	-25	-30	-35	-40	-45
5	36	31	25	19	13	7	1	-5	-11	-16	-22	-28	-34	-40	-46	-52	-57	-63
10	34	27	21	15	9	3	-4	-10	-16	-22	-28	-35	-41	-47	-53	-59	-66	-72
15	32	25	19	13	6	0	-7	-13	-19	-26	-32	-39	-45	-51	-58	-64	-71	-77
20	30	24	17	11	4	-2	-9	-15	-22	-29	-35	-42	-48	-55	-61	-68	-74	-81
25	29	23	16	9	3	-4	-11	-17	-24	-31	-37	-44	-51	-58	-64	-71	-78	-84
30	28	22	15	8	1	-5	-12	-19	-26	-33	-39	-46	-53	-60	-67	-73	-80	-87
35	28	21	14	7	0	-7	-14	-21	-27	-34	-41	-48	-55	-62	-69	-76	-82	-89
40	27	20	13	6	-1	-8	-15	-22	-29	-36	-43	-50	-57	-64	-71	-78	-84	-91
45	26	19	12	5	-2	-9	-16	-23	-30	-37	-44	-51	-58	-65	-72	-79	-86	-93
50	26	19	12	4	-3	-10	-17	-24	-31	-38	-45	-52	-60	-67	-74	-81	-88	-95
55	25	18	11	4	-3	-11	-18	-25	-32	-39	-46	-54	-61	-68	-75	-82	-89	-97
60	25	17	10	3	-4	-11	-19	-26	-33	-40	-48	-55	-62	-69	-76	-84	-91	-98

Wind (mph) *(vertical axis label)*

Frostbite Times   30 minutes   10 minutes   5 minutes

$$\text{Wind Chill (°F)} = 35.74 + 0.6215T - 35.75(V^{0.16}) + 0.4275T(V^{0.16})$$

Where, T= Air Temperature (°F) V= Wind Speed (mph)   *Effective 11/01/01*

Figure 19. Wind chill can make it feel colder than it is.

Heat

Heat is also relative to the person and what they are used to, at least to an extent. Last summer Grandpa Fred went to visit some retired friends in the town where he grew up in Texas. He noticed a few people running outdoors in 105 degree temperatures at 2:00 in the afternoon. The sun was blazing and without the slightest breeze. He was a bit dumbfounded that people ran in this heat. However, since he used to walk to school every day in the same heat, uphill both ways (hats off to Grandpa Fred), he figured he could handle it. He went out for his walk at 3:00 only to return at 3:15, red-faced and miserable. Fortunately, he was smart enough to know early on that he wasn't adapted to the climate and relocated his workout before he had serious problems.

Many of us would likely feel the same. In the cloudy Northwest where we rarely experience that level of heat for more than a few days each year, most of us wouldn't consider moving too far away from an air-conditioned gym — we spend so much of the year slogging through mud puddles that our bodies aren't as acclimated to the heat. But then again after months of rain the temptation for sun can be too much to resist for some of us. As with cold, planning ahead can help you avoid health risks:

- *Dress appropriately* to keep yourself cool, as well as protect your skin. Wear a hat and light-colored, light-weight clothing that fits loosely and allows sweat to evaporate. Remember, cotton keeps the sweat next to your skin, so look for materials that will pull it away.

Temperature (F)

Relative Humidity		80	82	84	86	88	90	92	94	96	98	100	102	104	106	108	110
	40	80	81	83	85	88	91	94	97	101	105	109	114	119	124	130	136
	45	80	82	84	87	89	93	96	100	104	109	114	119	124	131	137	
	50	81	83	85	88	91	95	99	103	108	113	118	124	131	137		
	55	81	84	86	89	93	97	101	106	112	117	124	129	137			
	60	82	84	88	91	95	100	105	110	116	123	130	136				
	65	82	85	89	93	98	103	108	114	121	128	137					
	70	83	86	90	95	100	105	112	119	126	134						
	75	84	88	92	97	103	109	116	124	132							
	80	84	89	94	100	106	113	121	129								
	85	85	90	96	102	110	117	126	135								
	90	86	91	98	105	113	122	131									
	95	86	93	100	108	117	127										
	100	87	95	103	112	121	132										

Caution	Extreme Caution	Danger	Extreme Danger

Figure 20. It can be unsafe to exercise in extreme heat.

- *Wear sunscreen.* Let's repeat that word — sunscreen, sunscreen, sunscreen. You almost never hear someone say that they wish they had worn less sunscreen, especially someone with a severe burn or blisters. Keep in mind that you will need to reapply often if you will be outside and active (sweating) for a long time. The more fair-skinned you are, the more often you should reapply regardless of how high your lotion's sun protection factor (SPF) is.

- *Exercise earlier* in the morning *or later* in the evening when the temperatures are lower if possible.

- Check your local weather channel or an online source for the *heat index.* The National Weather Service offers a guideline for what temperature and relative humidity (how it feels) could pose potential health problems. (Figure 20)

- *Stay hydrated.* Dehydration can cause loss of coordination, muscle cramps and fatigue, nausea and vomiting, headaches, and heat-related illness, such as heat stroke (see chart). It isn't as simple as aimlessly guzzling water, particularly if you're an athlete in competition. This can result in a feeling of fullness that impacts performance or even over-hydration (never drink more than 1 liter of fluid in an hour). The American College of Sports Medicine offers the following recommendations (Figure 21).

Exercising in the heat has its issues, particularly when humidity is high. Heat and humidity can raise your core body temperature. Your body will try to cool itself by sending blood away from the muscles and toward the skin. This in turn increases your heart rate. Humidity can be a bit like trying to exercise in a sauna. The sweat stays trapped on your skin, which can raise the body temperature even higher.

Our bodies are designed to adapt to heat, but our natural cooling systems can only handle an overload for a certain period of time, particularly when we begin to sweat excessively or become dehydrated. Potential heat-related illnesses include: Heat Cramps — muscles feel painful and

Time	Additional Step	Time	Drinking Amount
Before	Check your urine color.	4 Hours Before 10–15 Minutes Before	16–20 fluid ounces of water or sports drink. 8–10 fluid ounces of water
During		Every 15–20 minutes (If exercise is less than 60)	3–8 fluid ounces of water, or sports beverage.
After	Weigh yourself again to determine how much fluid you've lost.		20–24 ounces of water or sports drink for every pound lost.

Figure 21. Be aware of your hydration level before, during, and after exercise.

spasms/contractions may occur, may feel firm to the touch, body temp may be normal; Heat Exhaustion — profuse sweating, cramps, dizziness, fatigue, headache, cool moist skin, pulse may be slow/weak; Heat Stroke — dry/hot skin with no sweating, rapid/weak pulse, confusion, possible seizures, body temp above 105, loss of consciousness;

Air Quality

Smog or other air pollutants are a significant problem in many parts of the country and can make outdoor exercise uncomfortable or hazardous to your health. As much as possible, make use of parks, trails, and other green spaces where vehicle emissions are lower, avoiding busy roads where you'll breathe a lot of vehicle exhaust. Areas with tall buildings and traffic lights are a hot spot as the starting and stopping of vehicles and restricted air movement from the structures can create a higher pollutant zone.

Check your local news channel before you head out and heed warnings that the quality of air may not be suitable on a particular day. The Air Quality Index (AQI) provides a good indication of when the air is healthy, marginal, or even hazardous to your health. It is calculated based on four primary concerns: ground level ozone, particle pollution, carbon monoxide, and sulfur dioxide (Figure 22).

Ozone, which is normally higher in the atmosphere, can become a problem on the ground in warmer months when the sun can form a chemical reaction with everyday air pollutants. *Particle* pollution can happen when the air accumulates an excess of fine or course particles, such as when a forest fire occurs, though cars, factories,

Move to indoor activities when the heat index is too high to keep your goals on target. If your tough, resilient, never-give-up Grandpa Fred won't exercise in a particular climate, there is no shame for you in doing a few miles on the treadmill or taking an aerobics class.

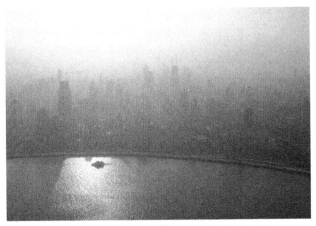

Figure 22. Poor air quality can affect your physical activity.

wood-burning fireplaces, and other sources can also produce particles. *Carbon monoxide* pollution is very common and its largest producers are the vehicles we drive. It develops when the carbon in our fuels does not burn completely, which happens more often in cooler months. *Sulfur dioxide* is a gas that comes from fuels that contain sulfur, such as coal and oil. This type of pollution is higher near industrial areas and power plants.

Air Quality Index Levels	Numerical Value	Color	Meaning
Good	0 to 50	Green	Air quality is considered satisfactory, and air pollution poses little or no risk.
Moderate	51 to 100	Yellow	Air quality is acceptable; however, for some pollutants there may be a moderate health concern for a very small number of people who are unusually sensitive to air pollution.
Unhealthy for Sensitive Groups	101 to 150	Orange	Members of sensitive groups may experience health effects. The general public is not likely to be affected.
Unhealthy	151 to 200	Red	Everyone may begin to experience health effects; members of sensitive groups may experience more serious health effects.
Very Unhealthy	201 to 300	Purple	Health alert: everyone may experience more serious health effects.
Hazardous	301 to 500	Maroon	Health warnings of emergency conditions. The entire population is more likely to be affected.

Figure 23. The AQI lets you know if it is safe to exercise outdoors.

Poor air quality can make it difficult to breathe as deeply as necessary, can damage the cells in your lungs, make you more at risk for infection, and even cause chest pains or permanent lung damage. The Environmental Protection Agency has established criteria as a guide (Figure 23).

Some individuals — such as people with asthma or other respiratory conditions, heart disease, children, the elderly, or people exposed to it often — may be more sensitive to issues with air quality. Change your outdoor run or bicycle ride to one on the treadmill or stationary bike when conditions are too risky for you.

The same rule applies to individuals with *seasonal allergies* that can make breathing uncomfortable. Take allergy medication or move your workout indoors if the pollen count is high. Most weather stations and weather-related websites offer pollen counts, particularly during the spring and summer months.

Higher altitudes can also pose a temporary challenge. The pressure in the atmosphere is reduced, which means less oxygen. Your body has to draw on its own supply more at higher altitudes than lower. This causes the body to circulate more blood and the heart to work harder. You may experience nausea, shortness of breath, headaches, or feel lightheaded.

Signs of Danger		Treatment
Heat		
Heat Cramps	Heat cramps are painful muscle contractions following exercise. They begin an hour or more after stopping exercise and most often involve heavily used muscles in the calves, thighs, and abdomen.	Rest and passive stretching of the muscle, supplemented by commercial rehydration solutions or water and salt, will rapidly relieve symptoms. Water with a salty snack is sufficient.
Heat Exhaustion	Most people who experience acute collapse or other symptoms associated with exercise in the heat are suffering from heat exhaustion — the inability to continue exertion in the heat.	Most cases can be treated with supine rest in the shade or other cool place and oral water or fluids containing glucose and salt; subsequently, spontaneous cooling occurs, and patients recover within hours.
Heat Stroke	Early symptoms are similar to those of heat exhaustion, with confusion or change in personality, loss of coordination, dizziness, headache, and nausea that progress to more severe symptoms.	Maintain the airway if victim is unconscious. Move to the shade or a cool place out of the sun. Use evaporative cooling: remove excess clothing to maximize skin exposure, spray tepid water on the skin, and maintain air movement over the body by fanning. Alternatively, place cool or cold wet towels over the body and fan to promote evaporation. Apply ice or cold packs to the neck, axillas, groin, and as much of the body as possible. Vigorously massage the skin to limit constriction of blood vessels and prevent shivering, which will increase body temperature.
Cold		
Frostbite	Frostbite is the term that is used to describe tissue damage from direct freezing of the skin. Frostbitten skin is numb and appears whitish or waxy.	Once the area has rewarmed, it can be examined. If blisters are present, note whether they extend to the end of the digit. Proximal blisters usually mean that the tissue distal to the blister has suffered full-thickness damage. For treatment, avoid further mechanical trauma to the area and prevent infection.
Hypothermia	When people are faced with an environment in which they cannot keep warm, they first feel chilled, then begin to shiver, and eventually stop shivering as their metabolic reserves are exhausted.	Modern clothing, gloves, and particularly footwear have greatly decreased the chances of suffering cold injury in extreme climates.

Figure 24. Watch for these dangerous symptoms.

The good news is that this is temporary. Your body will acclimate to the higher elevation and even thrive. The heart adjusts and does less work to gain oxygen, which is good. If you're only vacationing in the mountains a few days, you may not reap the benefits but over time your body will adapt and function well. In the meantime:

- Reduce the intensity or duration of your workout.

Surroundings

Be cautious of the rules that are in place to keep you safe, whether it is while you are biking, hiking, swimming, lifting weights at the gym, or any other activity. Adapt to your surroundings as needed. For example, if traffic is particularly heavy or the road you are on does not have a sufficient bike lane consider changing your

Health Issues

Individuals with a chronic health condition, disability (Figure 25), previous injury, or who are pregnant (Figure 26), should contact their physician for guidance with their fitness plan. Most people with health issues are still able to work up to moderate intensity activity, but that is a decision between you and your doctor (Figure 27).

Exercise During Pregnancy and Postpartum

For most women, moderate-intensity exercise is safe during pregnancy and the risks of pre-term delivery or pregnancy loss are very low, though it is always best to consult with your health care provider. Some evidence indicates that in addition to the physical benefits already discussed in this chapter, exercise can help prevent preeclampsia and gestational diabetes, and may even help reduce the length of labor though these studies are not conclusive.

It's important to keep in mind how active you were before you became pregnant. If you were sedentary, beginning a high-intensity program right away wouldn't be advisable. Start with light or moderate activity and listen to your body. Avoid exercises that are completed while lying on your back after your first trimester. At any point during pregnancy, avoid sports that are high contact, involve swift-moving objects, or present a fall risk. For example, playing basketball, horseback riding, and skiing should be avoided. Always check with your doctor beforeengaging in high-intensity exercises.

- Give your body time to adjust.

- Increase hydration and carbohydrate intake.

In Chapter 3 you will learn about how the heart and lungs work together to circulate blood and oxygen. Until your body adapts your heart rate will be elevated and you will need the additional fuel stores.

route to one that is more accessible or utilizing parks or trails. Follow the guidelines that have been established for your safety (such as particular rules in the weight room or pool) and be cautious of others who may be compromising them.

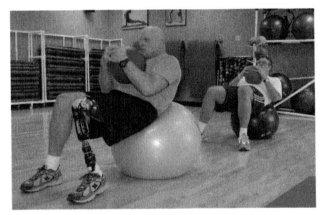
Figure 25. Exercising with a disability.

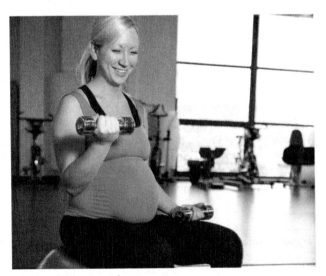
Figure 26. Exercising during pregnancy.

Injury	Symptoms	Solutions
Ankle Sprain	Tenderness, swelling, bruising, stiffness.	An ankle sprain should fully heal on its own between 2 and 12 weeks. If it does not, it is suggested to visit a doctor.
Groin Pull	Pain and tenderness on inner thigh, pain when bringing legs together	Ice your inner thigh, and compress it using an elastic bandage or tape. Stretching also assists tissue healing, with caution.
Hamstring Strain	Pain in the back of the thigh and lower buttock when walking, straightening the leg, or bending over.	Compress your leg, and rest it elevated. Avoid putting weight onto the injury.
Shin Splints	Ache or throb in shins after a short run or sprint.	Rest your body, ice the shin, and take anti-inflammatory painkillers.
ACL Tear	A feeling of looseness in the knee joint, inability to put weight on joint, swelling within first 24 hours.	A mild to moderate knee ligament injury may heal on its own, in time. To speed the healing, you can rest the knee. Avoid putting much weight on your knee if it's painful to do so. You may need to use crutches for a time.
Patellofemral-Syndrome	Pain in the knees, especially when sitting with knees bent, squatting, jumping, or using stairs. It is also common to have a popping or grinding sensation.	Taping or using a brace to stabilize the kneecap, avoid bending your knees for long periods of time, and rest them with ice.
Tennis Elbow	Pain focused on the outside of the arm, where your forearm meets your elbow.	Tennis elbow can usually be treated with exercise, physical therapy, and medications such as ibuprofen (Advil, Motrin), naproxen (Aleve), and aspirin.

Figure 27. Common injuries from exercise and their treatments.

After delivery and medical clearance from your doctor, exercise can help you get back to your pre-pregnancy state and improve your mood (important when your body is adjusting to changing hormone levels).

People with Disabilities

Many people with disabilities can benefit from physical activity, particularly since it can often help with improved ability to perform activities of daily living. Whether the disability is the result of an acute event, like a stroke or spinal chord injury, or something congenital, like cerebral palsy or muscular dystrophy, an exercise program can be developed to suit your individual abilities and needs.

It's important to understand your disability and what your body is capable of doing. Adapt the guidelines or establish a program in consultation with your health care provider. Some individuals are able to follow the federal guidelines for moderate intensity, while others have to make adjustments to ensure safety or to focus on their own specific needs. People with dementia, mental illness, or developmental disabilities may need supervision with activities.

Chronic Medical Conditions

Many people living with a chronic medical condition find that exercise can pose challenges. But refraining from physical activity often only compounds physical issues, leading to worsening or additional conditions.

Asthma

According to the CDC, 18.4 million American adults suffer from asthma. This is a chronic illness in which the airways of the body, responsible for carrying oxygen to and from the lungs, become irritated, swollen, and narrow. For people with asthma, certain irritants or allergies trigger an asthma attack, causing them to wheeze, cough, and experience shortness of breath and tightness in the chest. Some of these triggers include cigarette smoke, pet dander, mold, dust mites, and air pollution. Changes in the weather, colds, and even exercise can trigger an attack. These are usually treated with inhaled corticosteroids (long-term use) or bronchodilators (fast-acting).

Exercise itself does not cause asthma. As we begin to breathe heavier during exercise, we often do so through our mouth, which tends to bring in colder, dryer air. It is this cool air that acts as the trigger. Activities that are more likely to bring on an attack include any in cold, dry environments, such as hockey or skiing, and exercise that needs constant activity, such as long-distance running or soccer. Activities that are less likely include those that require short bursts of energy, like gymnastics, volleyball, and baseball, as well as walking, biking leisurely, or swimming in a warm, humid environment.

You can lessen the risk of triggering an attack by wearing a scarf over your mouth and nose during cooler weather, taking your medication prior to exercise, and doing a sufficient warm-up so the body (particularly the airways) has time to adjust to the intensity. Always keep your inhaler with you and consult your physician for other recommendations prior to beginning an exercise program.

Type 2 Diabetes

Exercise is highly recommended for individuals with type 2 diabetes because it can reduce weight and help control blood sugar levels. The precautions for exercising with diabetes relate to your blood sugar levels. Individuals who take insulin should discuss their exercise plans with their physician to determine how to monitor the amount of insulin they take. Your physician may recommend that you take less insulin or eat a small snack prior to exercise to avoid low blood sugar. Staying hydrated to keep the kidneys functioning well can also help reduce risk. Some individuals with type 2 diabetes who experience weight loss as a result of a healthy diet and exercise find that they need less insulin if any.

High Blood Pressure

High blood pressure, or hypertension, occurs when the blood pushes harder than normal against the artery walls. Regular physical activity reduces blood pressure. There are a few safety measures to keep in mind for people who've been diagnosed with high blood pressure:

- Take it slow at first. If you're just beginning an exercise program, don't attempt vigorous activity right away. Start with lower intensity and build up over time.

- If your blood pressure is uncontrolled, avoid lifting weights.

- Don't consume caffeine. Caffeine is a stimulant and it raises blood pressure.

- Stand slowly. Sudden changes in blood flow can cause slight dizziness, even in those without hypertension.

- Monitor your breathing. Always breathe during exercise and slow down if you become out of breath. You should be breathing a little heavy but still able to speak.

Dealing with Common Injuries

To avoid injuries, it's important to consider your current level of fitness, age, previous injuries, and increase activity gradually. Typically, the most common injuries are to our bones, joints, tendons, and ligaments, often related to repetition or overuse.

Sprains and Strains

A *sprain* is a tearing or stretching of your ligaments, the tissue that connects your bones together. A *strain* is the tearing or stretching of a muscle or tendon (the tissue that joins muscles to bone). A sprain in the ankle or a strain in the back can be quite common. To treat a sprain or strain, use the PRICE method:

- **P — Protection.** Immobilize the injured body part, such as with a splint, and don't put further pressure on it.

- **R — Rest** the injured body part. This is critical to heal the injury.

- **I — Ice** the area every few hours for no more than 20 minutes at a time for the first 24–48 hours. Ice can help reduce swelling and ease pain. Be sure to put a barrier between the ice and your skin to prevent skin damage.

- **C — Compression** of the injured area, such as with an elastic bandage, can reduce pain and limit swelling. Do not wrap so tightly as to cut off the blood flow to the area.

- **E — Elevate** the area so that it is above the heart and the blood flows away from it. This helps keep blood and fluid from building up in the injured area and reduces swelling.

If pain does not improve in a few days it may be more than a sprain or strain. If the pain worsens, increases when you move or apply pressure to the injured area, or won't move at all, see a physician right away.

Groin Pull or Hamstring Strain

The inner thigh area of your leg (groin) and the back of your thigh (hamstring) are also common areas to experience pulls and strains. These typically occur with side-to-side movements or from overstretching. These can also be treated using the PRICE method.

Shin Splints

Pain and swelling on the shin area of the leg (the inside, tibia area of your lower leg) usually results from overwork. Sudden increases to your level of activity are a common cause of shin splints. The muscles and tendons of the shin area simply aren't prepared. Your friend Kendal, the track star friend with the 6-minute mile, once broke her ankle and spent 2 months immobilized. After the doctors removed the cast and she had a bit of rang of motion back, Kendal eagerly returned to the track. Unfortunately she didn't build up as slowly as she should have (the state championships were getting close and she wanted to be ready). Much to her dismay, she developed a severe case of shin splints and was sidelined again for the rest of the season.

Any runner or competitive athlete will tell you that shin splints can be difficult to treat. In fact, they are much easier to prevent:

- Build intensity gradually, especially if you are a beginner or have had time off due to an injury. This is your first line of defense.

- Strengthen the surrounding area, such as the calf muscles and ankles. Resistance bands are excellent for this.

- Avoid running or jumping on concrete (such as sidewalks). Asphalt, dirt, tracks, treadmills, and wooden floors are much more forgiving and will absorb some of the shock.

- Invest in a good pair of shoes. If you've struggled with shin splints in the past, consider using an orthotic insert for better support. These can be purchased over-the-counter or customized for you at many specialty shoe stores. Use the STRETCH test in this chapter for help choosing the best shoe for you.

If you develop shin splints, treat them with ice, rest, and anti-inflammatory medication. Once they are feeling better, be sure to return to your exercise program slowly, giving your shins and the muscles surrounding them time to strengthen and work up to the higher intensity.

Some athletes find that wrapping the area or using compression sleeves helps give more support and lessen pain (Figure 28). If they do not go away, see your physician to make sure the injury isn't more serious, such as a stress fracture, or for a referral to physical therapy.

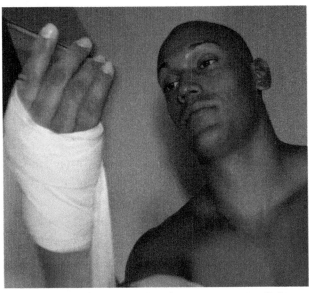

Figure 28. A compression bandage for temporary pain relief.

Knee Injuries

Knee injuries can occur from overuse or from sudden stops or directional changes, as well as from impact. The most common injury is the anterior cruciate ligament (ACL) tear. These can require surgery and should be addressed by a doctor. If the knee hurts, but you don't recall doing anything to it, it is most likely not serious and the pain will go away in a few days with ice and rest. If you experienced impact or felt (or even heard) the injury occur, watch for signs of significant swelling, redness, warmth of the area, significant tenderness or pain, and fever. See a health care provider if one of more of these occur.

Overcoming Barriers

There is no doubt that we live in a fast-paced age where we are on the move constantly and our schedules become quite busy. We've begun to rely on technology to solve this problem and have grown impatient with tasks and issues that can't be fixed with a simple Internet search. Our health and fitness is a physical practice that takes dedicated time and attention, not something we can manage with a click of a smart device (though there are supportive applications).

It's easy to find reasons not to exercise, such as lack of time, energy, motivation, resources, money, skill, knowledge, and support from our social influences. In Chapter 1, we discussed steps toward behavior change and learning what it means to enable and reinforce behavior. Many of our reasons not to exercise come down to our ability to make those changes and put the systems in place that will help us be successful. The following chart can give you some helpful suggestions:

It's important to know that physical activity can also be built into our activities of daily living. We can mow the lawn, do heavy gardening, bike to work, walk to the store, walk or jog with the dog, and make other adjustments to our routines that help us get our heart rate pumping and squeeze in activity to contribute to our 150 minutes. Try jumping rope or doing squats while you watch television, or doing lunges as you move from room-to-room. Read your homework on your stationary bicycle or stair climber. The possibilities are endless and the benefits well worth it.

Conclusion

This chapter gives you tools to understand what it means to be physically fit. We described:

- Definitions of physical activity, exercise, and fitness and what it means to be fit
- The benefits of being physically fit
- The guidelines for beneficial activity levels
- The data on how active we are as a nation
- Steps and considerations you can make to develop your own fitness plan

Your next steps should include assessing your own activity level, and using the information to create a fitness pan that includes daily physical activity. You can increase your lifespan and have a positive impact on your wellness by staying active throughout your life. This plan can help you take the first steps on that journey.

Chapter 3
Cardiorespiratory Fitness

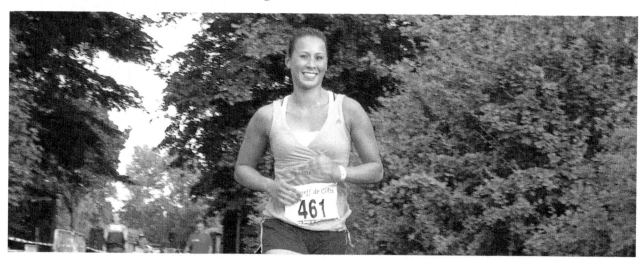

Cardiorespiratory fitness is one of the health-related components of our overall fitness. It is the ability of the heart and lungs to work together to perform sustained moderate to high levels of physical activity. Cardiorespiratory fitness contributes to an improved overall quality of life, longevity, and disease prevention.

Our level of cardiorespiratory fitness (CRF) is a strong predictor of our mortality. A low level of CRF endangers our heart and health as much as or more than smoking, high blood pressure, and type 2 diabetes. Even if you have a serious health condition like high blood pressure, a higher level of CRF can lower your chance of early death from that condition. There are so many reasons to have good CRF, as you'll soon see.

Good CRF also lets you perform physical activity normally, without needing to worry about becoming overtired or injured as a result. Imagine your beloved pet, your cat Larry, makes a break for it when you leave the door open while you get the mail. You could catch him, but will your body be up to the task? With good CRF, even unexpected physical activity is manageable for you. You don't have to worry about losing Larry forever because you couldn't chase after him.

This chapter defines the elements of the cardiorespiratory system, describes how chemical energy is produced in your body, and explains the dimensions of wellness that are most impacted by cardiorespiratory fitness. It also describes how to assess your cardiorespiratory fitness and outlines how to implement a cardiorespiratory fitness program in your own life.

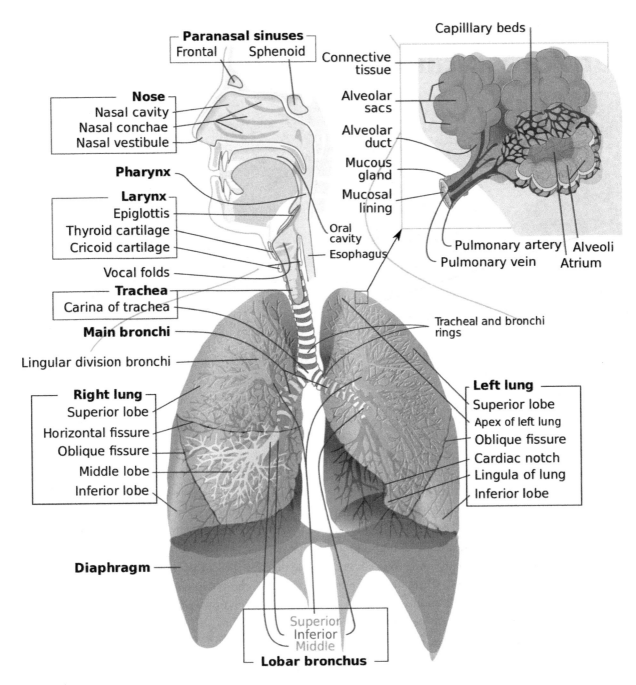

Figure 1. The respiratory system.

Cardiorespiratory Fitness

Cardiorespiratory fitness is the ability of our circulatory and respiratory systems to supply oxygen to our skeletal muscles during sustained physical activity. These systems work together to fuel the body during exercise, pumping oxygen and blood to our muscles. Our heart is a muscular organ. Like any other muscle, it needs exercise to stay fit and strong. Routine exercise strengthens the heart muscle and improves its efficiency, helping it do a better job of circulating blood to our lungs and throughout our bodies.

A stronger heart means more blood reaches our muscles, oxygen levels in the blood rise, and our capillaries (tiny blood vessels) widen, allowing them to carry more oxygen to the body and carry away waste. A stronger heart also means more efficient oxygen distribution to the muscles and less air depleted from our lungs.

Oxygen is important in cardiorespiratory exercise. The body needs to be able to effectively move oxygen and other nutrients around the body quickly when the heart rate is elevated. The cardiorespiratory system is made up of the vascular system and the respiratory system, both of which are responsible for moving oxygen around the body.

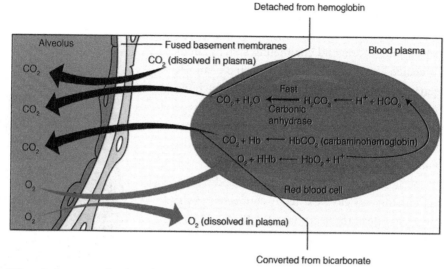

Figure 2. Oxygen and carbon dioxide exchange in the alveoli.

Cardiovascular System

The **cardiovascular system** is the organ system responsible for transporting blood to the rest of the body. This system — sometimes called the **vascular**, **blood-vascular**, or simply **circulatory system** — consists of the **heart**, and a system of **vessels (arteries)**, **veins**, and **capillaries** that distribute oxygen throughout the body through the blood. Our blood also carries other essential nutrients to the cells in our bodies and carries waste away. The average male has between five and six liters of blood in his body, while the average female has between four and five. Our blood, in some ways, is like the oil in a car. If it isn't at the appropriate level, clean, and well-circulated, our body can't function very well.

Heart Anatomy and Function

Understanding the heart's basic anatomy and function is important to understanding the body's cardiovascular and respiratory systems. All of its parts are connected, and each is necessary to keep the system — and your entire body — going.

Like an engine in a car, the core of the human circulatory system is the heart, which is responsible for generating the circulatory process. A heart is usually the size of a fist and is located under the ribcage between the lungs, in the center of the chest. Also like an engine, the heart has its own internal electrical system, a valve and pump system, and fluid lines. Your heart, however, works harder than your car's engine. It's always turned on. This relatively small source of energy keeps working even when you are parked.

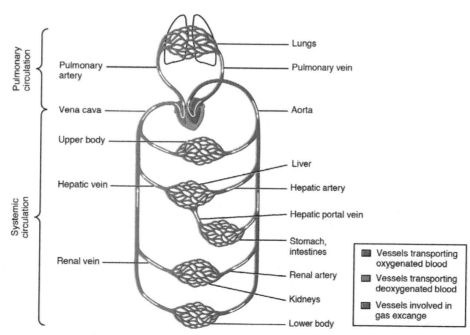

Figure 3. Circulation of oxygen and carbon dioxide.

Your heart has four chambers, two upper (the right and left atria) and two lower (the right and left ventricles). Its pumping action and channeling system circulates oxygenated blood where it needs to go and channels de-oxygenated blood to the various systems in the body responsible for waste (Figure 4). The system in charge of oxygenation of your blood is the **pulmonary system**, and the system in charge of distributing that blood to the rest of your body is called the **systemic system**.

Some of the primary arteries and veins (blood vessels) of your circulatory system are directly connected to the heart. The right side of the heart has the upper and lower vena cava, the largest veins in your body. They move oxygen-poor blood from your body through the right atrium of the heart. The superior vena cava handles the oxygen-poor blood from the upper parts of your body while the inferior vena cava handles the oxygen-poor blood from the lower parts. It then travels through the right atrium and right ventricle, then through the pulmonary arteries (one for each lung) and into your lungs.

From inside the lungs, the blood flows through many capillaries (tiny blood vessels that supply oxygen to tissues throughout the body), picks up additional oxygen, and sends the carbon dioxide waste to be released out of the lungs — a process called gas exchange (more to follow on this).

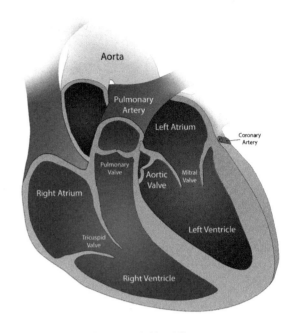

Figure 4. Diagram of heart with blood flow.

The oxygenated blood travels through your lungs and back into your heart through the pulmonary veins, through the left atrium and ventricle. From here, this oxygen-rich blood is pumped through the aorta (the main artery in the heart) and to the rest of your body.

Respiratory System

The vascular system works in tandem with the **respiratory system**. The respiratory system is composed of the airways, lungs, blood vessels, and muscles that enable you to breathe. Its primary function is to exchange gas between the external environment and your circulatory system.

In humans, this exchange balances oxygenation of the blood with the removal of carbon dioxide and other metabolic wastes from the blood. Gas exchange occurs in the **alveoli,** tiny air sacs in the lung covered with a mesh-like network of small blood vessels known as **capillaries**. Dissolved oxygen enters the **capillaries**, while carbon dioxide leaves through pulmonary circulation.

Airways are the small pipes through which air (and its oxygen) travels into the lungs and also through which the gaseous waste travels out. The airway system includes your nose and nasal cavities, mouth, larynx (voice box), trachea (windpipe), and various bronchial tubes and their branches. When you breathe, air enters through your nose or mouth, passes through your voice box, and

down your windpipe. It then separates into two paths of tubes into both your lungs.

Each lung and its associated blood vessels have a big job. They hold the responsibility of transporting oxygen inhaled from the atmosphere through your body, into the bloodstream, and releasing carbon dioxide out and back into the atmosphere.

The lungs, located near the backbone on either side of the heart, are the essential organs of the respiratory system. Once the air travels through the airway system, the exchange of gases is performed by the alveoli. These connect to a system of veins and arteries that move blood throughout your body.

The muscles near your lungs — the diaphragm, intercostal muscles, abdominal muscles, and muscles in the area around your collarbone and neck — help them expand and contract as you breathe. The diaphragm resides below your lungs, separating the chest cavity from the abdominal cavity, and is the primary muscle helping the lungs. The intercostal muscles are between your ribs and the abdominal muscles are beneath the diaphragm. Your abdominals help a lot when you are breathing fast, such as during exercise. When your other muscles aren't pulling their weight, if you have a lung disease, for example, the muscles around your collarbone and neck step in to pick up the slack.

Producing Energy

This energy source is called **adenosine triphosphate (ATP)**, and the systems that produce that energy are the ATP-Phosphocreatine (ATP-PCr) system, the glycolytic system, and the aerobic system. These contribute to energy production in most forms of exercise.

Adenosine triphosphate (ATP) is a molecule found in all of the cells in our body, one that carries energy. ATP acquires its energy when food molecules break down and then it releases this fuel as energy for other cellular processes. This is why scientists consider it our energy currency because it's the body's energy source for all muscle movement and fuels many of our metabolic functions as well. Later in this text you will learn about ways

ATP-PCr Energy System

The **ATP-PCr system** is used for fast or explosive movements and only operates for a short period of time. It provides energy from the ATP stored in all of the body's cells. Creatine-phosphate (PCr), also found in all cells, is a high-energy phosphate molecule that stores energy. ATP concentrations in the cell are reduced by the breakdown of ATP to a product called adenosine diphosphate (ADP) to release energy for muscle contraction. PCr is then broken down to release both energy and a phosphate to allow reconstruction of ATP from ADP.

The high-intensity bursts of activity that use ATP-PCr, such as a sprinting, standing up, throwing,

Glycolytic System

The active muscle cell's oxygen demand exceeds its supply when exercise is of high intensity. The cell must then rely on the **glycolytic system** to produce ATP in the absence of oxygen (anaerobic). This system can only use glucose, found in the blood's plasma and stored in both muscle and the liver as glycogen. The glycolytic energy system is the primary energy system for all-out bouts of exercise or movements lasting from 30 seconds to 2

Later in this chapter, we'll look at training adaptations in cardiorespiratory fitness that affect and are affected by your body's intake of oxygen. First, we still need to understand more about how the body converts oxygen into energy. Like a car converting fuel to energy and then torque to move itself forward, your body uses its fuel to create chemical energy, used by your muscles each time they move.

that fat and energy are stored. It's important to note that ATP does not store energy. Instead, it functions as the delivery driver. The body calls on other storage molecules, like fat and carbohydrates, when it needs energy. These break down into ATP which then delivers the energy where the body needs it.

The ATP-PCr, glycolytic, and aerobic systems each contribute to energy production in nearly every type of exercise, and they operate as you go about your day. The relative contributions of each system depend on factors like the intensity at the beginning of the exercise, your fitness level, and the availability of oxygen in the muscles.

jumping, or swinging a bat, don't require oxygen or build up lactic acid like prolonged activities do. The ATP-PCr system can produce energy at high rates during this type of exercise, and ATP and PCr stores, which are depleted in 10–20 seconds, will last just long enough to complete the exercise.

The ATP-PCr system also replenishes itself quickly, so after a few minutes you should be able to use it again, if you are doing a strength workout or interval training. If you are doing a movement that goes on after this system has exhausted its fuel, the muscles that are involved will use a different energy system to restore the ATP and PCr.

minutes, such as a 200-meter run. It can be accessed rather quickly, but if doesn't produce a large amount of ATP. This energy system is used at the beginning of an exercise session, or for typical movements like when you have to run a couple blocks to catch the bus, walk up several flights of stairs, or hurry to another classroom.

Lactate is the primary by-product of the anaerobic glycolytic energy system. At lower exercise intensities,

Energy System	Description	Type of Activity Powered	Fuels Used	Number of ATP Produced
ATP-PCr	The body needs a continuous supply of ATP for energy — whether the energy is needed for lifting weights, walking, thinking or even texting. It's also the unit of energy that fuels metabolism, or the biochemical reactions that support and maintain life. For short and intense movement lasting less than 10 seconds, the body mainly uses the ATP-PC, or creatine phosphate system. This system is anaerobic, which means it does not use oxygen. The ATP-PC system utilizes the relatively small amount of ATP already stored in the muscle for this immediate energy source. When the body's supply of ATP is depleted, which occurs in a matter of seconds, additional ATP is formed from the breakdown of phosphocreatine (PC) — an energy compound found in muscle.	Very high-intensity, short-duration (6-10 seconds) without the use of oxygen (i.e. anaerobic); active at the onset of all activity	Creatine phosphate Stored ATP	1
Anaerobic Glycolysis	The lactic acid system, also called the anaerobic glycolysis system, produces energy from muscle glycogen — the storage form of glucose. Glycolysis, or the breakdown of glycogen into glucose, can occur in the presence or absence of oxygen. When inadequate oxygen is available, the series of reactions that transforms glucose into ATP causes lactic acid to be produced — in efforts to make more ATP. The lactic acid system fuels relatively short periods — a few minutes — of high-intensity muscle activity, but the accumulation of lactic acid can cause fatigue and a burning sensation in the muscles.	High-intensity, short-to-moderate duration activities (10-90 seconds) without the use of oxygen	Blood Glucose Muscle & Liver glycogen	2
Oxidative Phosphorylation (Aerobic)	The most complex energy system is the aerobic or oxygen energy system, which provides most of the body's ATP. This system produces ATP as energy is released from the breakdown of nutrients such as glucose and fatty acids. In the presence of oxygen, ATP can be formed through glycolysis. This system also involves the Krebs or tricarboxylic acid cycle — a series of chemical reactions that generate energy in the mitochondria — the power plant inside the body cells. The complexity of this system, along with the fact that it relies heavily on the circulatory system to supply oxygen, makes it slower to act compared to the ATP-PC or lactic acid systems. The aerobic system supplies energy for body movement lasting more than just a few minutes, such as long periods of work or endurance activities. This system is also the pathway that provides ATP to fuel most of the body's energy needs not related to physical activity, such as building and repairing body tissues, digesting food, controlling body temperature and growing hair.	Low-to-moderate intensity, long duration (>90 seconds)	Blood glucose Muscle & Liver glycogen Adipose & Intramuscular fat	From carbohydrates: 36-39 From fat: >100

Figure 5. Energy production.

when the cardiorespiratory system can meet the oxygen demands of active muscles, blood lactate levels remain close to what they are when you're resting. This is because some lactate is used aerobically by muscle and is removed as fast as it enters the blood from the muscle.

As the intensity of exercise is increased, however, lactate enters into the blood from the muscle faster than it's removed from the blood, and blood lactate concentrations increase above resting levels. From this point on, lactate levels continue to increase as the rate of work increases, until the point of exhaustion. The point at which the concentration of lactate in the blood begins to increase above resting levels is referred to as the lactate threshold.

Lactate threshold is an important marker for endurance performance. As your fitness level increases, your lactate threshold increases. If you exceed your lactate threshold, you will begin to slow down. Distance runners set their race pace at or just slightly above their lactate threshold. The thresholds of highly trained endurance athletes occur at a much higher percentage of their maximum aerobic capacity, and thus at higher relative workloads, than do the thresholds of untrained persons. This key difference is what allows endurance athletes to perform at a faster pace.

Aerobic System

The **aerobic system** (or oxidative system) produces ATP directly from the oxygen in the bloodstream, and is therefore the most important system to cardiorespiratory fitness. This system uses oxygen to produce ATP within the mitochondria, which are special cell organelles within muscle. This process cannot generate ATP at a high enough rate to sustain an all-out sprint, but it is highly effective at lower rates of work (e.g., long distance running). ATP can also be produced from fat and protein metabolism through the aerobic system. Typically, carbohydrate and fat provide most of the ATP. Protein contributes only 5 to 10 percent at rest and during exercise under most circumstances.

You are using the aerobic system whenever you're doing prolonged physical activity, like a 10K run (about 6 miles), a session of Zumba, a moderate-paced walk with your dog, an indoor cycling class, or an elliptical workout. You are also using this energy system throughout your day, when you are doing something for longer than a couple of minutes.

This is the long-duration energy system. After 2–3 minutes of exercise the aerobic system becomes the primary to bring oxygen to the muscles. Aerobic energy pathways may take a while to use, but they are very efficient and have a significantly higher capability to produce ATP and for a much longer period. The net production of ATP for this system is 32 ATP molecules compared to 2 ATP molecules from the glycolytic system.

Another important factor is the number of mitochondria (the power sources of the cell) present in the muscles cells and the availability of oxygen. Regular training increases the number of mitochondria and the body's ability to use oxygen. Your body also has to have enough carbohydrates (glucose) present to fuel this system, or you'll start to tap into protein resources, which is tough on your body.

Energy Systems Working Together

Let's get back to our car analogy for a moment. Your car has many systems that function concurrently and in different ways depending upon whether you are idling, stuck in stop-and-go traffic, cruising through town, or speeding along the interstate. All the systems are functioning at each pace, but some systems have to do more than others based on your speed. Your body's energy systems function similarly, with one system dominating the others at a given time based on your body's needs (Figure 5).

Say that your housecat, Larry, makes a break for it when you leave the door open. Your first movement is a leap and failed grab in an attempt to catch the furry escape artist. At this point, your muscles use what ATP they have in them, just enough for a few seconds.

For your sprint to the fence where Larry is now crouched, about 80 meters away, your body calls upon the ATP-PCr system for help. Unfortunately, he climbs over the fence, heading toward an open field.

Fortunately, he stops to consider climbing a tree. You run after him and reach the tree in about 45 seconds. This action drew upon the glycolytic system. Apparently you are better at running than grabbing because you miss at yet another attempt to capture the beast. Now you are in for some aerobic exercise.

Larry is now running through the field, and so are you. Your aerobic system is supplying your muscles with oxygen. It takes you seven minutes of continuous running to catch up with Larry, who you only manage to apprehend because he stopped to pick up a field mouse. (Please note that this textbook discusses the benefits of improved agility that come with regular exercise.)

As you can see, good CRF plays a role in both your day-to-day activities and your success when exercising. In the scenario above, you could not have caught up to Larry without a bit of aerobic training. A seven-minute run, depending on speed, could be nearly a mile. You also drew upon your fat stores by accessing your aerobic system, which helps keep your body at a healthy weight. It's a good thing that you've been working on your CRF, or chasing Larry would have been almost impossible.

Benefits of Cardiorespiratory Fitness

Good cardiorespiratory fitness has benefits associated with wellness. Improvement in your daily functioning is just one piece of the large puzzle of benefits a good CRF level can create. These benefits could be physical, emotional, intellectual, and even environmental.

Physical Benefits

Physical benefits include reduced risk of disease and illness, increased life expectancy, and healthier body composition. There are many factors that contribute to both your wellness and your risk of disease. CRF is a key component because it requires aerobic exercise, in addition to a healthy diet (see Chapter 7). Exercise leads to a whole host of physical improvements.

Lower Risk of Disease and Illness

Cardiorespiratory fitness reduces your risk of developing diseases, particularly those associated with your heart, or can help you keep these issues manageable. CRF keeps blood moving through your body efficiently, widening capillaries, and enabling all the parts of your body to get more oxygen and carry away waste. This, along with a healthy diet, helps keep plaque and blood clots from forming in your arteries and causing significant damage or death. The following is a brief list of what good CRF can do:

- Reduce your blood pressure and reduce your risk of hypertension

- Reduce the triglyceride levels in your blood (these are bad fats)

- Raise HDL levels (good cholesterol)

- Help manage your insulin and blood sugar levels, lowering your risk of type 2 diabetes

- Reduce your risk of osteoporosis and certain forms of cancer

- Reduce your risk of becoming overweight or obese, or help you lose weight, reducing your risk of many other chronic diseases and illnesses.

As mentioned earlier, low levels of CRF often lead to increased mortality rates. In other words, a lack of aerobic exercise can lead to an earlier death, likely due to the development or poor management of disease. Bottom line — in general, people with good cardiorespiratory fitness live longer lives.

They also enjoy a better **body composition**. We discussed this briefly in Chapter 2 and will provide even more detail in Chapter 6. A healthy body composition essentially means that you are not carrying excess fat and have enough muscle to succeed in your activities. Excess fat is a health risk to your organs, joints, and metabolic systems. Too much fat and not enough muscle strength can also impact your ability to perform day-to-day activities, increase fatigue, and lower your self-esteem.

Emotional Benefits

Emotional benefits include better stress management, decreased likelihood of depression, and improved self-confidence and mood. Studies indicate that we can manage symptoms of depression and anxiety through exercise. Low levels of chemicals in the brain called neurotransmitters can lead to feelings of sadness, anxiety, and a general loss of interest in your life. These chemicals include dopamine, which is the chemical that triggers your reward centers in your brain. Exercise boosts these levels, making you feel happier. It also gives you a sense of control over your life that can increase your confidence level.

Stress is also easier to manage when we are healthy and exercising. The complications that arise from illness or disease can seriously interfere with your life and how you function. Not only does a high CRF level reduce the risk of this added stressor, but it also means that you are exercising. This means downtime from daily stressors, time to focus on yourself, and a distraction from those worries in life that can negatively impact you. Exercise can be a powerful outlet for managing stress, especially if you find a form of exercise that you enjoy or that gives you satisfaction. We'll look at stress management in more detail in Chapter 8.

The improved **body composition** discussed earlier also contributes to your emotional health. Many of us do not like to admit that our body composition impacts our life. We don't like the idea of being superficial in how we judge our appearance. But body composition is more about physical satisfaction with your health.

Yes, it is important to keep your expectations realistic and appropriate, but feeling healthy, comfortable, and confident is not superficial. It's tangible.

Your friend Jane, for example, has struggled to maintain a healthy body composition for years. Last fall, a mutual friend ran in a 10k fun run, and that inspired Jane to try it, too. But a few months later, when Jane signed up for a similar event, she found she couldn't finish the race, and didn't really have any fun like she was supposed to. She set a goal for her fitness: she would finish the race at the 5k fun run this coming fall. She started jogging each morning, increasing her cardiorespiratory fitness over time. By the time the race came around, she not only finished, but she completed the race without stopping to walk! The tangible accomplishment of finishing the race made Jane realize that she could use her body in ways she didn't think were possible, improving her self-esteem.

Cardiorespiratory exercise helps with managing and improving body composition by raising your overall daily caloric expenditure, burning calories during training sessions, and elevating your resting metabolic rate. Exercise alone isn't enough to make these changes. They have to be coupled with dietary changes.

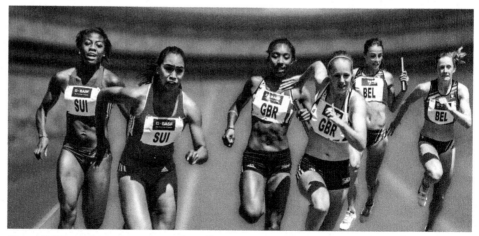

Figure 6. Competitive sports can motivate fitness.

Intellectual Benefits

Good cardiorespiratory fitness can also stimulate us on an intellectual level. When we exercise, our muscles release certain proteins that have a regenerative effect on the brain. The National Institute of Health supported research on a particular protein released during exercise called cathespin B. This protein is thought to directly impact the memory centers of our brain. Participants in the study found that after two weeks of regular exercise, their memories tested better than before they began the exercise routine. In this way, exercise is like a smart pill. You retain more information and generate new neurons in your brain to help you think critically and see improvement in your cognition.

Environmental Benefits

The environmental benefits of cardiorespiratory fitness include better ability to use physical activity as transportation. This decreases production of environment-harming pollutants, such as carbon monoxide. A person cycling or walking to the store or work pollutes very little. Not only are they more active and less sedentary, great for their health, but they also lower their carbon footprint on the planet.

Challenges to Improving Cardiorespiratory Fitness

There may be certain challenges along the way, particularly during times of illness or if a chronic disease is present. Chapter 2 discussed some of the methods for exercising with asthma, during pregnancy, with a previous injury, during extreme temperatures, and with poor air quality. Individuals who suffer from heart or lung diseases, common colds, or are older in age may have particular challenges for practicing cardiorespiratory fitness. There are, however, strategies for developing or maintaining CRF for people with certain health conditions.

General Considerations

There are general considerations for each and every person as during aerobic exercise:

- Check with your health care provider prior to exercise if you have an injury, chronic disease, or chronic pain.

- Listen to your body. If you experience chest pains, nausea, dizziness, become lightheaded, or feel significant pain in any part of your body, take a break. If the pain persists, stop. If you suspect you are having a heart attack, call 911.

Before an asthma episode

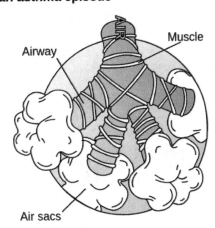

After an asthma episode

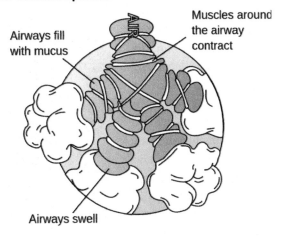

Figure 7. How asthma affects the lungs.

Specific Considerations

Some individuals have special circumstances to consider both as they develop an exercise program and as they perform exercise. The following information can offer some general assistance for certain conditions.

Bronchitis is a condition in which the bronchial tubes, the tubes that carry air to your lungs, become inflamed (Figure 8). Individuals with bronchitis often have a cough that produces mucus, wheezing, shortness of breath, a low fever, and discomfort or pain in their chest. Bronchitis can be acute — the result of an infection, virus, or pollutant — or chronic, meaning long-term. Chronic bronchitis is an ongoing, serious

condition. Both emphysema and chronic obstructive pulmonary disease (COPD) are forms of chronic bronchitis. It occurs if the lining of the bronchial tubes is constantly irritated and inflamed, causing a long-term cough with mucus. People with chronic bronchitis are more susceptible to viruses and bacteria. Smoking is the main cause of chronic bronchitis.

Exercise can improve chronic bronchitis symptoms. Yes, you may be out of breath, but you are working your respiratory muscles and circulating blood, with its valuable oxygen, throughout your body. Activities that boost cardiorespiratory fitness will help lessen shortness

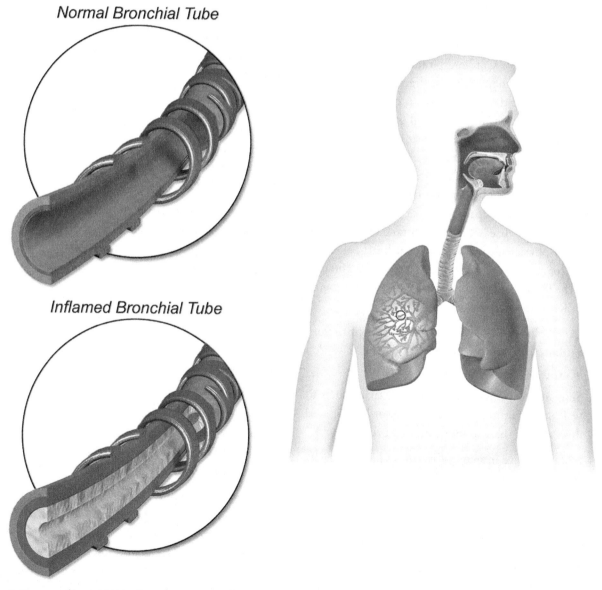

Normal Bronchial Tube

Inflamed Bronchial Tube

Figure 8. Progress of bronchitis in airways.

of breath, improve the body's use of oxygen, improve energy levels, and improve overall cardiovascular health. Stretching, aerobic exercise, resistance training, and even swimming are good activities for people with forms of chronic bronchitis, though you should always remember to build intensity gradually and listen to your body.

If you wear oxygen, be sure to consult your physician about when to use it during exercise. Some general breathing techniques are:

- Inhaling when you begin an exercise and exhaling during the most difficult part

- Taking slow breaths and pace your breathing

- Pursing your lips when breathing out

There are many different types of **heart disease**, such as congestive heart failure, coronary artery disease, and atrial fibrillation. **High blood pressure** is also associated with heart risk. Cardiorespiratory fitness can cause improvements in many cases of heart disease, though it may not reverse the disease itself. It can help manage symptoms by increasing blood and oxygen flow (and making your heart more efficient at its job), strengthening the heart and body, and lowering blood pressure and cholesterol levels that add insult to injury when it comes to the disease. It can help you be more active with fewer incidents of chest pain and other related symptoms.

As with any disease, it is important to first check with your physician to make sure your heart is healthy enough for exercise and what, if any, restrictions you may have. The following tips offer a basic guide to improving your CRF with heart disease:

- Do aerobic exercises for maximum benefit to your cardiorespiratory system. Make your heart work a little harder each time but not too hard.

- Start slowly. Choose an aerobic activity such as walking, swimming, light jogging, or biking, and do it at least three to four times a week.

- Always do five minutes of warm-up before exercising. Allow time to cool down after you exercise. For cool-down, you can do the same activity but at a slower pace.

- Take rest periods before you get too tired.

- Know your resting heart rate and an acceptable rate during exercise.

- Know your limits. If you experience any symptoms, such as chest pain, nausea, dizziness or lightheadedness, irregular heartbeat or pulse, or shortness of breath then stop and rest. Write down your symptoms, what you were doing when they occurred, and their duration so that you can share them with your health care provider.

- Stand slowly when moving from a lying, sitting, or bending position to reduce the chance of dizziness.

- If you take medication, such as nitroglycerin, for chest pain, be sure to have it handy. If you take medication for blood pressure, be sure to consult your physician about potential side effects prior to exercise.

Aging can sometimes seem like a barrier to cardiorespiratory exercises. Senior citizens often have a chronic illness, less muscle strength, weakened joints and bones, problems with balance, reduced flexibility, and even dementia. An older person who has maintained a good level of CRF throughout their life will likely have fewer limitations and be in much better physical condition. Even for someone who has limitations, cardiorespiratory training will offer many of the health benefits this chapter has addressed. The National Institute on Aging offers the following tips:

- Do a little light activity to warm up and cool down before and after your endurance activities.

- Be sure to drink plenty of liquids when doing any activity that makes you sweat.

- Dress in layers when exercising outdoors so you can add or remove clothes if you get cold or hot.

- To prevent injuries, be sure to use safety equipment.

- Walk during the day or in well-lit areas at night, and be aware of your surroundings.

- Build up your endurance gradually. If you haven't been active for a long time, it's important to work your way up over time. Start out with ten minutes at a time and then gradually build up.

- Try to build up to at least 150 minutes (two and a half hours) of moderate endurance activity a week. Being active at least three days a week is best. Remember, these are goals. Some people will be able to do more. It's important to set realistic goals based on your own health and abilities.

- When you're ready to do more, build up the amount of time you spend doing endurance activities first, then build up the difficulty of your activities. For example, gradually increase your time to 30 minutes over several days to weeks by walking longer distances. Then walk more briskly or up steeper hills.

Even adults with walkers or wheelchairs can get aerobic exercise. Wheeling is active and can be done around a track. Walking is walking, regardless of whether or not a walker is used. Treadmills, set on a safe speed, can be a good option. The important thing to remember is to know your capabilities and limits, and gain assistance when you need it.

Fighting a **cold or flu** can have a negative impact on your day and may make exercise difficult. Consider the following tips for how and when to continue with your program:

- It is usually safe to exercise if your symptoms are all above the neck, such as a runny nose or nasal congestion, or a slight sore throat. Consider reducing your intensity until you feel better and be sure to hydrate well.

- Do not exercise if you have symptoms below the neck, such as chest congestion, a hacking cough, or stomach upset.

- Do not exercise with a fever, or if you are achy and fatigued.

Women often find it a challenge to exercise during their **menstrual cycle**. Hormonal changes and blood loss can sometimes cause mild dizziness and fatigue. This is in addition to the pain of cramps and discomfort of bloating. Exercise during this time, however, does more to relieve the symptoms than aggravate them. The endorphins released during exercise serve as a temporary pain blocker and can also help relieve moodiness. Sweating can have some slight relief for bloating as well. Take acetaminophen or another pain reliever, wear comfortable clothing, and use your workout to improve your condition.

If the pain is too much, take the day off. Most women do not have periods that debilitate them, so if yours is sidelining you, see your doctor.

Regardless of your particular challenges remember, inactivity will likely make it worse not better. Good cardiorespiratory fitness will help you avoid additional problems and complications, and can improve your quality of life by making symptoms more manageable. Your doctor will let you know what is and isn't safe.

Cardiorespiratory Fitness Training

You can improve your cardiorespiratory fitness through training, beginning with self-assessments, goal setting, and creating a training plan. This section will show you how to assess your cardiorespiratory fitness, what kind of goals you should set, and suggest some different training methods and exercises to help meet your goals.

Your CRF can be assessed through the Rockport Walking Test and other VO_2 max tests, resting heart rates, and blood pressure.

The Rockport Walking Test and VO₂ Max

Experts at the University of Massachusetts at Amherst's Department of Exercise Science developed this one-mile test to measure a person's aerobic capacity (or VO_2 max) based on the participant's age, weight, and gender. All that is needed to complete the test is a level, one-mile track, a stopwatch, a scale, and comfortable clothes and shoes.

Procedure:

- Weigh yourself

- Take about 5–10 minutes to lightly warm up and stretch

- Start the timer and walk one mile as quickly as you can (do not run or speed walk)

- As soon as you complete the mile, take your pulse while walking slowly to cool down. To do this, locate your radial or carotid artery and count the number of beats for 15 seconds, then multiple that number by 4.

- Calculate your VO$_2$ max using the following formula:
- 132.853 – (0.0769 x weight) – (0.3877 x age) + (6.315 x 1 if male, 0 if female) – (3.2649 x time) – (0.1565 x heart rate)

Example:

If a 30 year-old man weighing 180 pounds finished the mile in 10.55 minutes (or 10 minutes 33 seconds) and had a heart rate of 160 beats per minute (bpm), his estimated VO$_2$ max would be as follows:

0.0769 (180 – 0.3877) (30+6.315) (1 – 3.2649) (10.55 – 0.1565) (160 = 54.21)

Use the following (Figure 9) table to determine where you are and set your goals.

The Rockport Walking Test is generally considered a safe and effective way to measure your aerobic capacity for most individuals. With level terrain, no running, low impact to the body, and no set time or pace established for completion, even inactive individuals can make use of this method to determine their cardiovascular fitness level.

The 1.5 Mile Test

This test is a lot like the Rockport. A level track or road that enables you to complete 1.5 miles, comfortable clothes and shoes, and a stopwatch are all that are needed. For this test, however, the participant will run, walk, or a combination of the two, as quickly as possible for the entire distance.

Cardiovascular endurance is measured based on how long it takes the individual to complete the run. Law enforcement and other government agencies often use this test to determine a potential employee's ability to meet the physical demands of the profession.

Maximal Oxygen Uptake Norms for Men (ml/kg/min)						
	18–25	**26–35**	**36–45**	**46–55**	**56–65**	**65+**
Excellent	>60	>56	>51	>45	>41	>37
Good	52–60	49–56	43–51	39–45	36–41	33–37
Average	47–51	43–48	39–42	35–38	32–35	29–32
Average	42–46	40–42	35–38	32–35	30–31	26–28
Average	37–41	35–39	31–34	29–31	26–29	22–25
Poor	30–36	30–34	26–30	25–28	22–25	20–21
Very Poor	<30	<30	<26	<25	<22	<20
Maximal Oxygen Uptake Norms for Women (ml/kg/min)						
	18–25	**26–35**	**36–45**	**46–55**	**56–65**	**65+**
Excellent	>56	>52	>45	>40	>37	>32
Good	47–56	45–52	38–45	34–40	32–37	28–32
Average	42–46	39–44	34–37	31–33	28–31	25–27
Average	38–41	35–38	31–33	28–30	25–27	22–24
Average	33–37	31–34	27–30	25–27	22–24	19–22
Poor	28–32	26–30	22–26	20–24	18–21	17–18
Very Poor	<28	<26	<22	<20	<18	<17

Figure 9. VO$_2$ max ranges.

3-Minute Step Test

The 3-minute step test requires stepping up and down on a 16.25-inch step for 3 minutes at a constant rate. At the completion of the activity, heart rate is measured for 15 seconds. The lower the heart rate, the better the ability to recover from an aerobic task, a good indication of CRF.

Resting Heart Rate

Your resting heart rate (RHR) is measured by the number of times your heart beats per minute (bpm) while you're at rest. In other words, it tells you how hard your heart needs to work when you are exerting almost no effort. This can be a good indicator of your CRF. A normal RHR is between 60–100 bpm, though studies suggest that people on the higher end of this range (above 80) are often at greater risk of heart-related diseases.

A high number could mean that you are already showing signs of disease and need to see your health care provider. A low number usually means your heart is very efficient. Highly trained athletes, such as long-distance runners, may have a rate as low as 40 bpm, or even lower. A person who is inactive and has a low heart rate should also see a health care provider.

Blood Pressure

Blood pressure is the force of blood pushing against the walls of the arteries as the heart pumps blood. Your blood pressure indicates how hard your heart is working. High blood pressure, or **hypertension**, happens when the force of your blood is too high. Health care workers check blood pressure using a gauge, a stethoscope or electronic sensor, and a blood pressure cuff (sphygmomanometer) (Figure 10). With this equipment, they measure:

- Systolic Pressure: blood pressure when the heart beats while pumping blood

- Diastolic Pressure: blood pressure when the heart is at rest between beats

They write blood pressure numbers with the systolic number above the diastolic number. Pressure is measure in

To measure your RHR, you just need a timer or stopwatch.

Procedure:

- Place your index and middle finger on one of your pulse points. They are located on either the inside of your wrist, below the thumb-side of the hand, or on either side of your neck adjacent to your Adam's apple.

- Set a timer or use a stopwatch to clock 30 seconds. Count the number of heart beats that occur during this period and double it. That is your RHR.

Many factors can influence your RHR, such as blood pressure medication and activity. It's best to measure it at different times of the day, but not within a few hours of exercising. For a good baseline, try measuring your RHR when you first wake up in the morning.

millimeters of mercury, or mmHg. For example, 110/70 mmHg. Normal blood pressure for adults is defined as a systolic pressure below 120 mmHg and a diastolic pressure below 80 mmHg. It is normal for blood pressures to change when you sleep, wake up, or are excited

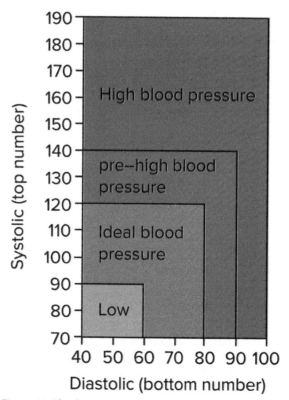

Figure 11. Blood pressure ranges.

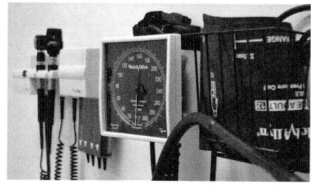

Figure 10. Blood pressure cuff.

or nervous. It is also normal for your blood pressure to increase during activity. However, once the activity stops, your blood pressure returns to your normal baseline range. Abnormal increases in blood pressure are defined as having blood pressures higher than 120/80 mmHg. Chapter 9 offers more discussion on high blood pressure.

Your health care practitioner can check your blood pressure. It is best not to drink coffee or smoke cigarettes for 30 minutes prior to the test. You should also use the restroom before the test, and sit down for at least 5 minutes before starting.

Goal Setting

Based on what you learn from the above assessments, you can set goals to achieve improvements in your problem areas. Each goal should follow the SMART goal principles of being specific, measurable, achievable, relevant, and time-based. For example, if your assessment reveals that you have high blood pressure, here is a SMART goal you could set for yourself:

Specific — I want to lower my blood pressure.
Measurable — From 140/90 to 130/80 mmHg.
Achievable — This is a small improvement.
Relevant — So that I feel healthier and reduce risk.
Time-based — At the end of three months.

In addition to setting SMART goals, you should also set smaller goals on the way to your large goals. The example above is a smaller goal on the way to healthy blood pressure. The goal now is closer to the healthy rate, but it isn't all the way there. This lets you celebrate the progress without feeling discouraged by the time it might take to reach your larger goal of a healthy blood pressure. Taking things in stages is wise, and small goals help you do that.

Moderate Activity 3.0 to 6.0 METs (3.5 to 7 kcal/min)	Vigorous Activity Greater than 6.0 METs (more than 7 kcal/min)
Walking, hiking, roller skating	Walking at 5 mph or faster, jogging or running, walking and climbing up a hill, mountain climbing
Bicycling 5 to 9 mph on level terrain	Bicycling more than 10 mph on uphill terrain
Aerobic dancing, water aerobics	Aerobic dancing step aerobics, water jogging
Calisthenics, yoga, general home exercises	Calisthenics — push ups, pull ups, karate, jump rope, jumping jacks
Weight training and bodybuilding with free weights	Circuit weight training
Boxing with punching bag	Boxing in ring, sparring, wrestling — competitive
Ballroom dancing, line dancing, square dancing folk dancing, modern dancing, disco, ballet	Professional ballroom dancing, square dancing, folk dancing, clogging
Table tennis — competitive, tennis — doubles	Tennis — singles
Softball, basketball — shooting baskets	Football game, basketball game, soccer game, rugby
Volleyball	Beach volleyball
Frisbee, juggling, curling, cricket	Handball, racquetball, squash
Downhill skiing, Ice skating	Downhill skiing — racing, ice skating, cross-country skiing, sledding, ice hockey
Swimming — recreational	Swimming — steady paced laps, water jogging, water polo water basketball
Canoeing or rowing a boat, rafting, sailing, paddle boating	Canoeing or rowing — 4 or more mph
Fishing, hunting	
Horseback riding	Horseback riding — competitive, polo

Figure 12. Activities by activity level.

The FITT Principle

The FITT principle (see Chapter 2) is a set of rules that should be followed to benefit from any form of fitness training program. Your cardiorespiratory fitness should involve this principle, following a plan that can strengthen your heart and lung capacity to function well:

Frequency — 3–5 days per week of aerobic activity depending upon intensity. Moderate-intensity walking is usually safe to do every day, but the body needs time to rebuild, repair, and restore energy between high-intensity workouts. Exercising more than 5 days per week may not yield additional benefits for everyone and could lead to overuse injuries, but this varies with the individual. Incorporating different types of cardio can help avoid overuse injuries, especially if a person wants to train more than three days a week. Training less than three days a week makes it challenging to improve fitness level. Some, however, is always better than none.

Intensity — The more intense your exercise, the faster your heart will beat. Based on your age, you can calculate your target heart rate, and then exercise with an intensity that raises your heart rate to the target. Target heart rate is measured as a percentage of your maximum heart rate (MHR) which is the fastest your heart can beat, also based on your age. If you are just starting an exercise program, you should target approximately 55–65% of your MHR and 65–90% of your MHR if you have been regularly exercising for a while.

You can calculate your MHR by subtracting your age from 220. To find your target heart rate, multiply your MHR by 0.55–0.90, depending on your experience level. You can also consult (Figure 13).

A person who has been inactive may want to begin targeting the lower end of their target heart rate zone, while an active person may see their heart rate closer to 90% of MHR. You can check your heart rate during exercise. To do so, take a short break at your peak performance (or at intervals throughout) but keep walking to stay warm. Test just as you did for your RHR. Use the chart to see if you are in your target zone.

For example, Claudia, who is 40 years old, has been measuring her resting heart rate each morning when she wakes up (a good way to get a baseline), and her average is 64 bpm. When she goes on her 5k jog on Mondays, Wednesdays, and Fridays, she turns around at the crosswalk at Dearborn and River Road — right at the halfway point — and checks her heart rate. Walking back toward home at first, she measures 145 bpm during her run using a fitness band that takes her pulse. 145 bpm is right at 80% of MHR, perfect for her routine and experience level. There are forms of technology available to help measure your heart rate. Some are in the form of watches and others as straps that can be worn across the chest. They are available at many fitness stores and online.

Claudia used to think that you could only burn fat by exercising at a low intensity. This is a myth. Advanced

Age	Previously Sedentary. Target Heart Rate Zone: 55–65%	History of Regular Exercise to Athlete. Target Heart Rate Zone: 65–90%	Maximum Heart Rate: 100%
20	110–130 beats per minute (bpm)	130–180 beats per minute (bpm)	200 beats per minute (bpm)
25	107–126 bpm	126–175 bpm	195 bpm
30	104–123 bpm	123–171 bpm	190 bpm
35	102–120 bpm	120–166 bpm	185 bpm
40	99–117 bpm	117–162 bpm	180 bpm
45	96–113 bpm	113–158 bpm	175 bpm
50	93–110 bpm	110–153 bpm	170 bpm
55	90–107 bpm	107–149 bpm	165 bpm
60	88–104 bpm	104–144 bpm	160 bpm
65	85–101 bpm	101–140 bpm	155 bpm
70	82–98 bpm	98–135 bpm	150 bpm

Figure 13. Target and maximum heart rate by activity level.

equipment in physiology labs does show that fat stores contribute a greater percentage of fuel used to power lower-intensity exercises, but that is offset by the total calorie expenditure in high intensity exercises. For example, in a one-hour exercise session, you chose a low-intensity exercise, and 60% of your burned calories came from fat stores, but you only burned 100 calories. In a high-intensity exercise of the same time, only 40% of your burned calories came from fat stores, but you burned 500 calories. So, at low-intensity you burned 60 fat calories, while at high intensity, you burned 200 fat calories. See the difference?

You can also determine your optimal heart rate by using the **Heart Rate Reserve** (HRR) method. Start by determining your MHR (use the chart above or subtract your age from 220 as an estimate). Subtract your heart's resting rate from your maximum. Test during performance as above. For Claudia, her HHR is 116 bpm (220 − 40 = 180 − 64 = 116).

As an alternative, to measure your intensity you can also use the **talk-test** or relative intensity. The talk test is a simple way to measure relative intensity. In general, if you're doing moderate-intensity activity you can talk, but not sing, during the activity. If you're doing vigorous-intensity activity, you will not be able to say more than a few words without pausing for a breath.

Another alternative is the **Rate of Perceived Exertion** (Figure 14). The Borg Rating of Perceived Exertion (RPE) is a way of measuring physical activity intensity level. Perceived exertion is how hard you feel like your body is working. It is based on the physical sensations a person experiences during physical activity, including increased heart rate, increased respiration or breathing rate, increased sweating, and muscle fatigue. Although this is a subjective measure, a person's exertion rating may provide a good estimate of the actual heart rate during physical activity.

Health care providers generally agree that perceived exertion ratings between 12 to 14 on the RPE scale (Borg Scale) suggests that physical activity is being performed at a moderate level of intensity. During activity, use the scale to assign numbers to how you feel (focus only on your level of exertion not any injuries you may have). Self-monitoring how hard your body is working can help you adjust the intensity of the activity by speeding up or slowing down your movements.

Through experience of monitoring how your body feels, it will become easier to know when to adjust your intensity. For example, a walker who wants to engage in moderate-intensity activity would aim for a level of "somewhat hard" (12–14). If he describes his muscle fatigue and breathing as "very light" (9 on the scale) he would want to increase his intensity. On the other hand, if he felt his exertion was "extremely hard" (19) he would need to slow down his movements to achieve the moderate-intensity range.

#	Level of Exertion	Activity
6	No	Lying in bed or sitting in a chair, relaxed. Little or no effort.
7	Very, very light	
8		
9	Very light	
10		
11	Fairly Light	
12	Somewhat hard	Target range: Cardiorespiratory exercise or moderate activity.
13		
14		
15	Hard	
16		
17	Very hard	Vigorous exercise or high intensity interval training. Maximal effort.
18		
19	Very, very hard	
20	Maximum exertion	

Figure 14. The Borg scale.

ACSM	HHS
• Adults should get at least 150 minutes of moderate-intensity exercise per week. • Exercise recommendations can be met through 30–60 minutes of moderate-intensity exercise (five days per week) or 20–60 minutes of vigorous-intensity exercise (three days per week). • Adults should train each major muscle group two or three days each week using a variety of exercises and equipment. • Very light or light intensity is best for older persons or previously sedentary adults starting exercise. • Adults should do flexibility exercises at least two or three days each week to improve range of motion. • Each stretch should be held for 10–30 seconds to the point of tightness or slight discomfort. Repeat each stretch two to four times, accumulating 60 seconds per stretch.	• All adults should avoid inactivity. Some physical activity is better than none, and adults who participate in any amount of physical activity gain some health benefits. • For substantial health benefits, adults should do at least 150 minutes (2 hours and 30 minutes) a week of moderate-intensity, or 75 minutes (1 hour and 15 minutes) a week of vigorous-intensity aerobic physical activity, or an equivalent combination of moderate- and vigorous-intensity aerobic activity. Aerobic activity should be performed in episodes of at least 10 minutes, and preferably, it should be spread throughout the week. • For additional and more extensive health benefits, adults should increase their aerobic physical activity to 300 minutes (5 hours) a week of moderate-intensity, or 150 minutes a week of vigorous-intensity aerobic physical activity, or an equivalent combination of moderate- and vigorous-intensity activity. Additional health benefits are gained by engaging in physical activity beyond this amount. • Adults should also do muscle-strengthening activities that are moderate or high intensity and involve all major muscle groups on 2 or more days a week, as these activities provide additional health benefits.

Figure 15. ACSM and HHS activity guidelines.

Time — The federal guidelines for physical activity recommend 150 minutes of moderate-intensity activity per week or 75 minutes of vigorous-intensity. More is recommended for weight management or loss, as a reminder. For additional and more extensive health benefits, adults should increase their aerobic physical activity to 300 minutes (five hours) per week of moderate-intensity, or 150 minutes per week of vigorous-intensity aerobic physical activity, or an equivalent combination of moderate- and vigorous-intensity activity. Additional health benefits are gained by engaging in physical activity beyond this amount.

Moderate intensity — 30–60 minutes of continuous activity, five times per week.

Vigorous intensity — 20–60 minutes of continuous activity, three times per week.

Time, intensity, and frequency are closely tied together. For vigorous workouts, less time is required to achieve similar benefits as moderate-intensity workouts. Vigorous workouts are not recommended until a person has established a solid cardiorespiratory foundation. Cardiorespiratory sessions can be broken up into multiple ten-minute sessions. Remember, a person can benefit from some activity even if they are not able to meet the time guidelines identified here.

In terms of the duration of your entire program, research suggests that at least six weeks is required to see noticeable improvement, and as much as a year or more before a peak in fitness is reached (Figure 15).

Type — Cardiorespiratory endurance activities include rhythmic movements of large muscle groups. With that in mind, there are many options for cardio training. People often ask, "What is the best type of exercise?" The answer is simple: one that you will actually do. It should be accessible, affordable, and something that you can enjoy. Try different activities to see which ones you enjoy the most. It is helpful to choose a variety of exercises to avoid overuse injuries and stay motivated. This could be running, aerobics class, bicycling, swimming,

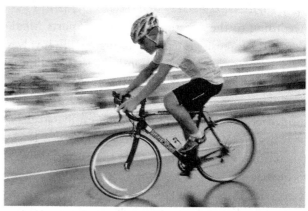

Figure 16. Cycling can be a moderate or vigorous activity.

walking, rowing, cross-country skiing, hiking, basketball, volleyball, dancing, or any activity that elevates your heart rate to the target zone and utilize your large muscles (Figure 16).

Cardiorespiratory exercise can be done indoors, outdoors, on a team, solo, or in a group. You might find that you enjoy a competitive form of exercise where you are playing a game or sport, or you may learn that you find a run outdoors satisfying. It may be worth taking a Physical Education course to explore an exercise mode more in-depth and gain hands-on experience.

Healthy Ways to Meet Guidelines

Training for CRF should follow the guidelines from the American College of Sports Medicine and the US Department of Health and Human Services' 2008 Physical Activity Guidelines for Americans. Fortunately, there are many ways to meet these guidelines safely and offer variety in your training. This will keep you focused and interested in enhancing your CRF.

Cross-Training

Cross-training is when a person takes advantage of different methods of training to develop a specific aspect of their fitness. To improve CRF, varying the type of aerobic activity you perform gives you many options. It can also help you work a variety of muscles and reduce your risk of injury. It is a good method of balancing a healthy training frequency while correctly resting other areas of your body when needed. You can vary not only your aerobic activities, but also your other types of activity, those that work your muscles and improve flexibility. You can play soccer one day, and lift weights and do yoga the next. What you choose depends on your goals and interests.

Your friend Kendal, the track enthusiast, actually does not run every time she works out. She has had issues with shin splints over the years and finds that she can work her CRF in other ways and still be ready to run during competition. She runs three days, and then on the other two she bicycles, takes a low-impact aerobics

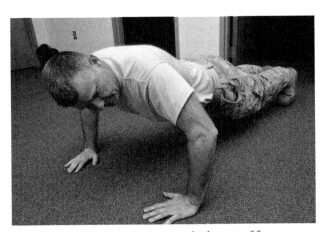

Figure 17. Cross-training improves multiple areas of fitness.

class, does kickboxing, or even occasionally swims laps. This helps her work a variety of muscles, keeps her from getting bored, and also reduces the risk of overusing her sensitive shins.

High Intensity Interval Training (HIIT)

According to the American College of Sports Medicine, High Intensity Interval Training (HIIT) involves repeated episodes of high-intensity activity followed by varied recovery times. These intense segments can range from five seconds to eight minutes and are performed at 80% to 95% of a person's estimated maximal heart rate. The recovery periods may last for as much time as the workout periods and are usually performed at 40–50% of a person's estimated maximum heart rate. The workout continues with the alternating work and relief periods totaling 20–60 minutes.

These workouts can be performed with nearly any type of activity, including cycling, walking, swimming, elliptical cross-training, and even in many group exercise classes. They provide similar fitness benefits as continuous endurance workouts, but in shorter periods of time. This is because HIIT workouts tend to burn more calories than traditional workouts, especially after the workout. The post-exercise period is called the excess post-exercise oxygen consumption (EPOC). This is generally about a two-hour period after a workout where the body is restoring itself to pre-exercise levels, using more energy.

Benefit	Description
Helps build endurance	High Intensity Interval Training (HIIT) adapts to the cellular structure of muscles which enables you to increase your endurance while doing any type of exercise.
Burns calories and fat in a shorter period of time	Studies show that 15 minutes of HIIT burns more calories than jogging on a treadmill for an hour.
Effective energy use	Through HIIT your body learns how to efficiently use the energy that comes from your body's energy system.
Boosts metabolism	HIIT helps you consume more oxygen than a non-interval workout routine. The excess amount of oxygen consumed helps increase your rate of metabolism from about 90 minutes to 144 minutes after a session of HIIT.
Burn calories and fat hours after you leave the gym	When participating in such HIIT workouts your body's repair cycle goes into hyper drive.
No equipment necessary	HIIT workouts are extremely cost efficient because you need zero equipment! All you need is a little open space.
Lose fat and not muscle	Steady cardio is often associated with losing muscle. HIIT workouts, however, combine weight training (the weight being your body) and effectively allows dieters to preserve their muscle gain while still shedding weight.
Choose your own workouts	HIIT doesn't limit you to just running or biking. In fact, you can pick any cardio workout and make it an interval workout.
Good for heart health	With HIIT it's easier to push yourself to that level because of the rest interval that comes right after you reach that point.
Challenging	HIIT workouts offer a new challenge and beginners a quicker way to see results.

Figure 18. Benefits of HIIT training.

HIIT training has been shown to improve:

- Aerobic and anaerobic fitness
- Blood pressure
- Cardiovascular health
- Insulin sensitivity (which helps the exercising muscles more readily use glucose for fuel to make energy)
- Cholesterol profiles
- Abdominal fat and body weight while maintaining muscle mass

Developing a HIIT Program

The ACSM states that when developing a HIIT program, you should consider the duration, intensity, and frequency of the work intervals and the length of the recovery intervals. Intensity during the high-intensity work interval should range ≥80% of your estimated maximum heart rate (Figure 19). As a good subjective indicator, the work interval should feel like you are exercising "hard" to "very hard." Using the talk test as your guide, carrying on a conversation would be difficult. The intensity of the recovery interval should be 40–50% of your estimate maximal heart rate. This would be physical activity that feels very comfortable in order to help you recover and prepare for your next work interval. The talk test isn't much help here because you will be in EPOC, and breathing may still be heightened.

Age	Steady State Heart Rate	Interval Heart Rate
20	60–80 Beats Per Minute	100–170 Beats Per Minute
30	60–80 Beats Per Minute	95–162 Beats Per Minute
40	60–80 Beats Per Minute	93–157 Beats Per Minute
50	60–80 Beats Per Minute	90–153 Beats Per Minute

Figure 19. Steady state and interval heart rates by age.

The relationship of the work and recovery interval is important. Many studies use a specific ratio of exercise to recovery to improve the different energy systems of the body. For example, a ratio of 1:1 might be a three-minute hard work (or high-intensity) bout followed by a three-minute recovery (or low-intensity) bout. These 1:1 interval workouts often range about three, four, or five minutes followed by an equal time in recovery.

Another popular HIIT training protocol is called the "spring interval training method." With this type of program, the exerciser does about 30 seconds of a sprint or other activity with a near full-out effort, followed by four to five minutes of recovery. This combination of exercise can be repeated three to five times (Figure 20). These higher-intensity work efforts are typically shorter bouts (e.g. 30 second sprint intervals).

Time	Interval	Exertion Level (0–10)
5 min.	Warm-up	3–4
1 min.	Speed	7–9
2 min.	Recovery	5–6
1 min.	Speed	7–9
2 min.	Recovery	5–6
1 min.	Speed	7–9
2 min.	Recovery	5–6
1 min.	Speed	7–9
2 min.	Recovery	5–6
5 min.	Cool-down	3–4

Figure 20. Sample HIIT training program.

Safety Concerns

HIIT training can easily be modified for people of all fitness levels and special conditions, such as people who are overweight or have diabetes. However, people who are inactive or who may have an increased coronary disease risk should get medical clearance from a physician before starting HIIT or any exercise training. These risks could be due to family history, cigarette smoking, hypertension, diabetes (or pre-diabetes), abnormal cholesterol levels, and obesity.

Prior to beginning HIIT training, you are encouraged to establish a foundational level of fitness. This foundation is sometimes referred to as a "base fitness level," usually requiring consistent aerobic training (three to five times a week for 20 to 60 minutes per session at a somewhat vigorous intensity) for several weeks. Establishing appropriate exercise form and muscle strength are important before engaging in regular HIIT to reduce the risk of injury.

Regardless of your age, gender, and fitness level, one of the keys to safe participation of HIIT training is to modify the intensity of the work interval to your preferred level of challenge. Safety should always be your first priority. Focus more on finding your own optimal training intensities rather than on keeping up with other people.

HIIT workouts are more exhaustive than traditional endurance workouts. Therefore, a longer recovery period is often needed. Perhaps start with one HIIT training workout a week, with your other workouts being your normal workouts. As you feel ready for more challenge, add a second HIIT workout a week, making sure you spread the HIIT workouts throughout the week.

Choosing a Fitness Program

Each person should carefully determine their exercise intensity based on their SMART goals and the safety of their chosen intensity. The type of CRF exercise you choose should suit your fitness goals and your preference for activity type. If you don't like competitive sports, don't do them! Hate aerobics classes? No need to go — there are plenty of options to choose from, so pick something you prefer. If you develop an exercise plan that works with your personality and interests, it will be more fun. If it feels more fun, you'll find it easier to stick to your new program.

Also, the amount of time you spend in each cardiorespiratory fitness activity should reflect a consideration of the guidelines and safety for you. Someone who is already athletic might comfortably jump into a HIIT program, but a low-activity person exercising for the first time might want to try something easier, like starting a Couch-to-5K program, or joining a walking group.

Stages	Description
Stage 1	People new to cardiorespiratory exercise need to develop a baseline level of aerobic fitness to avoid over-training and exhaustion. Generally, exercising at an estimated maximal heart rate (HRmax) of 65 to 75% is a safe intensity for apparently healthy adults; or 12 to 13 on the Rating of Perceived Exertion Scale (RPE) 6–20 scale. During this training period you should strive to gradually increase the duration and intensity of exercise bouts.
Stage 2	Stage II is the introduction to interval training in which intensities are varied throughout the workout. You should use intervals ranging from 65 to 85% of HRmax; or 14 to 16 RPE. Stage II differs from high-intensity anaerobic interval training in that it uses more moderate to challenging work intervals (i.e., running, not sprinting) with varying lower-intensity recovery periods (i.e. light jogging). This format also tends to be more engaging and less boring than steady state aerobic exercise.
Stage 3	Stage III is a form of high-intensity interval training involving short, intense bouts of exercise (i.e. sprinting), interspersed with active bouts of recovery (i.e., light jogging). People training in stage III should use intervals ranging from 65 to 95% of HRmax; or 17 to 19 RPE. The time needed to transition to stage III training is variable, perhaps requiring 2 to 3 months or longer.

Figure 21. Sample cardiorespiratory training based on prior and current experience.

Scenarios: Fitness Training Plans

Here are two examples that show how people at different ages, levels of fitness, and levels of experience can safely become more active over time.

Scenario — Bill: A Man Who Has Been Inactive for Many Years. Bill wants to work his way up to the equivalent of 180 to 210 minutes (three hours to three hours and 30 minutes) of walking per week. On weekdays he has time for up to 45 minutes of walking, and he plans to do something physically active each weekend. He decides to start with walking because it is moderate intensity and has a low risk of injury.

- The first week, Bill starts at a low level. He walks ten minutes a day three days per week. Sometimes he divides the ten minutes per day into two sessions. He prefers to alternate rest days and active days. (Total = 30 minutes per week)

- Between weeks three and eight, Bill increases duration by adding five minutes a day and continues walking on three non-consecutive days each week. The weekly increase is 15 minutes. (Week three total = 45 minutes / Week eight total = 120 minutes or 2 hours)

- In week nine, Bill adds another day of moderate-intensity activity on the weekend, and starts doing a variety of activities, including biking, hiking, and an aerobics class. Gradually increasing the minutes of activity by week twelve, he is doing 60 minutes or more of moderate-intensity activity on the weekend.

Reaching his goal: Over three months, Bill has increased to a total of 180 moderate-intensity minutes a week.

Scenario — Kim: An Active Woman. Kim currently does 150 minutes (two hours and 30 minutes) a week of moderate-intensity activity. She wants to work up to at least the equivalent of 300 minutes (five hours) of moderate-intensity activity a week. She also wants to shift some of that moderate-intensity activity to vigorous-intensity activity. Her current 150 minutes a week includes:

- Thirty minutes of mowing the grass one day a week;

- Thirty minutes of brisk walking four days a week;

- Fifteen minutes of Zumba two days a week.

Over a month, Kim adds walking on another weekday, and she gradually adds 15 minutes of moderate-intensity activity on each of the five walking days each week. This provides an additional 105 minutes (one hour and 45 minutes) of moderate-intensity activity.

Over the next month, Kim decides to replace some walking with jogging. Instead of walking 45 minutes, she walks for 30 minutes and jogs for 15 minutes on each weekday, providing the equivalent of 300 minutes a week of moderate-intensity physical activity from her walking and jogging.

Reaching her goal: After these increases, Kim is doing a total of 180 minutes of moderate-intensity activity each week (walking and mowing the grass) and doing 75 minutes (one hour and 15 minutes) of vigorous-intensity jogging. One minute of vigorous-intensity activity is about the same as two minutes of moderate-intensity activity, so she is now doing the equivalent of 330 moderate-intensity minutes (five hours and 30 minutes) a week. She has more than met her goal.

Conclusion

Your next steps should include assessing your own CRF and using your results to create a CRF plan that includes raising your activity level and monitoring your intensity for safety. Try different cardiorespiratory activities so that you can find something that you enjoy, and try to work moderate activity into your life on most days of the week. You might find that if you take brief activity breaks or walk between classes, it's not that difficult to work this into your day.

If you are not ready to commit to an exercise program, consider ways that you can increase your activity throughout the day, such as walking to school or walking your dog. If you are already incorporating cardiorespiratory exercise, you might think about how you can take your workout to the next level and stay consistent throughout the years. Staying active with cardiorespiratory exercise can help your heart stay healthy and functioning longer. You will also likely find that you have increased energy to enjoy a good quality of life for many more years.

Chapter 4
Muscular Strength and Endurance

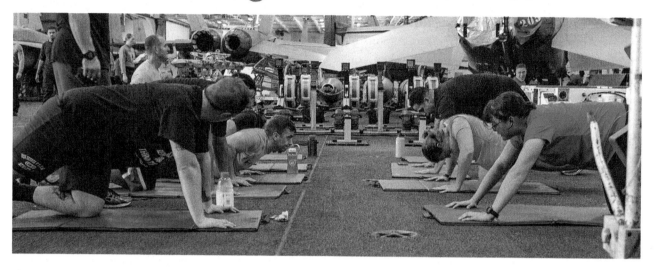

One component of fitness relates to the strength of our muscles and their capability to sustain that strength for as long as it is needed. We often depend on our muscles to perform without considering whether or not they are up to the challenge. We expect to be able to carry our 60-pound backpack all the way to class, even on days when we parked several extra blocks away from campus. Most of us just expect that we will be able to use our core muscles to go stand-up paddle boarding with some friends (Figure 1). On the other hand, many of us understand the concept of lifting weights at the gym and know that we can't lift just any weight. But in our day-to-day lives we don't think about our muscles having any limitations until we call upon them to complete a task and suddenly don't have the strength or stamina to get the job done.

Our lifestyle dictates just how much strength and energy we need to get through our day. Training for strength and endurance can have a significant impact. Each of the important muscle groups can be improved using targeted training techniques, and an understanding of the muscle and its functional components can help you along the way. This chapter will define muscular strength and endurance, describe some muscle types' structure and function, and show why muscular fitness is so important. It will then provide methods for you to assess your muscular fitness, set goals to improve it, and plan your own muscle strength and endurance training program.

Figure 1. Paddle boarding uses core muscles.

Muscular Fitness

Muscular fitness is measured by how often, for how long, and under how much resistance our muscles can contract without becoming fatigued. The primary function of our muscles is contraction, responsible for almost all of our body's movement. They control not only our obvious movements, like walking, bending, grasping objects, and running but also contract to maintain our posture, stabilize our joints, and even produce as much as 85 percent of the heat our body needs.

Muscles are a complex system with many parts to consider. The body contains various types of muscles — such as skeletal, cardiac, and smooth muscles — in addition to an array of fibers, tendons, ligaments, and other connective tissues that enable them to work on

our behalf. There are many working pieces involved in each and every contraction, voluntary and involuntary.

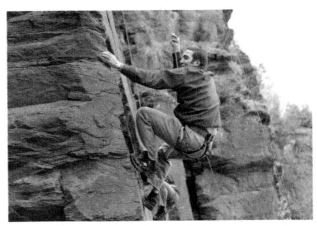

Figure 2. Rock climbing uses several muscle systems at once.

Muscle Strength

Muscular strength is the maximal amount of force a person can exert for a short period of time. The concept is simple — lifting something involves muscles strength. Lifting something heavy requires more strength. Your muscle's strength is what enables you to

hold up your end of that heavy sofa your friend wants you to help him move or lift that bag of trash you really should have taken out to the dumpster 2 days and 10 pounds ago.

Muscle Endurance

Muscular endurance is the ability of a muscle or group of muscles to repeatedly exert force against resistance. This is what enables you to do something several times without getting tired. Your strength enables you to pick up the end of that sofa for the friend who is always ask-

ing you to help him move, but your endurance is what determines how far you can carry it. Your muscular strength helps you lift the bag of trash, but your endurance will tell you if you will make it to the dumpster without having to set it down on the way.

Muscle Power

Muscular power is the maximum about of "work" that can be completed in a unit of time. "Work" is a concept from physics that specifically relates to energy transfer between the energy source and an object. Strength doesn't necessarily equal power. For example, high

upper-body strength might allow you to lift a lot of weight, but it doesn't necessarily mean you can throw a ball very far because of how that relies on speed in addition to strength. Power is the combination of forces that lets you transfer energy into something else.

Muscle Force

Muscular force is the measurable output of your muscles. To use another physics example, the downward force of gravity must be matched by the upward force

of your muscles if you are going to lift a weight off the ground. Your muscles have to be able to generate that much or more force.

Muscle Structure

Basic muscular structure comes in three types: skeletal, cardiac, and smooth.

Skeletal muscles are striated (having transverse streaks, appearing striped or grooved) and usually attached to bones (Figure 3). These are the muscles we control *voluntarily* through our central nervous system, responsible for moving our bones and supporting our skeleton. They make up 42% of the average adult male's body mass, and 36% of the average adult female's body mass. The muscles that control our arms (biceps and triceps) and legs (quadriceps and hamstrings) are examples of skeletal muscles, as are those controlling our abdomen, fingers, toes, eyes, nose, and any other part of the body with bone involvement that we move deliberately. Skeletal muscles attach to bones via **tendons** — strong, collagen-based cords. Bones attach to one another via **ligaments** and **cartilage** — other strong, collagen-based connective tissues.

Smooth muscles are non-striated muscles that operate bodily functions that you cannot control with intentional movements. These are *involuntary*, controlled by our autonomic nervous system. They are found in walls of hollow internal areas such as the iris of the eye, veins, trachea, and urinary and digestive tracts. These muscles make a slow, rhythmic contraction.

Cardiac muscles are striated muscles found in the walls of the heart, controlled by the autonomic nervous system . The heart is our muscular pump responsible for circulating blood (with its oxygen and nutrients) to all other parts of the body. The muscles contract in a strong, rhythmic manner, moving approximately five liters of blood per minute.

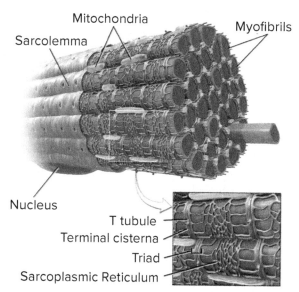

Skeletal Muscle Fiber

Figure 3. Skeletal muscle fibers.

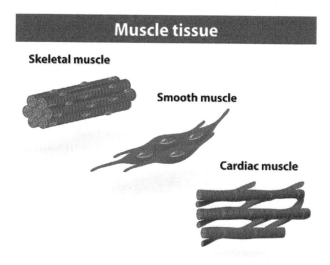

Figure 4. Structure patterns in different muscle types.

Strength Training on Skeletal Muscles

Strength training has specific effects on skeletal muscles, including hypertrophy — an increase in the size of the muscle, and atrophy — the shrinking or wasting away of the muscle. A little knowledge of how the muscles function can help us plan our training to maximize results.

As we age, in particular, our muscle mass becomes very important in helping us maintain our independence and health. A decrease in muscle mass in an older adult can lead to poor mobility, balance problems, illness, and even vision problems. A decrease in muscle strength can begin as early as age 30. By the age of 80, the average older adult has lost 30% of his or her muscle mass. Muscle strength declines even more rapidly than bone or muscle mass. The less active a person is, the earlier they will experience the issues that come with muscle loss.

To complicate this matter, the retirement age in the US has been increasing over the years, often due to economic reasons. People are often working beyond age 65. In fact, the Social Security Administration does not pay full benefits until age 66 for current retirees and people born after 1960 can expect to work until at least 67 for these benefits. Many people often choose to work even longer to save more for their retirement. The need to stay active and healthy as long as possible may be crucial. Strength training may mean more to you than just your health by the time you are in your sixties — it could mean your livelihood.

Muscle Physiology

Skeletal muscles are the type we can train for greater strength and endurance, so understanding more about their physiology will help us know why training yields improvements. Each contains different types of tissue — muscle, connective, nerve, and blood or vascular. The muscles can vary in size from tiny, such as those in the eye or ear, to large, such as those in the leg. Regard-less of size and location, their fibers play an important role in the function of the muscle.

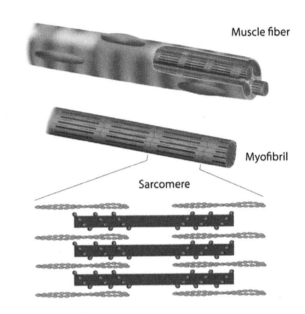

Figure 5. Myofibril structure.

Muscle Fibers

Skeletal muscles are made up of multiple bundles of cells called muscle fibers. Skeletal muscle fibers are cylindrical and have more than one **nucleus** (the "brain" of your cell, where DNA is stored) in their cells. These fibers are composed of **myofibrils**, and myofibrils are composed of action and **myosin filaments**. These are repeated in units called **sarcomeres**, the basic functional units of the muscle fiber. The sarcomere is responsible for the stri-ated appearance of skeletal muscle and forms the basic machinery necessary for muscle contraction. These bun-dles of fibers, like many other cells in the body, are delicate. They are covered in a layer of connective tissue that helps them hold up under frequent or even constant movement (Figure 6).

Each muscle cell could have thousands of sarcomeres. One sarco-mere contains many fila-ments called **actin** (thin) and **myosin** (thick). According to **sliding filament theory**, skeletal muscles function by the actin filaments of muscle fibers sliding past the myosin filaments during

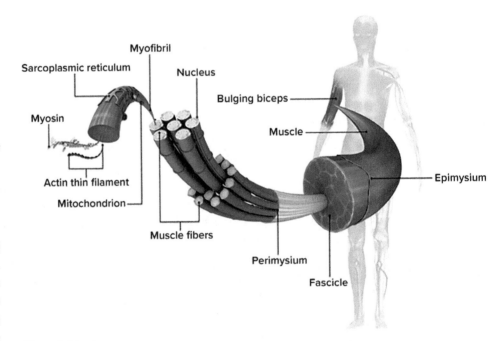

Figure 6. Muscle structure.

muscle contraction. Essentially, the friction shortens the muscle and causes the contraction (Figure 7). **Motor units** are the groups of fibers controlled by a particular neuron terminal from your brain. When a motor unit is activated, all of its fibers contract. The energy needed to make this movement possible, called ATP (see Chapter 3) is produced by **mitochondria** in the muscle cells.

Types of Muscle Fibers

There are two main types of muscle fibers: **slow-twitch muscle fibers** (type I) and **fast-twitch muscle fibers**, which come in two varieties — type IIa and IIx. Most of your muscles contain both types of fibers, though some parts of the body may contain more of one kind. There is no definitive evidence yet available to suggest that we can convert certain types of fibers from slow to fast or fast to slow, but exercising both will enable your body to be ready for different forms of activity.

Slow-twitch fibers are darker or redder in appearance because they contain a high number of capillaries. They also have a good amount of **myoglobin** that allows the muscle fiber to store oxygen. They are considered relatively fatigue resistant. The body uses them for activities such as long-distance running and bicycling (Figure 8). Certain parts of the body may have more slow-twitch fibers than fast-twitch. The muscles responsible for your posture, for example, may contain more because they must be frequently in a state of endurance.

Slow-twitch muscle fibers enable endurance, so cardiovascular training and activities that focus on prolonged endurance are important to their enhancement. Activities like long runs, swimming laps, and long bicycle rides are examples of slow-twitch enhancing exercises.

Fast-twitch muscle fibers handle short-term bursts of movement (Figure 9). These fibers typically generate energy through an anaerobic process, meaning they utilize carbohydrate combustion rather than oxygen to create fuel. Fast-twitch muscle fibers have fewer capillaries and aerobic enzymes. They contract quickly but fatigue faster than slow-twitch fibers because they use more energy. The body recruits them for activities that require shorter spurts of energy such as, sprinting, jumping, and catching objects. Muscles that are naturally responsible for quick movement on a regular basis, such as those in the eye, may have more fast-twitch fibers, but like slow-twitch, we can perform exercises that activate these particular fibers in all of our muscles.

Type IIa fast-twitch muscle fibers, also called intermediate fast-twitch, can use either aerobic or anaerobic metabolism to generate energy. Type IIa are relatively fatigue

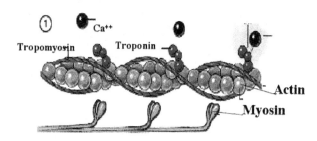

Figure 7. How sliding filament theory works.

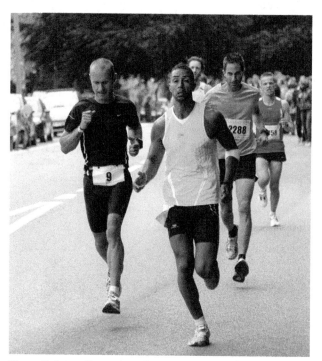

Figure 8. Long-distance running requires strong slow-twitch muscles fibers.

resistant. Essentially, they are a combination of slow-twitch (type I) and fast-twitch (type II). *Type IIx* fibers are the typical fast-twitch fiber that uses anaerobic metabolism and excels at rapid movement. These fibers fatigue rapidly. Using force and resistance against the muscles when training helps the body's readiness to recruit these fibers when needed. Lifting heavy or moderately heavy weights with shorter repetitions, for example, will activate these fibers as will doing sprints or agility drills.

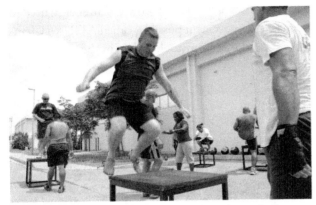

Figure 9. Bursts of movement require fast-twitch muscle fibers.

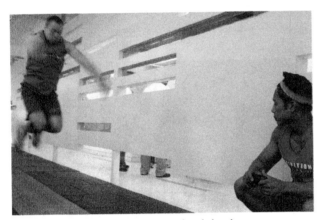

Figure 10. Muscles are used to propel and absorb momentum.

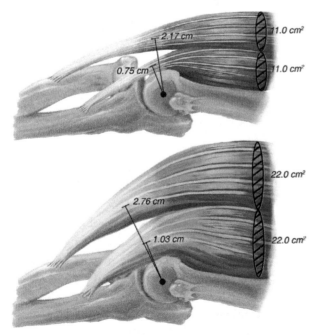

Figure 11. Muscle hypertrophy.

Hypertrophy is defined as the growth in the size of the organ or tissue by increasing its cells, in this case the muscles (Figure 11). It is often broken into two categories — sarcoplasmic and myofibril. Sarcoplasmic refers to the fluid in the muscle, whereas myofibril refers to the fibers. Both can increase during training, though it is the growth in the size (not quantity) of the myofibril that we generally see when our muscles gain strength. Fast-twitch muscle fibers are more likely than slow-twitch to undergo hypertrophy. This is why your friend Jake, whose genetic makeup likely includes more fast-twitch fibers, has a greater capacity to gain strength.

Atrophy occurs when proteins in the muscle fibers begin to break down and muscle mass decreases (Figure 12). Our bodies are designed to experience protein loss to a certain extent for cellular health, replacing unwanted proteins with new proteins. Shrinkage of the muscles, however, is rarely a positive thing and can occur as a result of poor nutrition, disease, or a lack of use. Our muscles are vital to the production of energy for our bodies. Extensive muscle loss puts us at risk for metabolic disorders, such as diabetes, and our bodies are ill prepared to handle any serious illnesses that may come our way, like cancer.

Genetics

Research suggests that your genes play a significant factor in the amount of each type of muscle fibers a person has. We all know people who seem naturally predisposed to developing muscle or have the lean make-up of a long-distance runner. Your long-time friend Jake, a power-lifter, seems like he's been buff since kindergarten (with Jake around, you never had to worry about bullies). He may have more fast-twitch muscle fibers and may have gravitated to this sport out of a natural ability to excel. Likewise, when your friend Kendal was in school, she always found stamina tests in P.E. to be child's play. She now runs three miles in under 16 minutes on her college's track team. Endurance activities may have come a bit more easily to her because her muscles contain more slow-twitch fibers.

Regardless of our individual make-up, exercising for both strength and endurance will still improve our overall performance. Someone who works to strengthen his fast-twitch muscle fibers, for example, may still be able to lift a heavier weight than someone who possesses more genetically but does not exercise them. If Jake ever slacks on his weight-lifting routine, and you really step yours up, who knows? Maybe you'll finally be able to arm-wrestle him and win.

Muscle Roles

Our muscles play different roles depending upon how they are used. They typically work as a team. A muscle providing the main force in a movement is considered the **agonist**, while the muscle that opposes it is the **antagonist**. For example, during a bicep curl, the bicep is doing most of the work and serves as the agonist, while the tricep muscle (the antagonist) relaxes. In an arm extension, their roles would reverse. The tricep would become the agonist and the bicep would be the antagonist. The antagonist doesn't always relax. Sometimes it works to slow down a motion to help maintain control. If the weight during a bicep curl is heavy, the tricep/antagonist will contribute a certain amount of tension for support.

We also have muscles that help out to keep our joints safe called **stabilizers**. These function as either

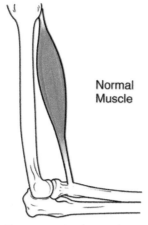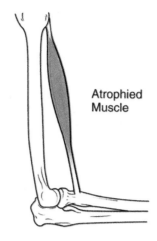

Normal Muscle

Atrophied Muscle

Figure 12. Muscle atrophy.

a **synergist**, which help movement by stabilizing the joint around which the movement occurs, or a **fixator**, which stabilize at the origin of the agonist and the joint it moves over. Our hips and shoulders joints, for example, have fixators for stability. In a bicep curl, the rotator cuff muscles serve to stabilize the movement and protect the shoulder. The muscles around the elbow (brachioradialis and brachialis) would be the synergists.

Benefits of Improving Muscle Strength and Endurance

We all can benefit from good muscle fitness and in more ways than one might imagine. Activities focused on muscle strengthening and endurance can yield many emotional and psychological benefits in addition to the physical.

Physical Benefits

As mentioned in Chapter 2, the benefits of exercise are extensive. Working on the strength and endurance of our muscles, in addition to the recommended 150 minutes of cardiovascular exercise contributes even more to our overall health and fitness than aerobic activity alone. The federal Physical Activity Guidelines recommend at least 2 days per week of muscle strengthening activity.

Recent studies indicate that only 29.3% of adult Americans meet these guidelines in 2011 — 34.4% of men and 24.5% of women. Young adults aged 18–24 meet these guidelines most often at just over 44%. This number drops nearly 10% for people aged 25–34 and the percentage continues to decline with the age of the population. Only 21.7% of adults over 65 meet the guidelines. Individuals who are overweight are even less likely to meet the guidelines at any age. It would seem that many Americans do not realize that including these exercises

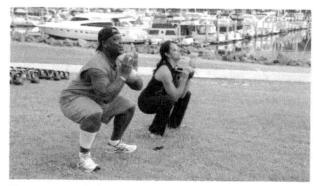

Figure 13. Muscle fitness leads to increased mobility.

into their routines results in vital strengthening needed for muscles and bones, leading to a significant impact in how they function throughout their lives, and helping improve or maintain physical functioning and avoid physical limitations (Figure 13).

Improved Performance of Physical Activities

Strength and endurance training enables us to complete our activities of daily living with greater ease. With our fast-paced lives, it can be difficult to find the time, and squeezing 2–3 days of this type of training can take a back seat to work, school, and household responsibilities.

Yet creating a plan to physically improve our bodies can make all the difference in the fulfillment of our responsibilities. Healthy muscle mass and muscle stamina enable us to get through our day-to-day tasks more quickly without fatiguing, whereas a decreased muscle mass will inhibit our functional ability. Climbing stairs, carrying boxes or loads of laundry, and just meeting the demands of our workload regardless of our profession or responsibilities becomes easier with increased strength, energy, and stamina.

Injury Prevention

If you've ever had a broken bone, sprained ankle, or simply taken a bad fall, you understand how quickly life becomes complicated. No one is immune to accidents, but the risk of certain injuries can be reduced with good muscle strength.

Improved Reaction Time

Consider how many accidents you have, or could have, avoided with quick reaction. Muscular strength and endurance lead to faster reaction times, and can help you catch yourself before a serious injury occurs. Reaction time is also important in athletics and certain types of recreation.

Improved Bone Strength

A reduction in the density of our bone minerals is one of the largest risk factors for fractures as we age. Like muscle, bone is living tissue that responds to exercise by becoming stronger. Young women and men who exercise regularly generally achieve greater peak bone mass (maximum bone density and strength) than those who do not. For most of us, bone mass peaks during our thirties. After that time, we can begin to lose bone. Women and men can help prevent bone loss with regular exercise. Strong muscles that can maintain stamina not only help to reduce the risk of falls but strengthen

Type	Benefit
Walking	Maintain a healthy weight. Prevent or manage various conditions, including heart disease, high blood pressure and type 2 diabetes. Strengthen bones and muscles. Improve mood. Improve balance and coordination.
Running	Lose weight. Boost confidence. Relieve stress. Eliminate depression.
Strength Training	Help keep weight off for good. Help protect bone health and muscle mass. Be stronger and fitter. Help develop better body mechanics. Play a role in disease prevention. Boost energy levels and improve mood. Burn more calories.
Weight Training	Increase physical work capacity and improve r ability to perform activities of daily living. Improve bone density. Promote fat-free body mass with decreasing sarcopenia. Increase the strength of connective tissue, muscles, and tendons. Improve quality of life.

Figure 14. Benefits of different training types.

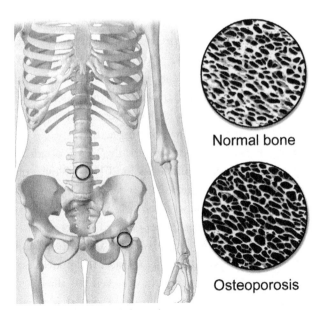

Normal bone

Osteoporosis

Figure 15. Osteoporosis bone damage.

Symptoms	Causes	Risk Factors
Back pain	Your bones are in a constant state of renewal. New bone is made and old bone is broken down. The higher your peak bone mass, the more bone you have "in the bank" and the less likely you are to develop osteoporosis as you age.	Sex
Loss of height		Age
A stooped posture		Race
A bone fracture that occurs much more easily than expected		Family history
		Body frame size
		Hormone levels
		Thyroid problems
		Dietary factors
		Steroids and other medications
		Seizures
		Gastric reflux
		Cancer
		Transplant rejection
		Medical conditions
		Lifestyle choices

Figure 16. Osteoporosis can have a severe impact on your body.

bone mass to lower the risk of fracture (Figure 15). This is especially important for older adults and people who have been diagnosed with osteoporosis (Figure 16) (see section on "Reduced Risk of Diseases").

Improved Balance and Alignment

Our skeletal muscles are connected to bone, tendons, and ligaments, all of which benefit from exercise and all of which help us keep our body in proper alignment under impact. Athletes in particular know the importance of training these muscles for injury prevention (Figure 17). When a muscle area and its connective tissue weaken, it isn't ready when it is called to use during sudden physical movements and is at an increased risk for damage.

Improved Body Composition

According to the National Institute on Aging, an increase in body fat, along with a decrease in lean muscle mass and bone density, often lead to common diseases and even disability, particularly as a person ages. Strength training can increase or maintain the amount of lean body mass and improve overall caloric expenditure. This can connect with weight management or weight loss, though it doesn't always result in lower body fat percentage. People with more muscle are able to burn more calories than people with less, even when at rest. Healthy percentages of body fat lower your risk of developing chronic diseases, such as type 2 diabetes, high blood pressure, and heart disease (see Chapter 6 on Body Composition and Chapter 9 on Chronic Diseases).

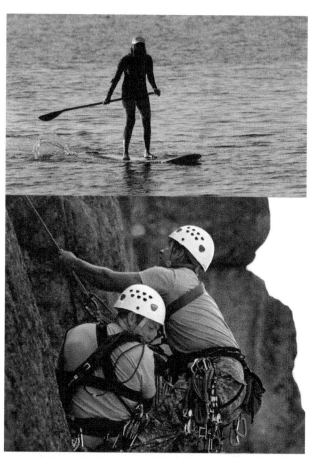

Figure 17. Athletic activities that require balance emphasize muscle strength.

Reduced Risk of Diseases

Research indicates that one of the leading causes of chronic disease and premature death is a lack of physical activity. As we age and begin to lose muscle and bone mass, along with strength, some of this loss can be avoided with regular strength and endurance exercises. In fact, maintaining skeletal muscle mass has been shown to produce positive health outcomes by providing energy reserves in the event of stress or illness.

These activities build or strengthen muscle and bone minerals, which reduces the risk of developing diseases such as *osteoporosis*, making us less prone to fractures. Osteoporosis is a disease that thins and weakens the bones. They become fragile and break easily, especially the bones in the hip, spine, and wrist. Women average 2–3% bone loss each year for the first 5–8 years after menopause, men 1% per year after age 50. For every 10% of bone mass lost the risk of fracture nearly doubles. Women, because they lose bone mass so quickly after menopause, are at a higher risk of osteoporosis.

Strength training increases metabolism, improves blood flow, and reduces fat in the body. Studies show that

Improved Athletic Performance

Improved muscular fitness can have benefits for recreational or serious athletes, in addition to making them less as risk for injury. Many sports involve strength or endurance training (or a combination of both) as a regular part of their fitness regimen. Studies indicate that improved strength and improved athletic performance go hand-in-hand. More strength means achieving greater power, faster. This means more explosiveness off the blocks for sprinters, more vertical jumping power

Additional Benefits

In addition to improved muscle and bone health with age, improved body composition, a higher metabolism (even when resting), and the avoidance of injury and physical limitations, strength and endurance training helps many other parts of our body that are less noticeable. Our posture, for example, can be improved. A strong core (torso) makes significant contributions in the way we manage nearly ever activity — sitting,

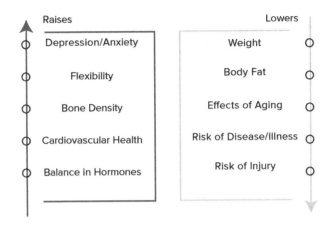

Strength Training Benefits

Figure 18. Strength training has benefits beyond strength.

it can help us avoid other issues as well, such as cardiovascular disease by lowering LDL cholesterol and raising HDL cholesterol, and by reducing blood pressure. It can also help prevent or aid in management of Type 2 diabetes, both prevention and management by improving the body's ability to process glucose.

for basketball players, more punch off the spring floor for gymnasts, and so on.

Muscular endurance training can be just as beneficial as strength. Even those athletes that seem as though muscle size and strength would be most important need endurance. Have you ever considered how much time football players spend in full gear, running up and down the field? They need the strength to carry the load, block, and tackle but need the stamina to do it safely and successfully.

standing, walking, doing chores, all of these become easier and less painful, particular in the lower back, when we maintain good muscle fitness. Even our digestion and sleep are improved through this type of physical training. This leads us to an overall improvement in our quality of life and our happiness.

Emotional and Psychological Benefits

Our confidence in our ability to handle our daily routine, the feeling of good health, and how comfortable we are with the appearance of our bodies can all impact our emotional and psychological wellness. The strength and endurance of our muscles can play an important role in helping us manage day-to-day difficulties with a positive attitude.

Improved Self-Esteem

These benefits shouldn't be thought of as non-physical, because they are caused by altered brain chemistry — specifically through changes with neurotransmitters and increased release of the endorphins mentioned earlier. Improved body image, contentment with health, and a general ability to manage your day with less stress boosts your confidence level.

Studies indicate that strength training significantly improves body image and overall comfort levels with an individual's activities of daily living. Confidence in our bodies extends well beyond what we imagine. More on this in Chapter 6.

Improved Psychological States

There have been many studies evaluating the effect of exercise on feelings of distress and personal well-being. On average, active Americans had significantly lower odds of feeling distressed and higher odds of having a more positive sense of their well-being than people who were inactive. In other words, active people are more likely to be satisfied with their lives and experience a positive psychological state.

Improved Energy

Strength and endurance training release endorphins, which hinder your body's ability to signal pain and give you a euphoric feeling. When your body reacts to stress and pain, such as when we push it physically beyond the limits it is used to, it releases endorphins to compensate. This is why runners experience what we call "runner's high." These endorphins, along with a higher metabolism, are what give you added energy.

Reduced Anxiety and Depression

Anxiety disorders, such as panic attacks, phobias, obsessive-compulsive disorders, and post-traumatic stress, impact over 16 million people in the US alone. According to the American Psychiatric Association, approximately 8 percent of women and 4 percent of men experience depression, costing the US around $83 billion annually in treatment. These issues can be debilitating, causing people to lose interest and a general ability to function in their lives and can even lead to suicide.

Physical activity, including strength training, in more than 100 population-based studies, has been shown to offer protection against symptoms related to these mental health concerns. Studies estimate that the odds of depression are lowered as much as 30–45% with regular activity. Moderate intensity resistance training, in particular, has been shown in clinical studies to reduce anxiety both immediately following a training session and long-term if the program persists. Even one session of weight training can reduce anxiety for approximately 2 hours after your workout, so imagine the results with a regular training plan in place.

Improving Muscular Strength and Endurance

To improve your muscular strength and endurance, you must first assess your current levels, set goals and plan your improvements, and then choose training exercises that target your improvement areas effectively while considering important safety and health factors.

The stage is set. The Olympic rings hover in the background and a barbell with a seemingly undefeatable amount of weight on either end sits menacingly in the center of the floor. A large, burly man with impressive arms and legs the size of tree trunks approaches the set of weights and breathes deeply. With his body perfectly positioned, the veins bulging from his neck, and a series of grunts he jerks the massive weight to his chest, then over his head, before dropping it to the floor with a resounding clang. This is a 1-RM, often used as a way to measure one person's strength against another.

In weight training, the one-repetition maximum refers to the heaviest weight you can lift with your maximum effort in a single repetition for any specific exercise. This could be a bench press, bicep curl, squat, or any other activity. Professional bodybuilders and weightlifters use this measurement competitively, but for the rest of us this serves as a good indicator to determine our current strength and track our progress. There are two methods for assessing your 1-RM.

Actual 1-RM

- Decide which muscle groups to test and which exercises you will perform to complete the test. The bench press and leg press are commonly done, but the test can be used to measure any muscle group.

- Complete a set of the exercise using a weight with which you can perform 15 repetitions.

- Add a small amount of weight and complete another set of up to 15 repetitions. Keep adding weight and completing sets until you reach a weight that you cannot lift for even one repetition. The weight prior to that is your 1-RM.

- Re-test at designated intervals (usually once per month) using the same methods and exercises.

It is important to note that the warm-up process for this should not be skipped. To choose a heavy weight and attempt to lift it without properly warming up can result in injury.

Estimated 1-RM

Estimating your 1-RM is a safer way to establish your current baseline, but if you do not lift weights routinely it may not be an option. If you know that you can routinely bench 200 pounds for 10 repetitions, you can use these numbers to estimate your 1-RM using the following formula:

$$1\text{RM} = w\left(1 + \frac{r}{30}\right), \text{assuming } r > 1$$

This is the Epley formula. There are several different formulas used and some deliver slightly different results, which is why the actual 1-RM test is more accurate. For this formula, if you could lift 200 pounds for 10 repetitions your 1-RM would be 267 pounds. A different formula, such as the Brzycki, might yield a slightly different number, but you will still get a reasonable baseline for measurement.

Once you've learned your current maximum capabilities, set a time to re-evaluate and measure your progress. Assessment of your muscular strength and endurance are an ongoing process of any training.

Setting Goals

Identifying the kind and amount of improvement you want to see in your strength and endurance is important to setting goals. Remember to use SMART goals to help you achieve improvements and avoid discouragement.

Improvements to Strength

Your goals can be based on how you function throughout your day or more specific to the activity you perform. Specific goals are easier to measure, track, and adjust. If your current 1-RM for a bicep curl is eight pounds, you may have a short-term goal of ten pounds and a long-term goal of 15. If you are currently able to do five consecutive crunches, you may have a short-term goal of 15 and a long-term goal of 30. If you currently run one mile before your muscles fatigue, you may have a goal of two miles as a way to build toward better muscle endurance.

Goals with activities of daily living may not be as easy to notice until we are called upon to perform. It could be that once each month your office receives a large box of copy paper and you have to call for help to have it carried in. Your goal may be to perform this task without assistance.

Improvements to Muscle Mass (Bodybuilding)

To set and measure specific goals in muscle mass, determining your Lean Body Mass (LBM), or the amount of weight you carry on your body that isn't fat, is helpful. You can also calculate your percent body fat. A trainer or dietician can help you do this with calipers. There are many ways you can assess your body fat and set goals around improving your body composition. See Chapter 6 for more information.

Improvements to Health

Consider your needs, daily activities, and current health. If you have an illness, such as type 2 diabetes, you may have a goal of reducing or eliminating your insulin intake. If your blood pressure is high, you may be hoping to lower it. If your body composition is an issue, determine a reasonable, healthy weight and set short-term goals for weight loss, remembering that these changes take time to achieve.

Types of Training

Your plan for muscular strength and endurance should include identifying what types of training exercises will best target your improvement goals and what types of equipment you will need to use. There are three main types of training: static exercise, isokinetic training, and dynamic exercise.

Static exercise, also known as isometric exercise, utilizes resistance rather than motion of the joints. Instead, it involves tension or contraction of the muscles as they push against an object or hold the object (or body position) steady (time under tension). Put your hands together in front of your chest with your fingers pointing upward and push your palms together until you feel your biceps contract. This is an example of static exercise. Essentially, it involves placing your body in a position where you are squeezing or flexing your muscle and holding that position for a predetermined amount of time, such as when you do a plank to work your abdominals (Figure 19). Other examples of static exercises include

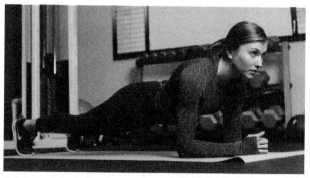

Figure 19. Planking takes muscle strength and endurance.

Type	Description
Muscle Power	Improving a muscle's explosive power, meaning its ability to perform a powerful movement in minimal time. Examples include launching into a fast sprint or jumping. Training for muscle power is generally used to help people improve their sporting performance. It involves doing one to six repetitions of each exercise at maximum speed.
Muscle Strength	All types of weight training will improve your strength. But this technique aims to improve absolute strength — meaning the ability to lift or push heavy weights. It involves one to six repetitions of each exercise performed relatively slowly.
Muscle Hypertrophy	This type of training aims to increase the amount of lean muscle in the body. It's especially useful for weight loss. It can also help with achieving a lean, toned look. For older adults, it can help counteract or reverse the age-related muscle loss that can lead to frailty.
Muscular Endurance	This kind of training helps muscles to be able to keep performing a movement for a prolonged period of time such as in Rowling. Training for muscular endurance involves doing 20 repetitions or more at a controlled speed, generally for one to three sets.

Figure 20. Different types of strength training help accomplish different things.

spine extension, glut bridge, wall sit, boat pose, and side plank.

Static training is effective in improving muscle endurance as well as strengthening muscle. This type of exercise can be done with weights as well in a variety of ways. If doing bicep curl repetitions, for example, you may do three and be unable to complete another, but you can hold the weight so that your bicep is in the flexed position for another ten seconds. If your muscles shake, that's normal. Static training forces your muscles to fatigue faster.

Isokinetic exercises are those where a special machine applies variable resistance to your limbs while in constant motion. One example of this is a stationary bike with increasing resistance to simulate inclines. It is more difficult for an athlete to overdo it or lose pace and sustain injury because the speed and resistance can be set where users can't exceed the limit.

Unlike static exercise, **dynamic training** involves the full range of motion of the muscle and movement of the joint. The muscle contracts through movement. The speed of contraction varies because muscle is weaker at its longest and shortest, and stronger in the middle of the range of motion. Because you are using the muscle's entire range of motion, the muscle is able to increase strength more effectively than static straining.

Dynamic training is the most common type and what we do during movement — based exercises, such as bicep curls, tricep dips, bench presses, squats, or crunches. This type of training offers a lot of variety and can be done almost anywhere. Dynamic exercises can be performed with free weights, machines, resistance bands, stability balls, kettle bells, and medicine balls.

Where static exercise holds the tension for a certain period of time, dynamic utilizes rhythmic repetition. When a muscle is shortened during a contraction it is considered **concentric.** When it is lengthened during a contraction, it is considered **eccentric.** In a bicep curl, the raising would be concentric and the lowering would be eccentric, working the entirety of the muscle. There is usually greater potential for a muscle to produce force during the eccentric contraction — a person can usually lower more weight than they can lift.

Both types of contractions have training benefits. Dynamic training works well for most individuals and is more effective for increasing strength, but for those with joint issues who struggle with full range of motion, static may be preferred for safety. A person could also incorporate static exercises into their dynamic strength routine to help increase muscular endurance and facilitate muscular fatigue as mentioned earlier.

Training Options

Many training options are available for each type of improvement, including weight training options, func-tional training options, plyometrics, and more. Your choices depend largely on your preferences, lifestyle, goals, and what is available to you. You can improve your strength with all of these training options.

Weight machines are available at nearly every gym and for home purchase (Figure 21). They are designed to isolate the muscle group and allow you to complete the movement without a spotter because the machine holds the weight for you through a series of cables and pulleys. You can work most muscle groups using various machines, such as the lat pull down, leg press, and rowing machine. The benefit is that they are easy and safe to use and isolate the muscle groups. The drawback is that they don't mimic normal human movement (which helps us with our day-to-day activities) or work smaller, stabilizing muscles. People who are lifting on their own prefer machines because they don't require a spotter and are less likely to sustain an injury. People who are doing strength circuits also often prefer machines.

If you're getting started, rehabilitating from an injury, or missing a spotter, weight machines might be a good choice.

Free weights require more assistance (Figure 22). You may need a spotter for many types of exercises. They do, however, allow you to use the full range of motion of the muscle, something that benefits you with your daily activities. They also tend to work those smaller, stabilizing muscles more and can promote greater strength gains. They offer more variety and allow you to combine muscle groups. Functional training, discussed below, usually incorporates free weights, along with other strength equipment. The ability to slightly change body position with free weights can help with strength development. You have to use your balance and coordination to properly strength train this way.

The drawback to free weights is that you really need a proper knowledge of good technique. Weight machines are easy because they usually have instructions on them and your exposure to injury is primarily from not knowing how much weight to attempt. You can work the same muscle groups with free weights as with weight machines, but free weights put more responsibility on the individual to know and maintain correct form in the activity. If you want to get the most out of your weight training, and you have available assistance and the knowledge to complete the task, free weights might be an excellent choice.

Functional training involves exercises that prepare the body for daily life. These exercises tend to focus on activities that build the muscles you use daily. For

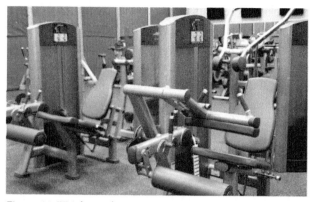

Figure 21. Weight machines.

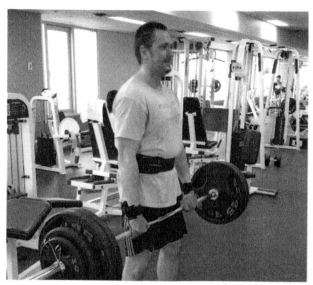

Figure 22. Free weights.

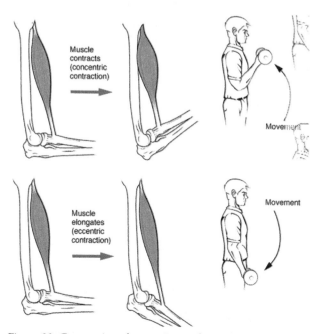

Figure 23. Concentric and eccentric muscle contraction.

example, throughout the day, we climb stairs, squat to pick up dropped objects, bend, turn, sit, stand, and so on. Many of these movements involve use of our core muscles, those that stabilize us. Exercises such as squats, lunges, abdominal work, and movements with medicine balls or stability balls force us to activate our core and improve our daily functioning.

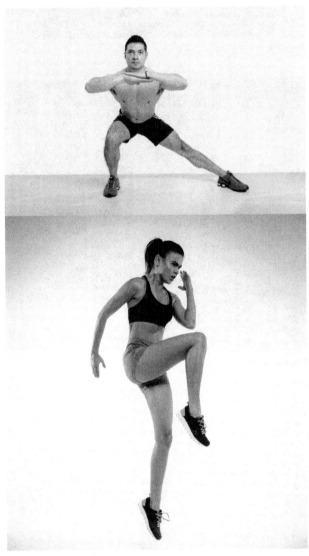

Figure 24. Strength movements.

Neuromotor exercise is a type of functional training recommended for two or three days per week. Exercises should involve motor skills (balance, agility, coordination, and gait), proprioceptive exercise training and multifaceted activities (tai chi and yoga) to improve physical function and prevent falls in older adults.

Core training is related to functional training but focuses specifically on core muscles. Like functional training, core training tends to encourages the core muscles to work as stabilizers, which is how they normally function, but core training may not include the entire body. Core muscles are hidden beneath the exterior musculature people typically train. These deeper muscles include the transverse abdominals, multifidus, diaphragm, pelvic floor, and many other deeper muscles.

These muscles support the upper and lower body through their daily movement. If your core is weak, your body may be unable to support your movement and you are more likely to sustain an injury or have lower back pain. Core exercises can include planks and side planks, deadlifts, bar exercises including toe-to-pull-up-bar leg lifts, or medicine ball chest passes.

Plyometrics focuses on speed, strength, power, and agility, often utilizing a series of jumps and leaps to build athletic performance. Jumping onto and off of boxes from different directions (box jumps and lateral box jumps), vertical leaps, broad jumps, and skater jumps (side to side movements that mimic ice or roller skating) are typical examples. These exercises train you to be quicker on your feet and more agile.

Other training methods and types of equipment include resistance bands, stability balls, Pilates, medicine balls, and no-equipment calisthenics. Many of these tools can be used at home with little to no assistance from anyone. If you can't or prefer not to pay for a gym membership, you can still train at little cost and with little space. Buy a Pilates DVD and some resistance bands, use your body for resistance, and put your knowledge to work (Figure 24).

FITT Principle

Training programs are widely available online. Here we cover the FITT Principle (see also Chapter 2) and the American College of Sports Medicine guidelines for implementing an effective training program.

Frequency

Adults should train each major muscle group two or three days each week using a variety of exercises and equipment. Adults should wait at least 48 hours between resistance training sessions.

Intensity

In muscular strength and endurance training, intensity refers to the amount of weight or resistance used. This is often calculated as a percentage of the one-rep maximum you are capable of.

For muscular strength training, a load equal to 60–70% of your 1-RM is recommended for beginners. Load of 80–100% of your 1-RM for advanced training. Lighter intensity is appropriate for older adults or people who are getting started. Intensity should be higher for people who have been exercising for some time or who want to build muscle mass.

For muscular hypertrophy, a load equal to 70–85% of your 1-RM is recommended for beginners and intermediate training. A load of 70–100% of your 1-RM is recommended for advanced training.

For muscular endurance, a different approach is needed. Overload is necessary to build endurance. The muscle needs to be stressed beyond its normal ability. Intensity in endurance training is about time instead of weight. Loads should therefore be lower, always less than 70% of your 1-RM. If you can easily do 8–12 reps, increase the weight on the next set. You want to choose a weight that you can do 8–12 reps (with proper form) that feels challenging. If it feels easy, increase the weight. If your form isn't good, reduce the weight.

Time

Training programs for muscular strength include the following exercises:

- 1–3 sets of 8–12 repetitions for beginner to intermediate training

- 2–6 sets of 1–8 repetitions for advanced training

- Rest period: 2–3 min for higher intense exercises that use heavier loads; 1–2 minutes between the lower intense exercises with light loads.

Training programs for muscular hypertrophy include the following exercises:

- 1–3 sets of 8–12 repetitions for novice to intermediate

Type

The type of exercise you choose will depend upon your fitness goals. Muscle movement exercises are possible for all muscle groups, and your chosen groups should be the focus of the exercises you choose (Figure 25).

A common myth of targeted exercise like this is fat reduction in a specific area, or "spot reducing." It is not possible to lose fat in a particular area by exercising that area only.

- 3–6 sets of 1–12 repetitions for advanced

- Rest period: 2–3 min for higher intense exercises that use heavier loads; 1–2 minutes between the lower intense exercises with light loads.

Training programs for muscular endurance include the following exercises:

- 2–4 sets of 10–25 repetitions

- Rest period: 30 seconds to 1-minute between each set

If you do not know what your 1-RM is, you can get started with a lighter weight and see how many reps you are able to do with proper form.

With a comprehensive strength program, you need to find a balance between muscle groups, exercising a variety of groups across the different days of your training. Some exercises move just one joint, while others require multi-joint movement. A good training program will include both (Figure 26).

Muscle Group	Free-Weight	Machine-Based	Body Weight
Chest	Supine Bench Press	Seated Chest Press	Push-ups
Back	Bent-over Barbell Rows	Lat Pulldown	Pull-ups
Shoulders	Dumbbell Lateral Raise	Shoulder Press	Arm Circles
Biceps	Barbell/Dumbbell Curls	Cable Curls	Reverse Grip Pull-ups
Triceps	Dumbbell Kickbacks	Pressdowns	Dips
Abdomen	Weighted Crunches	Seated "Abs" Machine	Crunches, Prone Planks
Quadriceps	Back Squats	Leg Extension	Body Weight Lunges
Hamstrings	Stiff-leg Deadlifts	Leg Curls	Hip-ups

Figure 25. Example resistance excercises.

Training Goal	Frequency	Intensity	Time
Muscle Strength (beginner)	2-3 days/week per muscle group	60-70% 1-RM	1-3 sets of 8-12 repetitions Rest: 1-3 minutes
Muscle Hypertrophy (beginnger)	2-3 days/week per muscle group	70-85% 1-RM	1-3 sets of 8-12 repetitions Rest: 1-3 minutes
Muscle Endurance (beginner)	2-3 days/week per muscle group	>70% 1-RM	2-4 sets of 10-25 repetitions Rest: 30 seconds to 1 minute
Muscle Strength (intermediate)	2-3 days/week per muscle group	60-70% 1-RM	Rest: 1-3 minutes
Muscle Hypertrophy (intermediate)	2-3 days/week per muscle group	70-85% 1-RM	1-3 sets of 8-12 repetitions Rest: 1-3 minutes
Muscle Endurance (intermediate)	2-3 days/week per muscle group	>70% 1-RM	2-4 sets of 10-25 repetitions Rest: 30 seconds to 1 minute
Muscle Strength (advanced)	2-3 days/week per muscle group	80-100% 1-RM	2-6 sets of 1-8 repetitions Rest: 1-3 minutes
Muscle Hypertrophy (advanced)	2-3 days/week per muscle group	70-100% 1-RM	3-6 sets of 1-12 repetitions Rest: 1-3 minutes
Muscle Endurance (advanced)	2-3 days/week per muscle group	>70% 1-RM	2-4 sets of 10-25 repetitions Rest: 30 seconds to 1 minute

Figure 26. Sample strength training program.

Considerations

Some considerations people must face when improving muscular fitness are their biological sex, age, and other genetic factors. Not everyone has the same capabilities, limitations, or capacity for muscle, and our physical make-up dictates, to some extent, how we will train.

Gender

Women who want to maintain their health and lifelong independence should incorporate strength training into their fitness plan (Figure 27). They benefit from improving their muscular fitness in similar ways that men do. Women in particular may consider benefits related to improving bone density and reducing their risk of osteoporosis.

Some women may be hesitant about strength training for fear of developing a bulky appearance. Due to the androgenic hormonal differences between biological males and females, women are generally unable to develop large muscles. Some women may be genetically predisposed to gaining larger muscles than others, but most will not be able to achieve the same muscle size as a man. Consider some of the fittest, most muscular female athletes — swimmers and gymnasts. Compared to the average woman, they are quite muscular. Yet given the

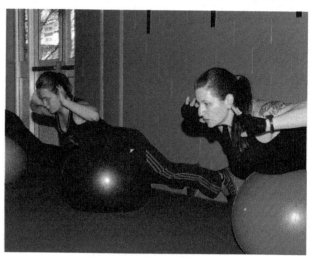

Figure 27. Women using balance in strength training.

number of hours they train, anywhere from 20 to 30 per week or more, their muscles still to do not achieve the same size of their male counterparts, in general.

For women who do want to improve their muscle mass, they would want to follow guidelines for increasing strength that are similar to the guidelines for men — moderate to heavy load, high volume with short rest periods.

Age

As mentioned earlier, our ability to build muscle size (hypertrophy) declines as we age, starting around 25–30. But that doesn't mean that we don't feel the benefits to our health and their impact on our functional level. People can improve their strength and endurance at any age. Studies show that strength and endurance training is effective in developing and maintaining independence, preventing illness and injury, maintaining a healthy weight, and improving motor skills.

A major consequence of muscle wasting is an increased risk of falling. The Centers for Disease Control reports that

falls are the leading cause of unintentional injury-related death for elderly adults. The statistics about falls and risk of fracture are striking. The lifetime risk of a fracture for men and women is about 40%. In addition, one in four women will sustain a low-trauma fracture (i.e., a fracture caused by a fall from standing height or less) after age 50.

For this reason, elderly individuals need to be proactive with strength training to both strengthen muscle and improve balance but also cautious and, if inexperienced or showing signs of cognitive decline, supervised during exercise.

Genetics

Individuals respond to strength training in different ways. Studies indicate that no specific gene can be consistently linked to athletic performance or success. They suggest that genetics likely factor into a person's success with training, but it is still unclear which

parts of our genetic code impact that success. As mentioned earlier in this chapter, scientists believe that the amount of fast-twitch vs. slow-twitch muscles a person has plays a significant role in the types of activities at which we excel.

Body size, body composition, and muscle fiber development are linked to genetics, and each plays a role in the likelihood of physical strength training success. Hand grip strength has also been linked to genetic factors by scientists as recently as July 2017.

Guidelines

Exercise guidelines for any training program must consider the amount of rest and recovery time between sessions, the specificity and progressive overload of any exercises you perform, and the prevention of injuries during and after workouts.

Rest and Recovery

Adequate rest is very important to prevent muscle atrophy and contribute to hypertrophy. Different muscle groups are worked each time we strength train. If you work your upper body on Monday, you shouldn't work it again for 2 to 3 days. The fibers experience microscopic tears during training and they need time to rest and rebuild, which is what increases strength. If you are idle too long, however, you may experience shrinkage of the muscle.

The amount of rest depends on the level of soreness you experience. Two days is a general guideline, but three may be necessary for a particular muscle group if you are still sore.

Within 24 to 72 hours following exercise, it is common to feel **Delayed Onset Muscle Soreness** (DOMS), particularly after eccentric muscle contraction. During muscle strengthening, the minute tears the fibers experience are likely what causes the pain, although this is not entirely understood. Swelling, stiffness, and loss of strength is to be expected when you increase a particular activity and challenge your muscles beyond what they are used to and is also a sign of progress. A normal response to increasing overload can be DOMS. Adding intensity more gradually to your workouts, warming-up, and cooling-down effectively can help prevent soreness. There are also ways to lessen the soreness and keep you on target with your exercise program:

- Gentle stretching

- Staying hydrated

- Taking anti-inflammatory medications, such as ibuprofen

- Using massage, foam rollers, or heat and cold treatments

Ultimately, taking it easy, but not stopping your exercise can be the best way to combat soreness. You may not be able to go full force with your activity level due to soreness, but light exercise will help keep the blood circulating to your muscles and heal them more quickly than complete rest.

Specificity

The principle of specificity suggests that to improve something, you need to train it, which is why we target specific muscle groups in our exercise plan and progressively overload these targets, adding intensity to our workouts slowly and incrementally to achieve our goals (see also Chapter 2). The more you do a specific exercise, the better you will become at it. What you choose to train depends on your goals.

If you want to strengthen your core muscles for stand-up paddle boarding, you need to include core

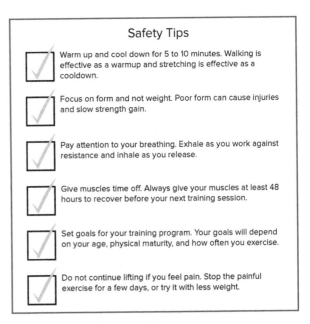

Safety Tips

☑ Warm up and cool down for 5 to 10 minutes. Walking is effective as a warmup and stretching is effective as a cooldown.

☑ Focus on form and not weight. Poor form can cause injuries and slow strength gain.

☑ Pay attention to your breathing. Exhale as you work against resistance and inhale as you release.

☑ Give muscles time off. Always give your muscles at least 48 hours to recover before your next training session.

☑ Set goals for your training program. Your goals will depend on your age, physical maturity, and how often you exercise.

☑ Do not continue lifting if you feel pain. Stop the painful exercise for a few days, or try it with less weight.

Figure 28. Safety is important in strength training.

movements regularly in your training. You will want to incorporate exercises for your abdominals, lower back, and hips, you will want to include functional movements that challenge the core muscles to hold your body in different positions.

Regardless of the type of activity, if you do not repeat it, improve at it, and gradually overload, you will see limited results. For example, if you lift weights to build strength in your arms only once every three weeks, you are not likely to experience a significant improvement. If you want to build strength in your arms but do only running, you may see some muscle definition, but since you have not specifically targeted the arms, you will not see the increase in strength you had hoped.

Safety

Safety and injury prevention is extremely important not only because it protects your health, but also because temporary lapses in your training program resulting from injury can cause reversibility, or the loss of your progress. In order to stay safe during workouts, be sure to warm-up before and cool-down after every workout, follow proper form and technique, use a spotter when lifting weights, breathe correctly, ensure the safety of your equipment, and use the right fuel for your developing muscles.

Warm-Up and Cool-Down

These activities are an important part of your exercise plan to reduce the risk of injury and lessen soreness. A strength warm-up may include a few minutes of light aerobic activity at a slower speed or lower intensity. This allows your heart rate to elevate gradually and the blood to begin flowing to your muscles.

When cooling down, spend a few minutes walking after you train to allow your heart rate time to return gradually to its normal, resting rate if it is elevated. Stretching the muscles you targeted while you are cooling down is ideal, because the blood is still flowing and the joints are still warm from the activity. This can also help reduce soreness and keep your training on schedule, in addition to improving flexibility.

Form and Technique

Strength and endurance training work well to improve your health, but the risk of injury increases when you aren't properly educated on the correct way to complete the activity. If you are just beginning a weight-training routine at the gym, it may seem like a good idea to watch the stranger next to you and see how he or she uses a particular piece of equipment, or to listen to your friend who came with you that had that one weight-lifting class in high school. A better approach is to spend some time educating yourself.

Most gyms have staff and trainers available to show you how to use equipment, not to mention detailed instructions hanging next to each apparatus. If you are training outside the gym, do your homework. Read the instruction manual that came with your medicine ball or spend some time on the Internet to find instructions from an expert in your chosen activity. The Mayo Clinic offers some general guidelines for weight training:

- Lift only the amount of weight that you can while still having correct form. You should be able to complete your set raise and lower it without dis-comfort. Some people are aiming for 5 while others are aiming for 15. If you cannot maintain good form, decrease the size of the weight. The better your form, the better your results.

- Go slow. Speed is not always an asset. Form is more important. Slow, controlled movements will yield better results and lower your risk of injury.

- Listen to your body and work within your limits. Doing more sets after you can no longer maintain your form will not lead to better results. Some individuals can do only one set, while others can do more. It depends on the activity, the body part you're training, and how many sets you complete. Doing more than you can handle may lead to injury.

- Listen to pain. If an activity hurts, try the movement in a different way to see if it feels differently. If not, stop. Try again in a few days with a smaller weight. If pain persists, talk to your health care provider.

- If you have an injury, focus on the muscle groups you are able to work.

Use a Spotter

When using heavy free-weights to strength train, it is important to have someone with you. A bit of fatigue, pulled muscle, or incorrect form could result in a lot of weight on your body unexpectedly. You may need help to place the weight in the starting or finishing position, if the weight tilts, or if you can't complete a lift. Using a spotter will reduce your chance of dropping the weight or getting injured.

Breathe

It is important to keep breathing when exercising. It may sound obvious, but some people have a tendency to hold their breath. There are dangerous implications on the heart and blood pressure for holding the breath while strength training. For your muscles to do their job, they need oxygen. How you breathe is important as well. When lifting weights, exhale as you lift and inhale as you lower (if you reverse the order, you may find it harder to do that next repetition without ready oxygen).

It is the same principle if the weight is your body.

Equipment Safety

In addition to knowing how to use the equipment safely, it's also important to ensure that the equipment is in good working order. If something is loose, broken, or making a strange noise, don't use it until it is repaired. Most equipment requires regular maintenance. You always want to

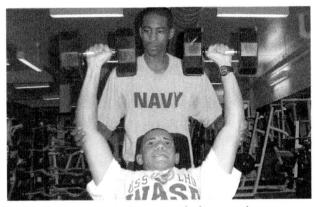

Figure 29. A spotter helps keep you safe if you overshoot your strength goals.

While doing crunches or push-ups, for example, exhale as you raise your upper body and inhale as you lower. For endurance activities, like running, athletes often find that a controlled, rhythmic pattern, breathing in through your nose and out through your mouth, often helps stamina and to prevent those nagging side cramps.

check that bands are not cracked, stability balls are adequately inflated and the proper size, weights are clear of cables or stacked to the right size, machines are locked into place, and weights are secured with collars (devices that secure weight to a barbell or dumbbell). People do lift without collars, but it is dangerous. Weights can easily slip off the bar if you lose your balance.

Dietary Supplements

For those individuals trying to build muscle or lose fat, some flawed training programs recommend the use of dietary supplements to help you achieve your goals, but they should be taken with great care because of the inherent risk and dangers associated with their misuse. We do not recommend using dietary supplements in this textbook for any reason.

The US Food and Drug Administration regulates these products but they are classified differently than drugs. Manufacturers are not required to prove the safety of their products prior to distribution, though the FDA can have products removed from the shelves if they later prove harmful. The FDA also do not evaluate whether or not these supplements prove effective in achieving what

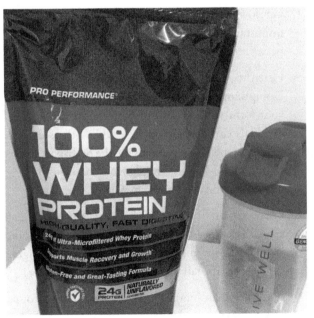

Figure 30. Protein supplements are not recommended.

they claim to achieve. Illegal supplements have other consequences, from health implications to legal risks.

Supplements range from those designed to boost energy, increase protein levels, or add amino acids to the body, to those designed to increase testosterone levels. All should be considered closely before being incorporated into your nutritional or training plan.

Creatine is an amino acid that occurs naturally in the body and stored mostly in our muscle cells. It is commonly found in the diet in red meat and seafood. Creatine can also be made in a laboratory and taken in the form of creatine supplements. When taken orally, creatine supplements can increase the creatine levels in the muscles, which help transport energy to the part of the body that needs it during contraction. It works well for activities requiring short bursts of energy, which is likely why trainers often recommend it for bodybuilders. It does not work well when combined with caffeine and could even have adverse effects if taken with other stimulants. The body can only store a certain amount of creatine, and taking in too much is not beneficial. The long-term risks of creatine use are unknown.

Protein powders are usually made from whey, soy, or casein (a milk protein), though whey is the most common. Whey protein is considered complete because it contains all 9 amino acids needed by the human body. Protein is essential to our body because it helps us convert food into energy and process toxins. We need approximately .36 grams per pound of body weight each day.

Though protein powders are generally considered safe, most people can get the protein they need from their diet. People doing increased strength training often need more protein and will add a protein powder to compensate. It is recommended that you increase your intake to 0.68–1.0 grams per kilogram of protein when trying to build muscle.

Protein supplements may not be dangerous, but they are an expensive way to consume protein. We recommend protein from real food sources. Protein supplements are generally considered safe, but there are healthier ways to consume more protein. And they may not be necessary, as most Americans do not need to increase their protein intake when strength training.

Testosterone boosters and **steroids** are sometimes used by athletes to increase their performance and muscular appearance, which may work in the short term. They can increase muscle size and help people recover faster. They are also illegal and dangerous. Anabolic steroids are a man-made version of testosterone, a male hormone. It seems ironic that these man-made, man-enhancing materials should actually (after long-term use) shrink testicles, enlarge male breasts, and lower sperm count, but they do. This is in addition to an increased risk of prostate cancer; kidney, liver, and heart damage; mood swings ("roid rage"), and irritability.

In women, ironically, we see a potential for male-pattern baldness, a deepened voice, facial hair, and an interrupted menstrual cycle. After long-term use, women become more "manly" and men lose certain aspects of their masculinity. Both are at risk for serious health problems. When steroids are used alongside other supplements, such as creatine and protein powders, there is an increased potential for kidney injury.

There are also various herbal supplements alleged to naturally boost the testosterone levels men lose as they age and, in theory, help improve or maintain muscle mass. The jury is still out on many of these supplements, but most seem to do little if anything to contribute to muscle growth. More information on supplements is available online from:

- National Center for Complementary and Alternative Medicine: nccih.nih.gov/

- National Institutes of Health Office of Dietary Supplements: ods.od.nih.gov/

- Federal Trade Commission: www.consumer.ftc .gov/articles/0261-dietary-supplements

- Food & Drug Administration Supplements: www.fda.gov/Food/DietarySupplements

Conclusion

Your next steps should be assessing your muscular strength and endurance and using what you find to create a muscle fitness plan that includes targeting areas of improvement and identifying training exercises. You may not be asked to assess your own fitness during this course, but you might consider activities that you do each day that may be easier or more enjoyable if you had greater muscular strength and endurance. Consider some ways you can adapt or change your other fitness programs to include muscle strength and endurance to stay challenged and motivated to improve your overall health and wellness.

Chapter 5
Flexibility

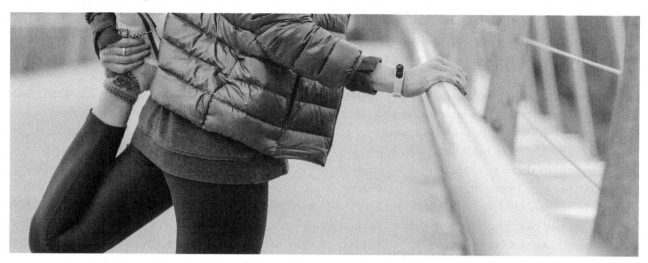

You're out for a run a few weeks before your vacation. You've always wanted to hike the Pacific Crest Trail (PCT) and decided that some initial trail running would be a good way to prepare for the terrain and build your cardiorespiratory stamina. It sounds like a good plan until you take a longer stride to avoid a puddle and tear your Achilles tendon. The good news is that your arms are about to get a major workout. The bad news? Crutches. Crutches don't hike the PCT. Your vacation will be a bit delayed.

With better flexibility you could have avoided such a scenario. Your body's flexibility is a key source of success and enjoyment of pain-free movement. You can achieve sufficient flexibility through training, making every other kind of fitness training (including runs and hikes) less prone to injury or pain.

This chapter defines and compares static and dynamic flexibility, shows why flexibility is so important, describes flexibility assessment, and details how to achieve better flexibility resulting in more satisfying exercises.

Defining Flexibility and Its Importance

Flexibility is your body's ability to execute a full range of motion, particularly involving muscles that cross joints and induce bending movements. Flexibility is specific to the joint being moved and depends upon variables, such as the rigidity of surrounding **tendons** and **ligaments**, the strong connective tissues between muscles and bones. You could be flexible in your legs, for example, but find that turning your head to check your blind spot in traffic is difficult because the range of motion in your neck seems limited. For this reason, flexibility exercises that target specific muscle groups or parts of the body are important in helping us function comfortably and safely.

You can lose your flexibility with inactivity, and regular stretching can improve your flexibility. You don't need to have a high amount of flexibility to notice

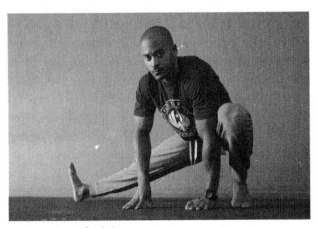

Figure 1. Static flexibility.

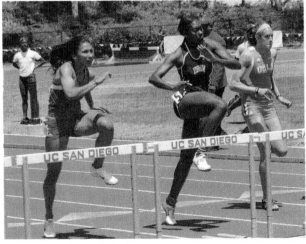

Figure 2. Dynamic flexibility.

health benefits. Flexibility is an often-overlooked aspect of fitness that is important for overall wellness.

There are two types of flexibility, static flexibility and dynamic flexibility. Static stretches impact our static flexibility **Static flexibility** is muscle movement conducted while staying relatively still with the rest of your body. How far you can reach, and hold the stretch, when bending to touch your toes is an example. It is a slow, steady stretch involving no motion other than the bend, no bouncing, pulsing, or quick repetitions (Figure 1).

Dynamic stretches impact our **dynamic flexibility**, or the absolute range of motion you can achieve through movement, such as swinging your arms across your body to see how far they can reach. In your toe touch, rather than holding the position you would do slow, controlled repetitions of the movement (Figure 2).

In our day-to-day lives, our bodies are often challenged in ways that involve both our dynamic and static flexibility. When we run, jump, hop off the curb, or have to reach out suddenly to catch something we are about to drop, our dynamic flexibility allows us to do that. It enables us to use the full range of motion of the joint. Really stretching to reach something or bending in any direction to pick something up, or even sometimes tying our shoes draws on our static flexibility to complete the task comfortably. Flexibility is important because flexible joints decreases your overall risk of injury and increases physical performance. Stretching works towards decreasing resistance in muscle tissue during any activity and helps increase blood and nutrients to tissues.

Flexibility can prevent stiffness, soreness and falls by helping to create balance around a joint in strength and flexibility. Flexibility exercises can also have benefits related to relaxation and stress management. Some types of joint pain, such as low back pain, can be improved with flexibility training.

Benefits of Flexibility

There are many benefits to flexibility that can keep us active and independent throughout our lives.

Joint Health — According to the US Department of Health and Human Services, joint pain can be one of the most common barriers to an active life, particularly as we age. Joint health is improved through maintaining flexibility and can help you avoid problems with your joints that contribute to poorer health, especially in older individuals (Figure 3). When our flexibility diminishes, our bodies begin to compensate in other ways. We stop performing activities that are uncomfortable, reducing our flexibility and activity level even more. Our posture, agility, and balance can be impacted from these limitations in our range of motion and our joints can develop chronic pain that is difficult, if not impossible, to reverse. A flexibility training program can also significantly reduce the risk of falls and related injuries, which is particularly important with aging.

If you've ever seen the hands of someone with arthritis whose joints have become contracted (bent in a certain direction), or someone disabled whose legs and feet will no longer straighten, keep that picture in your mind. Once contractures occur, research suggests that stretching does very little if anything to help because of the shortening of the ligaments and tissues. Flexible muscles and tissues at the joint enable it to move efficiently and keep it healthier longer.

Performance — Flexibility can improve performance, particularly when you focus on flexibility training that addresses the type of movement necessary for your preferred activity (your sport, hobby, or profession). To perform efficiently, whether it's throughout our normal day or during exercise, we need flexible joints to maintain balance and execute movements to the full extent needed to complete a task safely and effectively. Our flexibility has an impact on how much power we can exert during training or competition, or even when we need to respond to something in our daily lives (Figure 4). Tight muscles and tissues do not extend to their full capacity.

Imagine trying to sprint, either during a race or trying to catch your bus. Better yet, in all of those horror movies you've watched, did you ever see someone run from the chainsaw-wielding boogey man that didn't fall once or twice, even get caught? True, it's a movie, but you never see someone with martial arts training fall victim due to limited range of motion in these scenarios. Runners need increased flexibility in their legs and hips, for example. Swimmers need a full range of motion in their shoulders. For those of us that don't compete, we need good flexibility to keep our workouts consistent, comfortable, and efficient (and to keep us on our toes if we ever do need to make a run for it).

Injury and Pain — Flexibility can lead to reduced risk of injury and lower back pain, especially with the right kinds of stretches. Flexibility in our joints and

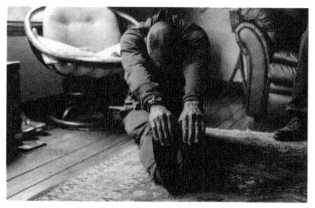

Figure 3. Stretching is important to maintaining mobility.

muscles enables us to maintain good posture and balance, which help us avoid other aches and pains, particularly in the back, shoulders, and neck.

How many times have you heard your mother tell you to stand up straight? She had good reason. If you take a moment to extend your back and abdomen and keep those shoulders back, you'll feel the stretch, and if

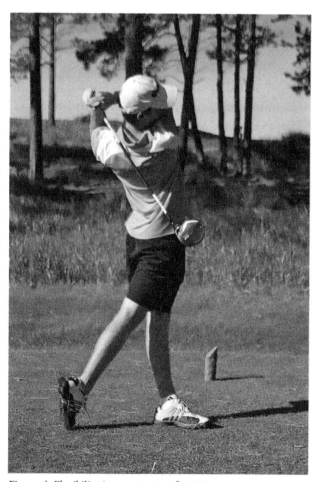

Figure 4. Flexibility impacts range of motion.

you tend to slouch, you'll feel the muscle exertion as well. We can make it easier on our bodies by keeping these muscles and joints that maintain our posture flexible. Poor posture can lead to poor balance, which can lead to injury. It can also cause our bodies to compensate in other ways, adapting to the poor position.

Your back is not the only body part susceptible to injury and pain. Your joints and connective tissues, as mentioned, can cause a great deal of chronic discomfort if not tended to properly. Your muscles, as well, need that range of motion in order to protect you to the best of their ability. Flexibility won't prevent every injury, but it can lower the risk of injuries, and it an important part of any rehabilitation from a previous injury.

Other Benefits

Reduced muscle tension — Stretching focuses on lengthening the muscle. Muscle tension is related to length. A longer muscle will be less tense.

Reduced blood pressure — It may seem strange, but when our bodies are stretched and flexible, our arteries are as well. Poor flexibility correlates to arterial stiffness. Stiff arteries are more prone to high blood pressure and cardiovascular disease.

Lowered breathing rate — If you've ever taken a yoga class, you know the importance of breathing. Part of stretching is knowing how to breathe as you stretch. This patterned breathing can be relaxing and, when done routinely, can lower your breathing rate, which is good for cardiorespiratory health.

Reduced stress and relaxation — Stretching forces us to relax our muscles. Routinely relaxing our muscles teaches our bodies to release tension. Stress is a form of tension. Flexibility training, in a sense, hard-wires our bodies to relax and relieve any form of tension it encounters. Additionally, illness and injury can be major forms of stress in our lives. The reduced risk of illness and injury the flexibility provides limits these as added stressors.

Relief from aches and pains — Stress can also cause psychosomatic responses in the body, causing physical symptoms of distress. Its reduction can make us feel better both emotionally and physically. Flexibility training stretches our muscles and connective tissues that, when tense, cause pain. This helps generate relief except when there is an injury (such as a fracture or torn ligament) present.

Relief from muscle cramps — Cramps happen when the muscle gets tight and contracts involuntarily. Stretching, which lengthens the muscle, can help relieve a cramp.

Improved mood — What happens when we reduce stress, relieve pain, limit our illnesses, and feel confident in our abilities? It stands to reason that we see an overall improvement in our mood.

Factors that Determine Flexibility

Flexibility is affected by a variety of factors, some that you can control and some that you cannot. Some factors, such as joint structure and function, cannot be changed. Other factors, such as muscle length at rest, can be changed. The goal in flexibility training is to have a full normal range of motion, not to create extreme flexibility. It's possible to have too much flexibility, just as it's possible to have too little.

Some challenges to flexibility are joint structure and function, connective tissue, nervous system regulation, injury and disease, genetics, biological sex, and age.

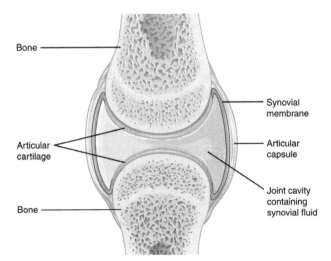

Figure 5. Joint structure.

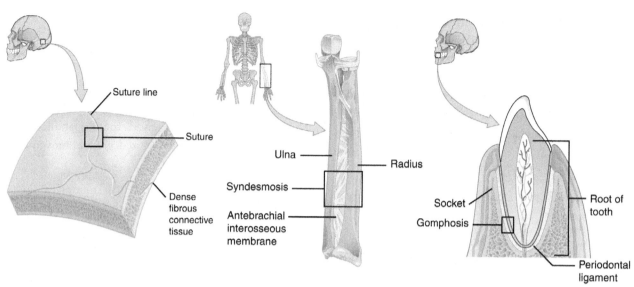

Figure 6. Ligament types.

Joint Structure and Function

Everywhere that two or more bones join together in our bodies, we have a joint. Joints can either be rigid, like the joints in your skull, or movable, like in your elbows and knees (Figure 5). Some joints have greater **range of motion** (ROM) due to their design than others. Some joints in the body have a lot of movement, some move a little, and others don't move at all. Joints are classified functionally by how they move, and structurally by how they are composed. We have three main types of joints: fibrous (synarthrodial), cartilaginous (synchondroses and sympheses), and synovial (diarthrosis).

Fibrous joints are immoveable, held together by fibrous connective tissue, like ligaments (Figure 6). How much fibrous tissue depends on how far the bones are from each other. The roots of your teeth, for example, are held into your jaw with fibrous joints, as well as the parts of your skull and other areas where the bones join but are not intended to move.

Cartilaginous joints are partially moveable. These bones connect to each other with cartilage. The vertebrae in our spines and the area where the ribs anchor are examples. Children have many temporary cartilaginous joints that we often refer to as growth plates. As they grow, bone replaces these and become permanent (Figure 7).

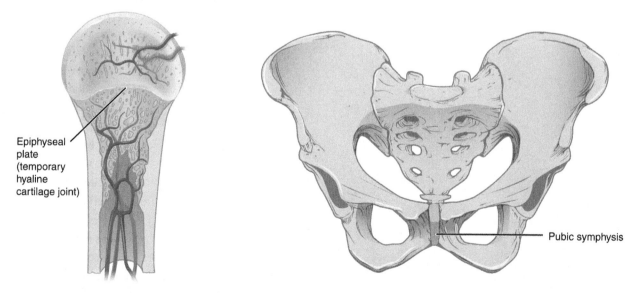

Figure 7. Ligament examples.

Synovial joints are very moveable and the ones we often think of when we envision a joint. Our knees, elbows, fingers, shoulders, and so on are synovial (Figure 8). They contain **cartilage** — hard connective tissues — membranes, and a joint cavity filled with lubricating fluid. The entire joint is surrounded by a collagenous type of capsule and a membrane that secretes the fluid into the joint to keep it moving efficiently. We have six different types of synovial joints:

- **Hinge** — Flexes and extends, such as your elbow and knee

- **Pivot** — Rotates one bone around another on its own axis, such as the first few vertebrae of your neck that enable your head to move

- **Ball and socket** — Flexes, extends, rotates, abducts (movement away from the body), and adducts (movement toward the midline of the body), such as your shoulder and hip (Figure 9)

- **Saddle** — Flexes, extends, rotates, abducts, adducts, and circumducts (360 degrees of movement), such as your thumb

- **Condyloid** — Flexes, extends, rotates, abducts, adducts, and circumducts, such as your wrist

- **Gliding** — Gliding movements, such as those that occur with the bones of your hand (intercarpal joints)

The shape of synovial joints determines in what way and degree a joint can move. Some synovial joints, such as the elbow and knee, allow movement in one direction. Other synovial joints, such as the hip and shoulder, allow movement in all directions. Joints that allow for a greater amount of movement have a higher risk of injury, as they tend to be more flexible. Flexibility varies by joint because the structure varies between joints. There is no single test to measure flexibility.

Joint structure and function can be a challenge to flexibility because not all of your joints are intended to have great range of motion. Many joints can move in almost any direction, while others, like your knees and elbows, only bend one way. We see athletes, such as gymnasts, on television and stand in awe of the way they tumble and bend.

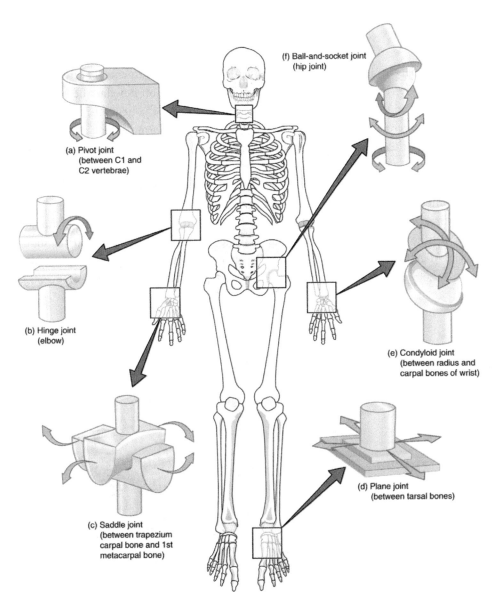

(f) Ball-and-socket joint (hip joint)

(a) Pivot joint (between C1 and C2 vertebrae)

(b) Hinge joint (elbow)

(e) Condyloid joint (between radius and carpal bones of wrist)

(c) Saddle joint (between trapezium carpal bone and 1st metacarpal bone)

(d) Plane joint (between tarsal bones)

Figure 8. Different joint types structure and function.

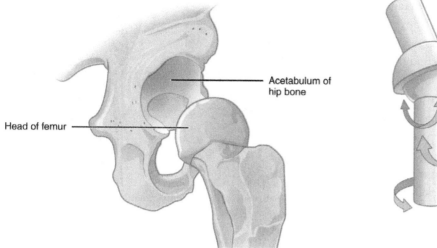

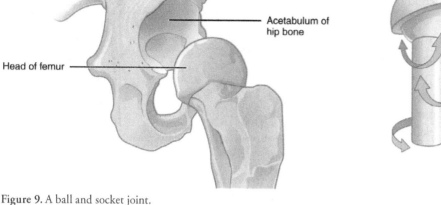

Acetabulum of
hip bone

Head of femur

Figure 9. A ball and socket joint.

We assume that their backs are quite flexible. In reality, many of those movements are accomplished through the flexibility of the shoulders, which have a greater range of motion. We may want to be able to bend our backs or any other part of our body in a certain way, but our joints will only allow us to perform certain tasks safely. Any time we move a joint beyond its natural capacity, we risk injury.

Connective Tissue and Nervous System Regulation

Our connective tissues are vital to the range of motion we experience in our joints and muscles. Collagen and elastin are types of proteins found in our connective tissues that allow them to stretch and then bounce back.

Over time, connective tissues can lose water and collagen or experience a build up of too much collagen that affect the way our body stretches. Different tissues vary in the way they can return to their original length or maintain a new length. **Ligaments**, for example, respond to stretching but do not have a fixed memory of their original shape. Some injuries can pose a risk of them acquiring a length that becomes unsafe or painful. Deep connective tissue, such as **fascia** and **tendons**, are present for stability and to prevent too much movement but can also limit range of motion.

These tissues provide stability for a joint, preventing the joint from moving too much. They also limit range of motion to prevent injury. If a person has increased

their muscle mass without also increasing their flexibility, the structures around the joint can be too tight and will limit movement. If a person's normal way of moving or daily activities emphasizes one particular muscle group or body part, those joints affected may be limited in their range of motion. Sitting is an example of this, where the hamstrings can be shortened and there may be lower back pain. This causes an imbalance between the different structures. Typically, the way to manage this is by strengthening and stretching the different areas around the joint.

Our muscles, tendons, and ligaments have **stretch receptors** that activate when the body part is lengthened or compressed by sending a message to the brain or spine through our nervous system. They are called **proprioceptors**. These facilitate the perception of our body. These allow us to move our bodies during our daily activities without having to watch our movements.

Injury and Your Joints

Injuries can challenge your flexibility. If you've ever broken a bone and been in a cast or brace for even a few weeks, you understand how difficult it can be to move your muscles and joints in the part of your body that has spent so much time not moving. Imagine, for example, that you break your ankle. You spend a few days waiting for the swelling to go down before the doctor can immobilize the joints

and bones so that the ankle can heal correctly. You then spend the next four weeks or so, if the break is minor, in a cast.

This means that not only is your ankle not getting exercise, but the rest of your body isn't getting much either. There are only so many things you can do on crutches. Your upper body and abdominals may get a workout, but the rest of your body suffers. When the cast is removed, things don't just go back to normal. It can take a long time for the ankle to be ready for strenuous exercise and even longer before it stops swelling the minute you even look at your running shoes. Naturally, your flexibility will be impacted. You find that you have to actively work to regain that range of motion.

Repeated injuries to a particular joint can lead to arthritis in the area, even at a young age. It is not uncommon for athletes to play through the pain in an attempt to compete, but this can lead to long-term complications. It's important to know how to manage and heal from a particular injury to get you back in action quickly yet safely. Your doctor should be able to advise you on what activities are safe and effective and when you can perform them.

Disease and Your Joints

Certain diseases that affect the joints can be challenging to your flexibility, creating a complicated situation for exercising. Consider a disease such as arthritis. A person with arthritis may find moving his or her joints a challenge yet movement is one of the things that help reduce the pain and swelling.

Joint diseases, such as arthritis, can limit range of motion, causing pain and swelling, and making both exercise and daily activities difficult. **Osteoarthritis** is one of the most common forms and occurs most often in older people, or in people who are inactive or over-active with certain joints (Figure 10). As cartilage wears down, our bones begin to rub together when we move them. This is why we often hear of someone having a knee or hip replacement. The pain can become unbearable and the movement so difficult that an artificial version of the joint becomes necessary. This can happen not only as a result of natural aging but also due to an injury that damages the cartilage, even in younger individuals.

Rheumatoid arthritis is considered an autoimmune disease, one in which the body's immune system attacks the tissues surrounding the joint, confusing healthy tissue with bacteria. This can be very painful, resulting in not just the pain, swelling, and limited range of motion associated with osteoarthritis, but also fatigue, fevers, and damage to other organs in the body. It is not yet understood what triggers the autoimmune conditions of rheumatoid arthritis (Figure 11).

Gout is another form of arthritis that can be quite painful. It occurs most often in men and frequently

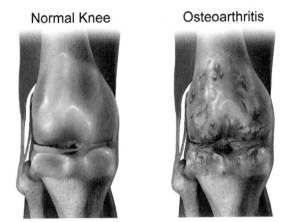

Figure 10. Osteoarthritis is inflammation of a joint.

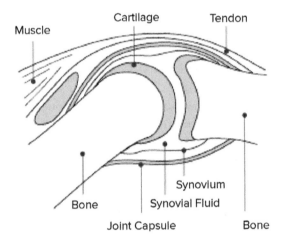

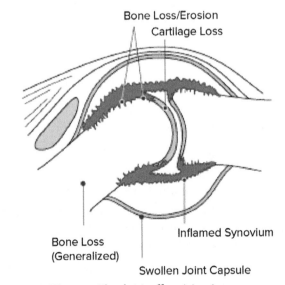

Figure 11. Rheumatoid arthritis affects joint tissues.

will begin in a big toe, though it can affect other joints as well. The attacks can be sudden — a man waking from his sleep with his big toe red, swollen, and throbbing with pain. People who are overweight or eat too many foods high in purines, chemical compounds that are broken down into uric acid in the body, are more prone to gout. Foods such as meat (particularly fatty red meat) and certain types of fish are high in purines. A high amount of these foods can make it difficult for our bodies to process the uric acid. Instead they forms uric crystals and store them in some of the joints of the body (Figure 12).

Years ago people sometimes referred to gout as a rich man's disease. People who were poorer back then did not have access to inexpensive fast food (like we do today) when they could not afford steak. Instead, they relied on what they could afford to raise, grow, and purchase. They were not as likely to consume foods high in uric

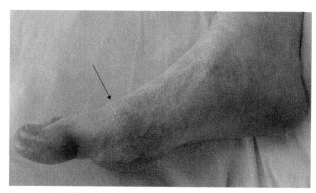

Figure 12. Affected foot in a gout patient.

acid nor be overweight. In the US today, however, anyone is at risk for gout regardless of income level.

Other diseases that can impact the functioning of our joints include fibromyalgia, lupus, diabetes, and psoriasis. Any disease that affects the joints or muscles will limit the range of motion of the individual and complicate attempts to exercise.

Exercising with Joint Pain

It's important to keep moving if you have joint pain or limited flexibility. Inactivity can lead less range of motion, increased stiffness, more pain, and in older individuals it can lead to contractures, a shortening or harden of muscles, tendons, or other tissues, causing joints to become rigid. Weak, rigid muscles mean more pressure on the joint itself. Exercising and stretching the muscles around the joint is crucial in managing pain and preventing further loss of mobility.

Some types of joint-related diseases require learning to exercise through pain, and other require doing something different so that there is not pain. In other words, sometimes, activities that cause pain can make joint problems worse, and sometimes the pain will not be made worse. Talk with your health care provider if you have a joint disease or joint injury to find out how you can safely stay active.

Genetics

Some people are genetically more flexible than others. Genetics can affect the connective tissues of our bodies, such as our tendons and ligaments, which can impact flexibility.

There are also individuals born with **hypermobility**, or what we might call being "double-jointed." Their

joints are particularly moveable and they are able to move them into positions that would injure the rest of us. This, however, is not always a good thing. Many people with hypermobility never experience any physical problems, but others become prone to pain, stiffness, joint dislocation, and have a higher risk of injury.

Biological Sex

There are many factors that affect flexibility, but females are generally more flexible than males. This is likely due to the amount of the hormone estrogen in the body. Estrogen encourages muscle lengthening and joint laxity or looseness. In fact, women are most flexible when pregnant because their estrogen levels

peak at this time. Testosterone (male hormones) has the opposite effect, which is why men may have more challenges in flexibility training. Testosterone makes muscles larger. This is good for strength, but it can limit range of motion, which is why men need the additional flexibility exercises.

Use and Age

It's easy to think that joint issues are only related to age because of how common it can be. But even in youth, how we use our bodies has the largest impact on our flexibility. This often happens to younger adults because of changes in lifestyle. For example, a sedentary occupation can lead to decreased energy for physical activity. Over time, if we are not doing activities that utilize our range of motion, our muscle fibers degrade and connective tissue undergoes a type of scarring usually associated with a healing injury.

This is called fibrosis. The excessive tissue begins to limit mobility and impede the muscle's ability to regenerate. There isn't much we can do to prevent age-related fibrosis. However, staying flexible to prevent injury-related fibrosis can help keep joints movable to a degree that will allow effective movement.

Assessing Your Flexibility

Flexibility can be assessed using several joint-specific measurements and simple ability tests that can help you target less flexible joints for training. Here you'll find several tests to help you assess the flexibility of different joints. Be sure to warm up for five to ten minutes before completing any assessment.

Assessment: Sit-and-Reach

The sit and reach test measures the flexibility of our lower back and hamstrings. You will need a sit-and-reach box with the footline set at 26 cm, and a partner.

- Sit with your bare feet flat against the box.

- With your hands parallel to the box, lean forward toward the ruler portion of the box as far as possible. Keep your hands side by side. Your legs should be straight, but do not lock your knees.

- Exhale and drop your head between your arms as you reach to extend the stretch as far as you are able.

- Hold for 2 seconds.

- Have your partner measure your distance

- Repeat

On the following page, find the rating that corresponds with your score on the chart (Figure 13).

Age (years)	15–19	20–29	30–39	40–49	50–59	60–69
Men						
Excellent	≥39 cm	≥40 cm	≥38 cm	≥35 cm	≥35 cm	≥33 cm
Very good	34–38 cm	34–39 cm	33–37 cm	29–34 cm	28–34 cm	25–32 cm
Good	29–33 cm	30–33 cm	28–32 cm	24–28 cm	24–27 cm	20–24 cm
Fair	24–28 cm	25–29 cm	23–27 cm	18–23 cm	16–23 cm	15–19 cm
Needs Improvment	≤23 cm	≤24 cm	≤22 cm	≤17 cm	≤15 cm	≤14 cm
Women						
Excellent	≥43 cm	≥41 cm	≥41 cm	≥38 cm	≥39 cm	≥35 cm
Very Good	38–42 cm	37–40 cm	36–40 cm	34–37 cm	33–38 cm	31–34 cm
Good	34–37 cm	33–36 cm	32–35 cm	30–33 cm	30–32 cm	27–30 cm
Fair	29–33 cm	28–32 cm	27–31 cm	25–29 cm	25–29 cm	23–26 cm
Needs Improvment	≤28 cm	≤27 cm	≤26 cm	≤24 cm	≤24 cm	≤22 cm

Figure 13. Sit-and-reach results by age and gender.

Assessment: Shoulder Flexibility

You will need a partner and either a ruler or tape measure for this test.

- Raise your right arm over your head

- Bend at the elbow and reach between your shoulders as far as you can with your palm against your back.

- Extend your left arm toward the ground

- Bend at the left elbow and raise your hand between your shoulders as far as you can with your palm against your back.

Assessment: Hamstring Flexibility

For this assessment, you need a goniometer or other joint measurement tool (optional) and a partner.

- Lie on your back with your arms at your sides.

- Bend one knee, keeping the foot flat on the floor and extend the other leg straight.

- Raise the extended leg so it is at least at a 90-degree angle, perpendicular to the floor.

- Your partner should measure the distance between the fingers of your right and left hand, or the amount of overlap, to the nearest quarter of an inch. If your fingers meet or overlap, the number is positive. If your fingers do not meet, the score is a negative number.

- Repeat, reversing the arms

Your score is the average of the two measurements. Find your rating in the table that corresponds with your measurement.

- Compare the range of motion in the raised straight leg relative to a 90-degree position. If a partner and a measuring instrument are available, you can obtain a more precise measurement of the joint angle.

- Repeat with the other leg

If you can't raise your leg so that it is vertical to your hips, your hamstring flexibility is below average. Beyond perpendicular would be above average.

Flexibility Training

Stretching has been considered an effective tool to boost performance levels, improve range of motion, and lower the risk of injury for many years. Flexibility training techniques include static, ballistic, and dynamic stretching, as well as proprioceptive neuromuscular facilitation (PNF) and myofascial release.

Static stretching, as mentioned earlier, involves only the motion of the bend. You should stretch until there is a slight tension, or just beyond, and hold it until you feel a slight discomfort. The benefits occur during the hold (usually about 20–60 seconds), which allows the muscle group time to relax and lengthen. The stretch is repeated and held 2–4 times for ideal improvement to flexibility. Normally, the length of the stretch can be improved a little with each repetition. This improves muscle elasticity and joint mobility.

Static stretching is often preferred for beginners because of the low risk of injury, providing you aren't attempting to place your body into an unnatural position. We've all seen those people that can sit on the floor and pull their foot behind their head, but nothing is gained for them but attention and, potentially, pain. But static stretching is not just for beginners. It's effective for everyone — and it's not as time consuming as some of the other methods.

Static-active stretching is done through the strength of the agonist muscle. The individual would assume a position and hold it with no other assistance. For example, from a standing position, bend your knee bringing your leg behind your body, actively engaging the force of your hamstrings (the agonists). Hold it there, engaging no other power than the strength of the hamstring. This means that your quadriceps (antagonists) — now lengthened — are being stretched while the hamstring is being strengthened. The hold for this type of stretch would be approximately 20 seconds as it can be a bit demanding. Many of the movements in yoga and Pilates are static-active.

Static-passive stretching utilizes some form of assistance with the stretch, either an object, a partner, gravity, or your own body (Figure 14). This is a type of relaxed stretching and is more commonly performed than static-active. For example, place your foot on top of a bar, bench, or chair with your leg extended at a 90-degree angle and slowly bend toward your knee as far as you can, holding the stretch for 10–30 seconds.

Whether active or passive, static stretching is great on warm muscles for cooling-down *after* a workout and for stretching tired or sore muscles. Studies show that static stretching *before* intense activity or athletic competition can *limit* performance in most age groups. In adults over 65, static stretching is good at any point during exercise.

Ballistic stretching requires momentum, and quick, bouncy movements. By propelling a limb, for example, we use the speed to push it past its normal range of motion. Repeatedly kicking or swinging your leg up to touch your toes to your hand extended high in the air would be an example.

This type of stretching can improve flexibility, but it is riskier. It does not allow the muscle time to relax and adjust to the stretched position. It is often used with certain types of athletics to prepare the body for specific movements, especially in sports where there is kicking, throwing, running, batting or other ballistic movements.

Dynamic stretching, mentioned earlier in the chapter, involves controlled repetitions of the movement through the range of motion. For example, a slow lunge down and up would stretch the quadriceps. Standing while slowly extending one leg out in front at a time is a dynamic hamstring stretch. The movements in dynamic stretches are never extended past the normal range of motion of the joint. Unless you work for the circus, it isn't necessary for most of us to be able to pull our ankles past our ears.

Dynamic stretching is beneficial for athletes and as a warm-up to aerobic activity or competition because it engages the joint in a range of motion more similar to what we experience in our active lives and can improve performance. Keep your movements controlled and intentional.

Proprioceptive neuromuscular facilitation (PNF) is a more advanced form of stretching and requires both the stretching and the contraction of the muscle. A person would stretch the muscles, like they would in a static stretch, then contract the muscle group while under some form of resistance to prevent movement, such as against an object or with the help of a partner (Figure 15). The contraction would be held for a certain amount of time (six seconds, for example). The person would then release the contraction, staying in a static stretch for 20 or 30 seconds, then rest and repeat. PNF not only stretches the muscle group but also serves as a form of strength training.

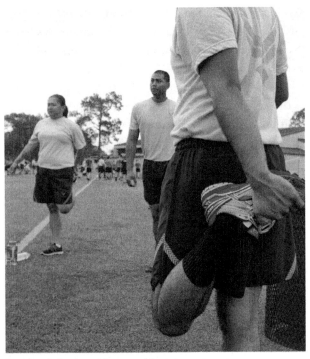

Figure 14. Static-passive stretching.

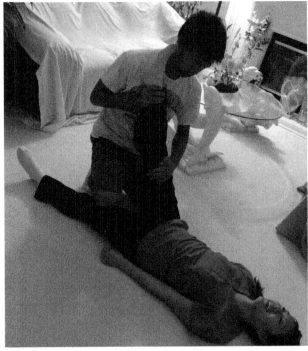

Figure 15. PNF stretching.

Myofascial release uses stretching, compression, direct pressure and other techniques to release restricted areas of fascia, ideally creating a biochemical and mechanical change that allows for more efficient movement. Foam rollers and other niche products assist in targeting and releasing the tissue.

Because of amount of stretch that it provides, don't do this prior to high-intensity exercise. Studies have shown, however, that doing PNF before jogging or other moderate or low-intensity exercises actually increases performance. It also serves as an excellent post-workout activity to improve range of motion and strength. It is, however, time consuming and often requires a partner.

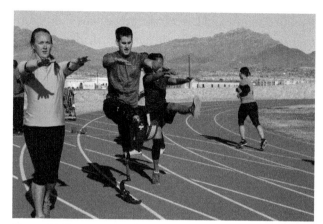

Figure 16. Dynamic stretching.

Planning a Flexibility Program

The FITT Formula can be applied to a flexibility training program in the same manner we apply it to other aspects of fitness. This will enable you to create a plan that will be effective and safe. When working on our flexibility, the following guidelines can be helpful:

Frequency — Stretching should be done at least two or three days each week, though more often is safe. People who are new to stretching should start with 2 days a week and gradually increase the frequency. Building it into your exercise program can make the process simpler and increase the benefits of your workout. For example, if you perform a cardiovascular activity four days per week, dynamic stretching as part of your warm-up will help prepare your body and improve performance, and static stretching afterwards can be part of your cool-down improve flexibility.

Intensity — Each joint in our body has a different capacity for range of motion. How far you stretch depends on what you feel. You should experience slight tension, but not pain. Once you feel tension, move slowly and slightly past it to challenge the body part. The tension helps you establish your threshold and set goals with your stretching. You have to use your own perceptions to determine

the appropriate intensity level for stretching. As you hold a stretch, try to relax and breathe comfortably. If you can't, you might be attempting to stretch too far.

Time — The amount of time for each stretch will depend upon the type of movement performed, whether static, dynamic, or PNF. A static stretch should be held for 15–60 seconds on average, two to four times. If you're a beginner, you may need to hold it for a shorter period of time. Rest between stretches for 30 seconds. A PNF would also be held for the length of time of the contraction (five to six seconds or more) and approximately 30 seconds afterwards, for two to five repetitions. It should take you approximately 10–15 minutes to complete a flexibility training routine.

Type — You should establish a routine to work each major muscle group, though choosing the type of stretch will depend upon your specific needs, skill level, and goals. Make sure to include stretching exercises for the neck,

F	Frequency of Exercise	How Often	Minimum two to three times a week. Best to do some stretching daily.
I	Intensity of Exercise	How Hard	You should stretch to the point where you feel tension, not pain.
T	Time of Exercise	How Long	15–30 minutes total. Static stretches of warm muscles; 15–60 seconds, three sets
T	Type of Exercise	Which Exercises	After warm up: dynamic stretch, prepares body for exercise. After cool down: static stretch, most improvement gains for flexibility.

Figure 17. The FITT Formula in flexibility training.

shoulders, upper and lower back, pelvis, hips and legs. If your range of motion is limited in a particular area, say your shoulders, you may choose to put more focus there. It can be helpful to assess flexibility in different joints to help set up a program that will be beneficial. If you're a beginner, you may choose static stretching over PNF or dynamic. If you prefer group activities, you may choose to join a yoga class instead of a 10–15 minute training program (Figure 18). Stretching exercises can be static, dynamic, PNF or a combination.

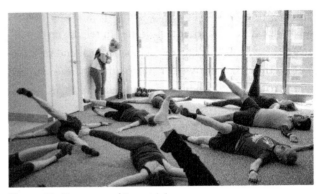

Figure 18. Group stretching activity.

Applying Training Principles

Like applying the FITT Formula, training principles like specificity, progressive overload, adaptation, and reversibility can be used to enhance your flexibility training program.

Specificity — After you've determined the flexibility of a certain muscle/tendon group, choose stretches that will focus on your major muscle groups, adding additional stretches for those that have a lower range of motion.

Progressive Overload — Each time you push your body past that point of tension a bit more, you are overloading. You may notice that when you initially assessed your hamstrings, your fingers only reached your ankles but now they reach the top of your shoe. Rather than trying to reach your shoe, you focused on the point of tension and going beyond it. Eventually, you may reach your heels.

Adaptation — As your flexibility improves, your muscle/tendon groups should see increased range of motion, resting muscle length, and greater force during muscle contractions. This will enable you to establish new target areas or set new goals if you choose.

Reversibility — It may take time to notice, but if you stop training your flexibility will eventually decrease. This also happens gradually with age, which is why maintaining a program is so important.

Safety

Some considerations for flexibility training are safety, warm-up and cool-down, stretches to avoid, and avoiding back pain. Any form of exercise can pose risks if we have a lack of knowledge or fail to listen to our bodies. As discussed, certain joints only move certain ways, so body awareness is important.

General Considerations

As with any physical activity, stretching has safety concerns that anyone should consider before attempting.

- During stretching, you should always breath smoothly and at a normal rate.

- If you've had an injury, particularly to your knee or hip, be sure to check with your doctor before beginning.

- Stretching should never hurt. Stretch to the point of tension not pain.

- Use controlled movements. Avoid bouncing or jerking while static stretching.

- Keep your joints soft. While your arms and legs can be straight, your joints should have a slight bend to avoid locking them in place.

- Modify stretches as needed. If you cannot perform a stretch in the recommended position, on the floor for example, try using a chair. If it causes pain or risk, make a slight adjustment.

STRETCH REPETITIONS, SETS, AND SESSIONS

Flexibility Exercise/ Stretch	# of repetitions per set	# of sets per session	# of sessions per week
Hamstrings	4 per side	1	After every aerobic or strength session
Alternative Hamstrings	4 per side	1	After every aerobic or strength session
Calves	4 per side	1	After every aerobic or strength session
Ankles	4 per side	1	After every aerobic or strength session
Triceps	4 per side	1	After every aerobic or strength session
Wrists	4 per side	1	After every aerobic or strength session
Quadriceps	4 per side	1	After every aerobic or strength session
Double Hip Rotation	4 per side	1	After every aerobic or strength session
Single Hip Rotation	4 per side	1	After every aerobic or strength session
Shoulder Rotation	4 per side	1	After every aerobic or strength session
Neck Rotation	4 per side	1	After every aerobic or strength session
Side Leg Raise	4 per side	1	After every aerobic or strength session

If you are not currently doing aerobic or strength activities, do flexibility and stretching at least 3 times per week for at least 20 minutes per session.

Figure 19. Sample flexibility training program.

Warm-Up and Cool-Down

Stretching should never be performed on cold muscles. Static stretches in particular can result in injury if done before the body is warm. This is why stretching after cardiovascular exercise or weight training makes sense. The purpose of warming up is to prepare the muscles for activity, raising the temperature of the muscles, and circulating the blood.

If planning to do cardiovascular exercise, such as running, begin at a lower pace for a few minutes to warm-up the muscles, then proceed to your chosen pace. A good time for static or PNF stretching is at the completion of your run. If doing dynamic stretching, do a slower-paced run, perform the dynamic stretches, then resume your run. If you are focusing only on flexibility training and are unable to walk or jog prior, dynamic stretching can be a good warm-up. If the stretching session was intense and involved movement (power yoga, for example), then it would be a good idea to end with gentler movement to slow down the breathing. Otherwise, stretching is in itself a great way to cool-down from more intense exercise.

Stretches to Avoid

Some stretches are no longer considered safe because they don't agree with the intended rotation of the joint. These should be avoided:

- Stretches that extend your neck backward. Years ago, it was considered good to put your neck through a 360-degree rotation, but now we know better. You can put your chin to your chest and raise it or put either ear toward your shoulder, but do not roll your head in a circle or stretch your head toward your back.

- Stretches that flex or extend your back in an un-supported way, such as standing straight leg toe touches (standing hamstring stretches), plows, donkey kicks, or seated hamstring stretches where both legs are extended. The range of motion of your back is only partial (cartilaginous) and these can put a strain on your lower back. They can also cause you to hyperextend your knee joint.

- Stretches that take your knee out of alignment with your ankle, such as deep knee bends or hurdler's stretches. Your form in exercises involving your knee is important in lunges, squats, and any other leg movements.

Posture and Low Back Health

Our posture is the position of our body when our torso is erect, such as when we are standing or sitting. Our back muscles can be injured by bad posture. Our **body mechanics**, or the way we use our body during movement, are important. If our mechanics cause injury, our backs can take a long time to heal and can be susceptible to chronic pain.

Your spine is divided into three sections, the **cervical spine** — the uppermost part of the spine in your neck — the **thoracic spine** in your chest, and the **lumbar spine** in your lower back. The spine is made up of bones called **vertebrae** and cushiony **discs** between them. These are all stacked on top of one another, forming a column that stands vertically when we are standing.

There are seven vertebrae within the cervical spine, numbered C1 to C7 from top to bottom, 12 vertebrae (T1 to T12) in the thoracic spine, and five vertebrae in the lumbar spine (L1 to L5). Some people have six lumbar vertebrae. The lumbar spine, which connects the thoracic spine and the pelvis, bears the bulk of the body's weight and are the largest vertebrae.

Almost 80% of people experience back pain at some point in their life. Men and women are equally affected by low back pain, which can range in intensity from a dull, constant ache to a sudden, sharp sensation that leaves the person incapacitated. Pain can begin abruptly as a result of an accident or by lifting something heavy, or it can develop over time due to age-related changes of the spine. Sedentary lifestyles also can set the stage for low back pain, especially when a weekday routine of getting too little exercise is punctuated by strenuous weekend workout.

Most back injuries occur with little knowledge of how we actually did it, but some typical causes of back pain are, poor posture or poor body mechanics, lifting a heavy object incorrectly, being in poor physical shape and/or overweight, having poor flexibility, having weak core muscles (abdomen/torso), twisting beyond the back's tolerated range of motion, making sudden movements that stress the back. You are also at greater risk for back injury during times of stress or fatigue.

You can prevent most back injuries by developing good habits when you are subject to these causes, like when lifting a heavy object. Some good habits include:

- Practicing good posture when standing or sitting. Keep your head up, shoulders back, pelvis straight, and stomach in (not sucked in). If sitting, keep your feet on the floor.

- Using good body mechanics. This will vary with the movement, but in general, knees (and all joints) should be slightly bent, pelvis in neutral position — not tipped either way. It can take practice and work learning what neutral is and getting the body to adjust to neutral, especially if a person has picked up poor posture habits over time.

- Never lifting more than you can handle or from a position that requires you to compromise your body mechanics. Ask for help or use a handtruck.

- Exercising, particularly your core muscles. Weak abdominals force your back to work harder to move your torso.

- Taking breaks when sitting or standing for long periods.

Exercises to Prevent and Manage Back Pain

For chronic sufferers, there are exercises that can help improve your core safely and reduce pain.

Partial crunches — Lie on the floor with your knees bent, feet flat on the floor, and your hands behind your head in sit-up position. Tighten your stomach muscles and raise your head and shoulders off the floor without bending your neck or pulling your elbows in. Keep your elbows back. Make the abdominals do the work, not your head or back. At no point should your feet or lower back leave the ground. Breathe out as you raise, hold for a second, lower, then repeat. Beginners should do approximately three sets of twelve crunches and work up from there as you gain strength.

Hamstring stretches — Lie on the floor with one knee bent. With the other leg, wrap a towel around the ball of your foot and extend it as straight as you can, pushing your heel toward the ceiling. Hold it for approximately 20 seconds, then repeat two to four more times per leg.

Back extensions — Lie with your stomach on the floor. Push with your hands so that your shoulders lift off the floor. You can rest on your elbows if it is comfortable. Hold the stretch for a few seconds, then lower.

Pelvic tilts — Lie on the floor with your legs bent and feet flat. Keeping your upper back on the floor, contract your pelvic and raise your hips and pelvis, keeping the muscles tight. Hold for around ten seconds, then slowly lower. Repeat eight to twelve times.

Bird dog — Begin on the floor on your hands and knees. Hands should be directly below the shoulders and knees below the hips. Keep your head so that you are looking down. Extend your right arm straight in front of you as you extend your left leg straight behind. Hold for seven or eight seconds. Repeat with the opposite side.

Wall sits — Stand in front of the wall and lean your back against it. Walk your feet out until you can slide down the wall into a squat, similar to sitting in an imaginary chair. The muscles in your thighs, abdomen, and buttocks should contract. Hold for ten to fifteen seconds. Gradually work your way to a one-minute hold.

Conclusion

Your next steps should be to assess your flexibility and set SMART goals for improving flexibility. Then design a training program that ideally targets joints that are most affected by the other training plans you has put in place so far.

Consider the impact that a regular flexibility program might have on your health. Think about improving your flexibility by incorporating different stretches into your fitness routine, and make sure that you are incorporating stretching into your cool-down routines. If you find yourself sitting for long periods of time, stand up and stretch. Practice the recommended sitting and standing postures that are described in this chapter. Adjust your workspace so that you have good alignment when doing schoolwork.

Chapter 6
Body Composition Basics

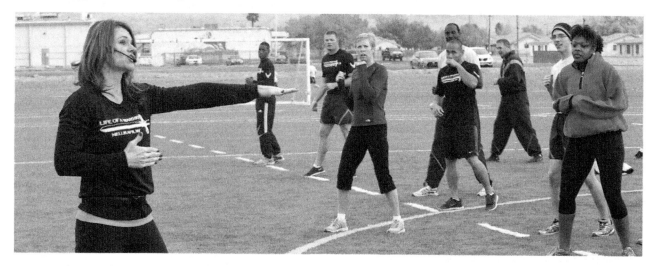

Body composition is the make-up of the body in terms of lean mass and fat mass, and there are different ranges that we can look at. There is a certain range that corresponds to the lowest amount of morbidity and mortality (disease and death), and there is a different range that is considered "athletic." Certain types of athletics have their own "ideal" level of body fat, weight, or weight-related standard that is very important, such as gymnastics, wrestling, and body-building. Most of us do not need to maintain the low level of body fat required of elite athletes, but we can all work to achieve a body composition that will help us maximize our quality of life.

Your sister Ann has been a gymnast since she was 3 years-old. She hasn't had any moments on the Olympic podium, but she's very competitive and her body shows it. She can do chin-ups, pushups, and crunches all day. You learned early in life not to pick on her.

A few months ago, she came to the realization that college gymnastics was not in her future and decided to retire from the sport. And, believe it or not, she asked for your help! After years of training with her team, burning so many calories during practices and building muscle using her body as resistance, she didn't know how to stay in shape without gymnastics. In the few months since her retirement, she had already grown concerned with some excess fat beginning to form, even though it's just a few extra pounds. She said she didn't know what to do to stay healthy. She wasn't even sure what healthy should "look" like. She had always "looked" like a gymnast.

The notion of an "ideal" body composition can sometimes be complicated by misinformation. In this age of instant information and constant advancement of knowledge, we frequently find ourselves so overwhelmed with evidence — testimonials of success stories, images of current notions of a healthy appearance, and the latest diet trend. We may find it difficult to know what is best for us.

First, let's look at one basic fact about obesity. Obesity continues to be a major public health problem in the US (Figure 1). It contributes to three of the top four causes of death (heart disease, cancer, and stroke) and is continuing to increase. Even ten extra pounds of fat can have adverse health effects, so understanding body composition basics is more important than many of us realize because of its impact on our risk of disease.

Second, lets challenge notions of the "ideal body." Weight, though it can be a good measuring tool at times, is not the only number to focus on. As you will learn in this chapter, body composition has other factors that go beyond the scale or your appearance.

This chapter defines body composition and the way fats are stored in the human body, describes the benefits of a healthy body composition and weight management, and illuminates the challenges many people face when attempting to change or maintain their body composition and weight. It also recommends methods for assessing, improving, or maintaining your body composition — through physical activity and healthy eating — which are the most effective long-term strategies for managing weight.

Definition of Body Composition

Body composition is the make-up of fat, muscle, bone, water, and other lean tissue in our body. Your body composition is usually defined simply as the percent of your body that is fat. For example, if you weight 160 pounds and you learn that your body fat percentage is 20%, then you have 32 pounds of fat in your body and 128 pounds of lean tissue.

Fat is not necessarily bad. In fact, our bodies need between 3–5% (in males) and 8–12% (in females) body fat, called our **essential fat**, to survive (Figure 2). Fat enables us to regulate the energy in our body, cushion and protect our organs, and store some of the essential nutrients our bodies need. Our bodies immediately use some of the food we eat for energy, which we measure in calories. Any calories not needed for use right away are stored for later use as adipose tissue.

Fat and Metabolism Basics

Excess fats are stored primarily as **triglycerides**. These are what the body breaks down when it needs extra energy, such as when we exercise. Until it's ready to be used, our bodies store fat in **adipose tissue**, which is considered an organ of the endocrine system. It is responsible for the balance and release of many hormones and for helping regulate metabolism and appetite, in addition to maintaining our body temperature. We have two types of adipose tissue, white and brown. It forms under the skin, around muscles, and vital organs. Most of our tissue is white. Brown tissue is most common in newborns. It generates heat by consuming energy, something infant humans and other mammals, particularly those that hibernate, need during times of inactivity. This tissue decreases as we age and is nearly non-existent by the time we reach adulthood.

Visceral fat is adipose tissue stored in the abdominal cavity and encompasses the organs there, such as the intestines, liver, and pancreas. This is different than the fat that we can see or feel directly under our skin, which is considered **subcutaneous fat**. Our bodies need a certain amount of this fat to store energy, regulate body temperature, and to protect the skin and organs. It can be found all over the body, but the largest amounts of subcutaneous fat are generally on the abdomen, hips, thighs, and buttocks.

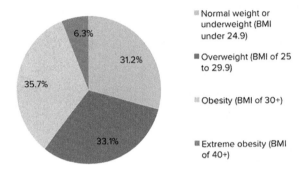

Overweight and Obesity among Adults Age 20 and Older, United States, 2009–2010

- Normal weight or underweight (BMI under 24.9)
- Overweight (BMI of 25 to 29.9)
- Obesity (BMI of 30+)
- Extreme obesity (BMI of 40+)

6.3%
31.2%
35.7%
33.1%

Figure 1. Overweight and obesity rates among adults.

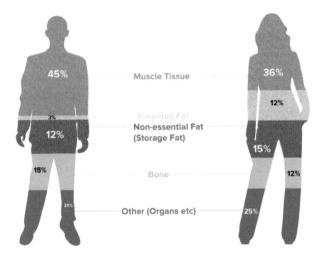

45%
36%
12%
3%
12%
15%
15%
25%
12%
25%

Muscle Tissue
Essential Fat
Non-essential Fat (Storage Fat)
Bone
Other (Organs etc)

Figure 2. Male and female healthy body composition differs.

Any amount of excess fat, regardless of type, can have a negative impact on your health. Many people think of subcutaneous fat when they think about excess fat because they can see it, but visceral fat can actually be more dangerous because of the way it can impact vital organs (Figure 3). People with an excess of visceral fat (abdominal obesity) are more prone to cardiovascular damage, colon cancer, diabetes, and several other chronic diseases.

Visceral fat is hormonally active and releases different bioactive molecules and hormones, such as adiponectin, leptin, tumor necrosis factor, resistin, and interleutin-6 (IL-6). These hormones play a role in risk for Type 2 diabetes, elevated glucose levels, hypertension, cardiovascular disease and certain malignancies.

It is a safe assumption that if you have a large amount of subcutaneous fat in your abdominal area that you likely have too much visceral fat as well. It is possible, however, to have visceral fat without significant abdominal fat — you may not even know it is there.

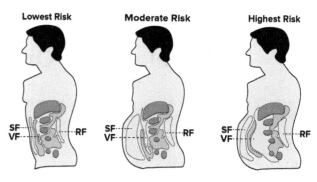

SF - Subcutaneous (superficial) belly fat
VF - Visceral (deep) belly fat
RF - Retroperitoneal (back) fat

Figure 3. Some fats are more dangerous than others.

Healthy Body Composition

Healthy body composition is an important factor when considering your weight, but it's not the only factor. For example, it doesn't tell us anything about a person's level of visceral fat. The misconception that weight is the primary determiner of someone's health is very common, but using weight to determine overweight or obesity doesn't take into account what is happening inside the body weight muscle mass, water and fat. As mentioned earlier, someone could be reasonably thin through most of their body, but have a substantial amount of visceral fat. Some-

one who lifts weights may weigh more overall than someone of comparable height but be in better health due to the way their body is composed, having a lower quantity of fat tissue.

How much body fat is the right amount? The American College of Sports Medicine suggests ranges for men and women by age (Figure 4). The human body has an essential fat threshold that never changes despite age. For men, this is 2–5%, and for women it's 10–13%. The ranges for excellent (athletic), average, and poor are included in this table, but more specific numbers are available.

Age (years)					
	20–29	30–39	40–49	50–59	60+
Male					
Essential Fat	2–5%	2–5%	2–5%	2–5%	2–5%
Excellent	7.1–9.3%	11.3–13.8%	13.6–16.2%	15.3–17.8%	15.3–18.3%
Average	14.1–17.5%	17.5–20.4%	19.6–22.4%	21.3–24%	22–25%
Poor	>22.4%	>24.2%	>26.1%	>27.5%	>28.5%
Female					
Essential Fat	10–13%	10–13%	10–13%	10–13%	10–13%
Excellent	14.5–17%	15.5–17.9%	18.5–21.2%	21.6–24.9%	21.1–25%
Average	20.6–23.6%	21.6–24.8%	24.9–28%	28.5–31.5%	29.3–32.4%
Poor	>27.7%	>29.3%	>32.1%	>35.6%	>36.6%

Figure 4. The ACSM's recommended body composition changes over the lifespan.

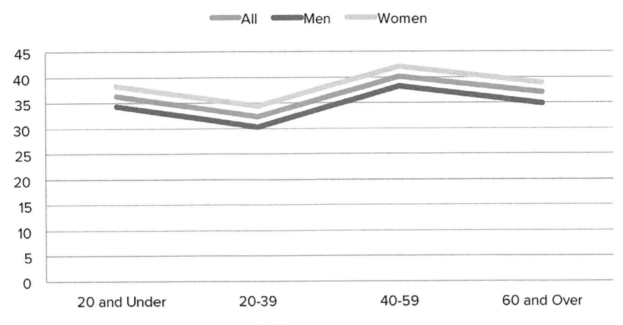

Figure 5. Obesity rates in the United States by age and gender.

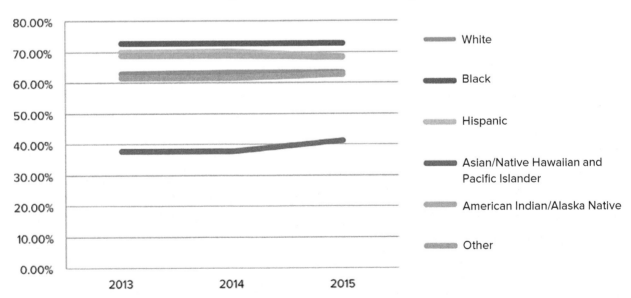

Figure 6. Overweight and obesity rates in the United States by race and ethnicity.

Overweight and Obesity

There are different ways to measure and define overweight and obesity, and these are detailed later in this chapter. The CDC defines overweight or obesity as weight that is higher than what is considered as a healthy weight for a given height as measured by the body mass index (BMI).

Based off of BMI data, over one third of US Americans are overweight (Figure 5). From 2011–2014 obesity rates were a little over 36% in adults, an increase from 1999 rates, and 17% in children, which has held stable. Among women, the rates were higher at 38.3% than men at 34.3%. Obesity rates were lowest among Asian adults (11.7%), followed by white (34.5%), Hispanic (42.5%), and black (48.1%) (Figure 6).

There are also disparities in weight related to geographic region. The southern United States has the highest prevalence of obesity at 31.5%, with Alabama, Louisiana, Mississippi, and West Virginia at 35% or more. The Mid West follows at 30.7%, the Northeast at 26.4%, and the West at 25.2%. Oregon is at 34.5%. Nationwide, the combined number of adults either overweight or obese is approximately 70%. Our nation is at a point where the prevalence of overweight and obesity is considered an epidemic that costs billions of health care dollars annually and many lives. Average life expectancy, though it has increased over the century, may soon begin to start decreasing.

Health Effects

When we store more fat tissue than we need, we begin to see a decline in our physical capabilities. Our activities of daily living fatigue us more quickly or we may find ourselves avoiding situations that involve a certain level of exertion. In other words, an unhealthy body composition places limits upon us, often slowly so that

Prevalence of Self-Reported Obesity Among U.S. Adults by State.

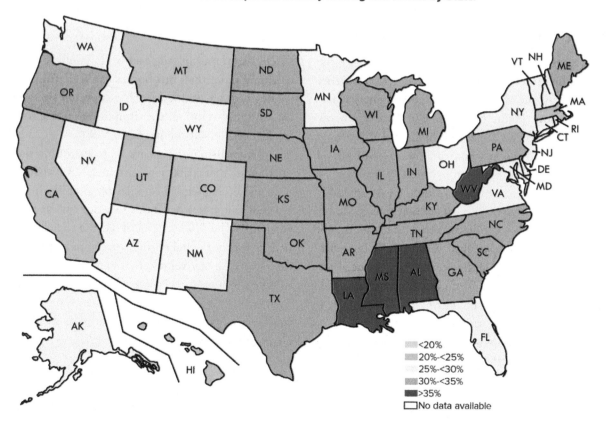

Figure 7. Obesity is most common in the midwestern and southern states.

we don't realize it right away. It may be months before we notice that we've been choosing the elevator over the stairs due to physical strain rather than convenience. Often, we simply aren't honest with ourselves about the shape we are in. We adjust to our bodies, then adjust again if we gain more fat, and tell ourselves that we are doing just fine and are happy. If you wait until you aren't fine, returning to health can get more and more difficult.

Underweight

It is possible for a person to have a body fat level that is too low. An adult with a BMI below 18.5 is considered underweight. A National Health and Nutrition Examination Survey in 2006 found that 1.8% of adults over 20 are underweight. In a nation of 235 million adults, that's roughly 4.2 million adults who are underweight, representing a serious problem.

This often is a result of malnutrition or health issues, but could also be the result of an eating disorder, such as anorexia nervosa or bulimia nervosa. As mentioned earlier, your body needs a certain amount of fat to function properly.

Excess adipose tissue increases our risk of experiencing a multitude of health-related issues, such as Type II diabetes, cardiovascular disease, cancer, stroke, depression, anxiety, high cholesterol, high blood pressure, gallbladder disease, sleep apnea, and osteoarthritis among others. All of these issues lead to fewer healthy years in our life, potentially with an obesity-related disability, and an increased risk of premature death. When we neglect our body composition, we aren't fine.

Too little fat can cause many problems. The resulting deficiencies in our fat-soluble vitamins A, D, E, and K can lower your immune system, causing you to be more prone to illness, weaken your bones (due to reduced bone mineral density), damage your vision, and even cause your blood to not clot properly. Body fat helps regulate insulin and hormones, and inadequate fat percentage can lead to diabetes and problems with reproduction or fertility in women and men, kidney problems, and loss of menstrual cycle. It can also impact your skin, causing it to sag or appear wrinkled. In serious cases, the body begins to break down muscle to get the energy it needs to function.

The Energy Balance Equation

Energy imbalances lead to fat storage. According to the National Institutes of Health, it is the concept of energy in and energy out, or what we consider an **energy balance equation** (Figure 8). We take in calories (energy in) through food and drink. Our bodies use this energy (energy out) to function, in areas from digesting food to breathing, and, of course, movement. When we take in more energy than we can use right away, our body stores it either as sugar in our liver and muscles, or as fat (triglycerides) in our adipose tissue. What we do not use right away stays put until we use it. If out energy out never increases to the point where we need the stores, it'll still be there. The longer this energy imbalance occurs (taking in more energy than we can use), the more fat tissue we accumulate.

This tissue develops in two ways — by multiplying and by enlarging. By the time we reach adolescence, our fat cells stop multiplying and begin swelling when we consume more than our bodies can use. This is when we begin to see an increase in our overall size and the formation of cellulite, the dimpling that occurs from swollen cells in subcutaneous fat.

Metabolism is the chemical process within the cells of our body that enable it to sustain life. As we discussed in previous chapters, our bodies are a bit like a car. We put fuel, oil, and other fluids into our car for it to run efficiently. The difference between the vehicle and our body is that our metabolism sorts and processes the fuel for us, unlike our vehicle that expects us to put each vital fluid in the correct place. Our metabolism is much smarter. It converts food/fuel into energy, proteins, fats, acids, carbohydrates, and even eliminates waste (no oil change necessary).

Energy Balance Equation

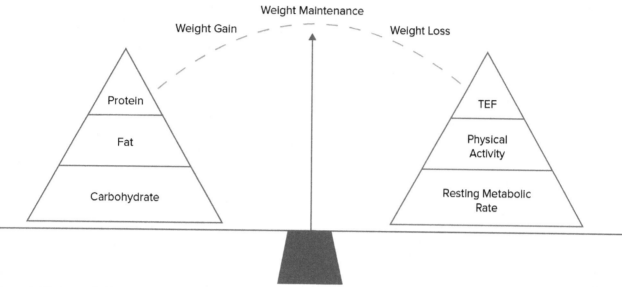

Figure 8. The energy balance equation.

RMR, BMR, and TEE

Just as our cars idle at a certain rate, we have a **resting metabolic rate** (RMR) at which this conversion occurs. This is the amount of energy the body needs to complete its physical processes, like breathing, brain function, and blood circulation — essentially, the energy it needs to expend to keep you alive or keep your motor running. This does not include calories burned during movement. There are factors that can affect your RMR, such as how active you are (fitness level), your age, biological sex, and weight loss efforts. Knowing your RMR can help you

determine how much energy you need to consume and how much exercise you need during the day. It is not perfect. There are limitations, as it doesn't explain why some people gain or lose weight easier, and it doesn't account for the different factors that influence RMR. However, it is a good starting point to help you measure progress with weight loss or weight management.

There are several different methods for measuring RMR. The following is the Mifflin-St. Joer equation:

- **Males:** (9.99 x weight in kilograms) + (6.25 x height in centimeters) – (4.92 x age) + 5

- **Females:** (9.99 x weight in kilograms) + (6.25 x height in centimeters) – (4.92 x age) – 161

For example: a male who weighs 150 pounds (68.03 kg), is 72 inches (182.88 cm) tall, and 25 years-old would have an RMR of 1705 calories per day.

(9.99 x 68.03) + (6.25 x 182.88) – (4.92 x 25) + 5 = 1705

For another example: a female who weighs 180 pounds, is 65 inches tall, and 44 years-old would have an RMR of 1472 calories per day.

(9.99 x 81.82) + (6.25 x 165.1) – (4.92 x 44) – 161 = 1472

(Note on the metric system: 1 pounds = .4536 kilograms and 1 inch=2.54 centimeters)

Components of Energy Expenditure

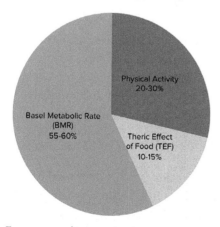

Figure 9. Energy expenditure categories.

Factor	Description
Body Mass	A person with greater body weight will have a higher resting metabolism than a smaller person.
Body Composition	Muscle burns more calories than fat, even at rest.
Age	Metabolism declines naturally in adults at a rate of about 2-3% per decade because of loss of lean muscle.
Gender	Men normally have a higher metabolism than woman due to body mass and body composition.
Hormones	Certain hormones can increase or decrease metabolism.
Nutritional Supplements	Certain supplements can increase or decrease metabolism.
Nicotine	Tobacco products can increase resting metabolism from 3-7%
Pharmaceuticals	Prescription and over the counter drugs can increase or decrease metabolism.
Fever and/or Infection	An increase in body temperature will increase metabolism.
Stress/Emotional Excitement	Good and bad stress could cause an increase in metabolism due to an increased utilization of stress hormones epinephrine and norepinephrine (catecholamines).
Exercise	Strength training can lead to a chronic increase in metabolism because of the increase in lean muscle mass.
Weight Loss	The two main reasons for a decrease in resting metabolism are that (1) a smaller body requires fewer calories and (2) during weight loss the body may try to conserve energy in response to a lower calorie intake.
Caloric Restriction	Restrictive diets consisting of less than 1000 calories per day can result in an acute decrease in resting metabolic rate.

Figure 10. Factors that affect metabolism.

Let's take into account how active these people are to get a more realistic number by estimating their Thermic Effective of Exercise (TEE):

Level Of Activity	Activity Factor	
	Male	Female
Sedentary — little to no activity	0.3	0.3
Lightly Active — you move a bit for work, stand and walk around a little with short bursts of moderate activity	0.6	0.5
Moderately Active — Same as above but add in 1.5 to 2 hours of moderate activity (e.g., jogging)	0.7	0.6
Very Active — You're active all day comparable to 9-13 miles of running (army recruits, full-time athletes, laborers)	1.1	0.9
Extremely Active — Equivalent of running 14-16 miles/day (lumberjacks, coal miners-heavy labor and exercise)	1.4	1.2

Figure 11. Activity levels by sex.

To calculate your TEE, multiply your RMR times the appropriate activity factor from the table above. For example, if our man in the previous example is lightly active, the activity factor to use is 0.6. His calculated RMR is 1705 calories per day, so his TEE is calculated as follows:

$$TEE = RMR \times activity\ factor$$

$$TEE = 1705 \times 0.6 = 1023\ calories/day$$

Add those calories to his daily total from RMR and we find he needs 2,728 calories each day to maintain his weight at his current activity level.

If the woman in our example is moderately active, the activity factor it the same at 0.6. Her calculated RMR is 1472 calories per day, so her TEE is calculated as follows:

$$TEE = 1472 \times 0.6 = 883\ calories/day$$

Add those calories to her daily total from RMR and we find she needs 2,355 calories each day to maintain her weight at her current activity level.

Basal metabolic rate (BMR) is often used interchangeably with RMR, but they are slightly different. Both are an estimate of the energy required by the body at rest, including breathing, circulation, maintaining body temperature, and building and repairing cells. BMR is more precise, but RMR is a more practical way of finding your metabolic rate because BMR is determined in a lab or clinical setting and you can calculate your own RMR.

The energy balance equation directly affects the way we process and store fat in our bodies. It is the concept of energy in and energy out. If we take in the exact amount of energy we need, burn as many calories as we consume, we have a *neutral* balance. If we consume more than our bodies can use, we have a *positive* balance, meaning we will gain fat. Using more than we consume during the day, our body utilizes stored fat, and we have a *negative* balance, meaning we will lose fat.

Training to lower your body fat percentage (the most common option) should be based on a reaching a negative energy balance by reducing the energy you take in from nutrition and increasing your energy out through physical activity. One pound of fat = 3,500 calories, and health professionals typically recommend a weight loss of one-half to two pounds per week of fat. To create a loss of one pound of fat each week, a person should have a deficit of 500 calories per day, ideally from a combination of increasing activity level and making changes in your nutrition. Sometimes it's not possible to do both, depending on individual circumstances. Some people, for example, aren't eating enough calories, or they might already have a high level of physical activity.

Most of the time, we can create that deficit from both activity changes and eating habit changes — gradual, sustainable changes. For example, most people can find 250 calories per day that they can reduce — changing your café mocha to non-fat can save a good number of calories. Adding 30 minutes of physical activity each day will usually burn at least a few hundred calories. This could yield one pound of fat lost in the week. If there is a day during the week that a person isn't burning the extra calories through physical activity, which is often the case, they would need to create a larger energy deficit through nutrition changes. And that can become more challenging, depending on their current habits.

Losing one-half to two pounds per week can be challenging for some people. It's a good idea to track progress regularly so that you can see if what you are doing is effective, and if you find that you aren't making gradual, steady progress, it's time to reassess and troubleshoot.

Gender	Age (years)	Activity Level		
		Sedentary	Moderately Active	Active
Female	2–3	1,000	1,000–1,400	1,000–1,400
Female	4–8	1,200	1,400–1,600	1,400–1,800
Female	9–13	1,600	1,600–2,000	1,800–2,000
Female	14–18	1,800	2,000	2,400
Female	19–30	2,000	2,000–2,200	2,400
Female	31–50	1,800	2,000	2,200
Female	51+	1,600	1,800	2,000–2,200
Male	2–3	1,000	1,000–1,400	1,000–1,400
Male	4–8	1,400	1,400–1,600	1,600–2,000
Male	9–13	1,800	1,800–2,200	2,000–2,600
Male	14–18	2,200	2,400–2,800	2,800–3,200
Male	19–30	2,400	2,600–2,800	3,000
Male	31–50	2,200	2,400–2,600	2,800–3,000
Male	51+	2,000	2,200–2,400	2,400–2,800

Figure 12. Calorie needs by age and gender.

The Set-Point Theory

Research in body composition is being done to better understand metabolism and the different mechanisms that can help with weight control, and there continue to be new insights. One theory is that each person's body is genetically predisposed or programmed to maintain a certain weight, it's natural weight. For example, if you're at this natural weight and you eat too much, your body will increase temperature and speed up metabolism to burn the extra calories. If you don't eat enough, you lose energy as your body slows down in an attempt to maintain this predetermined weight. This is why it can be challenging to lose weight. Your body will send you signals by increasing your hunger, telling you to eat, essentially fighting against you.

This theory can get a bit cloudy. In reality, we may have various "settling points" at which our body will become comfortable again. We often call them "plateaus" that are influenced by energy and macronutrient intakes. It can be difficult to get past them. But, our body's fight to maintain a set weight is there but may be weaker than we imagine. Consider how easy it is for your body to go the direction you *don't* want it to, even if it is unlike the weight you've traditionally maintained most of your life. Much of this is because of the nature of American diets and our constant exposure to enticing, high-calorie foods. We can get past our body's desire to maintain this set weight, and get past these different settling points, with a close attention to our energy balance equation and doing a fair assessment of our needs vs. wants. That's not to say it's always easy and, let's face it, we often want an easier approach.

Diet plans, programs, books, and TV shows will often claim you can achieve a higher weight loss — even as much as 10 pounds per week. If you consider that one pound of fat contains about 3,500 calories, you will realize that it's just not physiologically possible to lose 10 pounds of fat in one week. That would mean that you had an energy deficit of 5000 calories each day, which is not possible unless you were spending the entire day doing vigorous exercise. That wouldn't be safe, of course, and would be challenging even for a professional athlete.

It's important to also remember that we need to eat enough, too, so that we consume enough calories and essential nutrients for the body to do its many jobs. People often try to restrict their calorie intake too much, and their body will slow down metabolism in an effort to hold onto calories. Finding the right energy balance can be tricky. Health experts usually suggest finding out how many calories a person needs to maintain their body weight (using an energy expenditure formula like the ones described above), and then reducing calories by a couple hundred a day.

Benefits of Healthy Body Composition

A healthy body composition can have positive impacts on many factors related to our overall wellness, from the physical to the emotional and even economical.

Physical Benefits

By maintaining a health body composition, we reduce the risks of disease and premature death substantially and avoid placing limitations on our activities. We have more energy to complete tasks, greater stamina, and are more ready to participate in whatever comes our way. We become more functional members of our families and society.

Excess body weight also increases the risk of cardiovascular disease, type 2 diabetes, joint problems, sleep apnea, digestive problems, gallbladder and liver disease, asthma and other respiratory problems, and certain forms of cancer (breast, prostate, esophagus, endometrium, kidney, and others). Obesity can also reduce years of healthy life.

Emotional Benefits

The benefits are emotional as well as physical. You won't be happy just because you are physically fit. Having a healthy amount of body fat does not in itself reduce stress, but the exercise and healthy eating needed to achieve and maintain a healthy body does. As discussed in previous chapters, the body releases hormones during exercise that help your mood and energy levels. Not to mention, by reducing our risk of illness and disease, we reduce those stressors in our lives.

A healthy body composition can also help us maintain a positive body image. Individuals with a poor body image often struggle with anxiety, depression, and even eating disorders (more later in the chapter on this). Obese individuals can also experience social anxiety related to their weight that can be quite disruptive in their lives, such as an unwillingness to participate in social functions and seclusion. A healthy body composition won't solve all of our problems, but it can reduce those within our control.

Economical

The costs of poor health related to body composition are too big to ignore. According to the CDC, national estimates of health care costs related to obesity in 2008 were $147 billion. Illnesses related to obesity mean more trips to the doctor's office and potentially hospitalization. In addition to this, they estimate that the productivity costs related to obesity-related absenteeism due to health issues was $3.38 billion nationwide. Obese workers also experience "presenteeism," or a loss of productivity even while at work. This has the potential to cost a person his job and his livelihood.

Factors that Influence Body Composition

Our body composition can be affected by multiple factors. Our biological sex, ethnicity, age, environment, and even our genes play a role in how our bodies look, develop, and function.

Genetics

Your genetic makeup can affect your body composition. According to the Centers for Disease Control, lifestyle choices tend to play the largest role, but research suggests that our genes, which are responsible for giving our body cues for how to handle environmental changes, can have an impact.

Past studies of family members, twins, and adoptees offered indirect scientific evidence that a portion of the variation in weight among adults is due to genetic factors. For example, a key study that compared the body mass index of twins reared either together or apart found that inherited factors had more influence than childhood environment. In rare cases, obesity occurs in families according to a clear inheritance pattern caused by changes in a single gene. Affected children feel extremely hungry and become obese because of consistent overeating (hyperphagia). So far, rare variants in at least nine genes have been implicated in single-gene (monogenic) obesity.

In most obese people, no one genetic cause can be identified. Genome-wide association studies have found more than 50 genes associated with obesity, but most with very slight impact. The CDC suggests that most obesity seems to be multifactorial, that is, the result of complex interactions among many genes and environmental factors. Epigenetic research (study of gene expression) is ongoing in this area.

For most of us, the factors affecting our body composition are more multi-dimensional than just a genetic predisposition. Even in cases where suspect genes may be present, they are only expressed under certain circumstances. We may not be able to control many aspects of what we inherit, such as bone structure or the number of fast-twitch muscles in our bodies, but genetic tendencies related to the development of fat tissue can largely be managed.

Biological Sex

In general, women have a higher percentage of body fat than men and tend to store it around their hips and thighs, giving them more of a pear shape. This is likely due to hormones. Estrogen and testosterone respond differently in the body, with testosterone leading to more lean muscle mass. Men, though they may gain weight all over, are often seen with a larger accumulation of fat around the abdomen. More weight around the mid-section means more visceral fat, which is more dangerous to your health than the subcutaneous fat around your thighs.

Males are generally born larger, but most of the biological differences in body composition begin in puberty. As their hormone levels begin to change, males will see an increase in muscle mass, whereas females will gain fat. Hormones play a role again for women during and after menopause. This usually occurs between the ages of 45 and 55. The body's production of estrogen and progesterone, two hormones made by the ovaries, varies greatly during this transitional period that eventually leads to the cessation of a woman's menstrual cycle. The body begins to use energy differently during this period,

fat cells change, and women may gain weight more easily. They may also begin to see more of the visceral fat that men experience.

As testosterone declines with age, men see an even higher risk of visceral fat. In general, adult men tend to be overweight more often than women, approximately 38% in comparison to 28%. However, when overweight, women are more likely to be obese. Men have a naturally higher resting metabolic rate (RMR) than women, most likely due to the differences in lean body mass between the average man and woman. This could be why women's bodies are more likely to become obese. A higher RMR means that a man will have a higher metabolism and burn more calories even while at rest than a woman.

Age

Changing hormone levels are only one of the factors that affect our body composition as we age. Our muscle mass and bones also play an important role. As mentioned in previous chapters, these begin to deteriorate over time, particularly over age 60.

Each decade that a person is not involved in strengthening activities leads to 4–6 pounds of muscle lost. A 30 year-old person will have a greater quantity of bone and muscle than a 70 year-old with the same BMI. When we become elderly, much of our efforts in body composition relate to weight control and maintenance because our bodies have little ability to gain new muscle or strengthen bone. Obesity tends to be highest among middle-aged adults at around 40%, followed by older adults at 37%, and younger (age 20–39) at 32%.

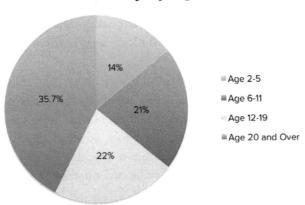

Figure 13. Obesity rates in the United States by age.

Ethnicity

Your race and ethnicity can also play a role in how your body is composed, though it is difficult to determine how much of this is related to sociocultural or socioeconomic differences as compared to inherited ones. These factors, which take into consideration malnutrition and lifestyle issues, impact the physical development and overall stat-

ure of an individual. There are, however, some tendencies among different groups. Blacks, for example, tend to have a larger musculoskeletal mass than whites, Hispanics, and Asians. Asians tend to have a smaller bone density than whites, Hispanics, or blacks. More research is needed to fully understand the dynamics.

Lifestyle and Environment

How we are raised, the environment in which we live, and our lifestyle choices are the largest factors in our body composition. Regardless of our biological sex, family history, race, or ethnicity, our health and those aspects of it that we can control often come down to this. We make **lifestyle** choices each and every day

that impact how we feel and how our bodies function, from our food intake and physical activity, to sleep, unhealthy habits, and even stress.

The type and amount of food we choose to eat dictates how much energy we need to burn. When the imbalance occurs, we store fat. Likewise, our choices related to exercise matter. This text has covered the need for physical activity at great length already, but its role in our body composition cannot go underemphasized.

Along with proper diet and exercise comes the need for enough rest for the body to regenerate. Sleep deprivation also leads to unhealthy eating habits. Research suggests that when we do not get enough sleep, our endocannabinoid (eCB) system is activated, similar to when a person smokes marijuana. Essentially, it triggers the reward center of the brain — a person lacking enough sleep will also lack the same control over their food choices as someone who is well-rested. They will even crave foods that make them feel better. Over time, this leads to gains in fat tissue. Imagine a person who both smokes marijuana and is sleep deprived? That could be a serious increase in caloric intake.

Our habits, such as smoking, excessive consumption of alcohol, and drug use can also contribute to our body composition. According to the US Surgeon General, people who smoke tobacco tend to store higher amounts of visceral adipose tissue than people who don't, putting them at greater risk for Type 2 diabetes and other chronic illnesses in addition to the higher percentage of body fat. Alcohol, like any other sugary drink with empty calories, contributes to body fat as well. In addition to adding excess calories, too much alcohol can slow our metabolism, making that energy out process even more difficult.

Stress seems to be a recurrent theme when we talk about health and increased body fat is a part of that. Some people quickly gain weight when they're stressed. According to the National Institutes of Health, a study has uncovered a potential molecular connection between stress and weight gain. A molecule called **neuropeptide Y** (NPY) is involved in the growth of the blood vessels necessary to support new tissue formation and is released from certain nerve cells during stress. Other research has shown that NPY and its receptors seem to play a role in appetite and obesity. Putting these results together, researchers think that NPY may be involved in new fat growth during stressful situations. In high fat, high sugar diets, researchers found that fat cells produced more NPY and more fat tissue.

Additionally, when your body is stressed it releases a hormone called **cortisol**. This triggers a release of insulin that lowers your blood sugar and causes you to look for sugar to put in your body. A study done among healthy female university students showed that as stress levels increased during the semester, levels of cortisol, binge eating, anxiety, and depression increased among many of the individuals. At the same time, their concern over their weight and shape decreased, and they showed less concern with eating habits. Over half the participants gained an average of 5 pounds. The increase in cortisol seems to have a direct connection to the other behaviors. Researchers consider the information critical in helping people understand the relationship between stress and eating behavior and the importance of stress management.

Beyond our lifestyle choices, our **environment** can affect our body composition as well. The CDC suggests that obesity is epidemic in populations of Americans that lead sedentary lives and consume high calorie foods. This is not always deliberate, but can result from a lack of infrastructure and resources.

Some environments do not contribute to a healthy lifestyle. Many neighborhoods do not have sidewalks, safe trails or parks, or access to health care. Our work and school environment, or wherever we spend our time, should also be taken into consideration. Access to or the availability of healthy food is crucial. If your workplace or neighborhood has greater access to fast food than to a grocery store, and nowadays most do, you will have to plan around your environment. This is difficult for many people who face challenges with transportation, money for whole foods, and time.

A "food desert" is an area with low access to healthy food. To qualify as a "low-access community," at least 500 people and/or at least 33% of the census tract's population must reside more than one mile from a supermarket or

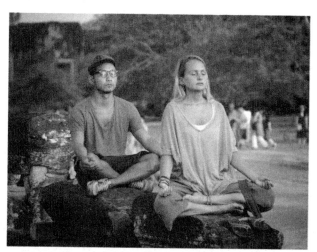

Figure 14. Stress management can lower cortisol levels.

large grocery store (for rural census tracts, the distance is more than 10 miles). Food deserts are typically low on whole food sources, but they could also be high on local quickie marts that provide a wealth of processed, sugar, and fat-laden foods that are known contributors to our nation's obesity epidemic

Some of our lifestyle choices have to do with our **family environment**. If you grew up eating doughnuts for breakfast rather than oatmeal, and burgers and fries at the drive-thru for lunch, you may not have learned the value of healthy, home-cooked meals. If you were raised to spend most of your leisure time watching television, a habit your still continue, you may not realize the impact your environment has on your health until you are away from it.

Even the **region of the country** in which you live can impact your body due to a lack of health education or an established community or family ideology that revolves around negative habits. If it is common in your community to fry most foods, or have frequent, large gatherings with food as the center, you may find it difficult to see this as a choice rather than a way of life.

This is what we term an "obesogenic environment" or "obesogenic society," one that encourages

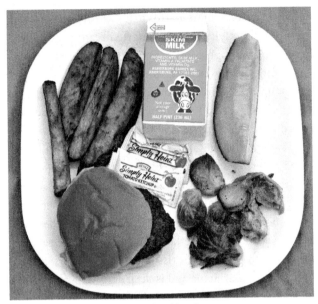

Figure 15. Washington, DC school lunch.

or contributes to obesity and makes weight management difficult. If many people in your home or community are overweight or obese and content to be so, they may not see or support the merits of a healthy body composition.

Body Image and Eating Disorders

Special considerations concerning body composition and weight include body image and eating disorders. Our body image is our perception of our physical body and our thoughts and feelings related to it, whether positive or negative. There are four aspects to body image:

- **Perceptual** — How you see or perceive your body. You may perceive yourself as under or overweight, though it may not be accurate.

- **Affective** — How you feel about your body (weight, shape, or individual parts), satisfied or dissatisfied.

- **Cognitive** — How you think about your body. This could be a preoccupation with your weight or body shape or a belief that you would be happier with yourself if you were thinner or had more muscle.

- **Behavioral** — How you behave as a result of your body image. This could be self-isolation or engaging in destructive behaviors (excessive exercising, vomiting, or not eating enough) in an attempt to change your body.

How do i know if i have a problem with eating disorders?

- I think my diet is out of control.

- I feel out of control when I eat.

- I feel scared around food.

- I am scared that if I eat normally I will gain weight.

- I am scared that I am fat but no one is telling me.

- I want to lose weight so people will like me more.

- I throw up sometimes after I eat.

- I throw up almost every time after I eat.

- I skip meals a lot or throw my lunch away.

- I don't eat foods I used to because they're fattening.

- I will not miss a day of exercise.

- I am scared to miss a day of exercise.

- I have lost more than 5 pounds this month.

- I think about food so much that it interferes with my life.

Eating Disorders	Characteristics	Symptoms and Dangers
Anorexia Nervosa	Emaciation, relentless pursuit of thinness, and unwillingness to maintain a normal, healthy weight Distorted body image (seeing oneself as overweight even when dangerously thin). Intense fear of gaining weight Extremely disturbed eating behavior Weight loss through excessive diet and exercise, use of self-induced vomiting, or misuse of laxatives, diuretics, or enemas Lack of menstruation	Thinning of bones Brittle hair and nails Dry and yellowish skin, growth of fine hair over body Anemia, muscle weakness and loss Severe constipation Low blood pressure, slowed breathing and pulse, lethargy Drop in internal body temperature Depression, anxiety, obsessive behavior Death from complications (cardiac arrest, electrolyte and fluid imbalances, suicide)
Bulimia Nervosa	Recurrent, frequent binge-purge cycles: eating an unusually large amount of food followed by compensatory purging (vomiting or use of laxatives or diuretics), fasting, or excessive exercise Feeling a lack of control over eating Fear of gaining weight Unhappiness with body size and shape Disgust or shame about eating behavior Normal weight or slightly underweight	Electrolyte imbalance Gastrointestinal problems (reflux disorder, irritation from laxative abuse) Worn tooth enamel and decaying teeth from exposure to stomach acids Chronically inflamed and sore throat Kidney problems from diuretic abuse Dehydration from purging fluids Depression, social withdrawal Death from complications
Binge Eating Disorder	Recurrent, frequent episodes of binge eating; no compensatory purging Feeling a lack of control over eating Disgust or shame about eating behavior Overweight or obesity	Risks from excess body weight, including high blood pressure and type 2 diabetes Depression

Figure 16. Characteristics, symptoms, and dangers of eating disorders.

- I spend my day thinking about where, when, and what I will eat.

- I like to think about food all the time. It is the best part of my life.

- I think I need help but I'm scared.

It can be challenging at times to develop and maintain a positive body image. In this day and age of constant media overload and photo-altered images of what is considered the "ideal" body, both men and women sometimes struggle to form an image of a truly healthy body. Our view of our body is often subjective rather than objective, as we are generally our own worst critics.

A **positive body image** exists when a person accepts and appreciates their body and treats it with respect. This has an impact on a person's overall self-esteem and leads to a more positive outlook and healthier behaviors. A **negative body image**, a sense of dissatisfaction with the body, can do the opposite, resulting in habits that can negatively affect your physical, emotional, and social health. Problems

can arise when a person has a negative body image, including stress, anxiety, depression, disordered eating, and other negative health habits. People with a negative image of their body are also more likely to attempt to change it with expensive and potentially risky surgeries.

Eating disorders, such as anorexia nervosa, bulimia nervosa, binge-eating, disordered eating, or eating disorders not specified are mental illnesses often associated with a poor body image. They occur most often in teens and young adults but can affect any age. Individuals with such an illness will go to extremes with food, severely limiting intake or severely overeating, depending on the disorder.

Among US children ages 13–18, 2.7% have eating disorders and more than half of them are girls. In adults, the numbers are slightly lower at .6% for anorexia, and .6% for bulimia, though a bit higher for binge-eating at 2.8% with all eating disorders being 2 ½ times more common in women than in men, though males do experience them as well. Research suggests that these disorders develop for a number of potential reasons, such as genetic, biological, psychological, and social factors. The risk factors are complex but most relate to a negative body image.

This can stem from a thin ideal perpetuated by society and peers (Figure 17). Friends, family, teachers, and even simple acquaintances can all have an impact on how we view ourselves. A lack of family support, a history of being overweight, or frequent comments focused on the individual's weight can contribute to this negativity. Probably the worst catalyst is the media and its representation of the human body. Altered photos of thin, "perfect" models and magazine covers with airbrushed, muscular abdominals and large biceps are constantly staring at us. Social media and "reality" television have added yet another level to our exposure to unrealistic images and expectations. Teens and young adults in particular spend a great deal of their time in front of these media outlets, adding more pressure for them to fit in with a false ideal.

Men, on average, are less likely to develop eating disorders, but they do report being dissatisfied with their appearance and bodies in similar numbers. Recent research has shown that men and women respond in nearly identical ways to questions regarding self-confidence "when [they are] with attractive persons of the other sex," "when the topic of conversation pertains to physical appearance," and "during certain recreational activities." Both men and women reported experiencing negative emotions between sometimes and moderately often. This shows that men and women are equally insecure in their bodies when the idea of "the body" is directly or indirectly confronted in social situations.

Anorexia Nervosa

Individuals with **anorexia nervosa** have a strong fear of gaining weight, which leads to them restricting their food intake and often exercising excessively. Sometimes they may assign rigid rules to their food intake, such as low-calorie limits or only eating food of one color. They see themselves as overweight even though they may be fine or underweight and don't eat enough food to maintain bodily functions (Figure 18). If left unresolved, this can lead to them becoming dangerously thin and the physical risks associated with it. Cardiovascular issues are a significant and potentially fatal risk. Anorexia can lead to low blood pressure, an irregular heartbeat, or even heart attack. They are also at risk for thinning

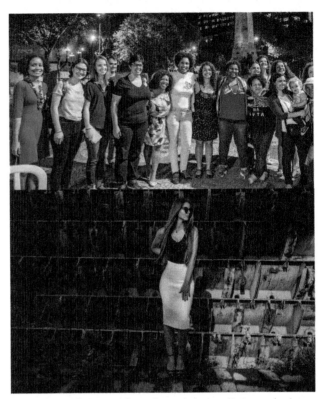

Figure 17. Body image often relies on an unrealistic standard.

Effects of Anorexia

Dizziness and/or fainting

Hair that thins, breaks, or falls out

Absence of menstruation

Dehydrations

Loss of bone calcium

Abnormal blood counts

Figure 18. Anorexia negatively affects the body in many ways.

bones, cessation of their menstrual cycle (in women), anemia, and kidney stones or kidney failure.

Symptoms of anorexia include weight loss, moodiness, missed periods, brittle hair and nails, yellow skin, weakness, dizziness, confusion, and a lack of desire to socialize. They often spend more time alone and avoid eating around others, or say they've eaten when they haven't. People with anorexia nervosa often restrict their food or weight as a means of controlling parts of their life they feel are out of control.

Anorexia nervosa is more common among women and girls, but recent studies show that many males are also being diagnosed. In women it may be a concern over weight, while in men they may over-diet and over-exercise to gain more muscle. Both are the result of an unrealistic image of what the body should look like.

This can be a very difficult illness to treat and generally involves psychological and behavioral therapy. In extreme cases, the person will need to be hospitalized to manage physical decline, treat the underlying mental illness, or both before it becomes fatal.

Bulimia Nervosa

Unlike anorexia, people with **bulimia nervosa** may be at a healthy weight because they do typically eat. They will sometimes eat a large amount of food and then attempt to get rid of it or thwart the weight gain by vomiting, taking laxatives, exercising a great deal, or fasting. This doesn't necessarily occur on a daily basis.

Someone with bulimia may participate in a binge as a result of stress or anxiety or in a response to hunger if they've been cutting back on their food intake. This would be followed by a purge, such as deliberately vomiting what they consumed. The purge does not always follow a large binge, however, but could occur as an emotional response to some stressor.

Again, this occurs more often in women and girls and is linked to a strong concern with body image. Over time, this can lead to stomach or intestinal damage from overeating and laxative use, ulcers and throat damage from vomiting, tooth decay, dehydration, and electrolyte imbalance which can lead to heart failure (Figure 19). Because people with bulimia often have a normal weight, or are overweight, it can be difficult to identify the problem. Symptoms include trips to the bathroom following eating, broken blood vessels in the eyes, damaged knuckles (from inducing vomiting), and acid reflux.

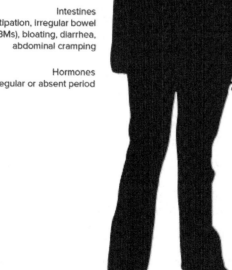

Blood
Anemia

Heart
Irregular heart beat, heart muscle weakened, heart failure, low pulse and blood pressure

Body Fluids
dehydration, low potassium, magnesium, and sodium

Kidneys
Problems from diuretic abuse

Intestines
Constipation, irregular bowel movements (BMs), bloating, diarrhea, abdominal cramping

Hormones
Irregular or absent period

Brain
Depression, fear of gaining weight, anxiety, dizziness, shame, low self-esteem

Cheeks
Swelling, soreness

Mouth
Cavities, tooth enamel erosion, gum disease, teeth sensitive to hot and cold foods

Throat & Esophagus
Sore, irritated, can tear and rupture, blood and vomit

Muscles
Fatigue

Stomach
Ulcers, pain, can rupture, delayed emptying

Skin
Abrasion of knuckles, dry skin

Figure 19. Bulimia negatively affects the body in many ways.

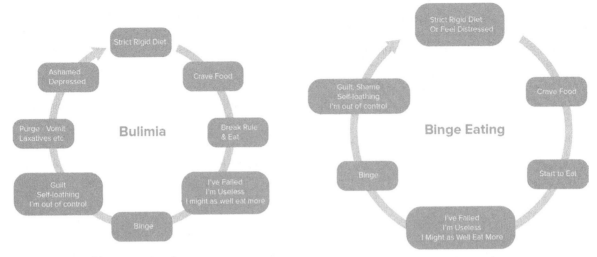

Figure 20. Bulimia and binge eating cycles.

Binge Eating Disorder

People who **binge eat** are often overweight or obese. They do not limit food or attempt to purge it. Rather they engage in episodes during which they eat large amounts of food within a short period of time (two hours, for example). They will eat until they are uncomfortable, even if they weren't originally hungry, often reporting a sense of feeling out of control (Figure 20). After bingeing, they often experience feelings of disgust and embarrassment.

Not everyone who is overweight or obese has a binge eating disorder, nor is every person with a binge eating disorder overweight. This can be a difficult illness to diagnose as people who binge eat often engage in the activity

when no one is around. It is also difficult because many of us have engaged in the activity at one time or another (though maybe not to the same extent) and may not see it as a problem if we are not around the person often. It is considered a disorder when a person binge eats at least once per week for approximately three months.

The individual may also have problems with substance abuse, depression, or other mental illnesses. People with a binge eating disorder are at higher risks of osteoarthritis, chronic kidney problems, high blood pressure and high cholesterol (both of which can lead to stroke and heart disease).

Disordered Eating

It is possible to have more than one eating disorder in a person's lifetime, particularly when we consider it as a mental illness that can sometimes be difficult to overcome. For some, particularly people who train heavily for a sport, their eating can become disordered in an attempt to control their weight and manage their performance, or even to keep their coaches happy. Crash diets, irregular eating patterns, and binge eating can often occur during this process in an attempt to find what works.

However, disordered eating can occur in any population. Dieting can be one form of it. Someone with this illness may become preoccupied with sticking to their diet, upset if they break the rules, and may avoid social situations where they may be expected to eat what is available. This can also lead to other eating disorders.

Here are some signs of an eating disorder:

- Skipping meals or making excuses for not eating.

- Adopting an overly restrictive vegetarian diet.

- Excessive focus on healthy eating.

- Making own meals rather than eating what the family eats.

- Withdrawing from normal social activities.

- Persistent worry or complaining about being fat and talk of losing weight.

- Frequent checking in the mirror for perceived flaws.

- Repeatedly eating large amounts of sweets or high-fat foods.

- Use of dietary supplements, laxatives or herbal products for weight loss.

- Excessive exercise.

- Calluses on the knuckles from inducing vomiting.

- Leaving during meals to use the toilet.

- Eating much more food in a meal or snack than is considered normal.

- Expressing depression, disgust, shame, or guilt about eating habits.

- Eating in secret.

Eating Disorders Not Specified (EDNOS)

Eating disorders not specified (EDNOS), or other specified feeding and eating disorders (OSFED), are those that don't fit neatly into one category. The person may have some symptoms of anorexia nervosa or bulimia nervosa, for example, but not often enough to be diagnosed with the disease or not yet having weight issues.

Over half of all cases seen at eating disorder treatment centers fall under this category.

The signs and symptoms are the same as other eating disorders. If left untreated, the person could develop a specified eating disorder or experience many of the same physical problems.

Body Dysmorphic Disorder and Muscle Dysmorphia

Body dysmorphic disorder and **muscle dysmorphia** are types of illnesses also related to a negative image about one's body and a distorted sense of what their body does and should look like. Body dysmorphic disorder occurs when someone has a fixation on a defect (even an imagined one) in his or her appearance, or on a certain part or characteristic of the body. For someone with this disorder, the flaw seems important and can consume daily thoughts. The person will often seek plastic surgery, or multiple plastic surgeries, to alter his or her appearance and correct the perceived flaw.

Muscle dysmorphia is more common among men and results in a fixation with becoming more muscular, no matter how much muscle they already have. It is generally grouped with eating disorders (a reverse anorexia) because food and exercise play a significant role in the formation of muscle. A person with this disorder may see their body as healthy even if muscular to the point of discomfort and deformation. Like any other disorder related to poor body image, body dysmorphic disorder and muscle dysmorphia can be treated with therapy and medical intervention.

Female Triad Syndrome

In women who train competitively for a sport, **female athlete triad syndrome** (Figure 21) can become a real risk. Participants in sports like gymnastics, figure skating, cross-country running, rowing and any other sport where having a low body fat is important to performance are at higher risk. In theory, excess body fat impacts training and performance whereas a lean body and good muscle tone will put an athlete at their peak. Rather than being at their best, the athlete will over train resulting in:

- **Disordered eating** — the push for a performance-ready body can lead to overly rigid or restrictive eating patterns and other eating disorders.

- **Low energy** — a lack of food means a lack of fuel. The body needs energy to run its systems. Without enough fat and carbohydrates the body will begin to break down protein in the muscles, which is counterproductive (energy balance equation).

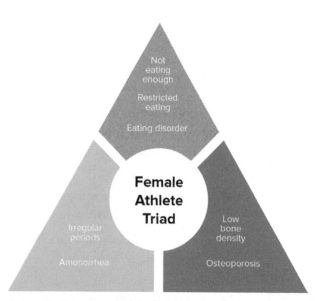

Figure 21. Components of the female athlete triad.

- **Amenorrhea (loss of periods)** — our bodies need fat to regulate hormones. Without enough body fat, a woman's menstrual cycle is interrupted.

- **Reduced bone mineral density (BMD)** — weakened bones can lead to stress fractures, osteopenia, and osteoporosis.

Coaches, parents, and the athletes themselves often become so focused on the competitive nature of the sport that they are willing to do whatever it takes to excel. At this point, their competitive nature has worked against them and caused a loss of performance.

The warning signs are similar to other eating disorders — decreased food intake, excessive exercise, and vomiting, along with fatigue and stress fractures. Health care practitioners must work as a team in conjunction with the family, athlete, and potentially coach to reverse these issues. Increased caloric intake and reasonable exercise are usually the first steps. Some athletes will be placed on oral contraceptives or other hormonal supplementation to resume their menstrual cycle, along with calcium, vitamin D and other vitamins and minerals to enhance BMD.

Like other eating disorders, this can be challenging to treat. These individuals are highly competitive and often unwilling to risk, ironically, being what they consider to be unhealthy. Mental health professionals often become involved. One approach in addition to counseling is to have the athlete sign a contract outlining their goals of treatment and their responsibilities related to their nutrition and exercise regimen as a condition of participation in their sport.

Treatment of Eating Disorders

Most people do get better with treatment and can go on to have a healthy, practical relationship with food and exercise. Doctors usually take an interdisciplinary approach that includes psychotherapy, nutrition therapy, support groups, and medicine, such as antidepressants. Some people who have eating disorders will need to be hospitalized to monitor their weight, ensure they are taking in enough food, and monitor their heart rate to ensure they are physically safe. Many areas have designated treatment facilities, or special programs within hospitals for people with eating disorders.

If you think you may have a problem with an eating disorder, the most important step is to speak to your doctor. He or she will ask you questions about your eating and exercising habits and run laboratory tests to rule out any other possible health problems. Honesty is the key. Since many people with eating disorders are secretive, they can go undiagnosed. It's important to be truthful with your health care practitioner about your behavior and feelings, even if it is awkward for you.

The National Eating Disorders Association offers the following tips for keeping a positive image:

- Wear comfortable clothes that you feel good in and that work for your body (not against it)

- Make a list of things you like about yourself that aren't related to your weight or body

- Consider yourself as a whole person, not just at your physical appearance

- Surround yourself with positive, supportive people

- Be a critical viewer of social media and other outlets — don't take things at face value

- Avoid negative or berating self-talk

- Set positive goals focused on health rather than a specific weight or size

- Avoid comparing yourself to others

- Say positive things to yourself every day

- Eat when you are hungry. Rest when you are tired

- Think back to a time when you felt good about your body

- Every morning when you wake up, thank your body for resting and rejuvenating itself so you can enjoy the day

- Every evening when you go to bed, tell your body how much you appreciate what it has allowed you to do throughout the day

Resources

There is a wealth of local, regional, and national resources to help people who have or may have eating disorders find treatment options and support for their condition. Help is available, and it should never be difficult to find it. Here are a few national resources available on the web:

- **Something-Fishy.org** — an online site raising awareness about eating disorders and collecting resources for treatment, recovery, and ongoing support

- **NationalEatingDisorders.org** — the National Eating Disorders Association's online resource hub, including resource collections at the state and local level

- **APA.org/helpcenter/eating.aspx** — the American Psychological Association's page on eating disorders, offering information and explanations of disordered eating from a clinical psychological perspective

Remember what your body is meant to do. This is the vessel that carries you your whole life. It has a big job. This is where focusing on body composition, rather than weight or appearance, comes into play. Our bodies really do serve an important purpose and their health should take precedence over any unrealistic image in our minds. Realistic goals and ideals can help you embrace this vessel and take care of it in a reasonable way.

Assessing Body Composition

Body composition can be assessed in several different ways, including body mass index, percent body fat measurements, and body fat distribution tests. According to the CDC, weight that is higher than recommended based on a person's height can be considered either overweight or obese (Figure 22).

Body Mass Index

One way to measure this is with the **Body Mass Index** (BMI) (Figure 23). This is a person's weight (in kilograms) divided by their height (in meters) squared. If the metric system is too much for you, you can also divide your weight (in pounds) by your height (in inches) squared, and then multiplying the result by 703.

For example: if your weight is 150 pounds and you are 5'5" (65"), your BMI would be 24.96, just inside the normal or healthy weight range.

$$150 \div (65^2) \times 703 = 24.96$$

This method makes it easy for the average person to determine their approximate body composition and the one used by many doctors. It does have some limitations. BMI does not take muscle into account nor does it directly measure fat, so it may not be accurate for someone who does strength training. Studies show that it can be a bit less accurate for men, who tend to have more lean mass, and for the elderly, who tend to have more of their weight as fat. However, it offers a good, general idea of how your body is composed in order to

Formula and Calculation
Kilograms and meters
Formula: weight (kg) / [height (m)]2 Example: Weight = 68 kg, Height = 165 cm (1.65 m) Calculation: 68 ÷ (1.65)2 = 24.98
Pounds and inches
Formula: weight (lb) / [height (in)]2 x 703 Example: Weight = 150 lbs, Height = 5'5" (65") Calculation: [150 ÷ (65)2] x 703 = 24.96

Figure 22. How to calculate BMI.

Body Composition	BMI Range
Underweight	0–18.5
Normal or Healthy Weight	18.5–24.9
Overweight	25.0–29
Obese	30.0–Higher

Figure 23. BMI ranges.

set initial goals and an easy way to track progress. It has also been shown to be a good, basic method of assessing disease risk.

There are other methods to determine body composition, such as skinfold thickness measurement, waist circumference, waist-to-hip ratio, bioelectrical impedance, underwater weighing, and dual energy x-ray absorptiometry (DXA) among others.

Our **body fat and lean mass percentages** are the amount of fat we have in our bodies compared to the amount of lean mass. Knowing how your body is composed and your percentage of body fat can be more useful because it does take fat into consideration, whereas your BMI does not. This eliminates

discrepancies over the amount of bone, muscle, and water versus the amount of fat in your body.

There are several methods for assessing percent body fat, including:

Underwater Weighing

Underwater weighing, also known as hydrostatic weighing, uses Archimedes principle of displacement to determine how much fat a person has (Figure 24). This suggests that there is a buoyant force exerted on the submerged object equal to the weight of the water that it displaces. Muscle and bone weigh more than fat, so when the person is submerged and weighed, professionals can compare their normal weight to the submerged weight. Someone with a lower percentage of body fat and more muscle will weigh more in the water. Someone with a higher percentage of body fat might weight less. This test is considered to be very accurate. The drawback is that the equipment is specialized and expensive, so it requires a trained professional. It is also time consuming and, for some participants, a source of anxiety if they are not comfortable under water.

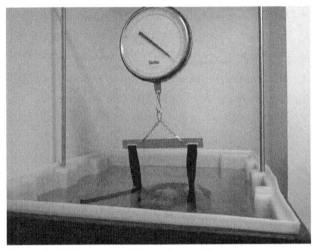

Figure 24. Underwater weighing.

Skinfold Measurements

In a **skinfold thickness test** a professional uses a special caliper to measure the amount of subcutaneous tissue the person has in 3, 4, or 7 sites on the body (abdominals, thigh, biceps, triceps, calf, scapula, and waist). It is easy to use once the person is trained and can be done anywhere. It may not work well for people who are quite obese or very lean due to the caliper's inability to grasp the tissue. If done correctly, it is fairly reliable though it does focus only on subcutaneous fat and cannot measure visceral (Figure 25).

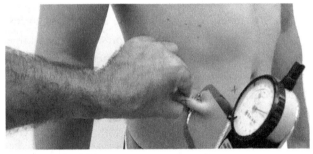

Figure 25. Skinfold measurement with a caliper.

Bioelectrical Impedance Analysis

Bioelectrical Impedance Analysis (BIA) measures resistance within the body to a small, electrical current (Figure 26). In doing so, it provides an estimate of the person's total body water by which it is able to estimate body fat. This can be done in several ways. One involves electrodes placed on the wrist and ankle. Another is with a machine. The participant stands on a special scale that sends the current through the body. Fat does not conduct electricity well and will make the flow of the current difficult. By measuring

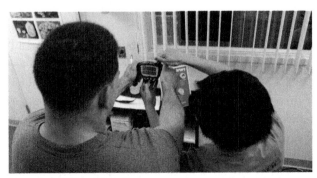

Figure 26. BIA test interface.

the resistance, the machine is able to determine body fat. It is fairly accurate if done correctly, but there are many variables that come into play, such as the amount of fluid in the body.

Bod Pod

The **Bod Pod** is an air displacement plethysmograph (ADP). Instead of using water, like in underwater weighing, the Bod Pod uses air (Figure 27). The participant is enclosed in a cocoon-like machine that measures the volume of air displaced by the body in order to measure the person's body volume. It is fairly accurate, though not quite as accurate as underwater weighing. How hydrated a person is during the test can affect results slightly as can their breathing pattern. This could be problematic for someone who is not fond of enclosed spaces and finds himself incapable of normal breathing. It works well for most ages and sizes and does not require a substantial amount of time. It's a better option than underwater weighing for people who cannot be submerged in water safely. Like underwater weighing, however, the equipment is expensive and not everyone has access to it.

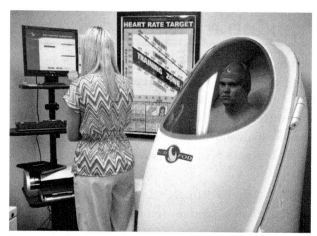

Figure 27. Bod Pod in use.

Our **body fat distribution** is the pattern in which our fat is stored over our body. For example, some people carry a lot of weight around their abdomen, while others carry it around their hips and thighs. By measuring certain areas of the body we can obtain ratios that help us determine our risks for certain diseases.

Waist Circumference

By measuring our waist, we can estimate the way fat is distributed. In women, a measurement over 35 inches is considered high risk, and in men a measurement over 40. A high circumference shows an elevated risk of cardiovascular disease, type 2 diabetes, and hypertension. In participants who are obese and will exceed the numbers, there is no way to measure incremental risk of disease (for example, there is no guide that says each inch equals a certain percentage of increased risk), but it offers a good guideline for most individuals, a tool by which to measure progress.

This doesn't mean that we can do crunches and try to focus on simply toning up our abdominals. It doesn't work that way. It means that we likely have more body fat overall (including visceral fat) than is healthy — not just what is around our waist — and need to work toward a healthier body composition to protect our health.

Waist-to-Hip Ratio

Measuring our waist-to-hip ratio is another method for determining abdominal fat and can be particularly helpful with identifying possible danger associated with visceral fat. Measure your waist at its most narrow point and your hips at their widest, then divide your waist measurement by your hip measurement. Women with ratios over 0.71 and men with over 0.83 are at risk for health issues.

Waist-to-Height Ratio

Comparing your waist to your height is another way to determine abdominal obesity. Measure your waist and height using the same units (inches, for example). This measures the way your body distributes fat. A healthy number is below 0.5.

Making a Plan and Setting Goals

Setting goals for changing body composition and creating a plan for weight management, such as lowering your body fat percentage or BMI, should involve measurable goals based on improving overall health or avoiding individual health risks. SMART goals should be used to make gradual improvements, often requiring a range of physical activity and nutrition changes to see results. Your goals need to be realistic, achievable, and specific to you, your needs, and your lifestyle. There is no one best way to do this — consider the energy balance equation and how it relates to your life.

Make a Commitment

Making the decision to improve or maintain your body composition, change your lifestyle, and become healthier is a big step to take. Start simply by making a commitment to yourself. Many people find it helpful to sign a written contract committing to the process. This contract may include things like the amount of weight (fat loss) you want to lose, the date you'd like to lose it by, the dietary changes you'll make to establish healthy eating habits, and a plan for getting regular physical activity.

Writing down the reasons why you want to lose weight can also help. It might be because you have a family history of heart disease or simply because you want to feel better in your clothes. Post these reasons where they serve as a daily reminder of why you want to make this change.

Take Stock of Where You Are

Consider talking to your health care provider. He or she can evaluate your height, weight, and explore other weight-related risk factors you may have. Ask for a follow-up appointment to monitor changes in your weight or any related health conditions.

Keep a "food diary" for a few days, in which you write down everything you eat. By doing this, you become more aware of what you are eating and when you are eating. This awareness can help you avoid mindless eating.

Next, examine your current lifestyle. Identify things that might pose challenges to your weight loss efforts. For example, does your work, school, or travel schedule make it difficult to get enough physical activity? Do you often find yourself surrounded by sugary foods? Think through things you can do to help overcome these challenges.

Finally, think about aspects of your lifestyle that can help you stay focused. For example, is there an area near your school or workplace where you and some friends can take a walk at lunchtime? Is there a place in your community, such as a YMCA, with exercise facilities for you and child care for your kids?

Set SMART Goals

Set some short-term goals and reward your efforts along the way. If your long-term goal is to lose 30 pounds of fat and to control your high blood pressure, some short-term eating and physical activity goals might be to start eating breakfast, taking a 15-minute walk in the evenings, or having a salad or vegetable with supper.

Remember to keep them specific. For example, "Exercise More" is not a specific goal. But if you say, "I will walk 15 minutes, three days a week for the first week," you are setting a specific and realistic goal for the first week. Remember, small changes every day can lead to big results in the long run.

Also remember that reasonable goals are *achievable* goals. By achieving your short-term goals day-by-day, you'll feel good about your progress and be motivated to continue. Setting unrealistic goals, such as losing 20 pounds in two weeks, can leave you feeling defeated and frustrated.

This also means expecting occasional setbacks. Setbacks happen when you get away from your plan for whatever reason — maybe the holidays, longer work hours, final exams, or another life change. When setbacks happen, get back on track as quickly as possible. Also take some time to think about what you would do differently if a similar situation happens.

Keep in mind everyone is different. What works for someone else might not be right for you. Just because your neighbor lost weight by taking up running, doesn't mean running is the best option for you. Try a variety of activities — walking, swimming, tennis, or group exercise classes to see what you enjoy most and can fit into your life. These activities will be easier to stick with over the long term.

Combining Healthier Nutrition and Physical Activity

When setting goals involving nutrition and physical activity, it is crucial to first understand your body's metabolism and energy balance. Once you've established your RMR or BMR, consider the strategies that will help you toward your goal.

It is often difficult to know how to approach your nutritional plan given the sheer abundance of possibilities available on television, through books, and online.

There is a constant change and flow of information in popular culture today. Many of the trendy diets may result in initial weight loss but are frequently unsustainable, resulting in people regaining any pounds lost and sometimes gaining even more. There are, however, some healthy nutrition strategies that focus on the basic concept of reducing energy in (Figure 28).

Type of Beverage	Calories in 12 ozs	Calories in 20 ozs	Difference
Fruit punch	192	320	128
100% apple juice	192	300	108
100% orange juice	168	280	112
Lemonade	168	280	112
Regular lemon/lime soda	148	247	99
Regular Cola	136	227	91
Sweetened lemon iced tea (bottled)	135	225	90
Tonic water	124	207	83
Regular ginger ale	124	207	83
Sports drink	99	165	66
Fitness water	18	36	18
Unsweetened iced tea	2	3	1
Diet soda (with aspartame)	0*	0*	0
Carbonated water (unsweetened)	0	0	0
Water	0	0	0
*Some diet soft drinks can contain a small number of calories that are not listed on the nutrition facts label.			

Figure 28. Calorie amounts in drinks.

Healthier Eating Habits

According to the *Dietary Guidelines for Americans 2015–2020*, a healthy eating plan:

- Emphasizes fruits, vegetables, whole grains, and fat-free or low-fat milk and milk products

- Includes lean meats, poultry, fish, beans, eggs, and nuts

- Is low in saturated fats, trans fats, cholesterol, salt (sodium), and added sugars

- Stays within your daily calorie needs

You don't have to give up your favorite comfort foods. Healthy eating is all about balance. You can enjoy your favorite foods even if they are high in calories, fat or added sugars. The key is eating them only once in a while, and balancing them out with healthier foods and more physical activity.

Here are some general tips for comfort foods:

- Eat them less often. If you normally eat these foods every day, cut back to once a week or once a month. You'll be cutting your calories because you're not having the food as often.

- Eat smaller amounts. If your favorite higher-calorie food is a chocolate bar, have a smaller size or only half a bar.

- Try a lower-calorie version. Use lower-calorie ingredients or prepare food differently. For example, if your macaroni and cheese recipe uses whole milk, butter, and full-fat cheese, try remaking it with non-fat milk, less butter, light cream cheese, fresh spinach and tomatoes. Just remember to not increase your portion size.

The point is, you can figure out how to include almost any food in your healthy eating plan in a way that still helps you lose weight or maintain a healthy weight.

Meal	Food Substitute Ideas
Breakfast	Substitute some spinach, onions, or mushrooms for one of the eggs or half of the cheese in your morning omelet. The vegetables will add volume and flavor to the dish with fewer calories than the egg or cheese. Cut back on the amount of cereal in your bowl to make room for some cut-up bananas, peaches, or strawberries. You can still eat a full bowl, but with fewer calories.
Lunch	Substitute vegetables such as lettuce, tomatoes, cucumbers, or onions for 2 ounces of the cheese and 2 ounces of the meat in your sandwich, wrap, or burrito. The new version will fill you up with fewer calories than the original. Add a cup of chopped vegetables, such as broccoli, carrots, beans, or red peppers, in place of 2 ounces of the meat or 1 cup of noodles in your favorite broth-based soup. The vegetables will help fill you up, so you won't miss those extra calories.
Dinner	Add in 1 cup of chopped vegetables such as broccoli, tomatoes, squash, onions, or peppers, while removing 1 cup of the rice or pasta in your favorite dish. The dish with the vegetables will be just as satisfying but have fewer calories than the same amount of the original version. Take a good look at your dinner plate. Vegetables, fruit, and whole grains should take up the largest portion of your plate. If they do not, replace some of the meat, cheese, white pasta, or rice with legumes, steamed broccoli, asparagus, greens, or another favorite vegetable. This will reduce the total calories in your meal without reducing the amount of food you eat. BUT remember to use a normal- or small-size plate — not a platter. The total number of calories that you eat counts, even if a good proportion of them come from fruits and vegetables.
Snacks	Most healthy eating plans allow for one or two small snacks a day. Choosing most fruits and vegetables will allow you to eat a snack with only 100 calories.

Figure 29. Healthy food substitution ideas.

Reflect, Replace, Reinforce

The CDC's recommendations for good nutrition are based on a systematic approach to each habit. They recommend you *reflect* on all of your specific eating habits, both bad and good, and your common triggers for unhealthy eating; *replace* your unhealthy eating habits with healthier ones; and *reinforce* your new, healthier eating habits.

Reflect

Create a list of your eating habits. Keeping a food diary for a few days, in which you write down everything you eat and the time of day you ate it, will help you uncover your habits. For example, you might discover that you always seek a sweet snack to get you through the mid-afternoon energy slump. It's good to note how you were feeling when you decided to eat, especially if you were eating when not hungry. Were you tired? Stressed out?

Highlight the habits on your list that may be leading you to overeat. Common eating habits that can lead to weight gain are eating too fast, always cleaning your plate, eating when not hungry, eating while standing up (may lead to eating mindlessly or too quickly), always eating dessert, and skipping meals (even just breakfast).

Look at the unhealthy eating habits you've highlighted. Be sure you've identified all the triggers that cause you to engage in those habits. Identify a few you'd like to work on improving first. Don't forget to pat yourself on the back for the things you're doing right. Maybe you almost always eat fruit for dessert, or you drink low-fat or fat-free milk. These are good habits. Recognizing your successes will help encourage you to make more changes.

Create a list of "cues" by reviewing your food diary to become more aware of when and where you're "triggered" to eat for reasons other than hunger. Note how you are typically feeling at those times. Often an environmental "cue" or a particular emotional state is what encourages eating for non-hunger reasons.

Circle the "cues" on your list that you face on a daily or weekly basis. Going home for the Thanksgiving holiday may be a trigger for you to overeat, and eventually, you want to have a plan for as many eating cues as you can. But for now, focus on the ones you face more often.

Ask yourself these questions for each "cue" you've circled:

- Is there anything I can do to avoid the cue or situation? This option works best for cues that don't involve others. For example, could you choose a different route to work to avoid stopping at a fast food restaurant on the way? Is there another place in the break room where you can sit so you're not next to the vending machine?

- For things I can't avoid, can I do something differently that would be healthier? Obviously, you can't avoid all situations that trigger your unhealthy eating habits, like your friend's birthday party. In these situations, evaluate your options. Could you suggest or bring healthier snacks or beverages? Could you sit farther away from the food so it won't be as easy to grab something? Could you plan ahead and eat a healthy snack before going?

Replace

Replace unhealthy habits with new, healthy ones. For example, in reflecting upon your eating habits, you may realize that you eat too fast when you eat alone. So make a commitment to share a lunch each week with a friend, or have a neighbor over for dinner one night a week. Other strategies might include putting your fork down between bites or minimizing other distractions (i.e. watching the news during dinner) that might keep you from paying attention to how quickly — and how much — you're eating.

Here are more ideas to help you replace unhealthy habits:

- Eat more slowly. If you eat too quickly, you may "clean your plate" instead of paying attention to whether your hunger is satisfied.

- Eat only when you're truly hungry instead of when you are tired, anxious, or feeling an emotion besides hunger. If you find yourself eating when you are experiencing an emotion besides hunger, such as boredom or anxiety, try to find a non-eating activity to do instead. You may find a quick walk or phone call with a friend helps you feel better.

- Plan meals ahead of time to ensure that you eat a healthy well-balanced meal.

Reinforce

Reinforce your new, healthy habits, and be patient with yourself. Habits take time to develop. It doesn't happen overnight. When you do find yourself engaging in an unhealthy habit, stop as quickly as possible and ask yourself: Why do I do this? When did I start doing this? What changes do I need to make? Be careful not to berate yourself or think that one mistake "blows" a whole day's worth of healthy habits. You can do it. It just takes one day at a time!

Portion Sizes

It is important to understand that the amount of what you eat matters. In order to know how much to eat, you need to understand what one serving of a particular food groups looks like. Dieticians often recommend that you use familiar objects to gage portion sizes. A piece of fruit, for example, is the size of your fist. A serving of meat should be about the size of a deck of cards. The best way is to read the label of what you are eating, not only to determine whether the food is healthy but also to find the measurement of one serving. The size and number of portions of a particular food will depend, again, on how many calories you should be consuming eat day.

You should also be trying to balance your food groups and eat foods low in saturated fats and sugars. One combo meal at a fast food restaurant may be 1500 calories. Choosing to eat only this during the day rather than three balanced meals plus healthy snacks would be the wrong approach to both energy intake and portion control. There is a lot more information about nutrition available in Chapter 7.

Physical Activity

There are many healthy, simple ways to boost physical activity and increase energy out. It is important to remember the FITT principle when planning your physical fitness program and adjust based on your goals. More information on healthy physical activities is available in Chapters 2–5.

General Strategies

To lose weight, increasing your activity level to 50 minutes of moderate or 25 minutes of high-intensity activity each day for modest gains. For more significant gains, increase to 300 minutes of moderate or 150 minutes of high-intensity aerobic activity each week.

Adding strength training to your routine can also help improve weight loss. Muscle helps boost your metabolism and improve your overall strength and stamina for your workout routines.

Add a sport or new exercise to your routine. If you enjoy soccer or   basketball, join a club and become more active in that way. Take up cycling, kickboxing, yoga or some other new activity that you haven't tried. The variety can keep you from getting bored and help you stay on track with your goals.

If you've not been physically active in a while, you may be wondering how to get started again. The CDC offers some good tips to help you begin:

- Look for opportunities to reduce sedentary time and to increase active time. For example, instead of watching TV, try taking a walk after dinner.

- Set aside specific times for physical activity in your schedule to make it part of your daily or weekly routine.

- Start with activities, locations, and times you enjoy. For example, some people might like walking in their neighborhood in the mornings; others might prefer an exercise class at a health club after work.

- Try activities with friends or family members to help with motivation and mutual encouragement.

- Start slowly and work your way up to more physically challenging activities. For many people, walking is a particularly good place to begin.

- When necessary, break up your daily activity goal into smaller amounts of time. For example, you could break the 30-minute a day recommendation into three 10-minute sessions or two 15-minute sessions. Just make sure the shorter sessions are at least 10 minutes long.

Moderate Physical Activity	Approximate Calories/30 Minutes for a 154 lb Person1	Approximate Calories/Hr for a 154 lb Person1
Hiking	185	370
Light gardening/yard work	165	330
Dancing	165	330
Golf	165	330
Bicycling (<10 mph)	145	290
Walking (3.5 mph)	140	280
Weight lifting	110	220
Stretching	90	180
Vigorous Physical Activity	Approximate Calories/30 Minutes for a 154 lb Person1	Approximate Calories/Hr for a 154 lb Person1
Running/jogging (5 mph)	295	590
Bicycling (>10 mph)	295	590
Swimming	255	510
Aerobics	240	480
Walking (4.5 mph)	230	460
Heavy yard work	220	440
Weight lifting (vigorous effort)	220	440
Basketball (vigorous)	220	440

[1]Calories burned per hour will be higher for persons who weigh more than 154 lbs (70 kg) and lower for persons who weigh less.Source: Adapted from Dietary Guidelines for Americans 2005, page 16, Table 4

Figure 30. Calories used by common physical activities.

Aggressive Weight Management

There are more aggressive approaches to weight loss or weight management than those described here, including diet programs, supplements, medications, and even surgery. These aren't all necessarily recommended by health professionals. Some of these may have signifi-cant science behind them and others have never truly been tested or proven to be effective over the long term. If you are considering a particular approach, speak to your doctor or nutritionist and do your homework before proceeding.

Diet Books and Programs

A few weeks ago, your friend Mary was scrolling through her social media feed and found the solution to all her weight problems, she was apparently eating bananas, a food the article claimed no one should ever eat. A few days later, she learned to never eat carrots because they had too much sugar. Next up was vinegar — all the celebrities drink vinegar to accelerate weight loss. No carbohydrates, then no meat, then no dairy, then only grass-fed animal products — one food was bad for the body, the next the environment, and so on. Before long, Mary was no health-ier and more confused than ever before.

There are more diet books and new programs available nearly every week, from those that focus on high protein or low carbohydrates to ones that encourage you to avoid meat entirely. Some even consider your blood type as a factor in how you eat and lose weight. Some might be quite practical and healthy while others make no sense at all. These methods are not a substitute for careful assessment of your current physical condition, planning, and training based on your goals.

As a general rule, be cautious of programs that offer rapid weight loss and quick fixes. There is no one food, no matter how super, that will magically remove fat any more than there is one food alone that will cause you to gain it. Plans with extreme restrictions on particular food groups, limits on food combinations, rigid and boring menus, and promises of fat loss without exercise are a dime a dozen and most likely not going to work. You may even end up missing out on vital nutrients in your diet. Consider whether you could really eat that way for the rest of your life. If you can't, it isn't for you.

If you want to participate in a structured program, look for a plan that promotes reasonable weight loss, such as one or two pounds per week. It should also discuss ways to keep weight off long-term, manage stress, change eating habits, deal with challenges, and get support. Losing body fat isn't a simple process — it requires knowledge and behavioral changes aimed at gaining or maintaining health. See Chapter 7 for more information.

Supplements

Many advertised supplements that claim to reduce your weight or build muscle contain ingredients that are untested or under-tested and possibly unsafe. The names of the ingredients can be so unfamiliar that without research you may be ingesting multiple forms of caffeine or other stimulants that could be hazardous. There simply isn't a quick fix for weight loss or muscle growth. Claims about rapid weight loss should be viewed with extreme skepticism. They can be dangerous. Even some vitamins and minerals are dangerous when taken in high doses.

Supplements are not regulated in the same way as medications or food. The manufacturers have the responsibility for testing their products and ensuring safety, not the FDA. If a product is found to be dangerous, it is removed from the market, which means it could be on the shelves for a while before the negative issues are reported. These companies are also under no obligation to prove whether their products work.

The following substances have noted safety concerns:

- comfrey
- chaparral
- lobelia
- germander
- aristolochia
- ephedra (ma huang)
- L-tryptophan
- germanium
- magnolia-stephania
- stimulant laxative ingredients

You should definitely avoid these substances. Check the labels of any supplement you are considering for these ingredients.

Medications

There are some over-the-counter medications on the market intended to help with weight loss, such as orlistat (xenical and Alli), lorcaserin (Belviq), phentermine, benzphetamine, diethylpropion, naltrexone combined with bupropion (Contrave), and others. These medications, depending upon the product, are designed to either slow the absorption of fat or suppress your appetite. They may help you lose five or ten pounds, on average, but unless combined with a healthy diet and fitness plan, consumers usually regain the weight once they stop taking the medication. Sometimes health care providers will recommend these in patients with BMIs over 30 and serious health issues in an effort to kickstart the weight loss process.

These should not be taken without first seeking the advice of a health care provider. Their Side effects can be serious, ranging from diarrhea, constipation, dry mouth, insomnia, and headaches to increased blood pressure, heart palpitations, depression, and even liver failure. Even if approved by your provider, typical use is limited to only short terms like a few weeks.

Surgery

In extreme situations, doctors will perform bariatric surgery to help a patient lose weight. Gastric bypass, gastric sleeves, and adjustable gastric bands are just a few but all are designed to limit the amount of food that gets to the stomach or the size of the stomach in general.

Gastric bypass, for example, involves the surgeon stapling the stomach into two sections, creating a small, upper pouch about the size of a walnut. The food goes directly into this pouch. It is so small that people can only eat about one ounce of food at a time. The doctor also connects a part of your small intestine directly to this pouch. This enables the food to pass through the body more quickly and the person to absorb fewer calories.

A gastric band is similar. The doctor places a band around the top of your stomach to create a small pouch. The doctor can adjust the band by injecting or removing a salt-water solution inside of it. A gastric sleeve, on the other hand, is permanent — surgeons remove most of your stomach. Again, the goal of these is to make you feel fuller, faster and eat less.

Most people can expect to lose 10–20 pounds the first month after surgery. Within a year, they may be able to lose half of the weight the need to as long as they continue to take in small portions. Bariatric surgery does not replace healthy habits, but may make it easier for someone to consume fewer calories and be more physically active. Most people regain some weight over time, but weight regain is usually small compared to their initial weight loss. The individual may need counseling in addition to surgery to help them manage any emotional issues that lead to overeating. The surgical approach is aggressive and can lessen your desire to eat but cannot stop you from reverting to old habits.

Doctors use surgery only when someone's health is seriously at risk due to excess fat, such as a BMI over 40 and/or serious weight-related illness, such as heart disease or type 2 diabetes. These surgeries are major and involve a significant recovery time. A patient can expect initial pain in addition to temporary drains and catheters, and a liquid diet until they are able to keep food down. They can also expect to pay a lot of money. On average, bariatric surgery costs between $15,000 and $25,000, depending on what type of surgery you have and whether you have surgery-related problems.

Liposuction

Liposuction is the removal of isolated areas of subcutaneous fat deposits. In this procedure, doctors will insert a tube (cannula) and a suctioning device through the patient's skin and into the area chosen for fat removal. This procedure will permanently remove fat cells from the targeted spots on the body. If a person gains a small amount of weight after liposuction, the remaining fat cells will grow. More than a 10% weight gain will result in new fat cell growth. The patient will see it in other parts of the body first, those that did not have the procedure. For example, if a person has fat removal on their abdomen, hips, and thighs they may see fat develop more in their face, arms, or chest. The liposuctioned areas will not grow as rapidly, but with continued weight gain they can still accumulate fat.

Liposuction comes with risks. Swelling and bruising is a given after treatment, but some people can also experience infections, skin sagging, and edema and seromas (fluid build-up). In some cases, patients may have an over-correction or under-correction. This means that too much or too little fat was removed from a spot, leaving the shape of the body part no longer contoured as it should be.

Usually only about five or six pounds can be removed safely in one treatment, so it isn't intended for someone with obesity. Like most surgeries, it is not a substitute for healthy eating and exercise. Someone who eats well, exercises, and maintains their weight will see better results than someone who is looking for a quick fix to an unresolved issue.

When You Are Trying to Gain Weight

Some people are interested in gaining weight and must consider healthy strategies for weight gain. This means you may need to increase your caloric intake (positive energy balance) by consuming more healthy foods. You also may need to incorporate strength training into your exercise program to build muscle mass. There are some simple tips that can help you add calories and gain weight in a healthy way:

- If you have a small appetite, try eating several small meals each day and drink fluids after meals so that they don't fill you up with.

- Add concentrated calories to your food, such as shredded cheese on your baked potato or almond butter on your toast.

- Prepare oatmeal and other hot cereals with milk instead of water and top them with fruits, nuts, or honey.

- Add healthy oils to salads, like olive oil, whole olives, avocados, nuts and seeds.

- Add 1–2 tablespoons of dry milk powder to soups, casseroles, liquid milk, and mashed potatoes.

- Choose nutrient-rich foods. Whole grains, fruits, vegetables, lean protein, nuts, seeds, and healthy fats are important to your diet. Try adding smoothies and shakes with fresh fruit and milk and maybe adding some flaxseed.

The important thing is to remember quality over quantity. Adding calories with candy bars may increase weight but not be beneficial to your health and body composition. It's also important to be realistic about your body type. Remember, it is about health not about looking a certain way that may not be realistic for you.

If you've tried to gain weight in a healthy way and are still struggling, there may be an underlying problem. Visit your health care provider if you are under weight and suspect you may have an illness or eating disorder causing the weight loss that needs to be addressed.

Conclusion

Your next steps should include assessing your body composition, setting goals for improving your health based on body composition or BMI, and planning a healthy energy balance for achieving your goals. It's important to keep weight management in perspective and focus on health. Do an honest appraisal of your body image. Is it accurate and fair, or is it negative and unhealthy? If you feel that you might have disordered eating or a disturbance in body image, you should get help from the sources listed in this chapter.

Chapter 7
Nutrition

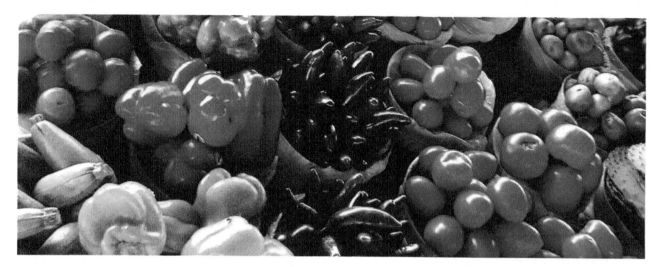

Nutrition is an essential part of a healthy life and contributes to several areas of wellness. The effects range from more serious, like whether or not a person can avoid, delay, or treat diseases (like diabetes, hypertension, or gout) to the more immediate, such as the effect hunger has on mood. Remember when you were small and your mom carried around snacks in her bag for you and your siblings? Well, it wasn't just for you to have a treat — it was to keep you from becoming unmanageable if you became hungry.

What you eat affects your health on many levels, which is why you need to understand nutrition and make educated choices. Your nutritional intake should be aligned with health guidelines and other health and fitness goals you may have. We're all a little different, so you'll probably discover that you can take some general guidelines and experiment until you find the nutrition plan that works for you.

This chapter first defines nutrition and essential nutrients then presents guidelines for health nutrition and potential plans for meeting those guidelines. The chapter concludes with a discussion of several common dietary concerns and how they affect individuals.

Nutrition and Its Essential Elements

Nutrition is the process of gaining essential nutrients and energy from the foods we consume, those we need for our bodies to function properly. It is connected to wellness due to the long-term effects both healthy and unhealthy nutrition can have on our quality of life. Combined with physical activity, your diet can help you to reach and maintain a healthy weight, reduce your risk of chronic diseases (like heart disease and cancer), and promote your overall health.

Deficiencies, excesses, and imbalances in diet can produce negative impacts on health. About half of all American adults — 117 million individuals — have one or more preventable chronic diseases, many of which may lead to various health problems such as obesity, osteoporosis, and diabetes. Many are related in large part to poor quality eating patterns. These include cardiovascular disease, high blood pressure, type 2 diabetes, some cancers, and poor bone health. More than two-thirds of adults and nearly one-third of children and youth are overweight or obese. These high rates of overweight and obesity and chronic disease have persisted for more than two decades and come not only with increased health risks, but also at high cost. For more information on chronic disease, see Chapter 9.

Many Americans do not meet the recommended guidelines for essential foods and nutrients and exceed what is recommended on foods that can be detrimental to their health in large quantities, such as saturated fats, sugars, and sodium. Before you plan your nutrition, it is important to be aware of nutritional requirements and the essential nutrients that are used by the body to meet those needs (Figure 1).

Calories Per Day*			
Height	**Activity Level****	**Men**	**Women**
5 ft. (60 in.)	Sedentary	1,950–2,200	1,700–1,850
	Low active	2,150–2,400	1,900–2,100
	Active	2,400–2,700	2,150–2,300
	Very active	2,650–3,000	2,400–2,600
5 ft, 6 in. (66 in.)	Sedentary	2,200–2,500	1,900–2,100
	Low active	2,400–2,750	2,150–2,300
	Active	2,700–3,050	2,400–2,600
	Very active	3,000–3,400	2,700–2,950
6 ft. (72 in.)	Sedentary	2,450–2,800	2,150–2,350
	Low active	2,700–3,050	2,350–2,600
	Active	3,000–3,400	2,650–2,900
	Very active	3,350–3,850	3,000–3,300

*Values show the range for 20-year-olds with a body mass index (BMI) between 18.5 and 25.0. For each year above age 20, subtract 7 cal/day for women and 10 cal/day for men.

** Activity levels: Sedentary (activities of daily living); low active (activities of daily living plus the equivalent of 30 min/day of moderate activity); active (activities of daily living plus the equivalent of about 60–90 min/day of moderate activity); very active (activities of daily living plus the equivalent of about 150–240 min/day of moderate activity). Thirty minutes of vigorous activity is equivalent to about 60 min of moderate activity.

Figure 1. Estimated calorie needs per day by height, activity level, and sex.

Nutrition and Energy

Our body needs energy to operate all of our vital organs and systems. We measure this energy as **calories**, units of energy that we take in through food. Scientifically, it is defined as the energy required to heat 1 kilogram of water by one degree Celsius. The total number of calories a person needs each day varies depending on a number of factors, including the person's age, biological sex, height, weight, and level of physical activity.

In addition, if you want to lose, maintain, or gain weight, the number of calories you should consume will change. Remember the energy balance equation from Chapter 6. A positive balance (more in, less out) means we gain weight, neutral balance (equal in and out) means we maintain our weight, and negative balance (less in, more out) means we lose. We need to understand how many calories our body needs to power its systems and then determine what we need to take in to reach our goal.

Your height and weight impact your Resting Metabolic Rate (RMR), or the number of calories you need. If you are physically smaller, for example, you might need fewer calories to function, whereas a professional athlete might consume a few thousand calories in a day. Estimates range from 1,600 to 2,400 calories per day for adult women and 2,000 to 3,000 calories per day for adult men.

In the table on the next page (Figure 2), you can see an idea of average height and weight needs for calorie intake. Within each age and sex category, the low end of the range is for sedentary individuals. The high end of the range is for active individuals. Due to reductions in basal metabolic rate that occur with aging, calorie needs generally decrease for adults as they age. Data is based on a male of 5'10" and 154 pounds and a woman of 5'4" and 126 pounds.

Keep in mind that these are just guidelines and would need to be adapted somewhat based on your height and weight. They would also need to be adjusted based on goals related to weight gain or loss. In Chapter 6, we discussed identifying your RMR or BMR as a means of identifying your daily needs, which would be another option for determining average energy intake when you add physical activity to calculate your energy needs.

It's important to note that we don't need to count calories each day, but it can be beneficial to track your diet periodically to gain a sense of how close you are to meeting the nutrient recommendations and help to identify patterns of eating and overall caloric intake. Tracking your food intake during the week and during the weekend may tell you if your food habits vary, which is true for many people. Calories alone aren't enough, however. Your body needs essential nutrients to survive, too. Most people get plenty of calories but not enough essential nutrients.

Calories Per Day for Males			
Age	Sedentary	Moderately Active	Active
18	2,400	2,800	3,200
19–20	2,600	2,800	3,000
21–25	2,400	2,800	3,000
26–30	2,400	2,600	3,000
31–35	2,400	2,600	3,000
36–40	2,400	2,600	2,800
41–45	2,200	2,600	2,800
46–50	2,200	2,400	2,800
51–55	2,200	2,400	2,800
56–60	2,200	2,400	2,600
61–65	2,000	2,400	2,600
66–70	2,000	2,200	2,600
71–75	2,000	2,200	2,600
≥76	2,000	2,200	2,400

Calories Per Day for Females			
Age	Sedentary	Moderately Active	Active
18	1,800	2,000	2,400
19–20	2,000	2,200	2,400
21–25	2,000	2,200	2,400
26–30	1,800	2,000	2,400
31–35	1,800	2,000	2,200
36–40	1,800	2,000	2,200
41–45	1,800	2,000	2,200
46–50	1,800	2,000	2,200
51–55	1,600	1,800	2,200
56–60	1,600	1,800	2,200
61–65	1,600	1,800	2,000
66–70	1,600	1,800	2,000
71–75	1,600	1,800	2,000
≥76	1,600	1,800	2,000

Figure 2. Calorie needs per day by sex, age, and activity level.

Energy Density vs. Nutrient Density

Not all calories are created equal. Some foods are heavy on calories but light on nutritional value, while some are packed with nutrients but not with calories. **Energy density** is the amount of energy or calories in a particular weight of food and is generally presented as the number of calories in a gram (kcal/g). Foods with a lower energy density provide fewer calories per gram than foods with a higher energy density. For the same amount of calories, a person can consume a larger portion of food lower in energy density than food higher in energy density.

Energy density values are influenced by the composition of foods. Water lowers the energy density of foods, because it has an energy density of 0 kcal/g and contributes weight but not energy to foods. Fiber also has a relatively low energy density (1.5–2.5 kcal/g). On the opposite end of the energy density spectrum, fat (9 kcal/g) is the most energy dense component of food, providing more than twice as many calories per gram as carbohydrates or protein (4 kcal/g). In general, foods with a lower energy density (i.e., fruits, vegetables, and broth-based soups) tend to be foods with a high water content, lots of fiber, or little fat.

We can also look at this from the concept of **nutrient density** (nutrient richness). These foods offer valuable calories because the energy comes from essential nutrients for your body without empty (not valuable) calories. The most nutrient-dense foods include vegetables, fruits, whole grains, seafood, eggs, beans and peas, unsalted nuts and seeds, fat-free and low-fat dairy products, and lean meats and poultry — all with little or no saturated fat, sodium, and added sugars.

Research indicates that consuming a low-energy-dense, nutrient-rich diet — one that is rich in fruits, vegetables, whole grains, lean meats, and low-fat dairy products — helps people lower their calorie intake. At the same time, eating low-energy-dense foods helps people control their hunger and maintain feelings of satisfaction and fullness. This is important when trying to stick to an eating plan. Making nutrient dense choices can be fairly simple. Look at a few foods side by side:

Typical Option	Lower Calorie Option
Regular hamburger patty (4 oz) = 235 calories	Lean hamburger patty (4 oz) = 167 calories
Medium croissant (2 oz) = 231 calories	Two slices of whole wheat bread = 138 calories
Slice of apple pie = 356 calories	Large apple (8oz) = 110 calories
Fried chicken w/skin and batter (3 oz) = 479 cal.	Roasted chicken breast, skinless (3 oz) = 141 cal.

Figure 3. Calorie comparisons of common foods.

Because the foods on the left have less fat, sugar, and added fillers, they contribute fewer calories at the same portion size. The basic nutrients may be comparable in the meats, but one is lean rather than fatty. The apple contains 3g of fiber and is rich in vitamins A and C compared to the slice of pie filled with sugar and fat. The whole wheat bread contains fiber, calcium, and potassium, while the croissant packs in nearly 6g of fat and lots of sodium.

Aside from choosing better versions of the foods we eat regularly, we can also seek out foods that pack a large nutrient punch. A large serving of kale, for example, has 2g of fiber, 3g of protein, and only 50 calories. Other foods that are standouts in the nutrient-rich class include salmon, liver, potatoes, berries, broccoli, almonds, and sweet potatoes.

Essential Nutrients

There are six classes of essential **nutrients** — carbohydrates, fat, protein, vitamins, minerals, and water. An "essential" nutrient refers to nutritional requirements that a person must meet through dietary intake because their body can't produce them or can't produce them in sufficient quantities for health.

Nutrients come in two types: macronutrients and micronutrients. **Macronutrients** (carbohydrates, fat, and protein) are the powerhouses, fueling your body to keep things running. Your body can't produce these nutrients on its own, so you must take them in through diet. **Micronutrients** are called that because our bodies need them in smaller amounts, such as milligrams and micrograms rather than grams. As these enter our digestive system, they are broken down in the stomach and then absorbed into the blood stream through the walls of our intestines (passive diffusion). Compared to macronutrients, micronutrients are absorbed very quickly.

Carbohydrates

Carbohydrates are one of the main types of nutrients, the most important (and quickest) source of energy for your body, and generally the largest source of calories in the diet. Common sources of carbohydrates include bread, pasta, cereal, grains, dairy products, fruits, vegetables, rice, and beans. There are 4 calories in 1 gram of carbohydrates. Carbohydrates are a pretty efficient source of calories, which your body needs to create energy. Carbohydrates consist of sugars, starches, and fibers.

Carbohydrates play a role in the functioning of the nervous system, metabolism, and muscles, and they are particularly important during exercise. Your digestive system changes carbohydrates into glucose (blood sugar) then your body uses this sugar for energy for your cells, tissues, and organs and to fuel your muscles, which is particularly important when we exercise. It stores any extra sugar in your liver and muscles for when it is needed. Without this nutrient, your body resorts to breaking down protein from your muscles.

Carbohydrates are considered either simple or complex, depending on their chemical structure. **Simple carbohydrates** include sugars found naturally in foods such as fruits, vegetables, milk, and milk products. They also include sugars added during food processing and refining. The sugars and starches in carbohydrates provide glucose, the main energy source for the brain, central nervous system, and red blood cells. Glucose also can be stored as glycogen (animal starch) in liver and muscle, or, like all excess calories in the body, converted to body fat. Simple carbohydrates break down very quickly into glucose and energy.

Complex carbohydrates include whole grain breads and cereals, starchy vegetables and legumes. These take longer to break down in your body, which means they don't elevate your blood sugar as quickly. This is particularly important for someone who is diabetic. Many of the complex carbohydrates are also good sources of fiber. Dietary fibers are non-digestible forms of carbohydrates. Dietary fiber is intrinsic and intact in plants, helps provide a feeling of satisfaction after meals, and is important in promoting healthy laxation. Diets high in fiber also have been linked to reduced risk of diabetes, colon cancer, obesity, and other chronic diseases.

Whole Grains

Whole grains are products made from the entire grain seed, usually called the kernel, which consists of the bran, germ, and endosperm (Figure 4). The bran is the outer shell of the grain that protects the seed — for us, it provides fiber, B vitamins, and trace minerals. The germ, which nourishes the seed, contributes antioxidants, vitamin E, and B vitamins to our diet. The endosperm provides energy in the form of carbohydrates and protein. If the kernel has been cracked, crushed, or flaked, it must retain the same relative proportions of bran, germ, and endosperm as the original grain in order to be called whole grain. Many, but not all, whole grains are also sources of dietary fiber.

We've heard on television, online, and now here in this text that whole grains are a valuable form of carbohydrate. The tricky part is actually making sure that the grains we are eating are in fact *whole*. We buy something brown or that looks grainy and think it must be healthy — the box says so! However, a lot happens to a grain

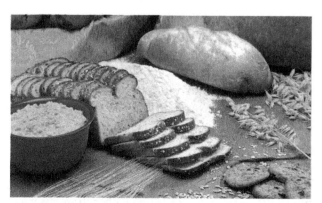

Figure 4. Whole grains can be found in many breads.

during the milling (refining) process. This is when our pristine-looking white bread and white flour achieves its appearance. But even those that look whole may not be. Often many of the components mentioned above are removed and other starches and flours are added in that we wouldn't consider whole. In fact, unless the word "whole" is in front of the ingredient, you may need to do a bit of investigation.

Flour can be one of the trickiest to determine. The US Food and Drug Administration (USDA) recommends looking for those labeled as:

- Cracked wheat
- Whole-wheat flour
- Crushed wheat
- Graham flour
- Entire-wheat flour
- Bromated whole-wheat flour
- Whole durum wheat flour

That covers the flour, but what about all of the other products that contain grains? Savvy consumers know that nowadays labels are designed to sell and can be deliberately misleading. Manufacturers want you to consider their cereal or their bread as healthy, especially with the push toward whole grains. But honesty is not always their policy. The USDA has some tips for this as well. Look for some common and usual names for whole grains:

- The word whole listed before a grain, for example, whole wheat
- The words berries and groats are also used to designate whole grains, for example, wheat berries or oat groats
- Rolled oats and oatmeal (including old-fashioned, quick-cooking, and instant oatmeal)
- Other whole-grain products that do not use the word "whole" in their description, but are a whole grain: brown rice, brown rice flour, wild rice, quinoa, millet, triticale, teff, amaranth, buckwheat, or sorghum

You may be wondering why whole grain is better than many refined grains. It comes down to nutritional content. Many refined grains lack the fiber and many other nutrients that are lost during the refining process. Some are "enriched," meaning a few nutrients will be added back in but rarely do they have the same health benefits. Whole grains are linked to lower body weight and lower incidences of heart disease, type 2 diabetes, and cancer — those nutrients missing from many refined products are important. The Dietary Guidelines for Americans recommend that at least half of your grain consumption be whole grains.

Gluten

Some grains — such as wheat, barley, rye, and spelt — contain a naturally occurring protein called **gluten**. This protein acts as a binder to keep the food together. It's what gives that stretchy consistency to dough when we make pizza, bread, and pastries. Yet this innocent little protein has been getting a bad reputation the last few years, getting blamed for any number of issues ranging from weight gain, headaches, and intestinal issues to poor cognition and attention deficit disorder.

Studies indicate, however, that gluten is a healthy protein for most individuals. Not only is evidence lacking to support many of the pop culture theories on gluten-free diets, gluten may actually serve as a pre-biotic, promoting the growth of good bacteria in our guts and helping out our gastrointestinal system. There has also been an increased risk of heart disease, type 2 diabetes, and stroke. Remember those diseases whole grains help you avoid? People often avoid many healthy grains in an attempt to avoid gluten, which results in an absence of beneficial whole grains in their diet.

For some individuals, gluten can be a serious health risk. **Celiac disease** is an autoimmune disorder that causes the body to sense gluten as a toxin. This leads to many side effects, including fatigue, bloating, constipation, diarrhea, weight loss, malnutrition, and intestinal damage. It is estimated that approximately 1% of the population has celiac disease, though it is commonly undiagnosed or misdiagnosed. There are other individuals that have milder reactions to gluten (gluten sensitivity) or allergies that involve skin reactions. For people with celiac disease or any form of gluten allergy, the only treatment is to avoid gluten. Most people, however, eat gluten their entire lives with no issues.

People with gluten sensitivity or Celiac disease must be careful to avoid gluten. Meat, fish, fruits, vegetables, rice, and potatoes without additives or seasonings do not contain gluten and are part of a well-balanced diet. You can eat gluten-free types of bread, pasta, and other foods that are now easier to find in stores, restaurants, and at special food companies. You also can eat potato, rice, soy, amaranth, quinoa, buckwheat, or bean flour instead of wheat flour.

Fiber

Dietary fiber, or fiber, is sometimes referred to as "roughage." It is a type of carbohydrate found in plant foods and is made up of many sugar molecules linked together. But unlike other carbohydrates (such as starch), dietary fiber is bound together in such a way that it cannot be readily digested in the small intestine.

There are two types of dietary fiber, and most plant foods contain some of each kind:

- **Soluble fiber** dissolves in water to form a thick gel-like substance in the stomach. It is broken down by bacteria in the large intestine and provides some calories.

- **Insoluble fiber** does not dissolve in water and passes through the gastrointestinal tract relatively intact and, therefore, is not a source of calories.

Soluble fiber can interfere with the absorption of dietary fat and cholesterol. This, in turn, can help lower low-density lipoprotein (LDL or "bad") cholesterol levels in the blood, reducing your risk of cardiovascular disease. Soluble fiber also slows digestion and the rate at which carbohydrates and other nutrients are absorbed into the bloodstream. This can help control the level of blood glucose (blood sugar) by preventing rapid rises in blood glucose following a meal.

Insoluble fiber provides "bulk" for stool formation and speeds up the movement of food and waste through the digestive system, which can help prevent constipation. Both soluble and insoluble fiber make you feel full, which may help you eat less and stay satisfied longer.

Soluble fiber is found in a variety of foods, including:

- Beans and peas

- Fruits

- Oats (such as oat bran and oatmeal)

- Nuts and seeds

- Vegetables

Insoluble fiber is found in a variety of foods, including:

- Fruits

- Nuts and seeds

- Vegetables

- Wheat bran

- Whole grain foods (such as brown rice and whole grain breads, cereals, and pasta)

The recommended healthy amount of fiber intake is 38g for men and 25g for women.

Most Americans do not get the recommended amount of dietary fiber. Dietary fiber is considered a "nutrient of public health concern" because low intakes are associated with potential health risks. The Dietary Guidelines for Americans recommends consuming a variety of nutrient-dense foods and beverages containing dietary fiber.

The FDA suggests using the Nutrition Facts Label as your tool for increasing consumption of dietary fiber. The Nutrition Facts Label on food and beverage packages shows the amount in grams (g) and the Percent Daily Value (%DV) of dietary fiber in one serving of the food. Food manufacturers may voluntarily list the amount in grams per serving of soluble fiber and insoluble fiber on the label (under Dietary Fiber), but they are required to list soluble fiber and/or insoluble fiber if a statement is made on the package labeling about their health effects or the amount (for example, "high" or "low") contained in the food.

The Daily Value for fiber is 25g per day. This is based on a 2,000 calorie diet — your Daily Value may be higher or lower depending on your calorie needs. When comparing foods, choose foods with a higher %DV of dietary fiber. The goal is to get 100% of the Daily Value for dietary fiber on most days. Keep in mind:

- 5% DV or less of dietary fiber per serving is low

- 20% DV or more of dietary fiber per serving is high

The FDA offers the following tips for bringing more fiber into your diet:

Look for whole grains on the ingredient list on a food package. Ingredients are listed in descending order by weight — the closer they are to the beginning of the list, the more of that ingredient is in the food.

- Switch from refined to whole grain versions of commonly consumed foods (such as breads, cereals, pasta, and rice).

- Limit refined grains and products made with refined grains (such as cakes, chips, cookies, and crackers), which can be high in added sugars, saturated fat, and/or sodium and are common sources of excess calories.

- Add beans (such as garbanzo, kidney, or pinto), lentils, or peas to salads, soups, and side dishes — or serve them as a main dish.

- Start your day with a bowl of whole grain breakfast cereal (such as bran or oatmeal) that is high in dietary fiber and low in added sugars. Top your cereal with fruit for sweetness and even more fiber!

- Choose fruit (fresh, frozen, dried, or canned in 100% fruit juice) as snacks, salads, or desserts.

- Keep raw, cut-up vegetables handy for quick snacks — choose colorful dark green, orange, and red vegetables, such as broccoli florets, carrots, and red peppers.

- Try unsalted nuts and seeds in place of some meats and poultry.

It is important to note that fiber should be increased gradually in the diet. Sudden, large increases can result in gas, bloating, and cramping. Take it one step at a time and drink plenty of water along with the higher fiber foods.

Added Sugars

The role of carbohydrates in the diet has been the source of much public and scientific interest. These include the relationship of carbohydrates with health outcomes, including coronary heart disease, type 2 diabetes, body weight, and dental caries. In most studies, however, little evidence has surfaced to support these theories or those related to poor cognition or behavior. Few studies have linked carbohydrates to obesity though some suggest the fiber content helps promote weight loss.

What *does* contribute to these diseases and works against weight loss, and your health in general, is **added sugar**. These are what give carbohydrates a bad name. Added sugars are sugar carbohydrates (caloric sweeteners) added to food and beverages during their production. This type of sugar is chemically indistinguishable from naturally occurring sugars, but the term "added sugar" has become increasingly used in nutrition and medicine to help identify foods characterized by added energy. They have no nutritional value, only adding "empty calories." Despite this, the average American consumes 22 teaspoons of added sugar each day.

Added sugars negatively impact your health a few different ways. First, the consumption of these empty calories often leaves your diet unbalanced. Earlier in this chapter we made a nutritional comparison between an apple and a piece of pie. The whole apple contained only the sugars naturally occurring in the food. The slice of pie contains a great deal of added sugars. A person who eats the slice of pie is filling up on a lot of empty calories compared to the person eating the apple. Our stomachs can only hold so much food. Each meal is a choice. If we choose the empty calories, and fill ourselves, we aren't likely to eat as many nutritionally dense foods.

If you ate a healthy diet *and* added sugar, would you be fine? Studies suggest no. How exactly excess sugar impacts the heart isn't yet clear, but individuals who consumed a healthy diet in addition to an excess amount of added sugar still had higher rates of heart disease.

You and your brother recently decided to eat "clean," removing most processed food and added sugar from your diet. You both did really well for the first few weeks because you focused only on whole foods, nothing out of a package

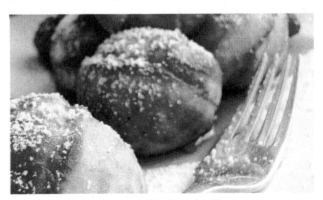

Figure 5. Added sugars can affect heart health.

or wrapper. But then you decided to take a road trip. You chose to plan ahead to avoid too many stops at fast food restaurants — great idea. But you needed to find foods that didn't take up so much cooler space — there's only so much room in your car and the Grand Canyon is a long way. While trolling the aisles, he begins picking out boxes of fruit and nut bars, and whole grain cereal. A little fruit, a little protein, some whole grains — no problem. Until you looked at the label. The bars contained honey and cane sugar. The box of whole grain cereal, though whole-wheat flour was the main ingredient, contained malt syrup and fruit juice concentrate. Are these the same as table sugar?

In short, yes! Added sugar goes by many different names. It doesn't matter how natural and unprocessed it sounds. The body doesn't differentiate between naturally occurring sugar and those that are added to the food. Looking at the total grams of sugar on the label is your best approach. Getting to know some of the names of different forms of sugar can also help when it comes to reading the labels and making choices. Some examples include:

- Agave nectar
- Glucose
- Brown sugar
- High-fructose corn syrup
- Cane crystals
- Honey
- Cane sugar
- Invert sugar
- Corn sweetener
- Maltose
- Corn syrup
- Malt syrup
- Crystalline fructose
- Maple syrup
- Dextrose
- Molasses
- Evaporated cane juice
- Raw sugar
- Fructose
- Sucrose
- Fruit juice concentrates
- Syrup

Recommended Carbohydrate Intake

Current dietary guidelines recommend consumption of carbohydrate-containing foods, including vegetables, fruits, grains (at least 50% of them whole), nuts and seeds, and milk products as part of a healthy diet. The recommended intake of carbohydrates is measured in grams, or in their percentage of your total calories, called the **Acceptable Macronutrient Distribution Ranges** (**AMDR**). These ranges take into account disease risk reduction and the intake of essential nutrients. The US Dietary Guidelines suggest that 45–65% of your calories comes in the form of carbohydrates.

How about that worrisome carbohydrate, added sugar? The American Heart Association recommends that we consume no more than six (women) to nine (men) teaspoons of added sugar each day. That's 100–150 calories or 24–36g at most. Just to give you an idea, that is the number of calories in one can of cola. The US Dietary Guidelines (2015–2020) have for the first time recommended that added sugar be limited to 10% of our diet.

Recommended Intake During Fitness Training

A person participating in a fitness training program, particularly when it involves endurance at a high level, may need additional energy for their muscles. This comes in large part from carbohydrates. These are the primary fuel sources for the body. Endurance athletes often have less body fat to draw from for energy during competition. This is ideal for health on a day-to-day basis, but when exercising it means your carbohydrate intake must be adequate to keep your body from robbing protein from your muscles to use as energy. Regardless of body fat, you need carbohydrates while training to maintain energy levels and performance. Great sources of quick energy include fruits (bananas and berries), brown rice, and yogurt.

The Academy of Nutrition and Dietetics recommends the following levels of intake:

Type of Training	Daily Carb Needs per Kilogram	Daily Carb Needs per Pound
Moderate duration and low intensity	5 to 7 grams per kilogram	2.3 to 3.2 grams per pound
Moderate- to heavy-training load and high intensity	6 to 10 grams per kilogram	3 to 4.5 grams per pound
Extreme training and high-intensity races (longer than 4 to 5 hours)	≥ 8 to 12 grams per kilogram	≥ 3.6 to 5.5 grams per pound

Figure 6. Additional carbohydrates are needed for fitness training.

Fats

Diet food, diet soda, fat-free this and fat-free that. These days there is a fat-free version of almost everything, from chips and soda to dairy products. Some are good (some foods don't really need fat to taste good), some have added sugar to mask taste and texture, and some are just wholly inedible. Often when we are trying to reduce our fat intake, we choke down foods that our dogs will not even steal a bite of. It might surprise you to learn that it's okay to eat fat, and that you even need it?

Fats are another of the three macronutrients, nutrients that we can only get from the food we eat. We need a certain amount of fat in our diets to stay healthy. They provide needed energy in the form of calories. In fact, they are the most concentrated source of energy in our diet. Fat has nine calories per gram, more than twice the number of calories in carbohydrates and protein, which each have four calories per gram. During exercise, your body uses calories from carbohydrates you have eaten. But after 20 minutes, exercise then depends on calories from fat to keep you going.

Fats do more than just provide energy. They help our bodies absorb important vitamins — called fat-soluble vitamins — including vitamins A, D and E. The fats you consume give your body essential fatty acids called linoleic and linolenic acid. They are called "essential" because your body cannot make them itself, or work

without them. Your body needs them for brain development, controlling inflammation, and blood clotting. You also need fat to keep your skin and hair healthy and to fill your fat cells, which insulate your body and help keep you warm.

Fats also make foods more flavorful and help us feel full. Let's be honest — they taste good. It is essential to eat some fats as part of a healthy and satisfying diet, though it is also harmful to eat too many. Fatty food's tastiness is paid for with a load of calories. This is why when eaten in large amounts, all fats, including healthy fats, can contribute to weight gain. Fats are vital to your health, but a fat-rich diet will give you way more calories than you need. Fats that aren't used for energy get stored in your body as (you guessed it!) fat.

The term "healthy fats" probably sounds like an oxymoron, but some types of fat are healthier than others. Choosing a small amount of healthy fats from plant sources (including nuts and seeds, good sources of omega-3 fats) more often than less healthy types from animal products can help lower your risk for heart attack, stroke, and other major health problems. Unhealthy fats increase your risk for these diseases and others, such as type 2 diabetes. Not only are you possibly tipping the scale on energy balance when you consume too much fat, but you could be affecting the inside of your body, even if your body composition is healthy.

Saturated Fat

All fats are made up of saturated and unsaturated fatty acids. Fats are called **saturated** or **unsaturated** depending on how much of each type of fatty acid they contain.

Imagine a building made of solid bricks. This building of bricks is similar to the tightly packed bonds that make **saturated fat**. The bonds are often solid at room temperature like butter or the fat inside or around meat. Saturated fats are most often found in animal products such as beef, pork, and chicken. Leaner animal products, such as chicken breast or pork loin, often have less saturated fat. We also typically find it in stick margarine, shortening, and coconut and palm oil, as well as in snack foods, chocolates, baked goods and other desserts, and deep-fried and processed foods.

Saturated fats raise your LDL (bad) cholesterol level. High LDL cholesterol increases your risk for heart attack,

stroke, and other major health problems. You'll learn more about cholesterol and its dangers in Chapter 9, but the most important thing to remember about it is that this soft, waxy substance can clog your arteries. Envision lighting a candle for a few minutes and then blowing it out. For a short time, the wax is in between hard and liquid, sort of soft and glue-like — it still runs a bit if you tip the candle but can't easily be washed away by other liquids. This is similar to what happens in your arteries when blood tries to pass build-ups of cholesterol. It gets in the way, interfering with blood flow and adding potentially life-threatening risk.

Saturated fats store well and take a long time to spoil, which is pretty important if you don't own a refrigerator, but a dubious claim-to-fame once it enters your body (any food that takes an unusually long time to spoil likely

	Butter (1 Tbsp)	Stick Margarine (1 Tbsp)	Soft/Tub Margarine (1 Tbsp)	Canola Oil (1 Tbsp)
Calories	100	100	60	120
Total Fat	11g	11g	7g	14g
Saturated Fat	7g	2g	1g	1g
Trans Fat	0g	3g	0.5g	0g
Cholesterol	30mg	0mg	0mg	0mg

Figure 7. Butter and margarine comparison.

contains more gifts from man than from nature). Unfortunately, saturated fats make up too high a percentage in the average American diet, which leads to numerous negative effects on overall health, especially cardiovascular health because of its impact on our arteries. The following data from the National Health and Nutrition Examination Survey (NHANES) tells us just how much saturated fat we consume compared to how much is recommended (Figure 8).

We can't avoid saturated fat completely. It would be almost impossible to remove every ounce of fat from your meat, and if you could, it would be more like jerky. Saturated fats, however, are not essential for life, so reducing them as much as possible is both safe and healthy.

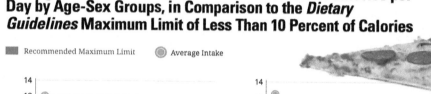

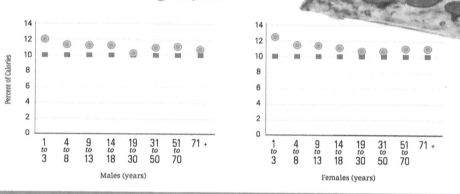

Figure 8. Most Americans eat more saturated fats than their daily maximum limit.

Unsaturated Fat

Imagine the links in a chain that bend, move, and flow. The chain links are similar to the loose bonds that make **unsaturated fat** fluid or liquid at room temperature like the oil on top of a salad dressing or in a can of tuna. Unsaturated fat typically comes from plant sources such as olives, nuts, corn, or seeds but is also present in fish. There are two types of unsaturated fats — monounsaturated and polyunsaturated.

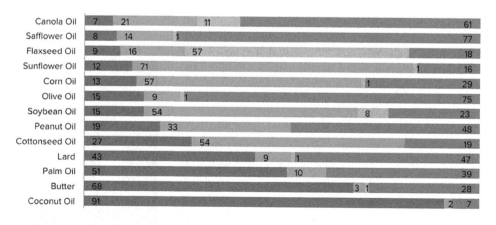

Figure 9. Cooking oils each have a different composition of dietary fats.

Monounsaturated fats are healthier forms of fat. Oils that are monounsaturated include olive, avocado, sunflower, safflower, canola, peanut, and most nuts. You may have heard people praise the merits of olive oil. There is a good reason for that. Eaten in moderate amounts and in place of saturated fats, monounsaturated fats can lower your LDL (bad cholesterol) levels, help your body regulate blood sugar, promote healthy cell regeneration, and improve your immune system. They also contain Vitamin E, which is great for your vision.

Polyunsaturated fats are also considered healthier and found in plants, salmon, vegetable oils, and some nuts and seeds. These contain omega-3 and omega-6 fatty acids. These are essential fatty acids that the body needs for brain function and cell growth. Our bodies do not make these acids, so you can only get them from food. **Omega-3 fatty acids** are good for your heart in several ways. They help:

- Reduce triglycerides, a type of fat in your blood
- Reduce the risk of an irregular heartbeat (arrhythmia)
- Slow the build-up of plaque in your arteries
- Slightly lower your blood pressure

Good sources of omega-3 acids include fatty fish — such as salmon, mackerel, and sardines — walnuts, flaxseeds, canola oil, and unhydrogenated soybean oil.

Omega-6 fatty acids may help:

- Control your blood sugar

Recommended Fat Intake

Reviews by the American Heart Association led them to recommend reducing saturated fat intake to less than 7% of total calories. This concurs with similar conclusions made by the US Department of Health and Human Services, which determined that reduction in saturated fat consumption to less than 10% each day would positively affect health and reduce the prevalence of heart disease (Figure 10).

The recommended AMDR for fat for adults is 20–35%. There are no specific guidelines on the exact amount of healthy fat we should consume, but of our recommended AMDR, we know that no more than 10% of that should be saturated. That means that we should work toward a range between 10% and 25% of our diet as unsaturated fats. The American Heart Association

- Reduce your risk of diabetes
- Lower your blood pressure

Good sources of omega-6 acids include vegetable oils, such as sunflower, safflower, corn, soybean, and walnut oils.

A note on fish and food safety: it's great to get more omega-3 acids into your diet, but some fish can be tainted with mercury and other chemicals. Eating tainted fish can pose health risks for young children and pregnant women. If you are concerned about mercury, you can reduce your risk of exposure by eating a variety of fish. Pregnant women and children in particular should avoid fish with high levels of mercury. These include:

- Swordfish
- Shark
- King mackerel
- Tilefish

If you are middle-aged or older, the benefits of eating fish outweigh any risks.

Most health experts agree that the best way to reap the benefits of omega-3 is from food. Whole foods contain many nutrients besides omega-3s. These all work together to keep your heart healthy. If you already have heart disease or high triglycerides, you may benefit from consuming higher amounts of omega-3 fatty acids. It may be hard to get enough omega-3s through food. Ask your doctor if taking fish oil supplements might be a good idea.

suggests that people try to consume between 5–10% of their daily calories from omega-6 fatty acids, which most people already do. They also recommend eating at least 2 servings a

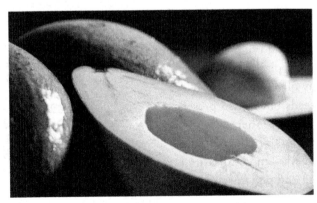

Figure 10. Avocados are rich in monounsaturated fat.

week of fish rich in omega-3s. For reference, a serving is 3.5 ounces (100g), which is slightly bigger than a checkbook.

If you're using more saturated fats than recommended, replacing the fats you regularly use with healthier options can be done with simple changes. Swap your partially hydrogenated oil with olive or canola oil. Try frying your morning eggs (if you just can't master poaching) in a small amount of olive oil rather than butter or bacon fat. Buy low fat dairy products (be careful to check the label for added sugar). Add some

nuts and seeds to your salad instead of processed croutons and bacon bits. You may be surprised at how easy and satisfying a few simple changes can be.

Higher Fat Foods	Lower Fat Alternative
Whole milk	Low-fat, reduced-fat, or fat-free milk
Sour cream	Plain low-fat yogurt
Cheese	Fat-free cheese, reduced calorie cheese
Ramen noodles	Rice or noodles
Pasta with white sauce	Pasta with red sauce
Regular ground beef	Extra-lean ground beef such as ground turkey
Pork	Pork tenderloin or trimmed, lean smoked ham
Whole eggs	Egg whites or egg substitutes
Regular margarine or butter	Light spread margarines, whipped butter

Figure 11. High fat foods can be substituted with healthier options.

Trans Fat

It's difficult to describe just how bad **trans fat** is for your body. Don't bother looking for recommended intake guidelines for trans fat — it's zero! Trans fat is the Frankenstein's monster of fat. Trans fatty acids are unhealthy fats that form when oils (even healthy oils) are hardened through a process called hydrogenation. Hydrogenated fats, or trans fats, are often used to keep some foods fresh for a long time. Trans fats are to fats like plastic is to garbage — it just doesn't biodegrade in any natural way.

This process began in the early-twentieth century with margarine and shortening. Once food manufacturers learned how to partially hydrogenate oils, it began

turning up in many processed (Figure 12) foods to extend their shelf life. Many restaurants (particularly fast food) used trans fat for years, enabling them to replace the oil in their fryers less often. Trans fats are under scrutiny for their health effects and many companies and food chains have begun to remove the fat from their products. Much of this came in response to measures by city and county governments to restrict trans fat usage within their communities. The USDA put its own efforts to work by requiring trans fat to be separated from other fats on food labels to fully inform consumers what they were putting in their bodies. In other words, it's a serious problem.

Saturated Fat	Trans Fat
High-fat cuts of meat (beef, lamb, pork)	Commercially baked pastries (cookies, doughnuts, muffins, cakes, pizza dough, pie crusts)
Chicken with the skin	Packaged snack foods (crackers, microwave popcorn, chips)
Whole-fat dairy products (cream/milk)	Stick margarine
Butter	Vegetable shortening
Palm and coconut oil (snack foods, non-dairy creamers, whipped topping)	Fried foods (french fries, fried chicken, chicken nuggets, breaded fish)
Ice Cream	Candy Bars
Cheese	Pre-mixed products (cake mix, pancake mix, chocolate drink mix)
Lard	

Figure 12. Where to find saturated and trans fats in common foods.

Trans fats can raise LDL cholesterol levels in your blood. They can also lower your HDL (good) cholesterol levels. In addition to high cholesterol levels, they cause inflammation that also can lead to heart disease, and stroke, and contribute to insulin resistance increasing your risk of type 2 diabetes. Research conducted at the Harvard School of Public Health suggests that even a small amount of trans fat, such as 2%, can increase your risk of heart disease by 23%. And those numbers are incremental. Every 2% increase adds an additional 23% risk!

How to Spot Trans Fat on Labels

According to the Food and Drug Administration, trans fat content must be expressed as grams per serving to the nearest 0.5g increment. If a serving contains less than 0.5g, the content, when declared, must be expressed as "0g." This means that even though the label indicates no trans fat, you could still be eating it and, as discussed, even small amounts can be detrimental to your health. Look at the ingredients on the label. Any substance listed as hydrogenated or partially hydrogenated is trans fat.

Proteins

Proteins, one of the three classes of macronutrients, are the building blocks of life. Every cell in the human body contains them. Proteins are large, complex molecules that play many critical roles in the body. They do most of the work in cells and are required for the structure, function, and regulation of the body's tissues and organs. You need protein in your diet for growth and development at every stage of life, from the womb to adulthood.

Proteins are made up of hundreds or thousands of smaller units called **amino acids**, which are attached to one another in long chains. There are 20 different types of amino acids that can be combined to make a protein. The sequence of amino acids determines each protein's unique 3-dimensional structure and its specific function.

Proteins can be described according to their large range of functions in the body:

As you can see, the amino acids from proteins have many jobs from building muscle and connective tissue fibers to making hormones and antibodies.

Their lowest priority is energy production. Proteins have 4 calories per gram, just like carbohydrates. Our bodies don't use this nutrient in the same way as it does carbohydrates. Proteins are constantly being broken down into acids, reassembled or rearranged, and used again. The muscle is the only part of the body that really stores any protein. This protein is only used for energy when other sources are depleted. When there is no available carbohydrate or fat storage to tap into, the protein in our muscles is used as a last resort. This is why we need to maintain a healthy amount of

Function	Description	Example
Antibody	Antibodies bind to specific foreign particles, such as viruses and bacteria, to help protect the body.	Immunoglobulin G (IgG)
Enzyme	Enzymes carry out almost all of the thousands of chemical reactions that take place in cells. They also assist with the formation of new molecules by reading the genetic information stored in DNA.	Phenylalanine hydroxylase
Messenger	Messenger proteins, such as some types of hormones, transmit signals to coordinate biological processes between different cells, tissues, and organs.	Growth hormone
Structural component	These proteins provide structure and support for cells. On a larger scale, they also allow the body to move.	Actin
Transport/ storage	These proteins bind and carry atoms and small molecules within cells and throughout the body.	Ferritin

Figure 13. Proteins serve many purposes in the body.

body fat and carbohydrate intake, particularly when we exercise regularly. However, any excess protein that the body cannot use for its daily functions converts to fat, just like everything else.

The human body needs a number of amino acids in large enough amounts to maintain good health. Amino acids are found in animal sources such as meats, milk, fish, and eggs though you do not need to eat animal products to get all the protein you need in your diet. They are also found in plant sources such as soy, beans, legumes, nut butters, and some grains (such as wheat germ and quinoa).

Complete, Incomplete, and Complementary Proteins

Dietary proteins are not all the same. They are made up of different combinations of amino acids and are characterized according to how many of the essential amino acids they provide.

Complete proteins contain all of the essential amino acids in adequate amounts. Animal foods (such as dairy products, eggs, meats, poultry, and seafood,) and soy are complete protein sources. They are not all nutritionally the same despite being a complete source of amino acids. The type of fat (saturated or unsaturated) and other nutrients they provide, for example, will vary depending upon the animal.

Incomplete proteins are missing or do not have enough of one or more of the essential amino acids, making the protein imbalanced. Most plant foods (such as beans and peas, grains, nuts and seeds, and vegetables) are incomplete protein sources. They are still high-quality foods both for protein and other nutrients. We just need to have a balance of various protein sources throughout the day to ensure we are getting all of the essential amino acids.

Complementary proteins are two or more incomplete protein sources that, when eaten in combination (at the same meal or during the same day), compensate for each other's lack of amino acids. For example, grains are low in the amino acid lysine, while beans and nuts (legumes) are low in the amino acid methionine. When grains and legumes are eaten together (such as rice and beans or peanut butter on whole wheat bread), they form a complete protein.

Good Sources of Protein

One ounce (30 grams) of most protein-rich foods contains 7 grams of protein. An ounce equals, for example:

- 1 oz of meat fish or poultry
- 1 large egg
- ¼ cup of tofu
- ½ cup of cooked beans or lentils
- 1 Tbsp peanut butter

Healthy sources of protein include:

- Turkey or chicken with the skin removed, or bison
- Lean cuts of beef or pork, such as round, top sirloin, or tenderloin (trim away any visible fat)
- Fish or shellfish
- Pinto beans, black beans, kidney beans, lentils, split peas, or garbanzo beans
- Nuts and seeds, including almonds, hazelnuts, mixed nuts, peanuts, peanut butter, sunflower seeds, or walnuts (just watch how much you eat, because nuts are high in fat)
- Tofu, tempeh, and other soy protein products
- Low-fat dairy products
- Whole grains — these contain more protein than refined or "white" products

You'll notice that the meat selections above are lean. The USDA recommends that most of your protein sources be lean selections to cut down on saturated fat. Trimming away fat, removing skin, and buying lean cuts of your favorite meats can help you do this. They also offer the following tips for varying your protein sources:

Choose seafood at least twice a week as the main protein food. Look for seafood rich in omega-3 fatty acids, such as salmon, trout, and herring. Some ideas are:

- Salmon steak or filet
- Salmon loaf
- Grilled or baked trout

Choose beans, peas, or soy products as a main dish or part of a meal often. Some choices are:

- Chili with kidney or pinto beans
- Stir-fried tofu
- Split pea, lentil, minestrone, or white bean soups
- Baked beans
- Black bean enchiladas
- Garbanzo or kidney beans on a chef's salad
- Rice and beans
- Veggie burgers
- Hummus (chickpeas spread) on pita bread

Choose unsalted nuts as a snack, on salads, or in main dishes. Use nuts to *replace* meat or poultry, not *in addition to* these items:

- Use pine nuts in pesto sauce for pasta.
- Add slivered almonds to steamed vegetables.
- Add toasted peanuts or cashews to a vegetable stir-fry instead of meat.
- Sprinkle a few nuts on top of low-fat ice cream or frozen yogurt.
- Add walnuts or pecans to a green salad instead of cheese or meat.

Meatless or Meat-Restricted Diets

Many people are choosing **vegetarian** or **vegan** diets to avoid animal proteins, either for health, personal, political, or environmental reasons. This means that many of the forms of protein they consume are considered incomplete. This does not mean, however, that they cannot maintain adequate nutrition levels. It does mean that they need to seek out a variety of proteins. One way to do this is to eat whole foods as much as possible, avoiding processed products that fill stomachs and crowd out good sources of nutrition. The following chart can give you an idea of the types of plant sources that are rich in protein:

Recommended Protein Intake

The amount of protein you need in your diet will depend on your size. The recommended daily intake of protein for healthy adults is .8g per kilogram (.36g per pound) of body weight. Studies suggest that the average American man consumes approximately 100g each day and the average woman 70g. A man weighing 200 pounds should be eating about 72g. The recommended AMDR for protein is 10–35% of your daily calories. Our country may be eating more protein than it really needs for good health.

Individuals looking to increase muscle mass through strength training may need to increase their protein intake. But they may be getting enough from food without any additional effort. You probably know proteins

Food	Serving	Calories	Protein (g)
Black Beans	.5 cup	114	8
Tofu	.5 cup	94	10
Soy Milk	1 cup	132	8
Peas	.5 cup	67	5
Spinach, cooked	.5 cup	41	3
Oatmeal	.5 cup	79	3
Pumpkin Seeds	1 oz	159	9
Sunflower Seeds	1 oz	140	6
Peanut Butter	2 tbs	188	7
Almonds	1 oz	163	6
Pistachios	1 oz	185	4

Figure 14. Foods with high protein content.

as the major component of muscle. Some people may think the way to build body muscle is to eat high-protein diets and use protein powders, supplements and shakes. However, most Americans already eat about 12–18%, or more, of their calories as protein. Before adding protein to your diet, and saturated fat along with it, keep track of the amount of protein you are already consuming to determine if the addition is really necessary.

Women who are pregnant or breastfeeding also need more protein (up to 0.59 grams per pound of body weight). The DRI for pregnant women is 71g a day, but this may change based on weight.

Health Risks

The medical community has raised many concerns about high-protein diets. There's no solid scientific evidence that most Americans need more protein. These diets operate on varying ideas about the consumption of carbohydrates, particularly grains and sugars. The general theory is that carbs create sugar, which creates fat — which creates problems. Less carbs means less fat (again, in theory). The exact approaches vary. These diets often (though not always) boost protein intake at the expense of fruit and vegetables, and particularly grains, so dieters can miss out on healthy nutrients — which could possibly increase their risk of cancer.

Many high-protein diets are high in saturated fat and low in fiber. Research shows this combination can increase cholesterol levels and increase the risk of heart disease and stroke. These diets generally recommend dieters receive 30% to 50% of their total calories from protein. Depending upon the type of protein consumed, this could lead to an amount of saturated fat far above and beyond the American Heart Association's recommendation of 7% and the recommended AMDR of no more than 10%.

In addition to an increased risk of heart disease, too much protein can impact other parts of your body. People on high-protein diets excrete more calcium through their urine than do those not on a high-protein diet. If a person sticks to a high-protein diet long term, the loss of calcium could increase their risk of developing osteoporosis. Additionally, people with kidney disease should consult a doctor before starting a high-protein diet. Research suggests people with impaired kidneys may lose kidney function more rapidly if they eat excessive amounts of protein — especially animal protein.

The jury is still out on the merits of low carbohydrate, high protein intake. Just as with the controversies over saturated fat, it's important to remember balance. As with anything in life, too much of a good thing is usually no longer good, with few exceptions.

Vitamins

When you were a child, your mom or dad probably gave you a sweet, crunchy, animal-shaped treat every morning — just one. Unlike your other snacks of fruit, cheese, or crackers, you only got a tiny bite of this snack. You were told it was good for you, so why couldn't you have more? The truth is that most healthy kids don't need a vitamin supplement if their diet is adequate.

Vitamins are a group of substances that are needed for normal cell function, growth, development, and to maintain life and health. How they are stored depends upon the type of vitamin (more later on this).

Vitamins have different jobs — helping you resist infections, keeping your nerves healthy, and helping your body get energy from food or your blood to clot properly. By following the Dietary Guidelines, you will get enough of most of these vitamins from food.

There are 13 essential vitamins. This means that these vitamins are required for the body to work properly. They are:

- Vitamin A
- Vitamin C
- Vitamin D
- Vitamin E
- Vitamin K
- Vitamin B1 (thiamine)
- Vitamin B2 (riboflavin)
- Vitamin B3 (niacin)
- Pantothenic acid
- Biotin (B7)
- Vitamin B6
- Vitamin B12 (cyanocobalamin)
- Folate (folic acid and B9)

Types of Vitamins

Vitamins are grouped into two categories, fat-soluble and water-soluble. **Fat-soluble** vitamins are stored in the body for long periods of time in the liver and fat tissues. Your body does not need these every day, and they are absorbed more slowly than water-soluble. They do need to be replaced in the body regularly. The four fat-soluble vitamins are vitamins A, D, E, and K. These vitamins are absorbed more easily by the body in the presence of dietary fat.

There are nine **water-soluble** vitamins. The body must use water-soluble vitamins right away. Any leftover water-soluble vitamins leave the body through the urine. Vitamin B12 is the only water-soluble vitamin that can be stored in the liver for many years.

Sources of Fat-Soluble Vitamins			
Vitamin A	Dark-colored fruit, Dark leafy vegetables, Egg yolk, Fortified milk and dairy products (cheese, yogurt, butter, and cream), Liver, beef, and fish	**Vitamin D**	Fish (fatty fish such as salmon, mackerel, herring, and orange roughy), Fish liver oils (cod's liver oil), Fortified cereals, Fortified milk and dairy products (cheese, yogurt, butter, and cream)
Vitamin E	Avocado, Dark green vegetables (spinach, broccoli, asparagus, and turnip greens), Margarine (made from safflower, corn, and sunflower oil), Oils (safflower, corn, and sunflower), Papaya and mango, Seeds and nuts, Wheat germ and wheat germ oil	**Vitamin K**	Cabbage, Cauliflower, Cereals, Dark green vegetables (broccoli, Brussels sprouts, and asparagus), Dark leafy vegetables (spinach, kale, collards, and turnip greens), Fish, liver, beef, and eggs

Figure 15. Source of fat-soluble vitamins.

Sources of Water-Soluble Vitamins			
Biotin	Chocolate, Cereal, Egg yolk, Legumes, Milk, Nuts, Organ meats (liver, kidney), Pork, Yeast	**Folate**	Asparagus and broccoli, Beets Brewer's yeast, Dried beans (cooked pinto, navy, kidney, and lima), Fortified cereals, Green, leafy vegetables (spinach and romaine lettuce), Lentils, Oranges and orange juice, Peanut butter, Wheat germ
Niacin (vitamin B3)	Avocado, Eggs, Enriched breads and fortified cereals, Fish (tuna and salt-water fish), Lean meats, Legumes, Nuts, Potato, Poultry	**Pantothenic acid**	Avocado, Broccoli, kale, and other vegetables in the cabbage family, Eggs, Legumes and lentils, Milk, Mushroom, Organ meats, Poultry, White and sweet potatoes, Whole-grain cereals
Thiamine (vitamin B1)	Dried milk, Egg, Enriched bread and flour, Lean meats, Legumes (dried beans), Nuts and seeds, Organ meats, Peas, Whole grains	**Pyroxidine (vitamin B6)**	Avocado, Banana, Legumes (dried beans), Meat, Nuts, Poultry, Whole grains (milling and processing removes a lot of this vitamin)
Vitamin B12	Meat, Eggs, Fortified foods such as soymilk, Milk and milk products, Organ meats (liver and kidney), Poultry, Shellfish	**Vitamin C (ascorbic acid)**	Broccoli, Brussels sprouts, Cabbage, Cauliflower, Citrus fruits, Potatoes, Spinach, Strawberries, Tomato juice, Tomatoes
NOTE: Animal sources of vitamin B12 are absorbed much better by the body than plant sources			

Figure 16. Sources of water-soluble vitamins.

Function and Sources

Each of the vitamins listed below has an important job in the body. A vitamin deficiency occurs when you do not get enough of a certain vitamin, which can cause health problems. For example, if you don't get enough vitamin C, you could become anemic. Vitamin A prevents night blindness. Not eating enough vitamin-rich foods — such as fruits, vegetables, beans, lentils, whole grains and fortified dairy — may increase your risk for health problems, including heart disease, cancer, and poor bone health (osteoporosis). See section on vitamin deficiency.

- Vitamin A helps form and maintain healthy teeth, bones, soft tissue, mucus membranes, and skin.

- Vitamin B6 is also called pyridoxine. Vitamin B6 helps form red blood cells and maintain brain function. This vitamin also plays an important role in the proteins that are part of many chemical reactions in the body. The more protein you eat the more pyridoxine your body requires.

- Vitamin B12, like the other B vitamins, is important for metabolism. It also helps form red blood cells and maintain the central nervous system.

- Vitamin C, also called ascorbic acid, is an antioxidant that promotes healthy teeth and gums. It helps the body absorb iron, maintain healthy tissue, and heal wounds.

- Vitamin D is also known as the "sunshine vitamin," since it is made by the body after being in the sun. Ten to 15 minutes of sunshine three times a week is enough to produce the body's requirement of vitamin D for most people at most latitudes. People who do not live in sunny places may not make enough vitamin D. It is very hard to get enough vitamin D from food sources alone. Vitamin D helps the body absorb calcium. You need calcium for the normal development and maintenance of healthy teeth and bones. It also helps maintain proper blood levels of calcium and phosphorus.

- Vitamin E is an antioxidant also known as tocopherol. It helps the body form red blood cells and use vitamin K.

- Vitamin K is not listed among the essential vitamins, but without it blood would not stick together (coagulate). Some studies suggest that it is important for bone health.

- Biotin is essential for the metabolism of proteins and carbohydrates, and in the production of hormones and cholesterol.

- Niacin is a B vitamin that helps maintain healthy skin and nerves. It is also has cholesterol-lowering effects.

- Folate works with vitamin B12 to help form red blood cells. It is needed for the production of DNA, which controls tissue growth and cell function. Any woman who is pregnant should be sure to get enough folate. Low levels of folate are linked to birth defects such as spina bifida. Many foods are now fortified with folic acid.

- Pantothenic acid is essential for the metabolism of food. It also plays a role in the production of hormones and cholesterol.

- Riboflavin (vitamin B2) works with the other B vitamins. It is important for body growth and the production of red blood cells.

- Thiamine (vitamin B1) helps the body cells change carbohydrates into energy. Getting plenty of carbohydrates is very important during pregnancy and breast-feeding. It is also essential for heart function and healthy nerve cells.

Antioxidants

Antioxidants are man-made or natural substances that may prevent or delay some types of cell damage, and counteract the damage of free radicals. Diets high in vegetables and fruits, which are good sources of antioxidants, have been found to be healthy. However, research has not shown antioxidant supplements to be beneficial in preventing diseases (Figure 17). Examples of antioxidants include:

- Beta-carotene
- Lutein
- Lycopene
- Selenium
- Vitamin A
- Vitamin C
- Vitamin E
- Vitamin A
- Vitamin C
- Vitamin E

Free radicals are highly unstable molecules that are naturally formed when you exercise and when your body converts food into energy. Your body can also be exposed to free radicals from a variety of environmental sources, such as cigarette smoke, air pollution, and sunlight. Free radicals can cause "oxidative stress," a process that can trigger cell damage. Oxidative stress is thought to play a role in a variety of diseases including cancer, cardiovascular diseases, diabetes, Alzheimer's disease, Parkinson's disease, and eye diseases such as cataracts and age-related macular degeneration.

Antioxidant molecules have been shown to counteract oxidative stress in laboratory experiments (for example, in cells or animal studies). However, there is debate as to whether consuming large amounts of antioxidants in supplement form actually benefits health. There is also some concern that consuming antioxidant supplements in excessive doses may be harmful. See discussion on the recommended intake of vitamins.

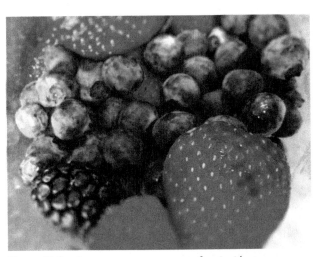

Figure 17. Berries are a common source of antioxidants.

Phytonutrients

Anti-oxidants are a type of phytochemical, or phytonutrients. These are chemicals produced by plants in order for them to stay healthy. For example, some phytonutrients protect plants from insect attacks, while others protect against radiation from UV rays.

Phytonutrients can also provide significant benefits for humans who eat plant foods. Phytonutrient-rich foods include colorful fruits and vegetables, legumes, nuts, tea, whole grains and many spices. They affect human health but are not considered nutrients that are essential for life, like carbohydrates, protein, fats, vitamins and minerals.

Among the potential benefits of phytonutrients are their antioxidant and anti-inflammatory properties. They may also enhance immunity and intercellular communication, repair DNA damage from exposure to toxins, detoxify carcinogens, and alter estrogen metabolism. The US Department of Agriculture (USDA) notes that consuming a phytonutrient-rich diet seems to be an "effective strategy" for reducing cancer and heart disease risks.

Many phytonutrients give plants their pigments, so a good way to tell if a fruit or vegetable is rich in phytonutrients can be by its color. Look for deep-hued foods like berries, dark greens, melons and spices. These foods also are rich in flavor and aroma, which makes them more palatable. But some phytonutrient-rich foods have little color, like onions and garlic, and you don't want to discount them. The different types of phytonutrients each do different things and offer different benefits.

Lignans can mimic the effects of estrogen, so lignans are considered phytoestrogens, though they can also affect the body in other ways. Like all phytonutrients, these are found in fruits and vegetables, especially kale, broccoli, flaxseeds, apricots, and strawberries. They are particularly abundant in seeds and whole grains. Lignans are associated with preventing hormone-related cancers because of their estrogen-like activity, and potentially other cancers, such as endometrial and ovarian.

Resveratrol has gotten a good deal of buzz in recent years because large concentrations of it are found in red wine. The best-known source of resveratrol is grapes. Resveratrol has particularly high concentration in grape skin and red wine. It is also found in peanuts, grape juice, cocoa, blueberries and cranberries. Some studies suggest that resveratrol may help slow cognitive decline and improve insulin sensitivity and glucose tolerance though more research is needed.

Carotenoids are the yellow, orange and red pigments in plants, such as carrots, yams, sweet potatoes, papaya, watermelon, cantaloupe, mangos, spinach, kale, tomatoes, bell peppers and oranges. The most common carotenoids are alpha-carotene, beta-carotene, beta-cryptoxanthin, lutein, zeaxanthin and lycopene. Carotenoids are associated with eye health, immune system activity, intercellular communication, and reduced risk of cancer and cardiovascular disease.

Ellagic acid, also called tannin, is found in raspberries, strawberries, blackberries, cranberries, grapes, pomegranates and walnuts. It can also be produced during the body's process of breaking down larger phytonutrients and is absorbed rapidly. It is associated with reducing inflammation, reducing blood pressure and arterial plaque, and may have properties that help your body remove carcinogens before they are metabolized.

Flavonoids are a very large group of phytonutrients known for its heart benefits, contributions to overall longevity, and reduction of cancer risk. Flavonoids are found across a large range of foods, such as apples, onions, coffee, grapefruit, tea, berries, chocolate, legumes, red wine, broccoli, cabbage, kale, leeks, tomatoes, ginger, lemons, parsley, carrots and buckwheat.

Food Storing and Cooking

It's apparent to you by now, perhaps painfully so, that you need to eat your vegetables. There are many lonely vegetables longing for homes, often because consumers don't know how to prepare them. For every person who loves kale, there are three others that detest it. The same goes for broccoli, asparagus, squash, and many other foods valued for their nutrition but questioned for their taste. Growing up, it is likely that someone in your home refused to have them on their plate (was it you?). Maybe your parent would make you try it and you would grudgingly swallow a small bite for permission to leave the table. Well, no offense to Mom, but maybe the problem was with the preparation, not the food.

How foods are cooked can have a big impact on their nutrient content and flavor. That's because many vitamins are sensitive to heat and air exposure (vitamin C, the B vitamins, and folate in particular). Loss of nutrients increases as cooking time increases and with higher temperatures(Figure 18).

Cooking methods that minimize the time, temperature, and amount of water needed will help to preserve nutrients. Steaming is a great way to cook vegetables quickly and retain valuable nutrients. Microwave cooking is also good because it uses minimal water, and the cooking time is very short. Stir-frying is another way to quickly cook a variety of vegetables.

It's useful to remember that cooking creates a chemical change in your food, using heat as a catalyst and, in some cases, will alter which nutrients you can more easily digest. Cooking, in some cases, makes otherwise inedible

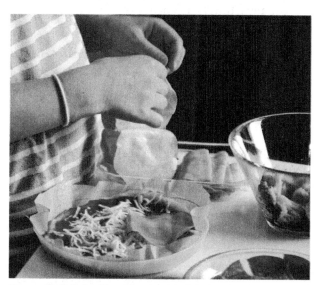

Figure 18. Safe food handling is critical during preparation and storage.

Myth	Fact
The only reason to let food sit after it's been microwaved is to make sure you don't burn yourself on food that's too hot.	In fact, letting microwaved food sit for a few minutes ("standing time") helps your food cook more completely by allowing colder areas of food time to absorb heat from hotter areas of food.
Leftovers are safe to eat until they smell bad.	The kinds of bacteria that cause food poisoning do not affect the look, smell, or taste of the food.
Once food has been cooked, all the bacteria have been killed, so I don't need to worry once it's "done".	Actually, the possibility of bacterial growth increases after coking because the drop in temperature allows bacteria to thrive. Keeping cooked food warmed to the right temperature is critical for food safety.
Marinades are acidic, which kills bacteria-so it's OK to marinate foods on he counter.	Even in the presence of acidic marinade, bacteria can grow very rapidly at room temperatures. To marinate foods safely, it's important to marinate them in the refrigerator.
If I really want my produce to be safe, I should wash fruits and vegetables with soap or detergent before I use them.	In fact, it's best not to use soaps or detergents on produce, since these products can linger on foods and are not safe for consumption. Using clean running water is actually the best way to remove bacteria and wash produce safely.

Figure 19. Common food handling myths and the facts.

foods edible, such as Taro, which is full of toxic crystals that need to be broken down before any of the plant can be consumed. Cooking also softens food, making it easier to chew and digest — imagine trying to eat rice without cooking it first!

Here are a few other tricks you can use to preserve nutrients:

- Leave vegetables in big pieces. That way fewer vitamins are destroyed when they are exposed to air.

- Always cover your pot to hold in steam and heat. This will also help to reduce cooking time.

- Use any leftover cooking water for soups and stews, sauces, or vegetable juice drinks.

- Eat fruits and vegetables raw whenever possible in salads and smoothies or as whole fruits and vegetables.

- Cook vegetables until crisp. Don't overcook.

- Use as little water as possible when cooking.

All of these tips awill help you retain the maximum amount of nutrients in your fruits and vegetables.

Let's talk a moment more about flavor, since this is often the largest objection. Many foods are, in fact, tastier when they are steamed. Having said that, if you need to add olive oil and lemon to your broccoli, sauté your asparagus or kale in a bit of olive oil and garlic, or add pine nuts to your steamed or sautéed spinach, go ahead. Throw some onion into the pot when you cook your green beans — it tastes great and there is no harm done. Even a *tiny* bit of olive oil, butter, salt, and pepper can make a world of difference as long as you aren't loading it with saturated fat (consider the pad of your thumb as a guide on butter). The most important factor, however, is to eat a healthy amount of fruits and vegetables each day.

If you need to store food, you have a lot of options. Right now, the best method for storing food while keeping the existing nutrients intact is by freezing. Research suggests there is no significant loss of nutritional value in frozen food, and it can be more convenient and cost effective than fresh if those issues are a factor for you. Canning is another good option, but the process requires cooking the food at a boil for a short time (so it doesn't give you botulism), which can alter the nutritional profile of the food. Older methods of preservation, like fermenting (kimchi, sauerkraut, etc.), drying, curing (usually meats and cheeses), smoking, storing in oil (like confit or olives), or storing in brine (pickles), have been around longer than recorded history and, like cooking, alter the flavors and nutritional values of your food.

Clean	Wash hands and surfaces often.
Separate	Don't cross-contaminate.
Cook	Cook to the right temperature.
Chill	Refrigerate promptly.
Shopping	Purchase refrigerated or frozen items after selecting your non-perishables. Never choose meat or poultry in packaging that is torn or leaking. Do not buy food past "Sell-By," "Use-By," or other expiration dates.
Storage	Always refrigerate perishable food within 2 hours. Check the temperature of your refrigerator and freezer with an appliance thermometer. Cook or freeze fresh poultry, fish, ground meats, and variety meats within 2 days. To maintain quality when freezing meat and poultry in its original package, wrap the package again with foil or plastic wrap that's recommended for the freezer. Canned foods are safe indefinitely as long as they are not exposed to freezing temperatures, or temperatures above 90 (F).
Preparation	Always wash hands with warm water and soap for 20 seconds before and after handling food. Don't cross-contaminate. Keep raw meat, poultry, fish, and their juices away from other food. After cutting raw meats, wash cutting board, utensils, and countertops with hot, soapy water. Using a solution of 1 tablespoon of unscented, liquid chlorine bleach in 1 gallon of water can sanitize cutting boards, utensils, and countertops. Marinate meat and poultry in a covered dish in the refrigerator.
Thawing	The refrigerator allows slow, safe thawing. Make sure thawing meat and poultry juices do not drip onto other food. For faster thawing, place food in a leak-proof plastic bag. Submerge in cold tap water. Change the water every 30 minutes. Cook immediately after thawing. Cook meat and poultry immediately after microwave thawing.
Cooking	Cook all raw beef, pork, lamb and veal steaks, chops, and roasts to a minimum internal temperature of 145 (F) as measured with a food thermometer before removing meat from the heat source. For safety and quality, allow meat to rest for at least three minutes before carving or consuming.
Serving	Hot food should be held at 140 (F) or warmer. Cold food should be held at 40 (F) or colder. When serving food at a buffet, keep food hot with chafing dishes, slow cookers, and warming trays. Keep food cold by nesting dishes in bowls of ice or use small serving trays and replace them often.

Figure 20. Food preparation and storage guidelines.

Recommended Vitamin Intake

The winter in the Pacific Northwest has set in and you find yourself craving some sunshine. After three weeks of straight rain and minimal sun, you're feeling weak, achy, and a bit gloomy. The weatherman says to start popping vitamin D because the sun will not be out any time soon. Do you run to the drug store? Is there a better way? Remember that tasty treat your mom used to give you in the morning? Did you need it?

Recommended amounts of vitamins vary by person, and the intake amount can be supplemented, but is not considered safe for everyone. Vitamin supplementation should only occur where deficiencies are evident, for example: men over 50 may need a B12 supplement and everyone who lives west of the Cascades in the Pacific Northwest can probably use some additional vitamin D. According to the 2015 Dietary Guidelines for Americans, individuals should aim to meet their nutrient needs primarily through healthy eating patterns that include nutrient-dense foods. These contain essential vitamins and minerals and also dietary fiber and other naturally occurring substances that may have positive health effects.

How much of each vitamin you need is very difficult to keep track of. You've seen the list so far and it's quite substantial. The bottom line is this — eat a large variety of healthy, nutrient-dense foods from all of the five food groups. These include proteins, fruits, vegetables, grains, and dairy. You only need to supplement if you have a particular illness or condition (like pregnancy), or have a true vitamin deficiency.

Vitamin Deficiency

Every vitamin has a purpose in your body. When you aren't getting enough of a particular vitamin in your diet, you could begin to feel adverse effects. In the US, we don't struggle with vitamin deficiencies in the same way that less developed countries do. Most of us have access to a variety of foods, so unless we are limiting our diet or have an underlying medical condition, we aren't likely to have a noticeable deficiency.

There are certain illnesses that could suggest a deficiency is present. One is anemia. Vitamin deficiency anemia is a lack of healthy red blood cells caused when you have lower than normal amounts of certain vitamins. Vitamins linked to vitamin deficiency anemia include folate, vitamin B-12 and vitamin C. This anemia can occur if you don't eat enough folate, vitamin B-12 or vitamin C, or if your body has trouble absorbing or processing these vitamins.

Not all anemias are caused by a vitamin deficiency. Other causes include iron deficiency and certain blood diseases. That's why it's important to have your doctor diagnose and treat your anemia. It can usually be corrected with vitamin supplements and changes to your diet.

One of the most common deficiencies is in vitamin D — not many foods have naturally occurring vitamin D. Our bodies also require a regular dose of sunlight to get vitamin D generating. This impacts our ability to absorb calcium, as well, which leads to bone weakness and diseases or injuries related to bones, such as osteoporosis.

Supplements

Many adults in the United States take one or more dietary supplements either every day or occasionally. We often take them without much thought. Supplements are not regulated by the FDA, so what you take over-the-counter may not be effective or may interact with other medications you are taking — and, again, that's if you need it at all.

Today's dietary supplements include vitamins, minerals, herbals and botanicals, amino acids, enzymes, and many other products. Dietary supplements come in a variety of forms — traditional tablets, capsules, and powders, as well as drinks and energy bars. Popular supplements include vitamins D and E; minerals like calcium and iron; herbs such as echinacea and garlic; and specialty products like glucosamine, probiotics, and fish oils (Figure 21).

According to the National Agricultural Library's Food and Nutrition Information Center, you should ask yourself one big question before taking a supplement — Do I really need them? First and foremost, nutritional needs should be met by eating a variety of foods as outlined in the Dietary Guidelines for Americans. In some cases, vitamin/mineral supplements or fortified foods may be useful for providing nutrients that may otherwise be eaten in less than recommended amounts.

If you are already eating the recommended amount of a nutrient, you may not get any further health benefit from taking a supplement. In some cases, supplements and fortified foods may actually cause you to exceed safe levels of intake of nutrients. (Note that fortified foods are those to which one or more essential nutrients have been added to increase their nutritional value.)

The Dietary Guidelines for Americans makes these recommendations for certain groups of people:

- People over age 50 should consume vitamin B12 in its crystalline form, that is, from fortified foods (like some fortified breakfast cereals) or as a supplement. Note that older adults often have a reduced ability to absorb vitamin B12 from foods. However, crystalline vitamin B12, the type of vitamin B12 used in supplements and in fortified foods, is much more easily absorbed.

- Women of childbearing age who may become pregnant and adolescent females should eat foods that are a source of iron (such as meats) and/or they

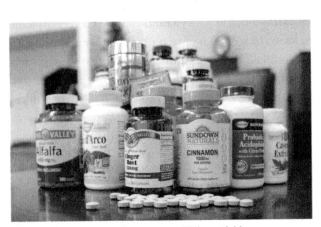

Figure 21. Dietary supplements are widely available.

should eat iron-rich plant foods (like cooked dry beans or spinach) or iron-fortified foods (like fortified cereals) along with a source of vitamin C.

- Women of childbearing age who may become pregnant and those who are pregnant should consume adequate synthetic folic acid daily (from fortified foods or supplements) in addition to food forms of folate from a varied diet.

- Older adults, people with dark skin, and people who get insufficient exposure to sunlight should consume extra vitamin D from vitamin D-fortified foods and/or supplements.

- People who smoke need more vitamin C due in part to increased oxidative stress. For this reason, it is recommended that these individuals need 35mg more vitamin C per day than people who don't smoke.

Vitamin or mineral supplements are not a replacement for a healthy diet. Remember that in addition to vitamins and minerals, foods also contain hundreds of naturally occurring substances that can help protect your health.

Tolerable Upper Intake Level (UL)

The **tolerable upper intake level** (**UL**) is the maximum usual daily intake level at which no risk of adverse health effects is expected for most of the individuals in a specific group based on stage of life. The risk of adverse reactions increases as intake exceeds the UL.

The term "tolerable" was chosen because it connotes a level of intake that can, with high probability, be tolerated biologically by individuals. It's not considered a

Safety

Many supplements contain active ingredients that can have strong effects in the body. Always be alert to the possibility of unexpected side effects, especially when taking a new product.

Supplements are most likely to cause side effects or harm when people take them instead of prescribed medicines or when people take many supplements in combination. Some supplements can increase the risk of bleeding or, if a person takes them before or after surgery, they can affect the person's response to anesthesia. Dietary supplements can also interact with certain prescription drugs in ways that might cause problems. Here are just a few examples:

The Food and Drug Administration recommends discussing these questions with your health care provider when considering whether you should take a vitamin/mineral supplement:

- Do you eat fewer than two meals per day?

- Is your diet restricted? That is, do you not eat meat, or milk or milk products, or eat fewer than five servings of fruits and vegetables per day?

- Do you eat alone most of the time?

- Without wanting to, have you lost or gained more than ten pounds in the last six months?

- Do you take three or more prescription or over-the-counter medicines a day?

- Do you have three or more drinks of alcohol a day?

If you answer yes to one or more of these questions, it may give you an idea of why you may be deficient. It is also a good idea to speak to your provider to determine what supplements are necessary if you cannot get the vitamin from your diet.

recommended level of intake. Currently, there is no research demonstrating a benefit for healthy individuals to consume quantities of nutrients above the recommended dietary allowance or adequate intake, except in a few specific cases. In short, you have no real reason to take nutritional supplements unless you have a diagnosed vitamin deficiency and are recommended to do so by your doctor.

- Vitamin K can reduce the ability of the blood thinner Coumadin® to prevent blood from clotting.

- St. John's wort can speed the breakdown of many drugs (including antidepressants and birth control pills) and thereby reduce these drugs' effectiveness.

- Antioxidant supplements, like vitamins C and E, might reduce the effectiveness of some types of cancer chemotherapy.

Keep in mind that some ingredients found in dietary supplements are added to a growing number of foods, including breakfast cereals and beverages. As a result, you may be getting more of these ingredients than you think, and more might not be better. Taking more than you need is always more expensive and can also raise your risk of experiencing side effects. For example, getting too much vitamin A can cause headaches and liver damage, reduce bone strength, and cause birth defects. Excess iron causes nausea and vomiting and may damage the liver and other organs.

Overdose

In large doses, some vitamins have documented side effects that tend to be more severe. The likelihood of consuming too much of any vitamin from food is remote, but overdosing (vitamin poisoning) from vitamin supplementation does occur. At high enough dosages, some vitamins cause side effects such as nausea,

Be cautious about taking dietary supplements if you are pregnant or nursing. Also, be careful about giving them (beyond a basic multivitamin/mineral product) to a child — your mom was right with just one. Most dietary supplements have not been well tested for safety in pregnant women, nursing mothers, or children.

diarrhea, and vomiting. When side effects emerge, recovery is often accomplished by reducing the dosage. The doses of vitamins differ because individual tolerances can vary widely and appear to be related to age and state of health. The majority of overdoses, though not fatal, happen in children under the age of six.

Minerals

Minerals are micronutrients that come from the Earth and cannot be made by us. Plants take in minerals from the soil, and we get most of the minerals in our diets from the plants or indirectly from the animals that eat them. In some areas mineral may also be present in the water we drink. Minerals from plant sources can also vary with the mineral content of the soil.

Minerals are important for your body to stay healthy. Your body uses minerals for many different jobs, including keeping your bones, muscles, heart, and brain working

properly. Minerals are also important for making enzymes and hormones. Most people get the amount of minerals they need by eating a wide variety of foods.

There are two kinds of minerals: macrominerals and trace minerals. You need larger amounts of **macrominerals**. They include calcium, phosphorus, magnesium, sodium chloride, and potassium among others. You only need small amounts of **trace mineral** such as iron, copper, iodine, zinc, chromium, and selenium.

Calcium

You have more **calcium** in your body than any other mineral, which is great because it has many important jobs. The body stores more than 99% of its calcium in the bones and teeth to help make and keep them strong. Bone itself undergoes continuous remodeling, with constant resorption and accumulation of calcium into new bone. The calcium not used by the bones is stored throughout the body in blood, muscle, and the fluid between cells. Your body needs calcium to help muscles and blood vessels contract and expand, to secrete hormones and enzymes, and to send messages through the nervous system.

Foods rich in calcium include:

- Dairy products such as milk, cheese, and yogurt

- Leafy, green vegetables

- Fish with soft bones that you eat, such as canned sardines and salmon

- Calcium-enriched foods such as breakfast cereals, fruit juices, soy and rice drinks, and tofu. Check the product labels.

The exact amount of calcium you need depends on your age and other factors. Women need between 1000–1300mg of calcium each day, and men between 1000 — 1200mg. Growing children and teenagers need more calcium than young adults. Older women need plenty of calcium to prevent osteoporosis.

The Tolerable Upper Intake Levels (ULs) for calcium established by the Food and Nutrition Board are 2500mg per day for people aged 19–50 and 2000 for those over 50. Getting too much calcium from foods is rare — excess intakes are more likely to be caused by the use of calcium supplements. Studies indicate that approximately 5% of women older than 50 years have estimated total calcium intakes (from foods and supplements) that exceed the UL by about 300–365mg.

Sodium Chloride

Sodium occurs naturally in most foods. The words "salt" and "sodium" are often used interchangeably, but they do not mean the same thing. Sodium is a mineral and one of the chemical elements found in salt. Salt (also known by its chemical name, sodium chloride) is a crystal-like compound that is abundant in nature and is used to flavor and preserve food. Milk, beets, and celery also naturally contain sodium, as does drinking water, although the amount varies depending on the source.

Sodium does have importance. It is an essential nutrient and is needed by the human body in relatively small amounts (provided that substantial sweating does not occur). Sodium is important for many body processes, such as fluid balance, muscle contraction, and nervous system function. As a food ingredient, sodium has multiple uses, such as for curing meat, baking, thickening, retaining moisture, enhancing flavor (including the flavor of other ingredients), and as a preservative.

Most of the sodium we eat does not come from the salt-shaker. It is added to various food products. It flies under the radar with names like monosodium glutamate, sodium nitrite, sodium saccharin, baking soda (sodium bicarbonate), and sodium benzoate — all forms of sodium. About 75% of dietary sodium comes from eating packaged and restaurant foods, whereas only a small portion (11%) comes from salt added to food when cooking or eating.

Condiments and seasonings such as Worcestershire

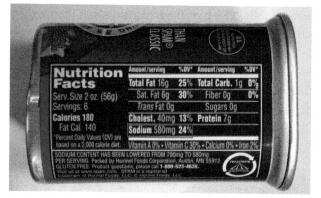

Figure 22. Nutrition Facts labels contain information about dietary content.

sauce, soy sauce, onion salt, garlic salt, and bouillon cubes contain sodium. Processed meats, such as bacon, sausage, and ham, and canned soups and vegetables are all examples of foods that contain added sodium. Fast foods are generally very high in sodium. Also, processed foods such as potato chips, frozen dinners and cured meats have high sodium content. Even breads, cheese, pasta, and pizza contain added sodium.

If you are eating a lot of high-sodium foods, expect health problems to develop in the not-too-distant future. The daily limit for sodium is 2,300 mg a day and about 90% of Americans eat too much. Your kidneys control how much sodium is in your body. If you have too much and your kidneys can't get rid it, sodium builds up in your blood. This can lead to high blood pressure. High blood pressure can lead to other health problems.

Potassium

Potassium is a type of electrolyte. It helps your nerves to function, muscles to contract, and your heartbeat to stay regular. It also helps move nutrients into cells and waste products out. A diet rich in potassium helps to offset some of sodium's harmful effects on blood pressure. Most people get all the potassium they need from what they eat and drink.

Foods rich in potassium include:

- Leafy greens, such as spinach and collards

- Fruit from vines, such as grapes and blackberries

- Root vegetables, such as carrots and potatoes

- Citrus fruits, such as oranges and grapefruit

Your kidneys help to keep the right amount of potassium in your body. If you have chronic kidney disease, your kidneys may not remove extra potassium from the blood. Some medicines also can raise your potassium level. If you have one of these issues, you may need a special diet to lower the amount of potassium that you eat.

Iron

Our bodies need **iron** for many functions. For example, iron is part of hemoglobin, a protein that carries oxygen from our lungs throughout our body tissues. It helps our muscles store and use oxygen. Iron is also part of many other proteins and enzymes.

Most of the elemental iron in adults is in

hemoglobin. Much of the remaining iron is stored in various forms in the liver, spleen, and bone marrow or is located in muscle tissue. Humans typically lose only small amounts of iron in urine, feces, the gastrointestinal tract, and skin. Losses are greater in menstruating women because of blood loss.

Foods rich in iron include:

- Red meat, pork and poultry
- Seafood
- Beans
- Dark green leafy vegetables, such as spinach
- Dried fruit, such as raisins and apricots
- Iron-fortified cereals, breads and pasta
- Peas

Your body absorbs iron best from meat. If you eat a primarily vegetarian diet, you may need to increase your intake of some of these other iron-rich foods. Vitamin C also helps improve the absorption of iron, so eating citrus foods as you eat iron-rich foods can help increase iron levels.

Your body needs the right amount of iron. People in the US usually obtain adequate amounts of iron from their diets, but infants, young children, teenaged girls, pregnant women, and premenopausal women are at risk of obtaining insufficient amounts. Men need approximately 8mg each day. Women need 18 until around age 50 when their iron needs decrease to 8. Pregnant women need more at 27mg per day.

If you have too little iron, you may develop iron deficiency anemia, a common type of anemia. In people with this condition, the blood lacks adequate healthy red blood cells. Red blood cells carry oxygen to the body's tissues. Without them, you could find yourself feeling fatigued and short of breath. Causes of low iron levels include blood loss, poor diet, or an inability to absorb enough iron from foods.

Too much iron, however, can damage your body and lead to iron poisoning. This usually occurs from taking too many iron supplements, though some people have an inherited disease called hemochromatosis, which causes too much iron to build up in the body. Sudden intakes of more than 20mg/kg of iron from supplements or medicines can lead to gastric upset, constipation, nausea, abdominal pain, vomiting, and faintness, especially if food is not taken at the same time. In severe cases (e.g., one-time ingestions of 60mg/kg), overdoses of iron can lead to multisystem organ failure, coma, convulsions, and even death.

Deficiencies in Vitamins and Minerals

Serious shortages in vitamins and minerals in the US aren't as common as in countries that lack sufficient access to healthy foods. We aren't immune to poverty and food concerns. We just don't experience them at the same level. Many of our foods are fortified with nutrients that we need, our school systems work hard to provide children with balanced diets, and our communities frequently strive to help people gain access to food in times of need. However, even those of us without any struggles to access a healthy diet can sometimes find ourselves coming up short for a variety of reasons. It could be a poor diet reliant on fast-food drive-thrus, a lack of understanding of what foods are healthy, an illness, poverty, or just inadequate planning.

According to the most recent US Dietary Guidelines, there are seven important nutrients in food that most Americans aren't getting in sufficient amounts:

- Calcium
- Potassium
- Fiber
- Magnesium
- Vitamin A
- Vitamin C
- Vitamin E

We can fix this primarily with good planning and attention to a healthy diet rich in lean protein, fruits, vegetables, whole grains, and low-fat dairy products, which will be discussed more in this chapter. If you think you may need a supplement for any vitamin or mineral, take a close look at your diet first and the consult your health care practitioner.

Water

Drinking enough water every day is good for overall health. As plain drinking water has zero calories, it can also help with managing body weight and reducing caloric intake when substituted for drinks with calories, like regular soda. The benefits of water are numerous as our body is highly dependent upon it. Nearly every part of our body contains and relies on it to function, from the transportation of nutrients, to the processing of waste, regulation of body temperature, and lubrication of our joints and tissues. Without it, we simply cannot function effectively.

Water Storage in the Body

Water is of major importance to all living things. In some organisms, up to 90% of their body weight comes from water. Up to 60% of the human adult body is water. Our brain, heart, lungs, skin, muscles, kidneys, and even bones all contain significant amounts of water.

Different people have different percentages of their bodies made up of water. Babies have the most, being born at about 78%. By one year of age, that amount drops to about 65%. In adult men, about 60% of their bodies are water. However, fat tissue does not have as much water as lean tissue. In adult women, fat makes up more of the body than men, so they have about 55% of their bodies made of water. Likewise, people who have an excess of body fat will have less water.

How do we know we are getting enough? It is understandable given the large role of water and its prevalence in our body that we need lots of it for good health. We lose a good portion, close to a liter, each day just from breathing, sweating, and through bowel movements. We lose another 1.5 by urinating. We lose even more than these averages if we're physically active.

Healthy people meet their fluid needs by drinking when thirsty and drinking with meals. Men need approximately 3.7 liters (15 cups) of fluid each day, and women 2.7 (11 cups). We can get some of this water from food. However, we should get about 80% of it or more from the liquids we drink. Men should drink 13 cups and women 9 cups each day. You need even more water when you're ill (having vomiting, diarrhea, or running a fever), exercising, or in a hot or humid climate. People with excess body fat have less water in their bodies, as mentioned, and so will need to drink a bit more (as a bonus, it helps you lose weight).

So how do you know if you are getting enough? Many of us experience mild forms of dehydration without even realizing it. Symptoms include but are not limited to:

- Fatigue
- Headaches
- Dizziness or lightheadedness
- Urine that is too yellow in color (it should be light yellow, like lemonade)
- Irritability and mood swings
- Constipation
- Urinary tract infections
- Dry skin and chapped lips

Where We Get Water

As noted above, about 20% of your water intake also comes from foods, with fruits and vegetables serving as better sources of water than grains. Cooked grains, like rice or oats, will have some water injected as part of the cooking process. Fruit, like watermelon, retains plenty of water (and they taste pretty good on a hot day!). Anything you drink contains water, as well, though it's good to be mindful of any diuretic side effects of your beverage, which can potentially lead to mild dehydration. A diuretic is a drink, like coffee or alcohol, or drinks with added sugar, that makes you urinate.

If you think you are not getting enough water, these tips may help:

- Carry a water bottle for easy access when you are at work of running errands.
- Freeze some freezer safe water bottles. Take one with you for ice-cold water all day long.
- Choose water instead of sugar-sweetened beverages. This can also help with weight management. Substituting water for one 20-ounce sugar sweetened soda will save you about 240 calories.
- Choose water when eating out. Generally, you will save money and reduce calories.
- Add a wedge of lime or lemon to your water. This can help improve the taste and help you drink more water than you usually do.

Assessing and Planning Your Nutrition

The benefits of healthy nutrition are most apparent in their relationship to body composition (see Chapter 6). Lowering your energy intake (fewer calories) is part of creating the negative energy balance needed to manage weight and obtain or maintain a healthy proportion of body fat and muscle. Much of this can be done with portion control and the selection of healthy foods, rather than strictly counting calories.

You can improve your nutrition by following the recommendations in the first section of this chapter, usually in conjunction with a combination of meal plans and careful assessments of your food's nutrient content. These plans focus on following some basic steps for meeting the established US Dietary Guidelines for nutrition:

- **Follow a healthy eating pattern across the lifespan.** All food and beverage choices matter. Choose a healthy eating pattern at an appropriate calorie level to help achieve and maintain a healthy body weight, support nutrient adequacy, and reduce the risk of chronic disease.

- **Focus on variety, nutrient density, and amount.** To meet nutrient needs within calorie limits, choose a variety of nutrient-dense foods across and within all food groups in recommended amounts.

- **Limit calories from added sugars and saturated fats and reduce sodium intake.** Consume an eating pattern low in added sugars, saturated fats, and sodium. Cut back on foods and beverages higher in these components to amounts that fit within healthy eating patterns.

- **Shift to healthier food and beverage choices.** Choose nutrient-dense foods and beverages across and within all food groups in place of less healthy choices. Consider cultural and personal preferences to make these shifts easier to accomplish and maintain.

- **Support healthy eating patterns for all.** Everyone has a role in helping to create and support healthy eating patterns in multiple settings nationwide, from home to school to work to communities.

Fortunately, there are several plans that are customizable for your individual needs, goals, and preferences. There are many ways to approach healthy eating, whether it is through a structured program, like the ones offered here or through an approach of your own. These are just a few but should help you on your path toward improving or maintaining nutritional balance in your life.

Using MyPlate to Plan

USDA's MyPlate is a tool to help you focus on the five food groups that are the building blocks for a healthy diet and help you determine the amounts from different food groups that should be represented in your daily eating plan.

Many individuals remember the Pyramids — the Food Guide Pyramid and MyPyramid — USDA's food guidance symbols before MyPlate, but not many people realize just how long USDA's history of providing science-based dietary guidance to the American public actually is. Starting over a century ago, USDA has empowered Americans to make healthy food choices by providing a number of publications, food guidance symbols, and, more recently, a suite of interactive online tools.

MyPlate (Figure 23) is a reminder to find your healthy eating style and build it throughout your lifetime. Everything you eat and drink matters. The right

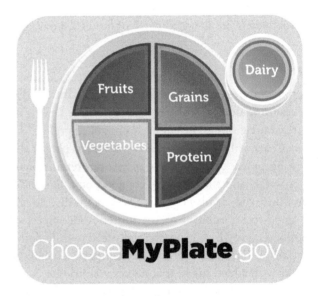

Figure 23. ChooseMyPlate is the latest federal nutrition program.

mix can help you be healthier now and in the future. This means:

- Focus on variety, amount, and nutrition.

- Choose foods and beverages with less saturated fat, sodium, and added sugars.

- Start with small changes to build healthier eating styles.

- Support healthy eating for everyone.

Eating healthy is a journey shaped by many factors, including our stage of life, situations, preferences, access to food, culture, traditions, and the personal decisions we make over time. MyPlate offers ideas and tips to help you create a healthier eating style that meets your individual needs and improves your health.

MyPlate helps you determine the types and portion sizes — based on your age, gender, and level of physical activity — you need for each of the five food groups. These are fruits, vegetables, grains, proteins, and dairy. My plate also contains recommendations for oils, but they are not a separate consideration.

Fruits

Any fruit or 100% fruit juice counts as part of the Fruit Group. Fruits may be fresh, canned, frozen, or dried, and may be whole, cut-up, or pureed.

In general, 1 cup of fruit or 100% fruit juice, or 0.5 cup of dried fruit can be considered as 1 cup from the Fruit Group.

Vegetables

Any vegetable or 100% vegetable juice counts as a member of the Vegetable Group. Vegetables may be raw or cooked; fresh, frozen, canned, or dried/dehydrated; and may be whole, cut-up, or mashed. Based on their nutrient content, vegetables are organized into five subgroups: dark-green vegetables, starchy vegetables, red and orange vegetables, beans and peas, and other vegetables.

In general, 1 cup of raw or cooked vegetables or vegetable juice, or 2 cups of raw leafy greens can be considered as 1 cup from the Vegetable Group. Recommended total daily amounts and recommended weekly amounts from each vegetable subgroup are shown in the two tables below.

These amounts are appropriate for individuals who get less than 30 minutes per day of moderate physical activity, beyond normal daily activities. Those who are more physically active may be able to consume more while staying within calorie needs.

Recommended Daily Fruit Amounts		
Women	19–30 years old	2 cups
	31–50 years old	1.5 cups
	51+ years old	1.5 cups
Men	19–30 years old	2 cups
	31–50 years old	2 cups
	51+ years old	2 cups

Figure 24. Recommended fruit amounts per day.

Recommended Daily Vegetable Amounts		
Women	19–30 years old	2.5 cups
	31–50 years old	2.5 cups
	51+ years old	2 cups
Men	19–30 years old	3 cups
	31–50 years old	3 cups
	51+ years old	2.5 cups

Figure 25. Recommended vegetable amounts per day.

Recommended Weekly Vegetable Amounts		Dark green vegetables	Red and orange vegetables	Beans and peas	Starchy vegetables	Other vegetables
Women	19–30 years old	1.5 cups	5.5 cups	1.5 cups	5 cups	4 cups
	31–50 years old	1.5 cups	5.5 cups	1.5 cups	5 cups	4 cups
	51+ years old	1.5 cups	4 cups	1 cup	4 cups	3.5 cups
Men	19–30 years old	2 cups	6 cups	2 cups	6 cups	5 cups
	31–50 years old	2 cups	6 cups	2 cups	6 cups	5 cups
	51+ years old	1.5 cups	5.5 cups	1.5 cups	5 cups	4 cups

Figure 26. Recommended vegetable amounts per week.

Vegetable subgroup recommendations are given as amounts to eat weekly. It is not necessary to eat vegetables from each subgroup daily. However, over a week, try to consume the amounts listed from each subgroup as a way to reach your daily intake recommendation.

Grains

Any food made from wheat, rice, oats, cornmeal, barley or another cereal grain is a grain product. Bread, pasta, oatmeal, breakfast cereals, tortillas, and grits are examples of grain products.

Grains are divided into two subgroups, Whole Grains and Refined Grains. Whole grains contain the entire grain kernel — the bran, germ, and endosperm. Examples of whole grains include whole-wheat flour, bulgur (cracked wheat), oatmeal, whole cornmeal, and brown rice. Refined grains have been milled, a process that removes the bran and germ. This is done to give grains a finer texture and improve their shelf life, but it also removes dietary fiber, iron, and many B vitamins. Some examples of refined grain products are white flour, de-germed cornmeal, white bread, and white rice.

Most refined grains are enriched. This means certain B vitamins (thiamin, riboflavin, niacin, folic acid) and iron are added back after processing. Fiber is not added back to enriched grains. Check the ingredient list on refined grain products to make sure that the word "enriched" is included in the grain name. Some food products are made from mixtures of whole grains and refined grains.

Recommended daily amounts are listed in this table below. Most Americans consume enough grains, but few are whole grains. At least half of all the grains eaten should be whole grains. In general, 1 slice of bread, 1 cup of ready-to-eat cereal, or 0.5 cup of cooked rice, cooked pasta, or cooked cereal can be considered as 1 ounce-equivalent from the Grains Group.

Recommended Daily Grain Amounts				
			Daily Recommendation	Daily minimum amount of whole grains
Women	19–30 years old		6 ounce equivalents	3 ounce equivalents
	31–50 years old		6 ounce equivalents	3 ounce equivalents
	51+ years old		5 ounce equivalents	3 ounce equivalents
Men	19–30 years old		8 ounce equivalents	4 ounce equivalents
	31–50 years old		7 ounce equivalents	3.5 ounce equivalents
	51+ years old		6 ounce equivalents	3 ounce equivalents

Figure 27. Recommended grain amounts per day.

Proteins

All foods made from meat, poultry, seafood, beans and peas, eggs, processed soy products, nuts, and seeds are considered part of the Protein Foods Group. Beans and peas are also part of the Vegetable Group.

Select a variety of protein foods to improve nutrient intake and health benefits, including at least 8 ounces of cooked seafood per week. The advice to consume seafood does not apply to vegetarians. Vegetarian options in the Protein Foods Group include beans and peas, processed soy products, and nuts and seeds. Meat and poultry choices should be lean or low-fat.

Most Americans eat enough food from this group, but need to make leaner and more varied selections of these foods. In general, 1 ounce of meat, poultry or fish, 0.25 cup cooked beans, 1 egg, 1 tablespoon of peanut butter, or 0.5 ounce of nuts or seeds can be considered as 1 ounce-equivalent from the Protein Foods Group.

Recommended Daily Protein Amounts		
Women	19–30 years old	5.5 ounce equivalents
	31–50 years old	5 ounce equivalents
	51+ years old	5 ounce equivalents
Men	19–30 years old	6.5 ounce equivalents
	31–50 years old	6 ounce equivalents
	51+ years old	5.5 ounce equivalents

Figure 28. Receommended protein amounts per day.

The USDA recommends several strategies for choosing healthy protein sources:

- Choose lean or low-fat meat and poultry. If higher fat choices are made, such as regular ground beef (75–80% lean) or chicken with skin, the fat counts against your limit for calories from saturated fats.

- If solid fat is added in cooking, such as frying chicken in shortening or frying eggs in butter or stick margarine, this also counts against your limit for calories from saturated fats.

- Select some seafood that is rich in omega-3 fatty acids, such as salmon, trout, sardines, an-

chovies, herring, Pacific oysters, and Atlantic and Pacific mackerel.

- Processed meats such as ham, sausage, frankfurters, and luncheon or deli meats have added sodium. Check the Nutrition Facts label to help limit sodium intake. Fresh chicken, turkey, and pork that have been enhanced with a salt-containing solution also have added sodium. Check the product label for statements such as "self-basting" or "contains up to __% of __", which mean that a sodium-containing solution has been added to the product.

- Choose unsalted nuts and seeds to keep sodium intake low.

Dairy

All fluid milk products and many foods made from milk are considered part of this food group. Most Dairy Group choices should be fat-free or low-fat. Foods made from milk that retain their calcium content are part of the group. Foods made from milk that have little to no calcium, such as cream cheese, cream, and butter, are not. Calcium-fortified soymilk (soy beverage) is also part of the Dairy Group.

In general, 1 cup of milk, yogurt, or soymilk (soy beverage), 1.5 ounces of natural cheese, or 2 ounces of processed cheese can be considered as 1 cup from the Dairy Group. The table below lists specific amounts that count as 1 cup in the Dairy Group towards your recommended daily intake.

The USDA recommends several strategies for choosing healthy protein sources:

- Choose fat-free or low-fat milk, yogurt, and cheese. If you choose milk or yogurt that is not fat-free, or cheese that is not low-fat, the fat in the product counts against your limit for calories from saturated fats.

- If sweetened milk products are chosen (flavored milk, yogurt, drinkable yogurt, desserts), the added sugars also count against your limit for calories from added sugar.

- For those who are lactose intolerant, smaller portions (such as 4 fluid ounces of milk) may be well tolerated. Lactose-free and lower-lactose products are available. These include lactose-reduced or lactose-free milk, yogurt, and cheese, and calcium-fortified soymilk (soy beverage). Also, enzyme preparations can be added to milk to lower the lactose content.

Calcium choices for those who do not consume dairy products include:

- Calcium-fortified juices, cereals, breads, rice milk, or almond milk. Calcium-fortified foods and beverages may not provide the other nutrients found in dairy products. Check the labels.

- Canned fish (sardines, salmon with bones) soybeans and other soy products (tofu made with calcium sulfate, soy yogurt, tempeh), some other beans, and some leafy greens (collard and turnip greens, kale, bok choy). The amount of calcium that can be absorbed from these foods varies.

Recommended Daily Dairy Amounts		
Women	19–30 years old	3 cups
	31–50 years old	3 cups
	51+ years old	3 cups
Men	19–30 years old	3 cups
	31–50 years old	3 cups
	51+ years old	3 cups

Figure 29. Recommended dairy amounts per day.

Oils

Oils are not a food group, but they provide essential nutrients. Therefore, oils are included in USDA food patterns. Some commonly eaten oils include: canola oil, corn oil, cottonseed oil, olive oil, safflower oil, soybean oil, and sunflower oil. Some oils are used mainly as flavorings, such as walnut oil and sesame oil. A number of foods are naturally high in oils, like nuts, olives, some fish, and avocados.

Foods that are mainly oil include mayonnaise, certain salad dressings, and soft (tub or squeeze) margarine with no trans fats. Check the Nutrition Facts label to find margarines with 0 grams of trans fat. Amounts of trans fat are required to be listed on labels.

Most oils are high in monounsaturated or poly-unsaturated fats, and low in saturated fats. Oils from plant sources (vegetable and nut oils) do not contain any cholesterol. In fact, no plant foods contain cholesterol. A few plant oils, however, including coconut oil, palm oil, and palm kernel oil, are high in saturated fats and for nutritional purposes should be considered to be solid fats. Solid fats are fats that are solid at room temperature, like butter and shortening. Many of these are the evil trans fats discussed earlier. Some common fats are butter, milk fat, beef fat (tallow, suet), chicken fat, pork fat (lard), stick margarine, shortening, and partially hydrogenated oil.

Some Americans consume enough oil in the foods they eat, such as:

- nuts
- fish
- cooking oil
- salad dressings

Others could easily consume the recommended allowance by substituting oils for some solid fats they eat.

To use MyPlate and customize your program, simply go to www.choosemyplate.gov and look through the tools, tips, resources, and quizzes that are available to you. Since record-keeping is such an important tool for success, you can download and use one of their easy-to-use daily checklists that are designed to fit a variety of ages and calorie requirements.

Recommended Daily Oils Amounts		
Women	19–30 years old	6 teaspoons
	31–50 years old	5 teaspoons
	51+ years old	5 teaspoons
Men	19–30 years old	7 teaspoons
	31–50 years old	6 teaspoons
	51+ years old	6 teaspoons

Figure 30. Recommended oils amounts per day.

Using Nutrition Labels to Plan

Nutrition labels on food provide specific information about serving sizes and daily percentages based on average calorie intakes. With a little practice, these labels are easy to use.

In the following Nutrition Facts label, we have colored certain sections to help you focus on those areas that will be explained in detail. You will not see these colors on the food labels on products you purchase.

Serving Size

The first place to start when you look at the Nutrition Facts label is the serving size and the number of servings in the package. Serving sizes are standardized to make it easier to compare similar foods; they are provided in familiar units, such as cups or pieces, followed by the metric amount, e.g., the number of grams.

The size of the serving on the food package influences the number of calories and all the nutrient amounts listed on the top part of the label. Pay attention to the serving size, especially how many servings there are in the food package. Then ask yourself, "How many servings am I consuming?" (e.g., 0.5 serving, 1 serving, or more). In the sample label, one serving of macaroni and cheese equals one cup. If you ate the whole package, you would eat two cups. That doubles the calories and other nutrient numbers, including the %Daily Values as shown in the sample label.

Daily Value

The % Daily Values (%DVs) are based on the Daily Value recommendations for key nutrients but only for a 2,000 calorie daily diet — not 2,500 calories. You may not know how many calories you consume in a day. But you can still use the %DV as a frame of reference whether or not you consume more or less than 2,000 calories.

The %DV helps you determine if a serving of food is high or low in a nutrient. A few nutrients, like trans fat, do not have a %DV, but trans fat should be avoided, anyway.

The %DV also makes it easy for you to make comparisons. You can compare one product or brand to a similar product. Just make sure the serving sizes are similar, especially the weight (e.g. gram, milligram, ounces) of each product. It's easy to see which foods are higher or lower in nutrients because the serving sizes are generally consistent for similar types of foods, (see the comparison example at the end) except in a few cases like cereals.

Use the %DV to help you quickly distinguish one claim from another, such as "reduced fat" vs. "light" or "nonfat." Just compare the %DVs for Total Fat in each food product to see which one is higher or lower in that nutrient — there is no need to memorize definitions. This works when comparing all nutrient content claims, e.g., less, light, low, free, more, high, etc.

You can use the %DV to help you make dietary trade-offs with other foods throughout the day. You don't have to give up a favorite food to eat a healthy diet. When a food you like is high in fat, balance it with foods that are low in fat at other times of the day. Also, pay attention to how much you eat so that the total amount of fat for the day stays below 100%DV.

A %DV is required to be listed if a claim is made for protein, such as "high in protein". Otherwise, unless the food is meant

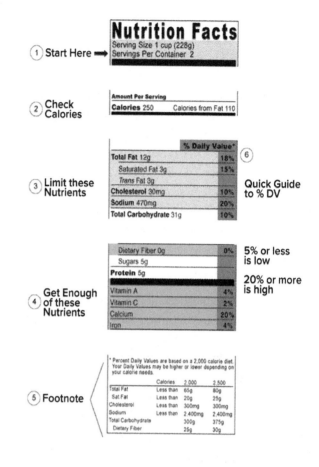

Figure 31. How to read a Nutrition Facts label.

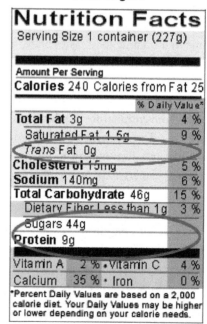

Figure 32. Comparison labels for plain and fruit yogurt.

for use by infants and children under 4 years old, none is needed. Current scientific evidence indicates that protein intake is not a public health concern for adults and children over 4 years of age.

No daily reference value has been established for sugars because no recommendations have been made for the total amount to eat in a day. Keep in mind, the sugars listed on the Nutrition Facts label include naturally occurring sugars (like those in fruit and milk) as well as those added to a food or drink. Check the ingredient list for specifics on added sugars.

The Accuracy of Food Labels

Nutrition labels have raised awareness of the energetic value of foods, and represent for many a pivotal guideline to regulate food intake. However, recent data have created doubts on label accuracy. Calories, especially, on food labels are subject to a wide margin of error, about 20% on either side.

Using Organic Food to Plan

Organic food is produced by methods that comply with the standards of organic farming. Standards vary worldwide, but organic farming in general features practices that strive to cycle resources, promote ecological balance, and conserve biodiversity. Organizations regulating organic products may restrict the use of certain pesticides and fertilizers in farming. In general, organic foods are also usually not processed using irradiation (exposing the food to radiation), industrial solvents, or synthetic food additives.

There is not sufficient evidence to support claims that organic food is safer or healthier than conventionally grown food. While there may be some differences in the nutrient contents of organically- and conventionally-produced food, the variable nature of food production and handling makes it difficult to generalize results. Claims that organic food tastes better are generally not supported by evidence.

However, there is widespread public belief that organic food is safer, more nutritious, and better tasting than conventional food, which has largely contributed to the development of an organic food culture. Consumers purchase organic foods for different reasons, including concerns about the effects of conventional farming practices on the environment, human health, and animal welfare.

In a recent analysis, detectable pesticide residues were found in 7% of organic produce samples and 38% of conventional produce samples. The FDA recommends washing produce before consuming, but some produce may retain more chemicals than others. These

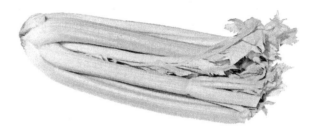

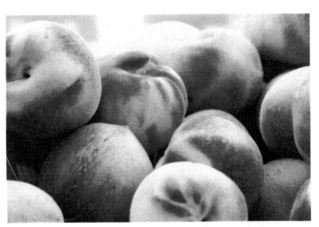

Figure 33. Celery and peaches are party of The Dirty Dozen.

are respectively called the "Dirty Dozen" and the "Clean 15" and are updated annually.

The fruits and vegetables on **The Dirty Dozen** list, when conventionally grown, tested positive for at least 47 different chemicals, with some testing positive for as many as 67. For produce on the "dirty" list, you could definitely go organic — unless you relish the idea of consuming a chemical cocktail. The Dirty Dozen list includes:

- Celery

- Peaches

- Strawberries

- Apples

- Domestic blueberries

- Nectarines

- Sweet bell peppers

- Spinach, kale and collard greens

- Cherries

- Potatoes

- Imported grapes

- Lettuce

All the produce on **The Clean 15** bore little to no traces of pesticides, and are considered safe to consume in non-organic form. This list includes:

- Onions

- Avocados

- Sweet corn

- Pineapples

- Mango

- Sweet peas

- Asparagus

- Kiwi fruit

- Cabbage

- Eggplant

- Cantaloupe

- Watermelon

- Grapefruit

- Sweet potatoes

- Sweet onions

Why are some types of produce more prone to sucking up pesticides than others? Many fruits and vegetables have an outer layer of defense, such as pineapples and corn. Others have no protection between the edible portion and the ground, pesticides, and hands of people picking the produce, such as strawberries.

Many people choose to eat all organic. However, this can be costly since organic produce tends to be a bit more expensive and can often have a shorter shelf-life. To watch cost, you can focus on eating The Clean 15 from conventional produce and buy organic for The Dirty Dozen. If you want to go organic, try shopping at markets focused on whole foods. These stores often (though not always) offer slightly cheaper prices on organic produce than your local chain.

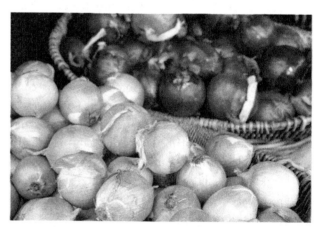

Figure 34. Onions are part of The Clean 15.

Meatless and Meat-Restricted Diets

There are a variety of diets limit your food intake of certain types of food. Vegetarian diets are probably the most well-known meat-restrictive diet, while also being one of the least understood. Others include vegan, lacto-vegetarian, lacto-ovo vegetarian, flexitarian, and pescatarian. Since a major problem with nutrition in the US is a lack of vegetables in the average diet, reviewing the different types of limited diets (none of which "limit" vegetables) are a good idea when making your nutrition plan.

Vegetarians avoid the consumption of animals, including seafood and animal flesh. Vegetarians will often still consume dairy products and products that may be made with eggs, such as pasta. There are many variations to this diet. Vegans, for example, will eat absolutely no animal products. They will avoid all meat, dairy, fish, eggs, and need to read the label on packaged goods to determine if any animal products are used in the ingredients. Lacto vegetarians will consume dairy, but no meat. Lacto-ovo vegetarians will consume both dairy and eggs.

Pescatarians will consume fish. The most recently introduced modification to the vegetarian diet is flexitarian. Many people consider themselves to be primarily vegetarian but choose to consume meat on occasion, making them a bit more flexible. These individuals, in general, avoid meat for health reasons rather than political ones.

Some nutrients should be of particular concern for individuals on these restricted diets because they are mostly found in foods that they do not eat, including Vitamins B-12 and D, Calcium, Iron, and Zinc. A common misperception is that vegetarians lack protein, but as we've learned already, protein is easy to get from plant sources. The FDA offers the following tips for getting enough nutrients and variety on a meat-restricted diet:

- Think about protein. Your protein needs can easily be met by eating a variety of plant foods. Sources of protein for vegetarians include beans and peas, nuts, and soy products (such as tofu, tempeh). Lacto-ovo vegetarians also get protein from eggs and dairy foods.

- Bone up on sources of calcium. Calcium is used for building bones and teeth. Some vegetarians consume dairy products, which are excellent sources of calcium. Other sources of calcium for vegetarians include calcium-fortified soymilk (soy beverage), tofu made with calcium sulfate, calcium-fortified breakfast cereals and orange juice, and some dark-green leafy vegetables (collard, turnip, and mustard greens, and bok choy).

- Make simple changes. Many popular main dishes are or can be vegetarian — such as pasta primavera, pasta with marinara or pesto sauce, veggie pizza, vegetable lasagna, tofu-vegetable stir-fry, and bean burritos.

- Enjoy a cookout. For barbecues, try veggie or soy burgers, soy hot dogs, marinated tofu or tempeh, and fruit kabobs. Grilled veggies are great, too!

- Include beans and peas. Because of their high nutrient content, consuming beans and peas is recommended for everyone, vegetarians and non-vegetarians alike. Enjoy some vegetarian chili, three-bean salad, or split pea soup. Make a hummus filled pita sandwich.

- Try different veggie versions. A variety of vegetarian products look — and may taste — like their non-vegetarian counterparts but are usually lower in saturated fat and contain no cholesterol. For breakfast, try soy-based sausage patties or links. For dinner, rather than hamburgers, try bean burgers or falafel (chickpea patties).

- Make some small changes at restaurants. Most restaurants can make vegetarian modifications to menu items by substituting meatless sauces or non-meat items, such as tofu and beans for meat, and adding vegetables or pasta in place of meat. Ask about available vegetarian options.

- Nuts make great snacks. Choose unsalted nuts as a snack and use them in salads or main dishes. Add almonds, walnuts, or pecans instead of cheese or meat to a green salad.

- Get your vitamin B12. Vitamin B12 is naturally found only in animal products. Vegetarians should choose fortified foods, such as cereals or soy products, or take a vitamin B12 supplement if they do not consume any animal products. Check the Nutrition Facts label for vitamin B12 in fortified products.

Other Dietary Plans

There really are a lot of diet plan options available in this day and age. Many of them, as previously discussed, are not backed by science. There are a few that have been around for quite some time and are supported by health professionals as providing a balanced, safe approach to a healthy diet.

The DASH Eating Plan

The **DASH** (Dietary Approaches to Stop Hypertension) eating plan is rich in fruits, vegetables, fat-free or low-fat milk and milk products, whole grains, fish, poultry, beans, seeds, and nuts. It also contains less sodium; sweets, added sugars, and beverages containing sugar; fats; and red meats than the typical American diet. This heart-healthy way of eating is also lower in saturated fat, trans fat, and cholesterol and rich in nutrients that are associated with lowering blood pressure — mainly potassium, magnesium, calcium, protein, and fiber.

The DASH plan does involve monitoring caloric intake, along with sodium and fats. The plan uses the following guideline for calories:

People on DASH are advised to choose and prepare foods with less sodium and salt, and not to bring the salt-shaker to the table. It's important to be creative — try herbs, spices, lemon, lime, vinegar, wine, and

salt-free seasoning blends in cooking and at the table. And, because most of the sodium that we eat comes from processed foods, be sure to read food labels to check the amount of sodium in different food products. Aim for foods that contain 5 percent or less of the Daily Value of sodium. Foods with 20 percent or more Daily Value of sodium are considered high. These include baked goods, certain cereals, soy sauce, and some antacids — many foods have added sodium (see minerals section of this chapter).

The Mediterranean Diet

The Mediterranean Diet contains more fruits and seafood and less dairy than does the traditional approach utilized by the FDA. People in Mediterranean countries have eaten this way for many years and have been known to have a lower incidence of heart disease and other illnesses, many of which are associated with lower cholesterol levels and more stable blood sugar. A Mediterranean diet focuses on:

- Eating primarily plant-based foods, such as fruits and vegetables, whole grains, legumes and nuts

- Replacing butter with healthy fats, such as olive oil and canola oil

- Using herbs and spices instead of salt to flavor foods

- Limiting red meat to no more than a few times each month

- Eating fish and poultry at least twice a week

- Drinking red wine in moderation (optional)

Possible Health Concerns

There may be health concerns with this eating style for some people, including:

- You may gain weight from eating fats in olive oil and nuts.

- You may have lower levels of iron. If you choose to follow the Mediterranean diet, be sure to eat some foods rich in iron or in vitamin C, which helps your body absorb iron.

- You may have calcium loss from eating fewer dairy products. Ask your health care provider if you should take a calcium supplement.

- Wine is a common part of a Mediterranean eating style but some people should not drink alcohol. Avoid wine if you are prone to alcohol abuse, pregnant, at risk for breast cancer, or have other conditions that alcohol could make worse.

It's Not as Hard as It Seems

College students and busy, working individuals can have crazy schedules that make eating healthy a challenge. Starting a new plan somewhat when you already have a full plate can be intimidating. It may be a bit time consuming initially, but even learning to make small, gradual changes can make a world of difference and help you adapt to a new, healthier way of eating.

You may also be concerned about giving up some of your favorite foods. A healthy eating plan that helps

you manage your weight includes a variety of foods you may not have considered. If "healthy eating" makes you think about the foods you **can't** have, try refocusing on all the new foods you **can** eat:

- Fresh, Frozen, or Canned Fruits — don't think just apples or bananas. All fresh, frozen, or canned fruits are great choices. Be sure to try some "exotic" fruits, too. How about a mango? Or a juicy pineapple or kiwi fruit! When your favorite fresh fruits aren't in season, try a frozen, canned, or dried variety of a fresh fruit you enjoy. One caution about canned fruits is that they may contain added sugars or syrups. Be sure and choose canned varieties of fruit packed in water or in their own juice.

- Fresh, Frozen, or Canned Vegetables — try something new. You may find that you love grilled vegetables or steamed vegetables with an herb you haven't tried like rosemary. You can sauté (panfry) vegetables in a non-stick pan with a small amount of cooking spray. Or try frozen or canned vegetables for a quick side dish — just microwave and serve. When trying canned vegetables, look for vegetables without added salt, butter, or cream sauces. Commit to going to the produce department and trying a new vegetable each week.

- Calcium-rich foods — you may automatically think of a glass of low-fat or fat-free milk when someone says "eat more dairy products." But what about low-fat and fat-free yogurts without added sugars? These come in a wide variety of flavors and can be a great dessert substitute for those with a sweet tooth.

- A new twist on an old favorite — if your favorite recipe calls for frying fish or breaded chicken, try healthier variations using baking or grilling. Maybe even try a recipe that uses dry beans in place of higher-fat meats. Ask around or search the Internet and magazines for recipes with fewer calories — you might be surprised to find you have a new favorite dish!

Remember Food Safety

One common challenge for people concerned with their nutrition is food safety, especially since they may be choosing and preparing food in new ways they might be unfamiliar with. This is especially true for people who aren't used to cooking, but want to take advantage of the health benefits of preparing their own food. Foodborne illness (sometimes called "foodborne disease," "foodborne infection," or "food poisoning") is a common, costly — yet preventable — public health problem. Each year, 1 in 6 Americans gets sick by consuming contaminated foods or beverages. Many different disease-causing microbes, or pathogens, can contaminate foods, so there are many different foodborne infections. In addition, poisonous chemicals, or other harmful substances can cause foodborne diseases if they are present in food.

The most common food safety concerns can be addressed with common sense healthy food handling, including proper cooking temperature, eliminating cross contamination, and consistent handwashing. Others are more difficult to avoid because of their connection to food safety issues that occur outside your control.

- Trichinellosis, also called trichinosis, is a disease that people can get by eating raw or undercooked meat from animals infected with the microscopic parasite Trichinella. Most often found in pork.

- Botulism is a rare but serious illness caused by a toxin that attacks the body's nerves. You can encounter botulism in improperly canned foods and shellfish. While rare, botulism is potentially lethal and proper food storage and preparation are important factors in its prevention.

- Salmonella, which is bacteria most often found in poultry (including eggs).

These different diseases have many different symptoms, so there is no one "syndrome" that is foodborne illness. However, the microbe or toxin enters the body through the gastrointestinal tract, and often causes the first symptoms there, so nausea, vomiting, abdominal cramps, and diarrhea are common symptoms in many foodborne diseases.

Prevention

When it comes to many of the vitamin-rich foods we are discussing — fruits, vegetables, grains, seeds, and beans — there isn't much you have to do to keep yourself safe, though there are some risks. With meats and dairy, however, we do need to pay attention. Food comes from many sources and is handled by many people under many conditions before we bring it to our home, even our produce. Years ago, our meats in particular were fed and cared for differently. We had to cook pork, for example, thoroughly to avoid trichinosis (in part because we used to let pigs control garbage problems — apparently they'll eat almost anything). Our standards are better now, but food-borne bacteria, like E. coli, salmonella, norovirus, and sometimes even trichinosis are still common:

- Wash your fruits and vegetables before preparing them.

- Watch for expiration dates, both at the time of purchase and at home.

- Never buy a package of food that has been torn or is leaking.

- Always refrigerate perishable food within two hours of purchase, and one hour if it's hot out.

- Cook or freeze meats within two days.

- Be sure to wrap meat tightly to avoid leakage and store meat in the refrigerator it has no opportunity to leak on other foods.

- Wash your hands and preparation surfaces before, during, and after cooking

- Any canned food that is dented, swollen, or has an elevated safety bubble (for jars) should be discarded.

Improper handling of food is the most common reason for foodborne illness, with the major culprit being cross contamination. Cross contamination is easy to avoid, however. First keep your meat and vegetables separated at all times. Do not use the same cutting board for meat preparation as you use for preparing vegetables, and wash your hands after every time you touch meat. If your utensils (like tongs) touch raw meat, make sure you wash them afterwards. As a general rule, when you are preparing food, you should wash your hands a lot.

The other main contributor for foodborne illnesses is improper cooking temperature. Chicken should be cooked to an internal temperature of 165 degrees Fahrenheit. Beef and pork should reach a minimum internal temperature of 145 degrees. To get the temperature correct, use a meat thermometer. Meat needs to rest for three to five minutes before eating to allow the cooking process to finish.

Food storage is another major factor contributing to foodborne illnesses. If you are keeping food hot, it needs to hold at or above 145 degrees. If you are keeping it cold, the food needs to be below 45 degrees. Anything in between is a great environment for bacteria to thrive.

Rapid temperature changes wreak havoc as well. For example, if you stick a pot of hot soup in your fridge with the cover on, you can expect to get sick after eating it the next day. Leave the cover off, so it can cool faster, and give it an occasional stir. That will get the food to a safe temperature faster.

There are a lot of easy techniques for keeping your food safe — make sure you learn them as you learn to prepare your own healthy, delicious meals.

Conclusion

Your next steps should be assessing your food intake based on nutrient content, using the guides available from MyPlate and other sources. Then, you can set SMART goals to achieve healthier nutrition in your life.

Changing your behavior can be difficult no matter what it is. Choosing to eat healthy is a choice, and one that takes much of the same kind of careful planning as a new fitness plan. It doesn't have to happen all at once, though. You might try swapping healthier snacks, eating a healthier breakfast, or planning a meatless dinner once a week. Consider ways you might incorporate more fiber into your diet or make sure that you are getting enough healthy fats and other essential nutrients. Assess your diet every once in a while, to make sure that you are making choices that are meeting your nutrient needs and fueling your body effectively.

Chapter 8
Stress Management

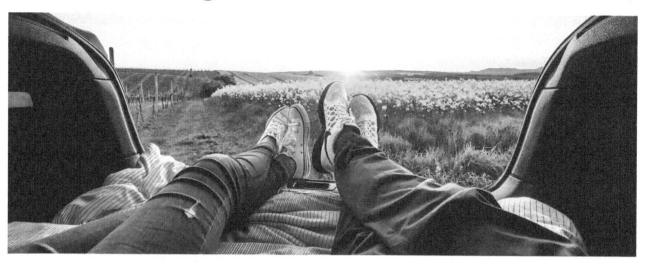

It's your first term in college and you're realizing that it's not as easy as you thought it would be. You registered for more courses than you could handle, your boss keeps scheduling you to work on days when you're supposed to be in class, your family keeps asking about your grades (You have to keep that scholarship!), and mid-term exams are next week. You need to study, but some days it seems like you barely have time to take a shower. And if that's not bad enough — you're broke! Welcome to college, right? You wonder — is it going to be like this all four years?

Everyone feels stressed from time to time and we all react differently to it. But what is stress? How does it affect your health? And what can you do about it? Stress is how the brain and body respond to any demand. Every type of demand or stressor — such as exercise, work, school, major life changes, or traumatic events — can be stressful.

It may not seem like it, but some stress can be beneficial by helping people develop the skills they need to cope with and adapt to new and potentially threatening situations throughout life. However, the beneficial aspects of stress diminish when it's severe enough to overwhelm a person's ability to take care of themselves and their family, or begins to impact their health. Using healthy ways to cope and getting the right care and support can put problems in perspective and help stressful feelings and symptoms subside.

One of the most critical elements of healthy emotional wellness is your ability to effectively manage your stress before it becomes overwhelming. This chapter begins by defining the different kinds of stress that we experience and some of its common sources. It then describes the ways that stress can affect your health. Finally, this chapter recommends stress management techniques to help you avoid the potentially dangerous effects of too much stress.

Understanding Stress

Have you ever been so nervous that you began to tremble or felt nauseous? Or been scared enough that your heart was pounding? Then you can understand how the body can react to what the mind experiences. When faced with danger, fear, or other forms of trial, our body tries to help. It begins to release hormones to prepare the body for action.

But it doesn't happen only in crisis situations. Stress is a physical and emotional reaction that people experience as they encounter changes in life. It's a normal feeling. But long-term stress may put your body in a state of "fight or flight" too often and may contribute to or worsen a range of health problems including digestive disorders, headaches, sleep disorders, asthma, and other physical symptoms, in addition to depression, anxiety, and other mental illnesses.

Everyone feels stressed from time to time. The American Psychological Association relates that in a recent study most participants reported suffering from moderate to high stress — 44 percent say that their stress levels have increased over the past few years. Concerns about money, work, and the economy are the most commonly reported sources of stress. Fears about job stability were reported by 49 percent of study participants. Millennials top the list of individuals with the most reported stress.

In a study focused on college students who sought counseling on campus, the numbers rose dramatically over a 13-year period, with many students indicating stress and anxiety as a major complaint. The CDC reports that there are a few particular stressors that college students typically face, including:

- Social and sexual pressures

- The temptation of readily available alcohol, drugs, and unhealthy food

- The challenge of getting enough sleep

- Stress from trying to balance classes, friends, homework, jobs, athletics, and leadership positions

Stress is common and a normal part of life. Some people may cope with stress more effectively or recover from stressful events more quickly than others. There

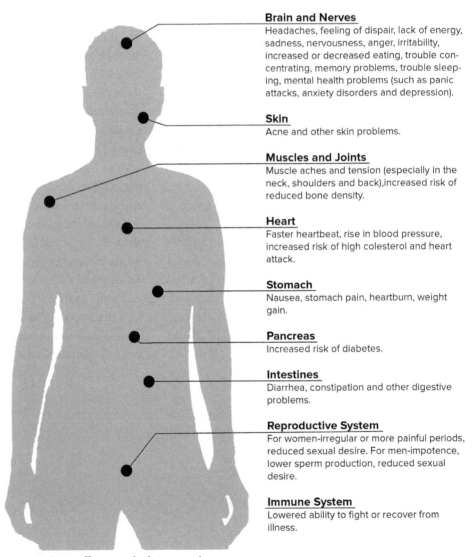

Brain and Nerves
Headaches, feeling of dispair, lack of energy, sadness, nervousness, anger, irritability, increased or decreased eating, trouble concentrating, memory problems, trouble sleeping, mental health problems (such as panic attacks, anxiety disorders and depression).

Skin
Acne and other skin problems.

Muscles and Joints
Muscle aches and tension (especially in the neck, shoulders and back),increased risk of reduced bone density.

Heart
Faster heartbeat, rise in blood pressure, increased risk of high colesterol and heart attack.

Stomach
Nausea, stomach pain, heartburn, weight gain.

Pancreas
Increased risk of diabetes.

Intestines
Diarrhea, constipation and other digestive problems.

Reproductive System
For women-irregular or more painful periods, reduced sexual desire. For men-impotence, lower sperm production, reduced sexual desire.

Immune System
Lowered ability to fight or recover from illness.

Figure 1. Stress affects your body in several ways.

are many factors that affect the way we manage stress. In learning to handle stress, it can be helpful to understand that there are different types — all of which carry physical and mental health risks (Figure 1).

Stressors are those things that cause us to become stressed. A stressor may be a one time or short-term occurrence, or it can keep happening over a long period of time. **Minor acute stressors** are short-lived, like the nerves before a class presentation or the concern that you may run out of gas on the freeway. **Major acute stressors** can be more traumatic, like a traffic accident, an argument with a friend, or experiencing an assault or natural disaster.

Chronic stressors are those that last long-term. This could be the result of routine stress related to the pressures of work, school, family, and other daily responsibilities. It could be brought on by a sudden negative change, such as losing a job, divorce, or illness — situations that we can't resolve quickly. Often they are situations in which we have a high level of demand but limited ability to make decisions or control the outcome. Some stressors can be both chronic and major, such as what soldiers experience in times of war.

Our body always attempts to maintain a level of **homeostasis**, balance within its physiologic systems. As we are faced with stressors, our body feels threatened and attempts to "right the ship," so to speak — keep it from tipping. Stressors can set off a chain of reactions in the body, primarily the release of hormones that control functions such as heart rate and breathing (more on this in a moment). The release of these hormones can result in a wide range of physical reactions to stress, including headache, dry mouth, difficulty swallowing, rapid heartbeat, nausea, cold hands, lack of concentration, difficulty sleeping, certain food cravings, and angry outbursts.

Types of Stress

Our body and mind experience different immediate and long-term affects based on the type of stress. There are six different kinds of stress, including eustress, distress, acute stress, episodic acute stress, chronic stress, and traumatic stress.

Eustress is stress that enhances function, physical or mental, such as through strength training or challenging work. It results from exhilarating, desired, or positive experiences — the type of stress you are likely to experience when there is job promotion, a move to a new and desired house, the birth of a child, an inheritance of a large amount of money, running a marathon, winning, and achieving.

Eustress is not defined by the cause of the stress, but rather how one perceives that stressor (e.g. a negative threat versus a positive challenge). This is considered good stress or adaptive stress. Eustress refers to a positive response one has to a stressor, which can depend on one's current feelings of control, the desirability of the change, as well as the location and timing of the stressor. It may temporarily be stressful because it's new, different, or maybe even unexpected, but we respond to it with motivation to work through the situation and adapt to it.

For example, if you move into a new apartment you may be excited about the change even though you have to pack, unpack, clean, and organize. Our bodies do not physically differentiate between types of stress and may still release hormones to compensate. The stress is there, but it's a positive form. The body adapts and achieves homeostasis (or eustasis). You still have the stressors to push through (the broken plates, the missing shoes, and the box of things you really should have thrown away) but you are excited and challenged.

Our bodies and minds need to face challenges and conquer them. This gives a sense of meaning and success in our lives, improving our overall sense of well-being and our health. Through these situations we learn how to manage stress in a positive way.

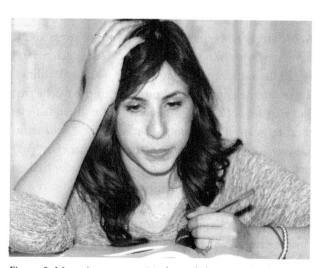

Figure 2. Managing stress positively can help you succeed.

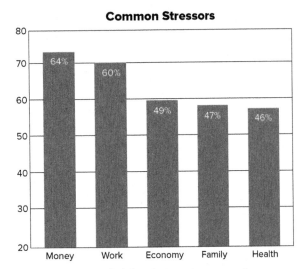

Figure 3. Percentage of adults who experience stress in these environments.

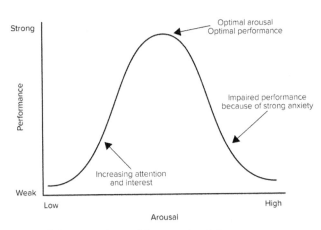

Figure 4. Stress can be good for you when it increases your performance.

Distress is a negative type of stress and works in an opposite way to eustress. It can be short- or long-term and something with which we struggle to cope or adapt. It may even feel overwhelming. Rather than motivating us, it can cause a decrease in our ability to perform.

Any negative stressor can lead to an overall feeling of distress (Figure 3). Divorce, job loss or excessive demands at work, difficult studies, illness, loss of a friend or family member, money problems, sleep problems, anything that the person perceives as negative and stressful can lead to distress. Just as with eustress, the stressor doesn't define distress. It is defined by the person's reaction to the stressor. Whether an individual experiences eustress or distress depends on the disparity between an experience (real or imagined), personal

Acute Stress

Acute stress is the more common form of stress and is associated with things in our everyday lives such as paying a bill on time, rushing to class, or making deadlines. These are the demands and pressures of the recent past and that we anticipate in the near future. It tends to be short-term stress that resolves without any serious damage to your health. Once you've turned in that essay, paid that bill, or made it to class the situation is resolved, at least for the moment. When the same things start over again the next day, and the next day, we begin to experience problems. Acute stress can actually be exciting and thrilling but too much can make you feel exhausted.

expectations, and the resources to cope with the stress. We experience distress when our resources to handle the stress are exhausted.

In a recent study, over 3% of adults reported experiencing serious psychological distress over a 30-day period. If we assume that the participants in the study are accurately representative of the nation as a whole, that's a significant number of people each month that can't handle the level of stress they experience, whose coping resources are overwhelmed or not readily available. That's because there are different types of distress — sometimes it is acute and other times chronic. Distress that is not resolved through coping or adaptation may lead to anxiety and/or depression, possibly making you mentally or physically ill.

Symptoms of acute stress can include emotional anguish, headaches, back pains and general muscular problems. They may also include irritable bowel syndrome (IBS), dizziness, and shortness of breath, chest pains, and heart palpitations, which can often be triggered by adrenaline.

Episodic acute stress is when we experience it more frequently. People that tend to suffer from this always seem to be in a rush, overscheduled (often deliberately), and always facing some form of stressor. They take too much on and tend not to be able to organize themselves to deal with demands and pressures.

Episodic acute stress can affect interpersonal skills and can make sufferers respond negatively towards others causing a deterioration of relationships at home and the workplace. Tammy's friends rarely spend time with her anymore, partly because she doesn't really have time for them, and partly because she's not very pleasant to talk to. Her tension level extends to those around her.

This type of prolonged over stimulation can lead to persistent tension, headaches or migraines, hypertension, and even chest pains. Tammy's lifestyle could have a negative impact on her health.

Chronic Stress

Chronic stress can wear a sufferer down making them feel "burned-out." It occurs when someone feels that they can't see a way out of the demands and/or pressures that are making them feel sad, miserable, and disheartened on a continual basis. Factors like poverty, chronic illness, an unhappy marriage, or a job that you hate but need, can lead to this type of stress.

Individuals experiencing chronic stress may even grow accustomed to feeling badly. They may notice acute episodes but have stopped trying to resolve the source of the chronic stress. They've given up hope and no longer look for answers. Sometimes they form an unhealthy ideology about the world or life, feeling like they'll never measure up or the world will always be harsh.

This form of stress can be very detrimental to a person's health, particularly when we become acclimated to it, sometimes even comfortable with it (its familiar). We may not feel any more stressed this month than we did last month, primarily because every month is the same. Over time, our bodies do feel the stress, placing us at greater risk for violent behavior, stroke, heart attack, and depression.

Traumatic Stress

Post-traumatic stress is associated with traumatic events. Traumatic events are marked by a sense of horror, helplessness, serious injury, or the threat of serious injury or death. Traumatic events affect survivors, rescue workers, and the friends and relatives of victims who have been involved. They may also have an impact on people who have seen the event either firsthand or on television. These can be traumatic experiences from someone's childhood, or wars, poverty, major accidents, shootings, sexual violence, or violent abuse.

A person's response to a traumatic event may vary. Responses include feelings of fear, grief, and depression. Physical and behavioral responses include nausea, dizziness, and changes in appetite and sleep pattern as well as withdrawal from daily activities.

Responses to trauma can last for weeks to months before people start to feel normal again. Most people feel better within a few months after a traumatic event, but for some problems become worse or last longer. The person may be suffering from **post-traumatic stress disorder** (PTSD).

Post-traumatic stress disorder (PTSD) is an intense physical and emotional response to thoughts and reminders of the event that last for many weeks or months after the traumatic event. The symptoms of PTSD fall into three broad types: re-living, avoidance and increased arousal.

Symptoms of **re-living** include flashbacks, nightmares, and extreme emotional and physical reactions to reminders of the event. Emotional reactions can include feeling guilty, extreme fear of harm, and numbing of emotions. Physical reactions can include uncontrollable shaking, chills or heart palpitations, and tension headaches.

Symptoms of **avoidance** include staying away from activities, places, thoughts, or feelings related to the trauma or feeling detached or estranged from others.

Symptoms of **increased arousal** include being overly alert or easily startled, difficulty sleeping, irritability or outbursts of anger, and lack of concentration.

Other symptoms linked with PTSD include panic attacks, depression, suicidal thoughts and feelings, drug abuse, feelings of being estranged and isolated, and not being able to complete daily tasks.

Stress in the US

Since 2007, the Stress in America™ survey has examined how stress affects the health and well-being of adults living in the United States. In 2015, reported overall stress levels increased slightly, with greater percentages of adults reporting extreme levels of stress than in 2014. Overall, adults report that stress has a negative impact on their mental and physical health. A sizable proportion do not feel they are doing enough to manage their stress.

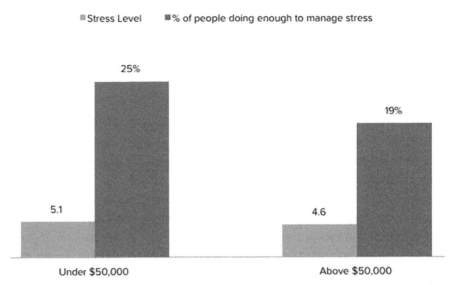

Income and Stress Levels

■ Stress Level   ■ % of people doing enough to manage stress

25%

19%

5.1   4.6

Under $50,000   Above $50,000

Figure 5. Income can be a predictor of stress levels.

In a recent survey, conducted by the American Psychological Association (APA), younger Americans report higher average stress levels on a scale of 1–10 than older individuals. Millenials and Gen-Xers reported stress ratings of 5.6 and 5.4, while Baby Boomers averaged 4.1 and Traditionalists (born before 1946) came in at 2.7. These younger groups are more likely to say their stress has increased in the past year compared with Boomers and Traditionalists.

Higher stress is disproportionately reported by Americans with lower incomes. Survey findings show that Americans whose total reported household income before taxes was less than $50,000 have an average stress level of 5.1, compared to 4.6 for Americans whose households made $50,000 or more. In addition, those with a total household income before taxes of less than $50,000 reported a higher percentage than their counterparts regarding not doing enough to manage stress (25 percent compared to 19 percent) (Figure 5).

College students are frequently feeling this high-stress environment. The transition to college life is a stressful period for young adults (Figure 6). Roles shift, identities change and additional stressors make students particularly prone to stress. Students are often attending school away from their homes and must meet expectations that they achieve academically while managing a new environment and learning to interact with others on a different level socially, culturally, and intellectually. These stressors continue throughout their time in college as other expectations and pressures arise (Figure 7). Often students work and attend school at the same time, begin new, long-term relationships, and take on adult roles. The increased life load, challenges with roommates and romantic partners, and generally learning to "adult" requires young adults to adjust, which can be a stressful experience.

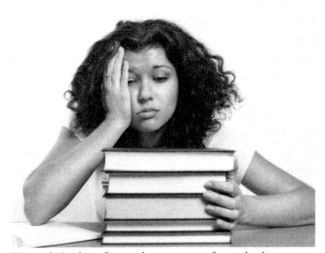

Figure 6. Students frequently report stress from school.

Leading stressors among college students

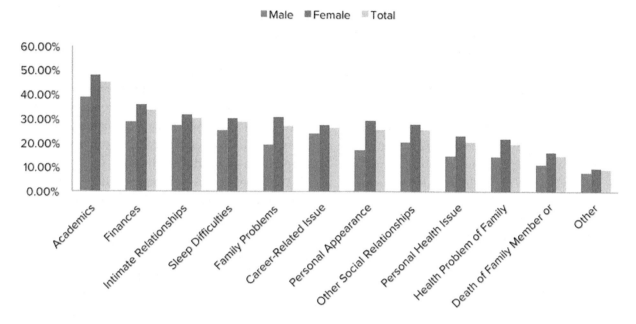

Figure 7. The most common sources of stress for students, by sex.

Higher education has been linked to a reduction in psychological distress in both men and women, and these effects persist throughout the aging process, not just immediately after receiving education. However, this link does lessen with age. The major mechanism by which higher education plays a role on reducing stress in men is more so related to labor-market resources rather than social resources as in women.

Sources of Stress

We can experience stress from any number of common sources, such as:

- Major life events (death of a loved one, job loss, moving to a new place, etc.)

- Daily hassles of life (commuting to work, paying bills, buying groceries, etc.)

- Job-related demands and expectations (deadlines, work schedules, etc.)

- Academic pressure (exams, essays, homework deadlines, etc.)

- Relationships and families (disagreements, parental expectations, family responsibilities, etc.)

- Environmental stressors (hot weather, long periods of rain, crowds, etc.)

- Bias and discrimination (racist jokes, being followed around a store, difficulty finding work, etc.)

Effects of Stress on the Body

Chronic stress can be difficult, even when it only occurs once in a while. A stressful situation, regardless of the source, can unleash the flow of stress hormones in an attempt to bring homeostasis to the body, making the heart pound, breathing quicken, muscles tense, and sweat begin to form.

This "**fight-or-flight**" response mentioned earlier in the chapter evolved as a survival mechanism, enabling people and animals to react quickly to life-threatening situations, and fight off the threat or get to safety. This may be great when you're trying to outrun a bear! But not so great when you're caught in traffic or racing to class — hardly life threatening. Sometimes the body can overreact to stressors that require you to neither fight nor flee, depending upon how you see the situation.

Unfortunately, chronic stress has long-term effects on physical and psychological health. Over time, this biological battleground, when experienced too often, can take a toll on the body. Chronic stress may contribute to high blood pressure, clogged arteries, and even cause changes in the brain that may contribute to anxiety, depression, and addiction.

Research suggests that chronic stress could also contribute to obesity. Sometimes when we're stressed we tend to overeat or pay less attention to the type of foods we consume. We also have difficulty sleeping and fitting exercise into our schedules, both of which can contribute to unhealthy weight gain.

We all look at the world through our own lens. People do not always react the same way to stress as one another, nor do we necessarily view a particular stressor the same way each time it occurs. Our response to stress can be different based on the nature of the stressor, biological factors, and our past experiences.

Stress Response

So, when you feel stress, what happens to make your body do the things it does? We've talked about this briefly, but let's look at it in more detail (Figure 8). When someone confronts an oncoming form of danger, the eyes and/or ears send the information to the amygdala, an area of the brain that contributes to emotional processing. The amygdala considers the images and sounds. If it suspects danger, it sends a distress signal.

Three glands "go into gear" and work together to help you cope with change or a stressful situation. Two are in your brain and are called the hypothalamus and the pituitary gland. The third, the adrenal glands, are on top of your kidneys. The amygdala first messages the hypothalamus. The hypothalamus is like your brain's remote control. It communicates with the rest of the body through the autonomic nervous system. This controls our involuntary body functions as breathing, blood pressure, heartbeat, and the dilation or constriction of key blood vessels. It has two parts the sympathetic and parasympathetic systems.

The hypothalamus is what sets off the biological chain reaction. It signals your pituitary gland that it is time to tell your adrenal glands to release the stress hormones called **adrenaline** (epinephrine), **noradrenaline**, and **cortisol**. These chemicals pump into your body through the bloodstream, increasing your heart rate and breathing and providing a burst of energy (increase of blood sugar) to take on the problem. Our breathing gets deeper, sending more oxygen to the brain, and heightening our sense and awareness. These chemicals can also control body temperature (which can make you feel hot or cold), keep you from getting hungry, and make you less sensitive to pain. Essentially, our sympathetic nervous system feels sorry for us, gets worried, and steps in to help.

This reaction can start before we are even fully aware of what's going on. It's instant! You've heard

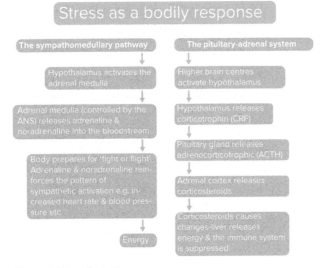

Figure 8. How the body reacts to stress.

stories of people completing super-human feats, lifting heavy objects and jumping out of the way of cars without thinking about it because of a rush of adrenaline. That's all courtesy of the body's ancient and inherent capacity for preservation.

Once the danger has passed, the nervous system changes channels. It shifts from heavy metal music videos to public broadcasting of the symphony. It activates our parasympathetic nervous system (this system tells the sympathetic system to calm down), which promotes a "rest and digest" response to calm the body.

But what happens when life continues to throw curves at you and if you have one stressful event after another? Your stress response may not be able to stop itself from running overtime, and you may not have a chance to rest, restore, and recuperate. This can add up and, suddenly, the signs of overload hit you — turning short-term stressors into long-term stress. This means that you may have even more physical signs of stress. Things like a headache, eating too much or not at all, tossing and turning all night, or feeling down and angry all

the time, are all signs of long-term stress. These signs start when you just can't deal with any more.

Another stress hormone, **oxytocin**, acts as a neurotransmitter when it's released during labor and breastfeeding. It can suppress other stress responses in women. Newer research on emotional impacts on mice have complicated its study as a positive hormone in men, but its positive impact on certain women remains.

Long-term stress can affect your health and how you feel about yourself, so it is important to learn to deal with it. No one is completely free of stress. The most important thing to learn about long-term stress is how to spot it. You can do that by listening to your body signals and learning healthy ways to handle it (Figure 9).

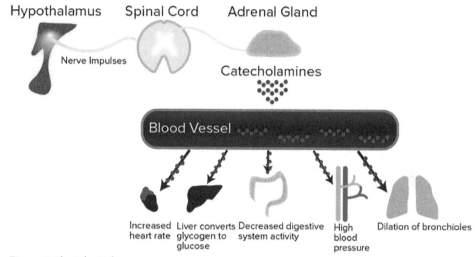

Figure 9. Physiological responses to stress.

Stress Emotions

Stress can intensify and create strong emotions in people, such as anger and fear. Like all your emotions, there is an appropriate time and place for each. But if it seems like you may be angry all the time, or you feel afraid of things that shouldn't cause fear, take some time to figure out what may be going on.

Everyone experiences **anger** from time to time. It's a normal emotion. But intense or prolonged anger can jeopardize employment, relationships, education, freedom, and even your health. Since antiquity, people have been aware of the harmful association between anger with health. Buddhism actually refers to this as one of the Three Poisons of the Mind, along with greed and foolishness.

Typically, when someone gets angry, there are responses that are physiological (becoming flushed, burst

of energy and arousal, etc.), cognitive (thoughts that occur in response to an event), emotional (feeling afraid, discounted, disrespected, impatient, etc.), and behavioral (sarcasm, swearing, crying, yelling, throwing, etc.). Problem anger occurs when someone experiences anger as a chronic irritability or a full-on rage as an emotion experienced too intensely or too often. The consequences of long-term anger issues can lead to arrest, injury (self or others), a negative impact to important relationships, or job loss. Some groups have a higher risk of experiencing problems with anger, including individuals who struggle with substance abuse, traumatic brain injury, PTSD, and personality disorders.

Uncontrolled anger is a significant problem. A person with anger management problems may do damage to themselves and others, sometimes irreparably (assaulting another person, for example, can do permanent physical damage and result in a felony charge). If a person realizes they may have a problem with anger, they should start by taking a moment to think about why, exactly, they are angry. They can ask themselves useful questions like "Have I eaten recently?" or "Is the thing I am angry about my actual issue?" Identifying the problem clearly and reasonably can make an angry person more capable of handling the issue in a healthy way. If the problem is ongoing, it's a good idea to learn more about anger management (Figure 10).

The goal of anger management is to reduce both your emotional feelings and the physiological arousal that anger causes. You can't get rid of, or avoid, the things or the people that enrage you, nor can you change them, but you can learn to control your reactions. Follow these guidelines to help manage moments of anger:

- Walk away when you're angry. Before you react, take time to regroup by counting to 10. Then reconsider. Walking or other physical activities can also help you work off steam. Plus, exercise increases the production of endorphins, your body's natural mood-booster. Commit to a daily walk or other form of exercise — a small step that can make a big difference in reducing stress levels.

- Practice relaxation. Breathe deeply, from your diaphragm; breathing from your chest won't relax you. Picture your breath coming up from your "gut." Slowly repeat a calm word or phrase such as

"relax," "take it easy." Repeat it to yourself while breathing deeply. Use imagery; visualize a relaxing experience, from either your memory or your imagination. Nonstrenuous, slow yoga-like exercises can relax your muscles and make you feel much calmer.

- Problem-solve realistically. It takes time to solve some problems. Set a plan or approach for how you will solve the problem and how you will face it rather than growing frustrated.

- Use cognitive restructuring focused on logic. Demand logic from yourself. Are you expecting more than is practical from yourself or someone else. Is what you expect reasonable? Practical? Tell yourself "I would like…" rather than "I demand…" or "I must have…" (Figure 11)

Like many horror movie aficionados, you may have learned that there is a certain value in **fear** — the temporary arousal, the sense of power that comes from being able to deprive the boogey man of his chainsaw, the heroic idea of saving yourself and others. In these situations you are scared but exhilarated, like being on a rollercoaster. The difference between these types of fear and those that happen in real life is the sense of an ending and knowledge of the outcome. We know the rollercoaster ride will end with us safely exiting a turnstile. We know the movie ends in 1 hour and 55 minutes, with the hero mostly intact.

And then there's the real world. We have a lot to fear from carcinogens, radiation, new technologies capable of spying on us and dominating the world — okay, maybe not world domination (yet). But we do often feel both lucky to have the industrial, technological, and scientific advances that we do and afraid of things we may not be

Anger	Description
Chronic	Prolonged anger, this can impact the immune system and be the cause of other mental disorders.
Passive	Doesn't always come across as anger and can be difficult to identify.
Overwhelmed	Caused by life demands that are too much for an individual to cope with.
Self-inflicted	Directed toward the self and may be caused by feelings of guilt.
Judgmental	Directed toward others and may come with feelings of resentment.
Volatile	Involves sometimes-spontaneous bouts of excessive or violent anger.

Figure 10. Anger is normal, but can be a problem.

Tips on Controlling Anger	
Relaxation	Breathe deeply, from your diaphragm. Use imagery. Try non-strenuous, slow exercises.
Cognitive Restructuring	Avoid words like "never" or "always" when talking about yourself or others. Use logic. Translate expectations into desires.
Environmental Change	Give yourself a break. Consider the timing. Avoid what you can.

Figure 11. Ideas for controlling anger.

able to control. Our sense of worry over one thing or another, real or imagined, can extend beyond a particular moment and become overwhelming.

Even when we are in actual danger, fear emotions might still cloud our judgment. There are hazards to our misperception of risk. The decisions we make when we are fearful are often over- or under-reactions to the actual risk factor at hand. Our heightened senses under stress — caused by adrenaline — can make unreal dangers seem real, and real dangers seem insignificant.

Why are so many people afraid so often? We no longer fear death or illness from many diseases (like smallpox or measles) — in many ways we are safer now than our world has ever been. In the US, most of us have access to food, clean water, and medical care (though this access may not be distributed evenly). But we do have new issues to deal with as a result of our advances — pollution, obesity, new pathogens, and potential hazards from technology — that we can't even yet fully comprehend. This is in addition to personal fears related to our family, relationships, or jobs.

Fear is, at its base, a response to risk. Those who study risk perception say that our responses to risks aren't simple. They aren't just an internal, rational analysis of the risk, but also intuitive, affective responses that apply our emotions, values, and instincts as we try to determine our level of danger. It helps us understand why our fears often do not match the facts.

The Characteristics of Risk

Risk perception researchers have determined that there are some consistent characteristics of risk that form the basis of our perceptions and our fears.

Trust — The less we trust the people or agencies who are supposed to protect us (e.g. government, friends, family), who are exposing us to risk in the first place, or informing us about the risk, the more afraid we will be. The more we trust, the less we fear.

Dread — Dread is relative to the level of risk. If we think it will kill us (like the boogey man really is going to catch us), we may be more afraid of this than a risk that is more real. We are more likely to die from heart disease but don't fear it as much. Likewise, we fear cancer more than other diseases because we measure the risk by the perceived level of suffering.

Yet there are many things in life that we dread other than disease. We dread giving that presentation, leaving our families for long periods, flying, hunting for a new job, attending a funeral, an any number of things about which our minds have determined risk — risk of death, sadness, failure, suffering, and so on.

Control — You may hate riding in the passenger seat of a car but love to drive — you feel safer when you're in control. If you feel you have some control over the level of risk that you will face, it will probably not seem as threatening as if it was determined by someone or something else that you can't control.

Natural or Man-Made — Risks created by man evoke more fear than natural ones. For example, we fear genetic modification and artificial intelligence more than the cross breeding of two different types of dogs. There is an element of the unknown to something man-made rather than something that has occurred since the beginning of time.

Choice — A risk we choose seems less dangerous than a risk we don't. You may have to give many speeches in class because you chose a Speech and Debate course. Giving an impromptu speech in front of your boss may feel higher risk.

Children — We have an inherent need to preserve our species and our offspring. We are far less likely to subject our children to risk than ourselves. For example, if you learn that the artificial sweeteners in diet soda are carcinogenic, you may forbid your child from drinking it, even if you continue to do so yourself.

Uncertainty — There is an old saying that "uncertainty is the mother of fear," or something along those lines. This seems to be true. The greater our uncertainty, the more cautious we are. We feel this way when we don't have all the answers to our questions (What will happen? Will this cause harm?), or the answers are confusing to understand (consider the language of academic journal articles). We are left uncertain and so are more afraid.

Novelty — New risks, like artificial intelligence or the Ebola virus, tend to be more frightening until we have lived with them for a while and learned enough to put the risks into perspective. Consider our initial reactions to HIV and AIDS — when they were new to us, we took precautions above and beyond what was really necessary. Once we learned how the disease was acquired and transmitted, our fears were somewhat lessened and we stopped isolating people with the disese.

Awareness — The more we are aware of a risk, the more we are likely to be concerned about it. Something gaining a particular amount of media exposure is more likely to cause concern (e.g. presidential elections, diseases, crime in a particular area, new drugs).

Vulnerability — Any risk seems greater if you think you or someone you care about could be a victim.

Risk-Benefit Trade Off — If we think something could benefit us from the risk, we see the risk as smaller or more worthwhile. Getting a flu shot, for example. We approach this like a cost-benefit analysis. Is the benefit worth the risk?

Catastrophic or Chronic — We are more likely to fear a mass attack, plane crash, or natural disaster than something like heart disease. These catastrophic incidents kill many people at once, often in a horrifying way. As we've learned, heart disease is the number one killer in the US, but most of us are likely less afraid of it than a large earthquake that could happen any time in the next several centuries west of Interstate 5 in Oregon. This is a good example of the dangers of misperceiving risk. We stock up on gallons of water and non-perishable food at the grocery store and visit the drive-thru for a combo meal on the way home.

Phobias

A **phobia** is a type of fear and can be an anxiety disorder (more later on this). It is a strong, irrational fear of something that poses little or no real danger. There are many specific phobias. Some of us have a fear of heights (acrophobia), enclosed spaces (claustrophobia), spiders (arachnophobia), or even leaving our homes (agoraphobia). If you become anxious and extremely self-conscious in everyday social situations, you could have a social phobia. Other common phobias involve tunnels, highway driving, water, flying, animals, and blood (Figure 12).

Common Phobias*	Percentage of US Population Affected**
Acrophobia (fear of heights)	7.5%
Arachnophobia (fear of spiders)	3.5%
Aerophobia (fear of flying)	2.6%
Astraphobia (fear of thunder and lightning)	2.1%
Dentophobia (fear of dentists)	2.1%
*Approximately 4 to 5% of the US population has one or more clinically significant phobias in a given year.	
**The average age of onset for social phobia is between 15 and 20 years of age, although it can often begin in childhood.	

Figure 12. Common phobias.

People with phobias try to avoid what they are afraid of. If they cannot, they may experience panic and fear, rapid heartbeat, shortness of breath, trembling, and a strong desire to get away or avoid the situation. These situations can be specific (certain animals vs. all animals), social (a fear related to a social challenge, like public speaking), or agoraphobic (fear of society in general and the inability to escape from a threat).

Overcoming Fear of Speaking in Public:

- Know your topic. The better you understand what you're talking about — and the more you care about the topic — the less likely you'll make a mistake or get off track.

- Get organized. Ahead of time, carefully plan out the information you want to present, including any props, audio or visual aids. The more organized you are, the less nervous you'll be.

- Practice, and then practice some more. Practice your complete presentation several times. Do it for some people you're comfortable with and ask for feedback.

- Challenge specific worries. When you're afraid of something, you may overestimate the likelihood of bad things happening. List your specific worries.

- Visualize your success. Imagine that your presentation will go well. Positive thoughts can help decrease some of your negativity about your social performance and relieve some anxiety.

- Do some deep breathing. This can be very calming. Take two or more deep, slow breaths before you get up to the podium and during your speech.

- Focus on your material, not on your audience. People mainly pay attention to new information — not how it's presented. They may not notice your nervousness.

- Don't fear a moment of silence. If you lose track of what you're saying or start to feel nervous and your mind goes blank, it may seem like you've been silent for an eternity. In reality, it's probably only a few seconds.

- Recognize your success. After your speech or presentation, give yourself a pat on the back. It may

Is it Fear or Anxiety?

We often conflate the terms "fear" and "anxiety" because our body's response to both of them is similar, if not the same, such as a fast heart rate and shakiness. Fear is a response to risk. **Anxiety** occurs even when the risk is not present. Anxiety is a worry about future events and fear is a reaction to current events. Often people who are anxious may not even know the source of their anxiety.

It's normal for people to feel anxious in response to stress. Sometimes, however, anxiety becomes a severe, persistent problem that's hard to control and affects day-to-day life — this is called an anxiety disorder. About 12% of people are affected by an anxiety disorder in a given year and between 5–30% are affected at some point in their life. They occur about twice as often in females as males, and generally begin before the age of 25. Anxiety disorders cost the US more than $42 billion a year, almost one-third of the country's $148 billion total mental health bill. More than $22.84 billion of those costs are associated with the repeated use of health care services — people with anxiety disorders seek relief for symptoms that mimic physical illnesses

not have been perfect, but chances are you're far more critical of yourself than your audience is.

Get support. Join a group that offers support for people who have difficulty with public speaking.

The most common are fear of spiders, fear of snakes, and fear of heights. Occasionally they are triggered by a negative experience with the object or situation. They often begin in childhood but can occur in response to any trigger at any time.

Specific phobias should be treated with exposure therapy where the person is introduced to the situation or object in question until the fear resolves. Medications (antidepressants, benzodiazepines, or beta-blockers) are not always useful with phobias or need to be combined with therapy. Specific phobias affect about 6–8% of people in the Western world and 2–4% of people in Asia, Africa, and Latin America in a given year.

Social phobia affects about 7% of people in the United States and 0.5–2.5% of people in the rest of the world. Agoraphobia affects about 1.7% of people. Women are affected about twice as often as men. Typically onset is around the age of 10 to 17. Rates become lower as people get older.

There are a number of anxiety disorders, including generalized anxiety disorder, specific phobia, social anxiety disorder, separation anxiety disorder, agoraphobia, and panic disorder. The disorder differs by what results in the symptoms. People often have more than one anxiety disorder. The most common are specific phobias, which affect nearly 12% and social anxiety disorders, which affects 10% at some point in their life. They affect those between the ages of 15 and 35 the most and become less common after the age of 55.

The cause of anxiety disorders is a combination of genetic and environmental factors. Risk factors include a history of child abuse, family history of mental disorders, and poverty. Anxiety disorders often occur with other mental disorders, particularly major depressive disorder, personality disorder, and substance use disorder. To be diagnosed, symptoms typically need to be present at least six months, be more than would be expected for the situation, and decrease functioning. Other problems may result in similar symptoms including hyperthyroidism, heart disease, caffeine, alcohol, or cannabis use, and withdrawal from certain drugs, among others, so your health care provider will rule out other potential catalysts.

For a person with an anxiety disorder, the anxiety does not go away and can get worse over time. The feelings can interfere with daily activities such as job performance, school, work, and relationships. It's not uncommon for someone with an anxiety disorder to also suffer from depression. Nearly one-half of those diagnosed with depression are also diagnosed with an anxiety disorder.

Overcoming Test Anxiety:

- Learn how to study efficiently. Your school may offer study-skills classes or other resources that can help you learn study techniques and test-taking strategies.

- Learn relaxation techniques. There are a number of things you can do right before and during the test to help you stay calm and confident, such as deep breathing, relaxing your muscles one at a time, or closing your eyes and imagining a positive outcome.

- Don't forget to eat and drink. Your brain needs fuel to function. Eat the day of the test and drink plenty of water.

- Get some exercise. Regular aerobic exercise, and exercising on exam day, can release tension.

- Get plenty of sleep. Sleep is directly related to academic performance. Preteens and teenagers especially need to get regular, solid sleep.

- Talk to your teacher. Make sure you understand what's going to be on each test and know how to prepare.

- Don't ignore a learning disability. Test anxiety may improve by addressing an underlying condition that interferes with the ability to learn, focus or concentrate — for example, attention-deficit/hyperactivity disorder (ADHD) or dyslexia.

See a professional counselor, if necessary. Talk therapy (psychotherapy) with a psychologist or other mental health provider can help you work through feelings, thoughts and behaviors that cause or worsen anxiety.

From the time a girl reaches puberty until about the age of 50, she is twice as likely to have an anxiety disorder as a man. Anxiety disorders also occur earlier in women and they are also more likely to have multiple psychiatric disorders during their lifetime than men. The most common to co-occur with anxiety is depression.

Differences in brain chemistry may account for at least part of these differences. The brain system involved in the fight-or-flight response is activated more readily in women and stays activated longer than men, partly as a result of the action of estrogen and progesterone.

The neurotransmitter serotonin may also play a role in responsiveness to stress and anxiety. Some evidence suggests that the female brain does not process serotonin as quickly as the male brain. Recent research has found that women are more sensitive to low levels of corticotropin-releasing factor (CRF), a hormone that organizes stress responses, making them twice as vulnerable as men to stress-related disorders.

Generalized anxiety disorder (GAD) is characterized by excessive worry about a variety of everyday problems for at least 6 months. For example, people with GAD may excessively worry about and anticipate problems with their finances, health, employment, and relationships. They typically have difficulty calming their concerns, even though they realize that their anxiety is more intense than the situation warrants.

Symptoms of Generalized Anxiety Disorder:

- Restlessness or feeling wound-up or on edge

- Being easily fatigued

- Difficulty concentrating

- Irritability

- Muscle tension

- Difficulty controlling worry

- Sleep problems (difficulty falling or staying asleep or restless, unsatisfying sleep)

People with **panic disorder** have recurrent unexpected panic attacks, which are sudden periods of intense fear that may include palpitations, pounding heart, or accelerated heart rate; sweating; trembling or shaking; sensations of shortness of breath, smothering, or choking; and feeling of impending doom.

Panic disorder symptoms include:

- Sudden and repeated attacks of intense fear

- Feelings of being out of control during a panic attack

- Intense worries about when the next attack will happen

- Fear or avoidance of places where panic attacks have occurred in the past

People with **social anxiety disorder** (sometimes called "social phobia") have a marked fear of social or performance situations in which they expect to feel embarrassed, judged, rejected, or fearful of offending others.

Social anxiety disorder symptoms include:

- Feeling highly anxious about being with other people and having a hard time talking to them

- Feeling very self-conscious in front of other people and worried about feeling humiliated, embarrassed, or rejected, or fearful of offending others

- Being very afraid that other people will judge them

- Worrying for days or weeks before an event where other people will be

- Staying away from places where there are other people

- Having a hard time making friends and keeping friends

- Blushing, sweating, or trembling around other people

- Feeling nauseous or sick to your stomach when other people are around

Evaluation for an anxiety disorder often begins with a visit to a primary care provider. Some physical health conditions, such as an overactive thyroid or low blood sugar, as well as taking certain medications, can imitate or worsen an anxiety disorder. A thorough mental health evaluation is also helpful, because anxiety disorders often co-exist with other related conditions, such as depression or obsessive-compulsive disorder.

Treatment for Anxiety

Anxiety disorders are generally treated with psychotherapy, medication, or both.

To be effective, **psychotherapy**, or "talk therapy," must be directed at the person's specific anxieties and tailored to his or her needs. A typical "side effect" of psychotherapy is temporary discomfort involved with thinking about confronting feared situations.

Cognitive Behavioral Therapy (CBT) teaches a person different ways of thinking, behaving, and reacting to anxiety-producing and fearful situations. CBT can also help people learn and practice social skills, which is vital for treating social anxiety disorder.

Two specific stand-alone components of CBT used to treat social anxiety disorder are cognitive therapy and exposure therapy. Cognitive therapy focuses on identifying, challenging, and then neutralizing unhelpful thoughts underlying anxiety disorders. Exposure therapy focuses on confronting the fears underlying an anxiety disorder in order to help people engage in activities they have been avoiding. This is used along with relaxation exercises and/or imagery.

CBT may be conducted individually or with a group of people who have similar problems. Often "homework" is assigned for participants to complete between sessions.

Some people with anxiety disorders might benefit from joining a **self-help or support group** and sharing their problems and achievements with others. Internet chat rooms might also be useful, but any advice received over the Internet should be used with caution, as Internet acquaintances have usually never seen each other and false identities are common. Talking with a trusted friend or member of the clergy can also provide support, but it is not necessarily a sufficient alternative to care from an expert clinician.

Stress management techniques and meditation can help people with fears and anxiety disorders calm themselves and may enhance the effects of therapy. Since caffeine, certain illicit drugs, and even some over-the-counter cold medications can aggravate the symptoms of anxiety disorders, these should be limited. More on stress management later in the chapter.

Medication does not cure anxiety disorders but often relieves symptoms. They are sometimes used as the initial treatment of an anxiety disorder, or are used only if there is insufficient response to a course of psychotherapy. In research studies, it is common for patients treated with a combination of psychotherapy and medication to have better outcomes than those treated with only one or the other.

The most common classes of medications used to combat anxiety disorders are antidepressants, anti-anxiety drugs, and beta-blockers. Be aware that some medications are effective only if they are taken regularly and that symptoms may recur if the medication is stopped.

For more information on dealing with anxiety, please locate the resources provided at the end of this chapter.

Mental Factors Affect Individual Stress

Several factors affect stress for individuals, including their personality type and traits, gender and biological sex, and cognitive patterns.

According to the American Psychological Association, **personality** refers to individual differences in characteristic patterns of thinking, feeling, and behaving. The study of personality focuses on two broad areas: One is understanding individual differences in particular personality characteristics, such as sociability or irritability. The other is understanding how the various parts of a person come together as a whole.

It is human nature to question aspects of personalities, our own and others. What may seem normal to one person may seem abnormal to another. Character traits, like strength or weakness, shyness or boldness, empathy or apathy, self-confidence or insecurity, and humbleness or narcissism are commonly understood on paper but often relative to the situation and highly variable within a person. What is normal in this situation for this person, and what is pathological? We like to think that we can determine a lot about people based on their "type" of personality.

Over thousands of years, we have developed a variety of categories to help describe personality types ranging from humors (different quantities of four fluids — blood, phlegm, yellow bile, and black bile — determined your personality type) to the Myers-Briggs (which also uses four personality indicators and combinations of those indicators to classify personality). The criticism for these approaches is that they are often considered a kind of oversimplification. Despite the controversy, identifying classifiable stress responses can give people some insight into how they respond to, or generate, stress and figure out a course of action that will help them deal with stress in a positive way.

Type "A"

In the mid 20th century, two cardiologists, Friedman and Rosenman, noticed a particular pattern among their patients. People who were more "intense" were more likely to have heart disease and high blood pressure. These are the classic **Type A** personalities. They are characterized as driven, highly competitive, self-critical, and deadline focused (always rushing). They are often seen as high achieving but short-tempered and impatient with themselves and sometimes others.

Type "B"

In theory, **Type B** individuals are the opposite of Type A. They are more tolerant of others, creative, relaxed, reflective, and have a lower level of stress. They tend to take the "go with the flow" attitude. This could be to the point of a lack of drive and competitiveness and no sense of urgency to meet deadlines. They are often more patient and adaptable to what happens around them. They also have a lower incidence of stress and disease.

Type "C"

The studies and categories have evolved over the years, with additional theorists bringing in additional categories to often include a C and D. **Type C** individuals have difficulty expressing emotions and will often suppress them. They tend to avoid conflict and desire social favorability. They often appear pathologically nice, overly compliant, and overly patient. They may not feel this patience — in fact, they may be angry, but they tend to keep it inside. Type C individuals often suppress their own needs and have difficulty speaking up for themselves. This makes them more prone to stress and stress-related illness, such as depression.

Type "D"

Individuals with a **Type D** personality tend to be very negative. They are critical of themselves, tense, and tend to worry a lot. It is frequently referred to as Type Distressed or Type Disease Prone. They are frequently dissatisfied with life, anxious, depressed, and irritable. And with this comes a higher risk for stress-related illnesses, such as heart disease.

We are not likely to fit one particular mold but the characteristics of each are important to note. If you're a clear Type A, you may be on your way to cardiac issues.

A Type B may be a bit too unmotivated for some professions and not particularly successful. The gloom and doom personality of Type D and self-effacing nature of C present their own complications. Consider those elements of each that you have and how they may impact your health.

Psychologists look at personality types as a means of determining what characteristics of an individual are likely to impact their level of stress. People rarely fall into neat, rigid categories when it comes to their personality. Your friend, Tammy, who we discussed earlier probably seems Type A and likely to be chronically stressed. And while many of her traits do fit that mold, she likely has more to her than what we see. Much of our ability to handle and adapt to stress comes down to particular **personality traits** within us that have a large role. Two in particular can help us reduce how often we will push our fight or flight response to its limits and learn to handle stress in a healthy way.

Psychological hardiness is defined as a compilation of attitudes, beliefs, and behavioral tendencies that consist of three components: challenge, control, and commitment. It comes down to resilience and our ability to cope with stress. The basic theories behind each component are:

Challenge — Hardy people see problems as challenges and opportunities to overcome an obstacle and succeed. They don't expect life to be easy. They accept change as part of life and are willing to work the problem at hand.

Control — Hardy people do not see themselves as victims of their stressors, nor do they accept them as something that they cannot control. They have an internal locus of control (see Chapter 1). They believe that their actions can improve the situation.

Commitment — People who are psychologically hardy have a purpose in life. Rather than getting by, they set a course of direction and move forward.

Studies suggest that psychological hardiness is often a predictor of success, the ability to adapt and cope, and a mentally healthy well-being. Some of this likely comes from training. It begins in childhood. Children who are taught to problem-solve as they grow become hardier adults.

However, even if your parents stepped in and managed your issues for you, or played the victim to their stressors themselves, this hardiness can still be learned. It comes down to shifting negative attitudes about yourself. Critical inner voices that are self-defeating or self-destructive are part of the problem. When you hear that voice that says "They aren't treating you fairly," or "Nothing you do works," recognize it as the language of a victim. We will discuss this more later.

It can also help to be honest about the negativity of those around you and how it may influence your thinking. For example, maybe you and your siblings always called your father "Daddy Downer." As far as Daddy Downer is concerned the world is always horrible, life is out to get him, and he is just keeping his head above water — every day is a race to the grave. Sounds miserable. Did you pick up any of this from your father? You don't need to judge him or change him but you should try to learn from him, or at least what not to do when it comes to negativity.

Avoid self-soothing behaviors that aren't productive. If you've grown accustomed to making yourself feel better by eating a pan of brownies or drinking excessively, it may be time to find healthier ways that are less about being a victim and more about being in control. Hardiness is about taking responsibility for your life with confidence rather than just letting it happen.

Shift-and-persist traits can also be quite valuable when it comes to learning how to manage stress. People with a low socioeconomic stats often have more challenges when it comes to access to medical care, safe living environments, and sometimes even having enough healthy food. Studies have shown that people facing such challenges are often at higher risk for disease.

Yet the shift-and-persist trait often thrives in many people who face challenges on a daily basis. Children in particular who grow up in difficult environments often learn to shift (adapt with and to the stress) and persist (hold on to life as something that has meaning, with optimism). They learn to accept that stress and challenges exist and work around them. They stare down adversity and stay focused on positive things in life. This takes them off the road to disease and depression and keeps them on a road that is likely to be healthier.

In fact, our environment and our culture can impact the way we view and handle stress. Some cultures promote an independent approach to stress management. Depending on how you were raised or the place you live, you may not feel comfortable asking for help or seeking support. Others may have a large network of individuals, a community of support ready to step in and help them manage. There are pros and cons to both, as we see with the shift-and-persist model and as you will see in a moment.

Gender and Biological Sex Impact Stress Response

As scientists discover that biological differences between male and female humans are less distinct than believed, there is oddly enough a genetic component to the fight or flight response.

The sympathetic nervous system functions differently in men and women. For men, the fight and flight response initiates that exact approach. When faced with danger or stress, the hormones circulate and men either stand and fight or seek safety. Women, on the other hand, are more likely to "tend and befriend" (Figure 13). Let's fight that boogey man one more time. He comes up behind your friends, Mary and Jack, with some form of menacing weapon wearing a ridiculously scary mask. Jack prepares to take him on. Mary begins to negotiate. "You don't really need to attack us," she says. "I can help you if you just put the machete down." The stress response specifically builds on attachment care-giving processes in females.

Theories suggest that women release more endorphins during stress that help alleviate pain and make them feel better about social interactions. Women release oxytocin as a stress hormone to combat negative feelings during labor and breastfeeding. There is also a theory that men have an extra gene, called the SRY gene, that increases the amount of norepinephrine released during stress, making the fight or flight response stronger than that of women. Testosterone and estrogen may play a role as well, with testosterone generating a more intense response.

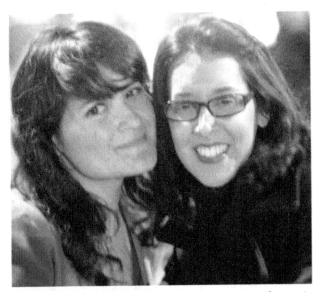

Figure 13. The tend and befriend stress management technique is more common among women.

You've read a bit already and will read more in Chapter 9, that our biological sex does make us more or less prone to certain diseases, both mentally and physically. Men are more prone to hypertension, aggressive behavior, and the abuse of drugs. Women tend to have more issues with chronic pain, depression, and anxiety disorders. Much of our risk of disease results from lifestyle choices, but sex hormones are likely a contributing factor. Often, these differences are more prevalent during reproductive years and then diminish after menopause.

Environmental issues and socially constructed roles are a significant contributing factor in how our bodies handle stress and develop health risks associated with stress. Women still often take on a greater responsibility for homemaking and caregiving (in addition to jobs outside the home). They still carry a larger load when it comes to housework, caring for children, and cooking than their male counterparts. Combine this with full-time work and you can understand how their stress load may be different.

However, while both men and women recognize the impact stress can have on physical health, men appear to be somewhat more reluctant to believe that it's having an impact on their own health. Likewise, men put less emphasis on the need to manage their stress than women do. Men see psychologists as less helpful and are less likely to employ strategies to make lifestyle and behavior changes. Yet men are more likely than women to report being diagnosed with the types of chronic physical illnesses that are often linked to high stress levels and unhealthy lifestyles and behaviors, signaling that there may be some important gender differences when it comes to stress management.

- Men (65 percent) and women (66 percent) say that they are generally satisfied with their lives. However, there are aspects of their lives that both find troubling. Fewer than half of men and women report they are satisfied with their financial security.

- Historically, women report higher levels of stress than men (5.4 vs. 4.8, respectively, on a scale of 1 to 10 where 1 is little or no stress and 10 is a great deal of stress).

- Compared to women, men are less likely to say they are doing an excellent or very good job handling relationships.

And they have different views on how they handle stress as well:

- Only 52 percent of men say it is very/extremely important to manage stress, compared to 68 percent of women. And 63 percent of men say they're doing enough to manage their stress, compared to 51 percent of women.

- One in four women acknowledge they are not doing enough when it comes to managing stress. Only 17 percent of men feel this way.

- Women are more likely than men to report using a multitude of strategies including reading, spending time with family or friends, praying, going to religious services, shopping, getting a massage or visiting a spa, and seeing a mental health professional (5 percent vs. 1 percent) to manage stress.

- On the other hand, men are more likely to report relying on playing sports as a stress management technique (14 percent vs. 4 percent).

- When it comes to the things they report as important and how well they are doing achieving them, women see a larger gap in their own performance than men do:

  a. Getting enough sleep — 40 percentage point gap for women vs. 24 percentage point gap for men

  b. Being physically active or fit — 33 percentage point gap for women vs. 21 percentage point gap for men

  c. Managing stress — 33 percentage point gap for women vs. 17 point gap for men.

Research shows that prolonged periods of stress and the release of fight or flight hormones can decrease proper cell function, thereby contributing to numerous emotional and physical disorders including depression, anxiety, heart attacks, stroke, hypertension, and immune system disturbances that increase susceptibility to infections.

Survey results suggest that the link between stress and physical health could be harder for men to recognize. Men are less likely than women to believe that it can have any impact upon their health, despite the fact that they are more likely than women to report having been diagnosed with the types of illnesses that are often exacerbated by stress. Women are more likely than men to say they've tried to reduce stress and implement strategies for behavior change.

There may be consequences for men in not recognizing the need to address the link between stress and physical health. Men are more likely than women to report having been diagnosed with chronic illnesses, such as high blood pressure, type 2 diabetes, and heart disease or heart attack.

Cognitive Patterns Impact Stress Response

There are many theories on how and why humans react to stress the way they do. Every person is unique in how they respond to a particular stressor, or even whether they view it as a stressor at all. In the latter half of the twentieth century, noted PhDs, Richard Lazarus and Susan Folkman, discussed a concept called the **Transactional Model of Stress and Coping**. This suggests that individuals, when faced with a stressor, go through a series of steps in an attempt to cope.

First, they conduct a primary appraisal the situation — Is this even significant? Does it impact me? Next, they conduct a secondary appraisal — How can I handle this and reach a favorable outcome? Do I have the resources to cope with this? Last, comes the coping mechanism, which is either problem-based or emotional. In a problem-based approach the individual senses their ability to cope and

handle the situation. In emotion-based coping, the individual may feel as if they don't have the control and may avoid the situation entirely or struggle to deal with it.

The basics of the concept suggest that the stress is between the person and the environment. Stress occurs when a person perceives that the demands exceed their ability to mobilize the resources needed to solve the problem. The essential point is that we all respond differently based on how we measure the stressor and how capable we feel of handling it.

Other theories suggest we take slightly different approaches when we encounter stress. **Attribution Theory** suggests that we naturally try to make sense of the problems around us — it is in our nature to establish a cause and effect relationship, even when one doesn't exist. There are two relevant parts to this theory:

Internal Attribution — We attach the cause of the behavior to some internal characteristic, rather than to outside forces. When we explain the behavior of others we look for internal attributions, such as personality traits. For example, we attribute the behavior of a person to their personality, motives, or beliefs. This could apply to the individual, as well, attributing the problem to his or her own personality.

External Attribution — We attach the cause of behavior to some situation or event outside a person's control rather than to some internal characteristic. When we try to explain our own behavior we tend to make external attributions, such as situational or environmental features.

For example, say that you took a test and did well on it. With internal attribution, you might be quite proud of yourself and discuss how hard you'd studied and how you earned that "A." If you had done poorly, you would remember how you went out with friends instead of studying and take responsibility for the "D." With external attribution theory, you may attribute your success or failures to your instructor, tutor, textbook, etc. Essentially, we look for the "Why?" behind the incident. It's in our nature to want to explain why things happen the way that they do.

Theories of how we react to stress can help us cope. They can help us determine what approach we may be taking in our assessment of a stressor and whether or not we are accurate and objective. Sometimes the first step in solving any problem is taking one backward to assess and get perspective.

Coping Strategies

Coping is the process of making a conscious effort to solve personal and interpersonal problems. When it comes to stress, we cope by attempting to solve, minimize, or tolerate the stress we are facing. To do this, we utilize **coping strategies** (Figure 14). All coping strategies are intended to resolve or reduce the stressor (adaptive) but some can be unhealthy or ineffective (maladaptive). Maladaptive behaviors can hinder or interfere with our ability to adjust to the situation.

Often, this occurs in an attempt to reduce anxiety but the result is not productive.

Say, for example, that you have an argument with a friend. You're really upset and worried that if you attempt to talk to her about it, you may yell or cry. Instead, you avoid her entirely, dodging her phone calls for nearly a month until she gives up. You avoided the anxiety of having an uncomfortable conversation but lost a friend in the process.

Coping Strategies	Examples of Strategies
Self-soothing	Something to touch (stuffed animal, stress ball) Something to hear (music, meditation guides) Something to taste (mints, tea, sour candy) Something to see (snow globe, happy pictures) Something to smell (lotion, candles, perfume)
Distraction	Take your mind off of the problem for a while with activities such as puzzles, books, artwork, crafts, knitting, crocheting, sewing, Sudoku, music, movies, etc.
Opposite action	Do something opposite of your impulse that is consistent with a more positive emotion.
Affirmations and inspiration	Look at motivational statements or draw motivational images. Watch or read something funny.
Emotional awareness	Identify and express your feelings with a list or chart of emotions, journal writing, drawing, or art.
Mindfulness	Use tools for centering and grounding yourself in the present moment, such as meditation, relaxation recordings, yoga, breathing exercises, or grounding objects (like a rock or paperweight).
Crisis plan	Develop a contact list of supports and resources for when coping skills aren't enough. This may include family, friends, therapist, hotline, crisis team/ER, 911.

Figure 14. Common coping strategies.

Emotion-Focused Strategies	
Being positive	Think of every situation in life as a learning experience and be positive irrespective of what happens. For example, if you failed to perform well in an exam, don't be intimidated by it when you face it again. Rather, be positive and find better ways to prepare for the exam. The next time around you will ace it. Negative emotions will only prevent you from dealing with situations effectively.
Don't let stressful events get the better of you	This is easier said than done, but once you realize that you're dealing with a stressful situation, quickly find a remedy. If you have to deal with several stressful situations at one time, just step back for a minute, take deep breaths and motivate yourself to deal with one issue at a time. Take control of the situation and you've already solved half the problem.
Communicate with others	Bottling up your emotions will only increase stress levels and lead to a big outburst. Always maintain good communication channels with the people around you. Talk or confide in someone about your stressful situation and discuss ways in which you can handle it. This will give you the comfort and strength needed to deal with difficult situations.
Be accepting	Accept the fact that no one in the world is perfect. Mistakes will always be made and it is impossible to control everything. Once you are accepting of yourself and others around you, you'll find that a lot of self-made stress is relieved.
Deal with mistakes	Mistakes are simply the steeping stones to a better future. Don't get disappointed with yourself or put yourself down when you make mistakes. Rather, learn from your mistakes so that your future decision making will be better.
Deal with success	Success can also be a huge stressor as one is always expected to perform at exceptional levels to maintain that success. Learn from your success and build on your competence to avoid unwanted pressures.
Be disciplined	Follow a good discipline in whatever you do. When you are consistent in your efforts you will be able to handle any situation with confidence.

Figure 15. Coping strategies that focus on emotional techniques.

The term "coping" usually refers to dealing with the stress that comes after a stressor is presented, but many people also use proactive coping strategies to eliminate or avoid stressors before they occur — strategies that may help you look at a stressor in a different light. How we choose to cope is determined by our personality traits and type, the social context, and the nature of the stressor presented.

While each theory has its merits and limits according to psychologists, there are some consistencies as to how we approach strategies. We tend to approach them in three distinct ways — through how we appraise the problem, how we problem-solve, and our emotions as we strategize.

Appraisal-Focused Strategies — The person attempts to change the way they look at the stressor, how they appraise the situation, and approach it differently, sometimes questioning his or her goals and values.

Problem-Focused Strategies — The person strives to deal with the cause of the stressor, work the problem, and in doing so remove the source of the stress and learning skills to manage it.

Emotion-Focused Strategies — The person focuses on the emotions he or she is having due to the stressor and attempts to modify them. This could be by releasing the emotions, distracting themselves, or actively trying to manage their mental state (Figure 15).

A typical person may engage in a mixture of these strategies when attempting to cope with a particular stressor. Their skill at this can change over time as they become more accustomed to actively learning to cope, or as they perceive a strategy as effective or ineffective.

Adaptive vs. Maladaptive Strategies

Positive coping strategies reduce stress and help the person learn from the situation. **Adaptive** coping strategies would be seeking support from a friend, taking care of your health, meditating, getting enough sleep, and maintaining a sense of humor. Sometimes coping strategies can be proactive. The person anticipates a particular situation to be stressful and determines ahead of time how they will cope with it. Adaptive coping strategies include:

Support — Talk to a friend, counselor, or family member for advice or assistance. Talk to someone who can do something concrete.

Accept — Accept that it has happened and that you must adapt and/or address it. Take responsibility for the problem if you are in control of it.

Reinterpret positively — Decide what you can learn from it. See it as an opportunity for growth.

Restraint — Give yourself time to think about it rather than making a hasty decision, possibly making the stressor worse.

Plan — Develop a plan to cope with either the stress or the stressor.

Suppress — Suppress any competing activities. Give yourself breathing room to concentrate on the situation.

Maladaptive or negative coping strategies may work to resolve the problem, but the result is dysfunctional and non-productive. They may offer a quick fix that either enables the person to disassociate the source of

stress from the symptoms, or they create another source of stress. Either way, the person doesn't learn to cope with the stress productively. The relief is short lived. This often occurs when we ignore or avoid a certain stressor, or we use alcohol, drugs, or some other mechanism in an attempt to forget about it. Maladaptive coping strategies include:

Avoid — Escape or avoid the problem by turning to other activities to take your mind off of it. Sleep a lot.

Disengage — Give up trying to cope.

Seek emotional support — Look for sympathy rather than assistance.

Vent — Focus on letting the emotions out and venting but not on adapting or resolving once the emotions are out.

Deny — Refuse to believe that it is happening.

Use alcohol or drugs — Use substances to forget the situation or make yourself feel better.

As you can see by the two lists, the first is focused on skills that actively manage the stress, the source of the stress, or both. The second list probably sounds familiar. How many times have you vented to a friend, felt better, and then ignored the problem at hand? This may be fine if the source of the stress was someone who cut you off in traffic. But what if it's something larger? What if you lose your job? Going out with friends for a few drinks and complaining about your boss may make you feel better for the moment, but once that's done you still need to assume an adaptive strategy, one that will be more productive.

Problem vs. Emotion

Let's get back to Lazarus and Folkman's Transactional Model for a moment. In a problem-focused approach, the person attempts to resolve the source of the stress. Examples of problem-focused strategies include many of the adaptive coping mechanisms you see above, such as:

- Getting help from someone

- Planning and researching to resolve the source of the stress (work the problem)

- Managing time — giving yourself some time to tackle the stress at its source

Emotion-focused strategies are a bit trickier. It's important to focus on those that will be productive. The idea is to attempt to reduce the negative emotional responses to stress. For example:

Seeking support — Sometimes the situation is out of your control (i.e. a death in the family). Getting support from friends and family can be the best and healthiest approach (Figure 16).

Distraction — Again, the goal is not to avoid. The goal is to calm yourself down if your emotions have gotten the better of you by focusing on something else.

Writing in a journal — Putting your emotions on paper in a private, tangible way can help you identify them and deal with them.

Meditation or prayer — For some individuals, taking time for relaxation and inner reflection can help them find a more calm and focused state.

The important thing to understand is that there are ways to manage stress that are healthy and that enable us to both handle it and learn from it.

Grow Your Social Network	
Cast a wide net	When it comes to your social supports, one size doesn't fit all. You may not have someone you can confide in about everything — and that's okay. Maybe you have a colleague you can talk to about problems at work, and a neighbor who lends an ear when you have difficulties with your kids. Look to different relationships for different kinds of support. But remember to look to people you can trust and count on, to avoid disappointing, negative interactions that can make you feel worse.
Be proactive	Often people expect others to reach out to them, and then feel rejected when people don't go out of their way to do so. To get the most out of your social relationships, you have to make an effort. Make time for friends and family. Reach out to lend a hand or just say hello. If you're there for others, they'll be more likely to be there for you. And in fact, when it comes to longevity, research suggests that providing social support to friends and family may be even more important than receiving it.
Take advantage of technology	It's nice to sit down with a friend face-to-face, but it isn't always possible. Luckily, technology makes it easier than ever before to stay connected with loved ones far away. Write an email, send a text message or make a date for a video chat. Don't rely too heavily on digital connections, however. Some research suggests that face-to-face interactions are most beneficial.
Follow your interests.	Do you like to hike, sing, make jewelry, play tennis, get involved in local politics? You're more likely to connect with people who like the things you like. Join a club, sign up for a class or take on a volunteer position that will allow you to meet others who share your interests. Don't be discouraged if you don't make friends overnight. Try to enjoy the experience as you get to know others over time.
Seek out peer support.	If you're dealing with a specific stressful situation — such as caring for a family member or dealing with a chronic illness — you may not find the support you need from your current network. Consider joining a support group to meet others who are dealing with similar challenges.
Improve your social skills	If you feel awkward in social situations and just don't know what to say, try asking simple questions about the other person to get the ball rolling. If you're shy, it can be less intimidating to get to know others over shared activities — such as a bike ride or a knitting class — rather than just hanging out and talking. If you feel particularly anxious in social situations, consider talking to a therapist with experience in social anxiety and social-skills training.
Ask for help	If you lack a strong support network and aren't sure where to start, there are resources you can turn to. Places of worship, senior and community centers, local libraries, refugee and immigrant groups, neighborhood health clinics and local branches of national organizations such as Catholic Charities or the YMCA/YWCA may be able to help you identify services, support groups and other programs in your community.

Figure 16. Coping strategies that focus on social techniques.

High Stress Is a Health Risk

Stress, and long-term or chronic stress in particular, can negatively affect several dimensions of wellness. Our bodies adapt to changes in state, including those changes caused by stress. **Chronic stress** is stress that lasts for a longer period of time. You may have chronic stress if you have money problems, an unhappy marriage, or trouble at work. Any type of stress that goes on for weeks or months is chronic stress. You can become so used to chronic stress that you don't realize it is a problem. If you don't find ways to manage stress, it may lead to health problems (Figure 17).

Signs of Too Much Stress	
1.	Your skin is breaking out in acne. Stress hormones cause acne to appear.
2.	You feel tired all the time. Stress causes your adrenal glands to become overtaxed with cortisol, causing you to feel worn out.
3.	Your hair is shedding. It is common to have hair that falls out or that is thinning all over during periods of stress.
4.	Your blood sugar feels low. High stress levels can affect your levels, making you feel weak and shaky.
5.	You feel achy and sore. This is especially true when you internalize all of your stress. This can also lead to headaches.
6.	You've experienced a fainting spell. When your blood pressure drops, it can make you feel woozy during times of stress.

Figure 17. Warning signs of heightened stress.

The fight or flight hormones released during stress make your brain more alert, cause your muscles to tense, and increase your pulse. In the short term, these reactions are good because they can help you handle the situation causing stress. This is your body's way of protecting itself.

When you have chronic stress, your body stays alert, even though there is no danger. Over time, this puts you at risk for health problems, including:

- High blood pressure
- Heart disease
- Diabetes
- Obesity
- Depression or anxiety
- Skin problems, such as acne or eczema
- Menstrual problems

If you already have a health condition, chronic stress can make it worse.

General Adaptation Syndrome (GAS) theorizes that during the fight or flight response, the body enters three different stages — alarm, resistance, and exhaustion (Figure 18). The initial stage is *alarm*. This is when the body first reaction and sets off that wonderful chain reaction of hormones, preparing you to react. The second stage is *resistance*. Our hormone levels are still high and we are still in a ready state, but we are no longer alarmed (at least not at the same level). At this point, we are ready to fight or flee (resist the stress). What we aren't able to do is take on an additional stressor very easily. The third stage is *exhaustion*. Once the body has remained in this ready state for a time, it begins to fatigue and become apathetic to the stress. This is when we can develop illness. Our bodies aren't meant to stay in this heightened state and other bodily systems begin to weaken, such as our immune system.

Allostatic load refers to the overload the body experiences when it reaches this state of exhaustion. "Allostasis" is essentially the body's attempt to create a new and poorer form of homeostasis. Homeostasis occurs when the body is comfortable with its environment — everything is as it should be. Too much time under stress and we can reach our allostatic load. Our body reaches a new normal, allostasis, in an attempt to adapt in the aftermath of a response to stress.

Short-term, sporadic stress can have an impact on health as well. Have you ever gotten sick to your stomach before a test or speech? Taken a sudden fall and found yourself dizzy even though you didn't hit your head? Our body can overreact at times, or just overwork in an attempt to help us out. Imagine what it does during major acute stress, like an earthquake or a large argument with your spouse.

Studies suggest that sudden emotional stresses, particularly anger, can trigger heart attacks, arrhythmias and even sudden death. This happens primarily in people who already have heart disease, but often people don't know they have a problem until acute stress causes a heart attack or other serious medical issues.

Seyle's General Adaptation Syndrome

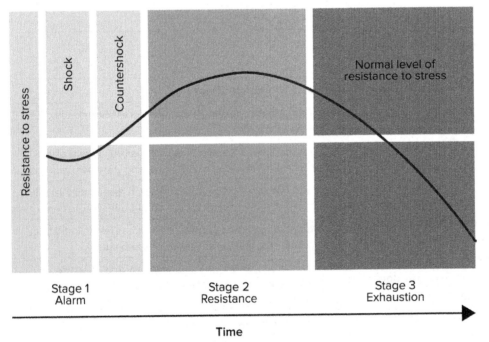

Figure 18. Seyle's path through the stages of stress.

Stress can start to interfere with your ability to live a normal, productive life. Over time, this can become dangerous. The longer the stress lasts, the harder it is on your mind and body. Fatigue and irritability are just the tip of the iceberg.

Chronic stress may cause disease. This can result from the exhaustion mentioned earlier or the unhealthy choices we often make when we aren't coping with stress effectively, such as smoking, drinking, eating poorly, not exercising, and not sleeping well. Situations where we are under high demand to perform but with limited decision-making powers (such as on the job) can increase our risk of health issues like ulcers and coronary heart disease, as can depression. Stress can also make it difficult to recover from an illness. Research suggests that cardiac patients with so-called "Type D" personalities — characterized by chronic distress — face higher risks of adverse outcomes.

Some emotional effects are less serious, like fatigue or irritability. Others are much more serious and can be dangerous.

Call a suicide hotline immediately if you are having thoughts of suicide. Contact your healthcare provider if you experience any of these symptoms:

- stress that is overwhelming or affecting your health

- new or unusual symptoms

- feelings of panic, such as dizziness, rapid breathing, or a racing heartbeat

- unable to work or function at home or at your job

- fears that you cannot control

- memories of a traumatic event

Your provider may refer you to a mental health care provider. You can talk to this professional about your feelings, what seems to make your stress better or worse, and why you think you are having this problem.

Depression

Sadness is a normal human emotion, but these feelings usually pass with a little time. **Depression** — also called "clinical depression" or a "depressive disorder" — is a mood disorder that causes distressing symptoms that affect how you feel, think, and handle daily activities, such as sleeping, eating, or working. To be diagnosed with depression, symptoms must be present most of the day, nearly every day for at least two weeks. Over 5% of Americans 12 years and older report being depressed and almost 10% of adults aged 40–59 (Figure 19).

Depression is a serious medical illness and an important public health issue. It can cause suffering for depressed individuals and can also have negative effects on their families and the communities in which they live. The economic burden of depression, including workplace costs, direct health care costs, and indirect costs to families is estimated to be over $200 billion annually.

Two of the most common forms of depression are:

- **Major depression** — having symptoms of depression most of the day, nearly every day for at least 2 weeks that interfere with your ability to work, sleep, study, eat, and enjoy life. An episode can occur only once in a person's lifetime, but more often, a person has several episodes.

- **Persistent depressive disorder** (dysthymia) — having symptoms of depression that last for at least 2 years. A person diagnosed with this form of depression may have episodes of major depression along with periods of less severe symptoms.

Some forms of depression are slightly different, or they may develop under unique circumstances, such as:

- **Perinatal or Postpartum Depression** is much more serious than the "baby blues" that many women experience after giving birth, when hormonal and physical changes and the new responsibility of caring for a newborn can be overwhelming. It is es-

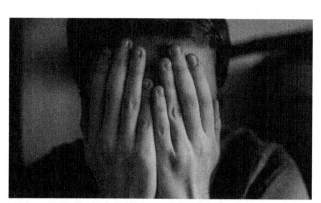

Figure 19. Depression is a serious condition.

timated that 10 to 15 percent of women experience postpartum depression after giving birth. Some women begin to see these mood changes during pregnancy, long before the birth of the child.

- **Bipolar disorder** is different from depression. The reason it is included in this list is because someone with bipolar disorder experiences episodes of extreme low moods (depression). But a person with bipolar disorder also experiences extreme high moods (called "mania").

- **Seasonal Affective Disorder (SAD)** is a type of depression that comes and goes with the seasons, typically starting in the late fall and early winter and going away during the spring and summer.

- **Psychotic Depression** occurs when a person has severe depression plus some form of psychosis, such as having disturbing false fixed beliefs (delusions) or hearing or seeing upsetting things that others cannot hear or see (hallucinations).

Some symptoms of depression include:

- Persistent sad, anxious, or "empty" mood
- Feelings of hopelessness or pessimism
- Feelings of guilt, worthlessness, or helplessness
- Loss of interest or pleasure in hobbies or activities
- Decreased energy, fatigue, or being "slowed down"
- Difficulty concentrating, remembering, or making decisions
- Difficulty sleeping, early-morning awakening, or oversleeping

- Appetite and/or weight changes
- Thoughts of death or suicide or suicide attempts
- Restlessness or irritability
- Aches or pains, headaches, cramps, or digestive problems without a clear physical cause and/or that do not ease even with treatment

Depression affects different people in different ways. Women have depression more often than men. Biological, lifecycle, and hormonal factors that are unique to women may be linked to their higher depression rate. Women with depression typically have symptoms of sadness, worthlessness, and guilt.

Men with depression are more likely to be very tired, irritable, and sometimes angry. They may lose interest in work or activities they once enjoyed, have sleep problems, and behave recklessly, including the misuse of drugs or alcohol. Many men do not recognize their depression and fail to seek help.

Older adults with depression may have less obvious symptoms, or they may be less likely to admit to feelings of sadness or grief. They are also more likely to have medical conditions, such as heart disease, which may cause or contribute to depression.

Younger children with depression may pretend to be sick, refuse to go to school, cling to a parent, or worry that a parent may die. Older children and teens with depression may get into trouble at school, sulk, and be irritable. Teens with depression may have symptoms of other disorders, such as anxiety, eating disorders, or substance abuse.

Depression Treatment

The first step in getting the right treatment is to visit a healthcare provider or mental health professional, such as a psychiatrist or psychologist. Your healthcare provider can do an exam, interview, and lab tests to rule out other health conditions that may have the same symptoms as depression. Once diagnosed, depression can be treated with medications, psychotherapy, or a combination of the two. If these treatments do not reduce symptoms, brain stimulation therapy may be another treatment option to explore.

Medication called antidepressants can work well to treat depression, many of which are designed to alter the levels of neurotransmitters (signaling chemicals) in the brain — essentially, they try to put your brain in a happier state. They can take 2 to 4 weeks to work and can have side effects (drowsiness, nausea, insomnia), but many side effects may lessen over time.

Psychotherapy helps by teaching new ways of thinking and behaving, and changing habits that may be contributing to depression. Therapy can help you understand and work through difficult relationships or situations that may be causing your depression or making it worse.

When medications and therapy are unsuccessful, **Brain Stimulation Therapies** (such as Electroconvulsive Therapy) are sometimes used. Brain stimulation therapies involve activating or inhibiting the brain directly with electricity. While these types of therapies are less frequently used than medication and psychotherapies, they hold promise for treating certain mental disorders that do not respond to other treatments.

In addition, people experiencing depression can add **self-help techniques** (Figure 20) they learn through research or via medical guidance. Some examples of self-help are improving diet, getting exercise, and making sure to seek out positive social interactions. Talking to people in your close social group, like friends and family, is a good idea and can help alleviate some of the burden

of depression. Being alone too much can have severe negative effects.

Major depression is one of the most common mental disorders in the United States. According to the World Health Organization (WHO; 2010), major depression also carries the heaviest burden of disability among mental and behavioral disorders. Specifically, major depression accounts for 3.7% of all US disability-adjusted life years (DALYs) and 8.3% of all US years lived with disability (YLDs).

Depression can become a significant problem if left untreated. If you are experiencing depression, or think you are, you can quickly find resources to help. Talk to your loved ones, a counselor, or make an appointment with your health care provider. Be honest with yourself if you recognize symptoms, and don't be embarrassed or assume the feelings will go away on their own. Seeking

Self Help with Depression	
Stick to your treatment plan	Don't skip psychotherapy sessions or appointments. Even if you're feeling well, don't skip your medications. If you stop, depression symptoms may come back, and you could also experience withdrawal-like symptoms. Recognize that it will take time to feel better.
Pay attention to warning signs	Work with your doctor or therapist to learn what might trigger your depression symptoms. Make a plan so that you know what to do if your symptoms get worse. Contact your doctor or therapist if you notice any changes in symptoms or how you feel. Ask relatives or friends to help watch for warning signs.
Avoid alcohol and recreational drugs	It may seem like alcohol or drugs lessen depression symptoms, but in the long run they generally worsen symptoms and make depression harder to treat. Talk with your doctor or therapist if you need help with alcohol or substance use.
Simplify your life	Cut back on obligations when possible, and set reasonable goals for yourself. Give yourself permission to do less when you feel down.
Don't become isolated	Try to participate in social activities, and get together with family or friends regularly. Support groups for people with depression can help you connect to others facing similar challenges and share experiences.
Structure your time	Plan your day. You may find it helps to make a list of daily tasks, use sticky notes as reminders or use a planner to stay organized.
Don't make important decisions when you're down	Avoid decision-making when you're feeling depressed, since you may not be thinking clearly.
Reach out to family and friends	Especially in times of crisis, to help you weather rough spells.
Get treatment at the earliest sign of a problem	To help prevent depression from worsening.
Consider getting long-term maintenance treatment	To help prevent a relapse of symptoms.

Figure 20. In addition to professional help, these tips can help you cope with depression.

help is the best strategy for yourself and for those you love.

In addition to seeking help or treatment, try to do things that you used to enjoy. Remember to go easy on yourself, give yourself some time to see improvements. Other things that may help include:

- Trying to be active and exercise

- Breaking up large tasks into small ones, set priorities, and do what you can as you can

- Spending time with other people and confide in a trusted friend or relative

Special Concern: Self-Injury and Suicide

Depression and forms of mental illness can sometimes feel overwhelming. Many people struggle with thoughts of suicide. The risk factors for suicidal behavior are complex. People of all genders, ages, and ethnicities can be at risk. Each suicide takes a substantial toll on individuals, families, and communities far beyond what the victim could anticipate. In the past, suicide was addressed by providing mental health services to people who were already experiencing or showing signs of suicidal thoughts or behavior. But we now understand that we have to address many problems before they get too far and increase access to as many resources as possible to avoid this risk. As with many other illnesses and diseases that have the potential to end badly, suicide is preventable.

Most suicidal individuals give **warning signs** or signals of their intentions. The best way to prevent suicide is to recognize these warning signs and know how to respond if you spot them. Major warning signs for suicide include:

- Talking about killing or harming oneself

- Talking or writing a lot about death or dying

- Increasing substance use

- Changes in mood

- Big changes in eating or sleeping patterns

- Seeking out things that could be used in a suicide attempt, such as weapons and drugs

- Loss of interest in day-to-day activities

- Neglecting his or her appearance and hygiene

- Persistent sad, anxious, or "empty" mood

- Feelings of hopelessness or pessimism

- Postponing important life decisions until you feel better — discuss decisions with others who know you well.

- Avoiding self-medication with alcohol or with drugs not prescribed for you

The resources at the end of this chapter offer more information on how to get help with depression.

- Feelings of guilt, worthlessness, or helplessness

- Loss of interest or pleasure in hobbies or activities

- Decreased energy, fatigue, or being "slowed down"

- Difficulty concentrating or making decisions

- Difficulty sleeping, early-morning awakening, or oversleeping

- Appetite and/or weight changes

- Thoughts of death or suicide or suicide attempts

- Restlessness or irritability

- Aches or pains, headaches, cramps, or digestive problems without a clear physical cause and/or that do not ease even with treatment.

A more subtle but equally dangerous warning sign of suicide is hopelessness. Studies have found that hopelessness is a strong predictor of suicide. People who feel hopeless may talk about "unbearable" feelings, predict a bleak future, and state that they have nothing to look forward to. These signals are even more dangerous if the person has a mood disorder, such as depression or bipolar disorder, suffers from alcohol dependence, has previously attempted suicide, or has a family history of suicide.

If you believe that a friend or family member is suicidal, you can play a role prevention by pointing out the alternatives, showing that you care, and getting a doctor or psychologist involved. If the threat is immanent, do not hesitate to call 911. If the threat is not immanent, let the friend express feelings, be cautious of using judgmental language, and encourage them to seek professional help.

The resources at the end of this chapter offer more information and assistance.

Special Concern: Violence

Violence and abuse can take on many forms — physical, emotional, and sexual. It can happen to anyone by anyone and can be a significant form of stress. One of the most common is **intimate partner violence** (IPV). In fact, one in every four women and one in every nine men are victims of either sexual violence, physical abuse, and/or stalking by an intimate partner with a negative impact, such as fear, physical injury, or needing to call for assistance. Nearly 23 million women and 1.7 million men have been victims of rape or attempted rape at some point in their lives.

The term "intimate partner violence" describes physical, sexual, or psychological harm by a current or former partner or spouse. This type of violence can occur among heterosexual or same-sex couples and does not require sexual intimacy.

Persons with certain risk factors are more likely to become perpetrators or victims of intimate partner violence. Those risk factors contribute to IPV but might not be direct causes. Not everyone who is identified as "at risk" becomes involved in violence. Some risk factors for IPV victimization and perpetration are the same, while others are associated with one another. For example, childhood physical or sexual victimization is a risk factor for future IPV perpetration and victimization. A combination of individual, relational, community, and societal factors contribute to the risk of becoming an IPV perpetrator or victim. Stress can increase the risk and side effects of violence.

Being abusive is not a clear-cut issue of problems with anger management. Abuse is about power. Understanding the multilevel intersecting factors below that contribute to abuse can help you identify various opportunities for prevention. People experiencing these risk factors are statistically more likely to be the perpetrators of abuse. It's not a guarantee of that behavior, but just as other health risks disproportionately affect people (disparities), so does abuse.

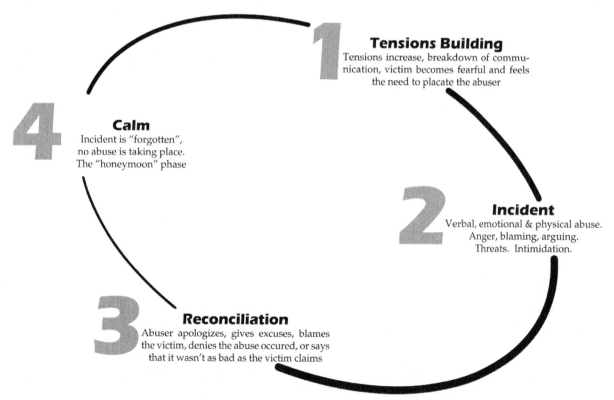

Cycle of Abuse

1 Tensions Building
Tensions increase, breakdown of communication, victim becomes fearful and feels the need to placate the abuser

2 Incident
Verbal, emotional & physical abuse. Anger, blaming, arguing. Threats. Intimidation.

3 Reconciliation
Abuser apologizes, gives excuses, blames the victim, denies the abuse occured, or says that it wasn't as bad as the victim claims

4 Calm
Incident is "forgotten", no abuse is taking place. The "honeymoon" phase

Figure 21. The cycle of abuse.

Individual Risk Factors

- Low self-esteem
- Depression
- Anger and hostility
- Low income
- Low academic achievement
- Young age
- Heavy alcohol and drug use
- Unemployment
- Prior history of being physically abusive
- Antisocial personality traits
- Borderline personality traits
- Stress
- Perpetrating psychological aggression
- Aggressive or delinquent behavior as a youth
- Being isolated from other people
- Emotional dependence and insecurity
- Belief in strict gender roles (e.g., male dominance and aggression in relationships)
- Desire for power and control in relationships
- Being a victim of physical or psychological abuse (one of the strongest predictors of perpetration)
- History of experiencing poor parenting as a child
- History of experiencing physical discipline as a child

Relationship Factors

- Marital conflict-fights, tension, and other struggles
- Marital instability-divorces or separations
- Economic stress
- Dominance and control of the relationship by one partner over the other
- Unhealthy family relationships and interactions

Community Factors

- Poverty and associated factors (e.g., overcrowding)
- Low social capital — lack of institutions, relationships, and norms that shape a community's social interactions
- Weak community sanctions against IPV (e.g., unwillingness of neighbors to intervene in situations where they witness violence)

Societal Factors

- Traditional gender norms (e.g., women should stay at home, not enter workforce, and be submissive; men support the family and make the decisions)

It can also be important to recognize signs of abuse in victims. People experiencing any form of abuse often don't realize it themselves or attempt to hide it from friends out of fear for their safety or fear of judgment. Take a look at some of the warning signs.

People who are being abused may:

- Seem afraid or anxious to please their partner
- Go along with everything their partner says and does
- Check in often with their partner to report where they are and what they're doing
- Receive frequent, harassing phone calls from their partner
- Talk about their partner's temper, jealousy, or possessiveness

People who are being physically abused may:

- Have frequent injuries, with the excuse of "accidents"
- Frequently miss work, school, or social occasions, without explanation
- Dress in clothing designed to hide bruises or scars (e.g. wearing long sleeves in the summer or sunglasses indoors)

People who are being isolated by their abuser may:

- Be restricted from seeing family and friends
- Rarely go out in public without their partner
- Have limited access to money, credit cards, or the car

People who are being abused may:

- Have very low self-esteem, even if they used to be confident
- Show major personality changes (e.g. an outgoing person becomes withdrawn)
- Be depressed, anxious, or suicidal

The impact of violence on an individual's health can be severe. In addition to the immediate injuries from an assault, the person may suffer from chronic pain, gastrointestinal disorders, psychosomatic symptoms, and eating problems, often from the stress of a difficult situation. Although psychological abuse is often considered less severe than physical violence, all forms of intimate partner violence can have devastating physical and emotional health effects. Domestic violence, for example, is associated with mental health problems such as anxiety, post-traumatic stress disorder, and depression. Women who are abused suffer an increased risk of unplanned or early pregnancies and sexually transmitted diseases, including HIV/AIDS. As trauma victims, they are also at an increased risk of substance abuse.

Women are particularly vulnerable to attacks when pregnant, and thus may more often experience medical difficulties in their pregnancies. Recent research has called for increased study of pregnancy-associated deaths. Women who are abused are more likely to have a history of sexually transmitted disease infections, vaginal and cervical infections, kidney infections and bleeding during pregnancy, all of which are risk factors for pregnant women. Abused women are more likely to delay prenatal care and are less likely to receive antenatal care. In fact, partner abuse may be a larger risk than other common gestational health concerns, such as hypertension and diabetes.

Anyone can abuse others. They come from all groups, all cultures, all religions, all economic levels, and all backgrounds. They can be your neighbor, your pastor, your friend, your child's teacher, a relative, a coworker — anyone. It is important to note that the majority of abusers are only violent with their current or past intimate partners. One study found 90% of abusers do not have criminal records and abusers are generally law-abiding outside the home.

There is no one typical, detectable personality of an abuser. However, they do often display common characteristics:

- An abuser often denies the existence or minimizes the seriousness of the violence and its effect on the victim and other family members.
- An abuser objectifies the victim and often sees them as their property or sexual objects.
- An abuser has low self-esteem and feels powerless and ineffective in the world. He or she may appear successful, but internally, they feel inadequate.
- An abuser externalizes the causes of their behavior. They blame their violence on circumstances such as stress, their partner's behavior, a "bad day," on alcohol, drugs, or other factors.
- An abuser may be pleasant and charming between periods of violence and is often seen as a "nice person" to others outside the relationship.

Red flags and warning signs of an abuser include but are not limited to:

- Extreme jealousy
- Possessiveness
- Unpredictability
- A bad temper
- Cruelty to animals
- Verbal abuse
- Extremely controlling behavior
- Antiquated beliefs about roles of women and men in relationships
- Forced sex or disregard of their partner's unwillingness to have sex
- Sabotage of birth control methods or refusal to honor agreed upon methods
- Blaming the victim for anything bad that happens
- Sabotage or obstruction of the victim's ability to work or attend school
- Controls all the finances
- Abuse of other family members, children or pets

- Accusations of the victim flirting with others or having an affair

- Control of what the victim wears and how they act

- Demeaning the victim either privately or publicly

- Embarrassment or humiliation of the victim in front of others

- Harassment of the victim at work

Support and Prevention of Violence

One of the things you can do if you suspect someone you know is a victim of abuse is to maintain contact with that person. Abusers often try separating their victims from friends and family, making them feel like they have no support network. Make sure you are supportive — it won't help to try and make someone feel guilty or bad if they don't leave the relationship. There are many factors that can make a victim return to an abuser multiple times. Many victims are told that if they attempt to leave their abuser they will be killed, making any attempt to leave a potential for increased violence. The important thing is that you remain available for your friend or family member. However, if you know someone may be in immediate physical danger, call 911.

You can take steps to help. Each of us has the power to reach out to someone we love and tell them that abuse is not their fault. Love shouldn't hurt. And safety is possible. Visit the resources at the end of this chapter for more advice and assistance.

Benefits of Stress Management

The risks of not managing stress should be apparent by now, but what about the benefits? Research suggests that individuals who learn to manage stress do much more than just avoid disease, particularly in comparison to people who haven't learned to manage it. Exercise, healthy eating, relaxation, positive thinking, etc., all help to improve our overall wellness. Some of the psychological and physiological benefits include:

Psychological Benefits

- Improved self esteem
- Improved self confidence
- Reduced anxiety levels
- Reduced risk of depression
- Less reliance on alcohol
- Improved coping skills
- Reduced anger levels

- Improved relationships
- Greater optimism
- Greater efficiency at work
- Improved concentration and memory
- Increased feeling of control
- Improved decision making
- Reduction in mood swings

Physiological Benefits

- Lower blood pressure
- Reduced risk of heart attack and stroke
- Reduced osteoporosis risk
- Lower risk for certain cancers
- Better immune system
- Fewer colds and flu
- Lower risk of type II diabetes

- Reduced risk of intestinal problems
- Higher energy levels
- Improved sleep pattern
- Improved cholesterol profile
- Reduced back pain
- Reduced muscle tension

Assessing Your Stress

A good plan for managing stress begins with assessing your stress level and anticipated stressors in your life, such as work, home, and recent stress events. There are a variety of tools for assessing stress, many of which are best used with the aid of an expert. If you use one on your own and are aware that you may be suffering from stress, it's a good idea to talk with someone who knows how to help.

A great way to assess stress is with the **Perceived Stress Scale**. The Perceived Stress Scale (PSS) is a classic stress assessment instrument. We've learned in this chapter that stress and our ability to cope with it is relative more to our perception of the stressor than the stressor itself. Understanding how you perceive stress can help you determine your risk for negative, health-related impacts and take appropriate strategies to manage it.

The tool, while originally developed in 1983, remains a popular choice for helping us understand how different situations affect our feelings and our perceived stress. The questions in this scale ask about your feelings and thoughts during the last month. In each case, you will be asked to indicate how often you felt or thought a certain way. Although some of the questions are similar, there are differences between them and you should treat each one as a separate question. The best approach is to answer fairly quickly. That is, don't try to count up the number of times you felt a particular way — rather indicate the alternative that seems like a reasonable estimate.

The PSS is interesting and relevant because your perception of what is happening in your life is most important. Consider the idea that two individuals could have the exact same events and experiences in their lives for the past month. Depending on their perception, their total score on the PSS could put one of those individuals in the low stress category and put the second person in the high stress category.

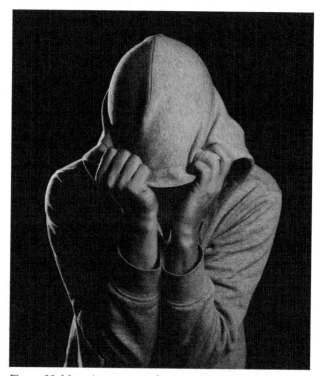

Figure 22. Managing stress can eliminate overwhelming moments.

Managing Your Stress

There are many techniques to effectively manage your stress and limit its negative effects, from preventative measures to reduce stress before it occurs to active stress management techniques that are useful during and after stress experiences. First, let's look at some effective tools to manage stress before it happens.

Time Management

There never seems to be enough hours in the day to get everything done. Between work, school, chores, errands, and family commitments, you could fill 24 hours with tasks. **Time management** becomes increasingly important when our workload is heavy. It enables you to arrange your schedule for many of the things you want and need to do and to decide which things are urgent and which can wait. Learning how to manage your time, activities, and commitments can be hard. But doing so can make your life easier, less stressful, and more meaningful.

- When you manage your time, you decide which tasks and activities are most important to you. Knowing what's important helps you decide how best to spend your time.

- There are three parts to time management: prioritize tasks and activities, control procrastination, and manage commitments.

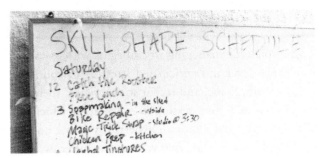

Figure 23. Manage your time to avoid stressful situations.

Prioritize Tasks

You're sitting at the kitchen table staring at the screen of your laptop. You know this paper won't write itself, but you become distracted by the large pile of laundry sitting in the basket a few feet away. You tell yourself you'll be able to concentrate better if the clothes get folded, so you tackle those. You head back toward the table but notice that there are several dishes in the sink, so you tackle those. Finally, you sit back down to get to work. You end up spending 30 minutes on social media and watching online videos of cats. The paper is due tomorrow.

We often become overwhelmed because we have too many tasks and no plan for how to approach them. Often we complete things that are less urgent because they are less difficult and end up pushing ourselves into a stressful situation. Start by making a list of all your tasks and activities for the day or week. Then rate these tasks by how important or urgent they are.

One method for doing this is offered by

Steven Covey in his book *The 7 Habits of Highly Effective People*. Covey's method focuses on breaking tasks into categories based on importance and urgency (Figure 31). Consider the importance, urgency, and "due date".

Quadrant 1 should be your highest priority, followed by quadrant 2. These get first priority because they are important. Quadrants 3 and 4 are typically the tasks that draw our time away from more meaningful tasks. Some of them are quite fun and can offer a nice break, but we don't want to spend too much time there until the first two quadrants have been cleared. You may have some tasks from quadrants 3 and 4 in your schedule with the majority being from quadrants 1 and 2.

	Urgent	**Non-Urgent**
Important	Quadrant 1: Examples: Things due today or tomorrow, dealing with emergencies or crises	Quadrant 2: Examples: Long-term projects, planning ahead, studying in advance, getting started early
Not Important	Quadrant 3: Examples: Interruptions, distractions, fun events that come up, social invitations	Quadrant 4: Examples: Time wasters, busy work, procrastination activities, aimless internet browsing

Figure 24. Covey's task prioritizer.

ABC Analysis

A technique that has been used in business management for a long time is the categorization of large data into groups. These groups are often marked A, B, and C — hence the name. Activities are ranked by these general criteria (Figure 32):

Each group is then rank-ordered by priority. To further refine the prioritization, some individuals choose to then force-rank all "B" items as either "A" or "C". ABC analysis can incorporate more than three groups.

"A" Status — "Must Do"	High priority, very important, critical items, with close deadlines or high level of importance to them
"B" Status — "Should Do"	Medium priority, quite important over time, not as critical as "A" items, but still important to spend time doing
"C" Status — "Nice to Do"	Low priority at this time, low consequences if left undone at this moment

Figure 25. ABC analysis.

Control Procrastination

Sure, somewhere in this world is someone who never procrastinates on a task. They see something that needs to be done and they're on top of it. Why put off until tomorrow what you can do today? Isn't that the saying? But most of us struggle with procrastination to some degree. When it adds stress to our lives, it becomes a problem — procrastination becomes one of the stressors we have to handle. Fortunately there are some ways to do that. The Academic Success Center at Oregon State University offers the following tips:

- Make a plan. Set goals and make use of a weekly schedule and a to-do list. These can keep you organized and help you stay committed to completing your tasks.

- Find motivation. Think of one or two good reasons for getting tasks done early, and write those reasons down. We often allow ourselves to procrastinate because we think "I can do this later." When that thought comes up, make sure you have an answer for why it's important to complete the task now.

- Make it easier on yourself. Schedule a date and time for starting your task, be specific about what you will accomplish, and find a location that is conducive to accomplishing your task.

- Identify your procrastination tendencies and your excuses. If you know that cleaning is a technique you use to procrastinate from homework, plan ahead for this. Set aside time for each task, pay attention when you get distracted, and redirect yourself to the reasons you want to complete the task now.

- Learn to say "no" when distractions arise. There will always be things that threaten to interrupt your productivity. Saying "no" to interruptions or distractions can keep you on track as you complete your task.

- Be patient. Procrastination is something you work to overcome over time by developing better habits. There will be areas of your life and times during the term when it will be harder to overcome this challenge. Recognize when you are making positive choices, and reward your successes.

Cognitive Strategies for Managing Stress

We've all uttered defeatist phrases that, rather than offering a solution, make us feel worse or even encourage us to give up on a resolution.

"I can't do it."

"It will never work."

"I'm lousy at this."

We often don't realize how significantly our language to ourselves can impact our emotions and our behaviors, and ultimately our level of stress. We can, however, change the way we talk to ourselves utilizing **cognitive strategies** to help us manage our stress.

Therapists teach cognitive strategies to their clients to encourage them to shift negative self-talk to talk which is positive, more likely to reduce stress and enable individuals to better manage their lives. They do this through a process of recognition, restructuring, and refocusing.

Step One: Recognize Negative Thoughts

There are some common forms of **negative thinking**. These include:

Filtering — This occurs when you highlight the negative parts of a situation and filter out all of the positive ones. For example, you got stuck in heavy traffic on your way home from work. You took a detour on some side streets to avoid it, stopped at a great market you'd never been to, and managed to pick up something unique for dinner. You were only 15 minutes later getting home than you had planned. That night at dinner while everyone is happy with the food, you focus only on being late and getting stuck in traffic, planning to leave work on time the next day.

Personalizing — You automatically blame yourself when something bad happens. For example, a friend you haven't seen in a while comes into town and doesn't call you. You assume it's because he doesn't like you and doesn't want to see you.

Catastrophizing — You automatically anticipate the worst. You get a "C" on an exam the first week of the term and just know that the class will be too difficult and you will fail.

Polarizing — Things are either black or white, good or bad, right or wrong. If you aren't perfect, you're a failure.

Step Two: Restructure Your Thoughts

When you hear the negative self-talk, rephrase it. Here are some good examples:

Negative Self-Talk	Positive Thinking
I've never done it before.	It's an opportunity to learn something new.
It's too complicated.	I'll tackle it from a different angle.
I don't have the resources.	Necessity is the mother of invention.
I'm too lazy to get this done.	I wasn't able to fit it into my schedule, but I can re-examine some priorities.
There's no way it will work.	I can try to make it work.
It's too radical a change.	Let's take a chance.
No one bothers to communicate with me.	I'll see if I can open the channels of communication.
I'm not going to get any better at this.	I'll give it another try.

Figure 26. Use positive self-talk to encourage positive stress management.

Step 3: Refocusing On the Present

When you are feeling overwhelmed, it may be because you are getting bogged down with too many things at once. Your future responsibilities are entering your present. Take time to set priorities and determine what needs to be done now, handled today or this week. Focus on the moment. Competitive athletes often have periods of "mental blocks." Gymnasts, for example, who have performed a particular skill many times will suddenly start freezing up. They mount the bars or the beam and when they try to begin a skill, they stop, over and over again. Sports psychologists have them break each move into steps and talk their way through each skill. This keeps them focused on what they are supposed to be doing at that moment, not on the dismount that is six skills in the future. Long-term goals are fine, but you cannot complete them if you ignore the little steps in life along the way.

We've talked a lot about setting SMART goals. This applies to nearly everything in life. Are you being realistic about what you can accomplish? Are you breaking goals into short-term and long-term? For example, it's great to have a goal to be a columnist for *The New York Times* and win a Pulitzer Prize for journalism. First you need to write a great article for the school newspaper, pass your journalism class, take several more, do well, get a degree, and a job at a local paper, and so on. Very few people win a Pulitzer Prize. You might, but it isn't a particularly realistic thing to focus on and shouldn't be a source of pressure. It may give you the tendency to see small setbacks as goal-threatening rather than opportunities to learn.

ABCDE Model for Effective Thought Remodeling

Albert Ellis, developer of Rational Emotive Behavior Therapy (REBT), devised the **ABCDE model** (Figure 27) to provide a way for people to examine their internal processes by learning to break down events into clear steps. The idea is to take the mystery out of the situation.

We are responsible for the images and thoughts in our minds and the emotions they generate. We can work ourselves into a frenzy over a situation, giving ourselves a stomachache or we can attach new meanings and interpretations that help us deal with something positively.

This gives us power over our emotions. We can do this with five steps, ABCDE.

For example and practice, think about a recent event that resulted in a strong emotional reaction. This should be an event where you would wish you had responded differently. Consider each of the five steps of the ABCDE model and write down your own experience each step of the way.

"A" — Adversity or Activating Event
Consider the event that triggered the emotional

response in you, whatever happened right before you began feeling an emotion such as anxiety, sadness, or anger. When you become more mindfully aware of events that typically trigger strong emotional responses, you can learn to watch out for these events in the future and be better prepared to deal with them more effectively.

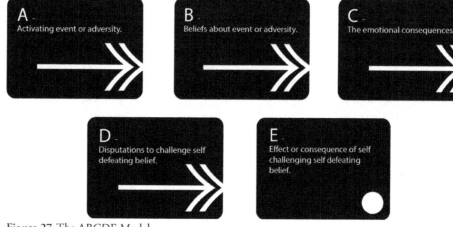

Figure 27. The ABCDE Model.

Example: A friend asks you if he can borrow your car again.

"B" — Beliefs

We all try to establish meaning for why something occurs. For the moment, avoid labeling your beliefs as "right" or "wrong" and simply recognize them. We often have irrational beliefs that create maladaptive emotional responses and generate problems. A belief is generally "irrational" when it lacks clear evidence, is overgeneralized, or is otherwise based on faulty reasoning.

Example: "He just hangs out with me to use my car."

"C" — Consequences

Consequences are more than just the outcome of the event. They can take behavioral and emotional forms. Sometimes we observe them externally, such as noticing that another person is angry with us or ignoring us. Other times, consequences are internal, such as experiencing anxiety or sadness.

Example: Regret, disappointment, and withdrawal from the friend. Refusal to hang out with the friend that borrows your car.

"D" — Disputing

This step involves actively disputing harmful belief systems through mindfully examining, questioning, and challenging them. First, locate the harmful beliefs in your stream of consciousness in such a way that you can examine them carefully. Then prepare to enter the "disputation phase" by asking yourself the following six questions:

- Does this belief fit with reality?

- Does this belief support the achievement of reasonable/constructive interests and goals?

- Does this belief help foster positive/healthy relationships?

- Does this belief make you feel better or worse?

- Does this belief seem reasonable and logical given the context in which it occurred?

- Is this belief generally detrimental or generally helpful?

These questions can help you separate realistic from dysfunctional thinking. Through mindfully examining your beliefs in this way, you are also increasing your own self-awareness and insight into the ways that you tend to think and behave.

Example:

- No, there are plenty of times when we've hung out and he hasn't asked to use my car.

- No, this belief actually defeats my interest in overcoming the anxiety related to his requests.

- No, my emotional reaction only served to harm the friendship.

- No, the belief that he's using me makes me feel weak and gullible.

- No, my friend really does need a car at times and can't afford one.

- In this case, it's generally detrimental. It only costs time and emotional energy, with no beneficial return.

"E" — Effects

Notice the effects that result from actively examining and disputing faulty thinking. Once you become realistically aware of your emotionally charged beliefs about a situation, you can begin to create adjust your line of thinking based upon more rational and reasonable beliefs.

Example: I know he's been down on his luck, and by using my car he may be able to improve his situation.

Keep in mind that the ABCDE model will not set aside normal, healthy emotions, such as appropriate loss, regret, realistic fears, or frustration. Not all emotions need to be changed. If your friend never calls you except when he wants the car, does not thank you, does not pitch in for gas, and does not respect your vehicle, your response might be appropriate and it may teach you to set healthy boundaries. Quite often, emotions are incredibly valuable and useful tools that are providing you with important information about the situation. Other times, when emotional responses are causing unnecessary suffering or are based in faulty thinking, mindfully applying the ABCDE model can shed light on a situation where you feel struck.

Problem-Solving Skills

You can't solve a problem successfully until you understand it. We can get so overwhelmed with a particular problem that we choose to just ignore it or worry over it, rather than try to fix it. Take time to analyze the problem. Write down a brief description of the problem you want to solve. Then ask yourself these questions:

- What is happening?

- Where and when is it happening?

- Is it happening around certain people or in specific situations?

- How do you feel about it?

Be specific and focus on issues rather than on whose fault it is. Now consider its severity and how much time you need to solve it realistically:

- Is the problem really that big? Would others think so?

- Will this matter in two years?

- Would solving it improve your life?

- Do you have control over any aspect of the situation?

You can't change everything. Focus on issues you can realistically change and that will improve your level of stress. Pick your battles.

Think about solutions, of all the ways you might solve your problem. Now isn't the time to judge whether one solution is better than another. Recall past problems that were similar that you were able to solve. Could a similar solution work for this problem, too? Don't be afraid to ask others for advice, particularly those that may be knowledgeable in the area.

If you're still having trouble, maybe your problem is too complicated. Break the problem down into smaller parts you can more easily handle. Then, brainstorm some ideas for taking on each part. Which has the most potential? Ask yourself:

- Do I realistically think it will solve the problem?

- How will using this solution make me feel in the end?

- What are the possible positive and negative consequences of this path?

Take another couple of minutes to think through your decision. Ask yourself:

- Do I have the resources and the drive to carry out this plan? Can I complete it?

- Will it create any new problems?

- What might go wrong? Can I adjust the plan to prepare for it?

A good long-term solution may temporarily create new problems. That doesn't mean you should give up the plan, just that you need to be ready to make adjustments or even switch to a plan B.

Healthy Relationships and Social Support

Hugs, kisses, and caring, supportive conversations are key ingredients of our close relationships. Scientists are finding that our links to others can have powerful effects on our health. Whether with romantic partners, family, friends, neighbors, or others, social connections can influence our biology and well-being.

Wide-ranging research suggests that strong social ties are linked to a longer life. In contrast, loneliness and social isolation are linked to poorer health, depression, and increased risk of early death.

Studies have found that having a variety of social relationships may help reduce stress and heart-related risks. Such connections might improve your ability to fight off germs or give you a more positive outlook on life. Physical contact — from hand-holding to sex — can trigger release of hormones and brain chemicals that not only make us feel great and reduce stress but also have other biological benefits.

When maintaining a relationship, any behavior that is positive and promotes deepening trust and closeness between people is a pro-social maintenance behavior. The more pro-social behaviors evident in a relationship, the more likely for strong bonds to be formed, and the relationship to prosper and continue. Positivity, openness, task sharing, supportiveness, humor, and working together are all examples of pro-social behavior (Figure 28).

Sometimes, our social bonds feel more like bondage. We can get into patterns of disrespectfulness, impatience, intolerance, being judgmental and using language and behavior toward each other that adds to our stress. There are ways that we can improve the positive aspects of our relationships starting with how we behave within our social networks, whether it is to treat those around you more respectfully or react to the anti-social behavior of others in a productive way. We've all heard the golden rule — treat others the way you want to be treated. There are many healthy ways to do this and, hopefully, reap the benefits of pro-social behavior in return.

Nurture Your Friendships	
Be kind	This most-basic behavior, emphasized during childhood, remains the core of successful, adult relationships. Think of friendship as an emotional bank account. Every act of kindness and every expression of gratitude are deposits into this account, while criticism and negativity draw down the account.
Listen up	Ask what's going on in your friends' lives. Let the other person know you are paying close attention through eye contact, body language and occasional brief comments such as, "That sounds fun." When friends share details of hard times or difficult experiences, be empathetic, but don't give advice unless your friends ask for it.
Open up	Build intimacy with your friends by opening up about yourself. Being willing to disclose personal experiences and concerns shows that your friend holds a special place in your life, and deepens your connection.
Show that you can be trusted	Being responsible, reliable and dependable is key to forming strong friendships. Keep your engagements and arrive on time. Follow through on commitments you've made to your friends. When your friends share confidential information, keep it private.
Make yourself available	Building a close friendship takes time — together. Make an effort to see new friends regularly, and to check in with them in between meet-ups. You may feel awkward the first few times you talk on the phone or get together, but this feeling is likely to pass as you get more comfortable with each other.
Manage your nerves with mindfulness	You may find yourself imagining the worst of social situations, and feel tempted to stay home. Use mindfulness exercises to reshape your thinking. Each time you imagine the worst, pay attention to how often the embarrassing situations you're afraid of actually take place. You may notice that the scenarios you fear usually don't happen. When embarrassing situations do happen, remind yourself that your feelings will pass, and you can handle them until they do. Yoga and other mind-body relaxation practices also may reduce anxiety and help you face situations that make you feel nervous.

Figure 28. Nurturing friendships ensures you have a social support system when you need it and boosts your self-confidence.

Speaking Up with Respect

To ensure that a relationship can be a healthy one, individuals need to be able to speak to one another honestly and assertively.

Assertiveness is the quality of being self-assured and confident without being aggressive. In the field of psychology and psychotherapy, this is a learnable skill and mode of communication. Being appropriately assertive affirms the person's rights or point of view without either threatening the rights of another (assuming a position of dominance) or submissively permitting another to ignore or deny your rights or point of view.

Assertiveness is based on mutual respect. This makes it an effective and diplomatic communication style. Being assertive shows that you respect yourself because you're willing to stand up for your interests and express your thoughts and feelings. It also shows that you're aware of and respect the rights of others and are willing to work as a team and solve problems together. It is direct but polite — this is the way you want people to speak to you.

There are two forms of communication that can have a negative impact on our relationships, depending on the situation — passive communication and aggressive communication. **Passive communication**, or passive behavior, is not always a bad thing. Sometimes people are shy and or have a tendency to just go with the flow, let the opinions and ideas of others take precedence over their own. There is a time to listen to others who may be more experienced or knowledgeable and take a back seat, allowing others to shine. But when you do it all the time, people can discount your opinions or disregard your wants and needs. It is easy to feel manipulated, angry, even emotionally abused — in other words, stressed.

Aggressive communication or behavior does not respect the personal boundaries of others and thus is liable to harm others while trying to influence them. If your style is aggressive, you may come across as a bully who disregards the needs, feelings, and opinions of others. You may appear self-righteous or superior — like a know-it-all. Very aggressive people humiliate and intimidate others and may even be physically threatening. You may think that being aggressive gets you what you want, and it might for a time, but it comes at a cost. Aggression undercuts trust and mutual respect. Others may come to resent you, leading them to avoid or oppose you.

When dealing with individuals who communicate aggressively. The following tips can help:

Follow the golden rule when you communicate with them. If you speak to them assertively (not passively or aggressively) they may notice that their own behavior is inappropriate. Don't stoop to their level.

Be careful not to take it personally. Aggressive individuals are often this way with everyone. If you personalize it, you may overreact and exacerbate the problem with anger or sadness.

Speak up. Don't be afraid to express your opinion, calmly.

Disengage when necessary. If they will not allow you to express your opinion or they are speaking in a disrespectful manner, let them know. Speak to them when they're ready to listen and have a mature exchange.

Respond with logic rather than emotion. Aggressive communication is often about dominance more than reasoning. Presenting logic and being constructive can make the lack of reasoning apparent and diffuse the situation.

Focus on how to solve the problem rather than whose fault it is. Again, this is about dominance and winning. Assertive communication deals with respect and resolution rather than assignment of blame.

Finding Supportive People

Whenever possible, it is important to surround yourself with supportive, positive people who respect you and your goals. Supportive people make you feel good about yourself because they sincerely care about your well-being. They are also understanding of your experiences. It's a good idea, for example, to make friends with people who are in college with you, because they can understand your time allowances and the goal you are working toward. You can find new friends in your classrooms and by doing things like joining clubs. Shared hobbies are a great way enhance your social circles, and people who share your interests are likelier to be as excited and supportive of your successes as you are.

Investing In Your Loved Ones

Making time for the people who care for you is important to your overall happiness and can reduce stress. By doing so, you give back to your community and you remind yourself that you have people who care about your goals and your well-being. This can seem hard to do if you are juggling college classes and work, but taking a little time to reinvest and recharge is worth it. Your family and friends can be an important support system and can need support from you as well. Strong, mutual, pro-social relationships can help lessen your stress and make many difficult situations feel worth it.

Spiritual Wellness

Spirituality means more than a belief in God. There are many different religions and belief systems that invest in the idea of a higher power. This higher power can mean many different things to different people. But, many of the habits of people that consider themselves as spiritual can be good for our health.

Meditation and prayer often take on similar forms — they involve internal reflection and release. For people who pray, it is often because they've taken the opportunity to be thankful, look for support or strength, consider the world and people around them, and release their problems to a higher power. In other words, they de-stress! You do not have to believe in a higher power to embrace your spiritual side. Taking time to meditate, reflect, and release negative energy out into the universe can be a positive, relaxing experience.

For many people, part of spirituality is a larger consideration for the environment and the community. Often, taking time to volunteer at a homeless shelter, planting trees, or simply helping out your neighbor can make you feel good about your purpose in life. That's a large part of what it means to be spiritual — identifying a sense of purpose.

Embrace your spiritual side in whatever form that takes. You'll enjoy a more relaxed, grateful, and reflective attitude on the people and world around you. Emphasizing the role of spiritual wellness in your life can help improve your self-esteem, give meaning to the activities you choose, and help you foster positive relationships.

Active Stress Management Techniques

The term has just begun and the pace is already picking up. It's your last few classes before transferring to a four-year university and you want that transcript to be pristine. The nursing program only takes students with a 4.0 and you have Biology this term — ugh! Your tendency might be to forget everything else in your life but that biology class. However, let's look at some active techniques that can be used to manage stress while it is happening (Figure 29).

Self Care Tips	
Avoid drugs and alcohol	They may seem to be a temporary fix to feel better, but in the long run drugs and alcohol can create more problems and add to your stress—instead of taking it away.
Find support	Seek help from a partner, family member, friend, counselor, doctor, or clergyperson. Having someone with a sympathetic, listening ear and sharing about your problems and stress really can lighten the burden.
Connect socially	After a stressful event, it is easy isolate yourself. Make sure that you are spending time with loved ones. Consider planning fun activities with your partner, children, or friends.
Take care of yourself	Eat a healthy, well-balanced diet. Exercise regularly. Get plenty of sleep. Give yourself a break if you feel stressed out—for example, treat yourself to a therapeutic massage. Maintain a normal routine
Stay active	You can take your mind off your problems with activities like helping a neighbor, volunteering in the community, and taking the dog on a long walk. These can be positive ways to cope with stressful feelings.

Figure 29. Tips for practicing good self care.

Physical Activity

This text has devoted many pages to the merits of physical exercise, from contributing to a healthy body composition to avoiding disease. But it is also vital for your

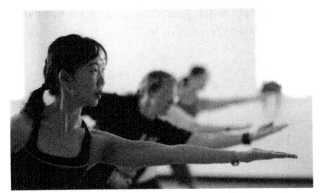

Figure 30. Meditation and yoga are just two techniques to improve stress management.

Nutrition

It may sound strange, but the foods we eat can impact our stress level (Figure 31). No, not just the three energy drinks you consumed that now have you anxious and jittery. The bag of potato chips that you hurriedly chased down with the sugary soda for lunch the last few days on your lunch break are impacting your stress as well. Worry and overwork can lead to unhealthy lifestyle habits, which causes more stress, leading to a very harmful cycle. When you are facing a very tight deadline at work or school, you might make poor choices about what to eat, relying on sugar and caffeine to get you through the day.

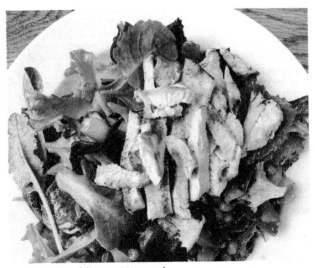

Figure 31. Healthy nutrition can boost your energy.

mental health and can reduce stress. Studies suggest that it is very effective at reducing fatigue, improving alertness and concentration, improving sleep, elevating and stabilizing mood, enhancing self-esteem, and enhancing overall cognitive function (Figure 30).

We've learned a lot about the body's reaction to stress. Exercise and other physical activities produce endorphins — chemicals in the brain that act as natural painkillers — which in turn can reduce stress. It also gives us energy. When we are stressed, we often feel a sense of fatigue and that burst of energy may be just what we need to rally our internal resources.

And, let's not forget that illness is a stressor, maybe one of the largest ones. When we stay healthy and keep our hearts pumping efficiently, we reduce our risk of chronic illnesses that can lead to chronic stress.

Unfortunately, these food choices can create more stress in the long run, as well as other problems. Below is a list of common bad habits people sometimes indulge in when overwhelmed and worried:

- Drinking Too Much Caffeine — You may find yourself drinking several cups of coffee, soda, or energy drinks.

- Eating Unhealthy Foods — Increased levels of cortisol make people tend to crave foods high in fat, sugar, and salt. This combined with a busy schedule often leads to foods with poor nutritional value.

- Skipping Meals — When you are juggling a dozen things at once, eating a healthy meal often drops down in priorities. You might find yourself skipping breakfast because you're running late or not eating lunch because there's just too much on your to-do list. Sometimes, we get so busy we simply forget to eat.

- Mindless Snacking — Stress also makes us prone to emotional eating, where we eat despite not being hungry but eat because it feels comforting.

- Forgetting Water — It's easy to forget to drink your water. A good portion of Americans drink no water, and get water only from soda or coffee.

- Fast Food — So many drive-thrus, so little time. It's easier to just drive through a fast food place or go to a restaurant than to go home and cook something. Unfortunately, this gets expensive and is often unhealthy.

- Crash Diets — Stress often leads to weight gain, which can lead to people to look for a quick fix in their busy schedule. Some people intentionally eat less food than they need, or try dangerous fad diets in order to lose the excess weight. Diets that aren't balanced with fruits and vegetables, protein, and

healthy carbohydrates can often be bad for your health in the long run, even if they look attractive short term.

Eating nutrient-rich food and a balanced diet and making sure you stay hydrated, are two simple practices that can keep your stress levels healthy and manageable. The bottom line, as you learned in Chapter 7, is that healthy food has a positive impact on our health, can help our self-esteem, and can prevent the stress of increased body fat and illness.

Sleeping Habits

We don't treat our need for sleep with respect. We love when we get enough but often see it as something we can catch up on later when our stress subsides. Sleep is a necessary human function that allows our brains to recharge and our bodies to rest. We need sleep to repair muscle and consolidate memory. Sleep is so crucial that even slight sleep deprivation or poor sleep can affect memory, judgment, and mood. In addition to feeling fatigued and sluggish, chronic sleep deprivation can contribute to health problems, from obesity and high blood pressure to safety risks while driving. Research suggests that most Americans would be happier, healthier, and safer if they were to sleep an extra 60 to 90 minutes per night.

Here are a few tips for improving your sleep habits:

- Keep a consistent sleep schedule. Get up at the same time every day, even on weekends or during vacations.

- Set a bedtime that is early enough for you to get at least 7 hours of sleep.

- Establish a relaxing bedtime routine (e.g. a warm bath).

- Use your bed only for sleep and sex — don't use electronics or watch TV in bed.

- Make your bedroom quiet and relaxing. Keep the room at a comfortable, cool temperature.

- Turn off electronic devices at least 30 minutes before bedtime.

- Don't eat a large meal before bedtime. If you are hungry at night, eat a light, healthy snack.

- Exercise regularly and maintain a healthy diet.

- Avoid consuming caffeine in the late afternoon or evening.

- Avoid consuming alcohol before bedtime.

- Reduce your fluid intake before bedtime.

As you can see, most of your healthy sleep routines overlap with other stress-reducing practices. What you gain from healthy sleep patterns are lowered stress levels, improved immune system health, improved cardiac health, and higher cognitive function.

Human sleep needs vary by age and amongst individuals, and sleep is considered to be adequate when there is no daytime sleepiness or dysfunction. You know you are getting enough sleep when you are able to wake up on your own and feel rested, usually at least 6 to 7 hours.

Relaxation

Relaxation techniques include a number of practices such as progressive relaxation, guided imagery, biofeedback, self-hypnosis, and deep breathing exercises. The goal is similar in all — to produce the body's natural relaxation response, characterized by slower breathing, lower blood pressure, and a feeling of increased well-being. Meditation and practices that include meditation with movement, such as yoga and tai chi, can also promote relaxation.

Breathing Exercises

Deep breathing exercises are usually done by breathing deeply through the nose (filling the lungs) and slowly exhaling through the mouth. Physically, it should feel like you are filling up with air, starting at the top of the belly and moving up above the heart. You can count breaths to help stay focused on breathing, and imagine that your inhalation fills you with energy and positive thoughts, while exhalation lets out stress and negative thoughts. To practice deep breathing, you can try diaphragmatic breathing (Figure 32). The technique is pretty simple:

- Lie on your back on a flat surface or in bed, with your knees bent and your head supported. You can use a pillow under your knees to support your legs. Place one hand on your upper chest and the other just below your rib cage. This will allow you to feel your diaphragm move as you breathe.

- Breathe in slowly through your nose so that your stomach moves out against your hand. The hand on your chest should remain as still as possible.

- Tighten your stomach muscles, letting them fall inward as you exhale through pursed lips. The hand on your upper chest must remain as still as possible.

- When you first learn the diaphragmatic breathing technique, it may be easier for you to follow the instructions lying down. As you gain more practice, you can try the diaphragmatic breathing technique while sitting in a chair, as shown below.

You can do this breathing exercise while sitting in a chair, too:

- Sit comfortably, with your knees bent and your shoulders, head and neck relaxed.

- Breathe in slowly through your nose so that your stomach moves out against your hand. The hand on your chest should remain as still as possible.

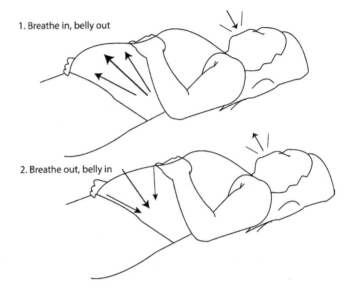

1. Breathe in, belly out

2. Breathe out, belly in

Figure 32. Deep breathing technique.

- Place one hand on your upper chest and the other just below your rib cage. This will allow you to feel your diaphragm move as you breathe.

- Tighten your stomach muscles, letting them fall inward as you exhale through pursed lips. The hand on your upper chest must remain as still as possible.

Note: You may notice an increased effort will be needed to use the diaphragm correctly. At first, you'll probably get tired while doing this exercise. But keep at it, because with continued practice, diaphragmatic breathing will become easy and automatic.

At first, practice this exercise five to ten minutes, three or four times per day. Gradually increase the amount of time you spend doing this exercise, and perhaps even increase the effort of the exercise by placing a book on your abdomen.

Progressive Muscle Relaxation	
Autogenic relaxation	Autogenic means something that comes from within you. In this relaxation technique, you use both visual imagery and body awareness to reduce stress. You repeat words or suggestions in your mind that may help you relax and reduce muscle tension. For example, you may imagine a peaceful setting and then focus on controlled, relaxing breathing, slowing your heart rate, or feeling different physical sensations, such as relaxing each arm or leg one by one.
Progressive muscle relaxation	In this relaxation technique, you focus on slowly tensing and then relaxing each muscle group. This can help you focus on the difference between muscle tension and relaxation. You can become more aware of physical sensations. In one method of progressive muscle relaxation, you start by tensing and relaxing the muscles in your toes and progressively working your way up to your neck and head. You can also start with your head and neck and work down to your toes. Tense your muscles for about five seconds and then relax for 30 seconds, and repeat.
Visualization	In this relaxation technique, you may form mental images to take a visual journey to a peaceful, calming place or situation. To relax using visualization, try to incorporate as many senses as you can, including smell, sight, sound and touch. If you imagine relaxing at the ocean, for instance, think about the smell of salt water, the sound of crashing waves and the warmth of the sun on your body. You may want to close your eyes, sit in a quiet spot, loosen any tight clothing, and concentrate on your breathing. Aim to focus on the present and think positive thoughts.

Figure 33. Progress muscle relaxation techniques.

Progressive Muscle Relaxation

Progressive muscle relaxation (PMR) is a recognized technique for the reduction of stress and anxiety. Muscle tension accompanies anxiety — you can reduce anxiety by learning how to release the tension in your muscles.

To do progressive muscle relaxation, a person can recline in a dark room and follow a simple progression through your muscles. Start by tensing and relaxing the muscles in your toes and progressively working your way up to your neck and head. You can also start with your head and neck and work down to your toes. Tense your muscles for at least five seconds and then relax for 30 seconds, and repeat (Figure 33).

Meditation

Meditation is a mind and body practice that has a long history of use for increasing calmness and physical relaxation, improving psychological balance, coping with illness, and enhancing overall health and well-being. Mind and body practices focus on the interactions among the brain, mind, body, and behavior. There are many types of meditation, but most have four elements in common:

- A quiet location with as few distractions as possible

- A specific, comfortable posture (sitting, lying down, walking, or in other positions)

- A focus of attention (a specially chosen word or set of words, an object, or the sensations of the breath)

- An open attitude (letting distractions come and go naturally without judging them).

Many studies have investigated meditation for different conditions, and there's evidence that it may reduce blood pressure as well as symptoms of irritable bowel syndrome and flare-ups in people who have had ulcerative colitis. It may ease symptoms of anxiety and depression, and may help people with insomnia.

In modern guided meditation, or mindfulness, you might be instructed to sit comfortably in a chair with your eyes "softly focused" on nothing in particular. Then you would be instructed to take several deep breaths — in through the nose and out through the mouth. After a few breaths, you close your eyes and begin to breath normally, focusing on the sensations in your body. If you start to get distracted by stressful thoughts, you could focus on your breathing, counting them in tens, with the odd number on the inhale and the even number on the exhale. After about ten minutes, you would be asked to open your eyes and recognize the feeling of relaxation you have before stretching and carrying on with your day.

This process can be as short as just a few minutes.

Visualization or "Guided Imagery"

For this technique, people are taught to focus on pleasant images to replace negative or stressful feelings. Guided imagery may be self-directed or led by a practitioner or a recording.

Guided imagery is based on the concept that your body and mind are connected. Using all of your senses, your body seems to respond as though what you are imagining is real. An example might be to imagine yourself at the beach, engaging all of your senses. Imagine the smell of the water, the sound of the waves and seagulls, the feel and texture of the sand and water on your feet,

If you feel you need to "ground" yourself and relax, a brief meditation exercise can provide a short break from a chaotic time.

and the taste of salt water on your lips. You may begin to feel chilly (if you picture an Oregon coast) or warm (if you image a real beach). This exercise demonstrates how your body can respond to what you are imagining.

You can achieve a relaxed state when you imagine all the details of a safe, comfortable place, such as your grandmother's house. This relaxed state may aid healing, learning, creativity, and performance. It may help you feel more in control of your emotions and thought processes, which may improve your attitude, health, and sense of well-being.

Other Relaxation Techniques

Other techniques include journaling, creativity, music, practicing gratitude, massage, humor, and other outlets. If you experience depression, for example, keeping a daily log of good experiences or moments of pleasure and happiness can be a useful tool that provides evi-

dence to your depressed mind that you experience good things. Learning to paint, craft, or play music can provide you with relaxing activities that also give you a sense of self-satisfaction.

Important Resources for Depression, Anxiety, Violence and Suicide Prevention

This chapter has focused a great deal on many of the issues in life that can lead to stress, the side effects of stress, and how we can improve our stress levels. Often times we need help to do this or face a situation that is

out of our control, even dangerous. It's important to understand that you aren't alone. There are individuals, instructors, and agencies available to help. The counseling office on the college campus can be a good first step.

Chemeketa Community College — Counseling Office

Our community college campus offers short term counseling services to all enrolled students. There are several ways to sign up for an appointment:

- Schedule through ChemekNET via MyChemeketa

- By phone at (503) 399-5120

- By email at counseling@chemeketa.edu

- In person at the Information Desk reception area in Building 2, Room 115 on the Salem Campus

- If you are on campus and need immediate assistance, go directly to Building 2 to the Counseling Services office or Public Safety.

- Chemeketa Public Safety: (503) 399-5023.

Resources for Anxiety and Depression

In addition to the campus resources above, psychiatric help is available from other local resources in Salem. If you need to speak to a mental health professional immediately, please call the 24-hour Psychiatric Crisis Center (PCC) at (503) 585-4949. To find help on the web for Salem area residents, go to www.salemhealth.org

Resources for Domestic Violence

Local resources for victims of violence are available in Salem at the Center for Hope and Safety crisis hotline: 503-399-7722, and the Canyon Crisis Center crisis hotline: 503-897-2327.

Resources for Suicide Prevention

If you're thinking about suicide, are worried about a friend or loved one, or would like emotional support, the National Suicide Prevention Lifeline is available at all times across the United States. You can contact:

- 1-800-273-TALK (8255) or go to www.suicidepreventionlifeline.org

- En español: 1-888-628-9454

- TTY: 1-800-799-4TTY (4889)

  The following websites can also offer advice or assistance:

- Centers for Disease Control and Prevention: www.cdc.gov/violenceprevention

National resources are available anywhere you are, and they can help you find mental health or crisis management services locally. The National Alliance on Mental Illness (NAMI) has a help line that can connect you with local branches. Call them at 1-800-950-NAMI (6264).

The Anxiety and Depression Association of America (ADAA) offers web resources for people suffering from these conditions and their supporters at adaa.org.

- The National Domestic Abuse Hotline: 1-800-799-7233

- TTY: 1-800-787-3224

- CDC Facebook Page on Violence Prevention: facebook.com/vetoviolence

- National Institute for Mental Health: nimh.nih.gov

- Substance Abuse and Mental Health Services Administration: samhsa.gov

- Suicide Prevention Resource Center: www.sprc.org

- Preventing Suicide: A Global Imperative: www.who.int/mental_health/suicide-prevention/world_%report_2014/en/

Resources for Sexual Assault, Dating Violence, Domestic Violence, Harassment or Discrimination Stalking

Students with these concerns can find Chemeketa's contact and resource information at the following links:

- Sexual Misconduct Website: www.chemeketa.edu/contactus/concerns/sexual_misconduct/

- Know Your Rights resource guide link: www.chemeketa.edu/contactus/concerns/sexual_misconduct/documents/know-your-rights_english_001.pdf

Conclusion

Your next steps should be to assess your stress levels and anticipated stressors, make a plan for how you will avoid experiencing stress with preventative management techniques and manage the unavoidable stress in your life with active stress management.

This chapter covered the basics of stress and how it is processed by the body and brain. You learned about the different kinds of stress and its sources, as well as how widespread stress is among adults in the US You also saw several techniques for identifying and managing the stress in your life, and were provided with a list of resources for addressing situations where you may feel out of control. You're not alone, and help is available, no matter the seriousness or cause of the situation.

Chapter 9
Chronic Disease

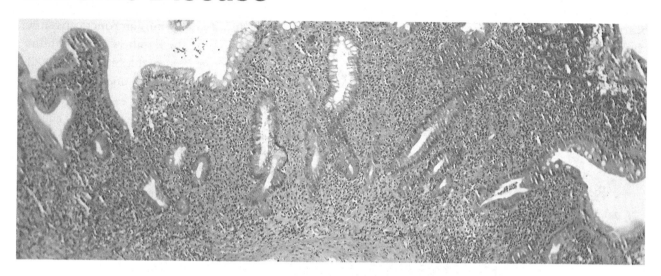

Eight of the top ten causes of death for Americans are chronic diseases. A chronic disease is any disease that lasts longer than three months. If you consider how miserable you feel with a simple cold that lasts a few weeks, imagine living with an illness on a daily basis for several years, even decades. The potential restrictions to your daily activities could easily impact the overall quality of your life. Chronic diseases generally cannot be prevented by vaccines or cured by medication, nor do they just disappear over time. These conditions affect millions of Americans, but you can prevent contracting many of these diseases with healthy behavioral choices.

US deaths from diseases in 2016:

- Heart disease: 633,842

- Cancer: 595,930

- Chronic lower respiratory diseases: 155,041

- Accidents (unintentional injuries): 146,571

- Stroke (cerebrovascular diseases): 140,323

- Alzheimer's disease: 110,561

- Diabetes: 79,535

- Influenza and pneumonia: 57,062

- Nephritis, nephrotic syndrome, nephrosis: 49,959

- Intentional self-harm (suicide): 44,193

While many of these diseases are more common in older adults, the risk for these diseases is rising among younger people as unhealthy behaviors become the norm, especially concerning nutrition and fitness. There are many reasons our bodies can become susceptible to disease, and yes, some of those are out of our control. Many of those reasons are not, however, and as you'll see in this chapter, you can do something about it with improved nutrition and fitness habits.

Some of the people we've described in this book, like Chuck in his armchair, were able to start a fitness program and turn their fitness around before any chronic diseases could take hold, but it's not hard to imagine what would happen to Chuck if he never decided to start his jogging routine. As you'll see in this chapter, his risk for heart disease, certain cancers, and diabetes increases with poor nutrition, physical activity, and body composition.

This chapter begins by defining several types of cardiovascular disease, the most common cause of death in America. It then defines cancer and diabetes, two other leading causes of death in the US. The chapter then shifts its focus to behaviors that can help you prevent these diseases in your life, starting by assessing your risks for chronic diseases and then recommending behaviors to lower those risks.

Cardiovascular Diseases

Cardiovascular diseases are conditions that involve narrowed or blocked blood vessels, dysfunctional heart muscles and valves, or irregular heart rhythm. Heart diseases are the number one cause of death in the US, causing nearly 24% of all deaths nationwide. In fact, 610,000 people die each year from heart disease and about 80 million Americans suffer from some form of it. The numbers are astounding and a bit scary. The disease does not discriminate — it attacks men and women equally, claiming credit for one in four deaths for both sexes. Approximately half of all victims had no knowledge they were ill before their death.

And if the mortality rates aren't scary enough, heart disease has also become quite costly to the nation, not just in lives but also in dollars. Annually, about one in every six US healthcare dollars is spent on cardiovascular disease (Figure 1).

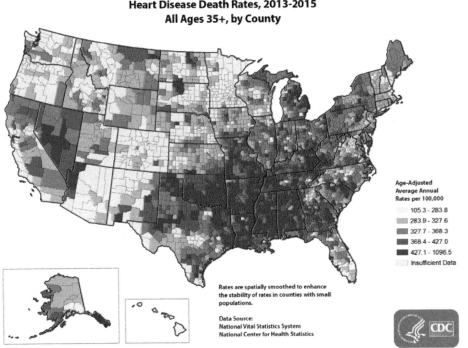

Heart Disease Death Rates, 2013-2015 All Ages 35+, by County

Age-Adjusted Average Annual Rates per 100,000
- 105.3 - 283.8
- 283.9 - 327.6
- 327.7 - 368.3
- 368.4 - 427.0
- 427.1 - 1096.5
- Insufficient Data

Rates are spatially smoothed to enhance the stability of rates in counties with small populations.

Data Source:
National Vital Statistics System
National Center for Health Statistics

Figure 1. Heart disease map of the United States.

Types of Cardiovascular Disease

The heart is a complex organ with a large job. This small yet mighty warrior has a complicated anatomy when we consider the number of other systems in the body it can affect, and the sheer magnitude of what can happen when it doesn't work properly. Understanding the risks and symptoms of various cardiovascular diseases is important for living your longest, fullest life possible (Figure 2).

Coronary artery disease (CAD) is the most common type of heart disease and claims 370,000 victims each year in the US It is the single leading cause of death in the nation. CAD develops in two major ways — atherosclerosis and arteriosclerosis — both inhibit blood flow in the arteries.

Atherosclerosis occurs when plaque (a hardened byproduct of cholesterol, fat, calcium, and other

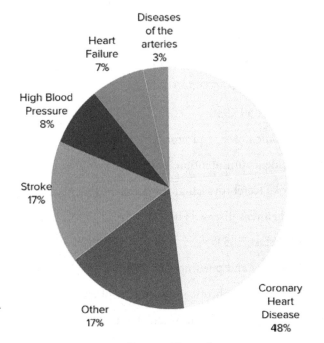

Figure 2. Comparing all types of heart disease.

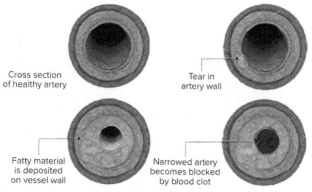

Cross section of healthy artery

Fatty material is deposited on vessel wall

Tear in artery wall

Narrowed artery becomes blocked by blood clot

Figure 3. Development of atherosclerosis.

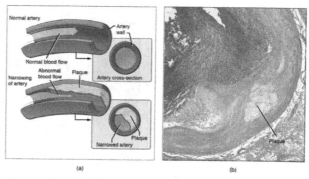

Figure 4. Plaque buildup.

substances) accumulates in the walls of the arteries that feed the heart and other parts of the body (Figure 3). This results in a narrower passage for the blood to navigate now that the plaque is partially blocking its way through the body. When the heart cannot get enough blood, the person may experience chest pain (see angina pectoris below), the most common symptom of CAD (Figure 4). Unfortunately for some people, a heart attack is their first symptom of CAD and the largest risk to the individual since it can result in death.

Arteriosclerosis occurs when the artery walls stiffen or harden (atherosclerosis is a type of arteriosclerosis). We commonly refer to this as "hardening of the arteries." This can be quite common among the elderly since our arteries, which are normally flexible, begin to stiffen with age. High cholesterol levels in the blood, a lack of exercise, and smoking can accelerate the process.

Atherosclerosis and arteriosclerosis have different impacts on our body depending upon which arteries experience the

most narrowing or hardening. For the coronary artery, we experience the symptoms of CAD already mentioned. If the peripheral artery narrows, we experience **peripheral artery disease** (PAD), which impacts blood flow to our legs, arms, head, and stomach but most often the legs (Figure 5). People with PAD often experience pain, cramping, or tiredness in these extremities.

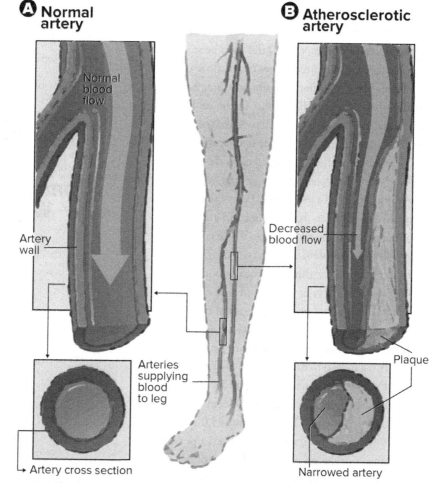

Ⓐ Normal artery

Normal blood flow

Artery wall

Artery cross section

Arteries supplying blood to leg

Ⓑ Atherosclerotic artery

Decreased blood flow

Plaque

Narrowed artery

Figure 5. Blood flow is blocked in an atherosclerotic artery.

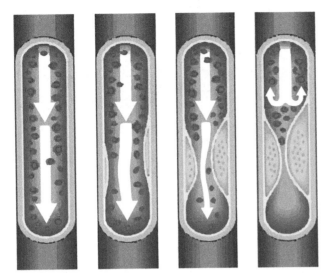

Figure 6. Blood clots cause serious problems.

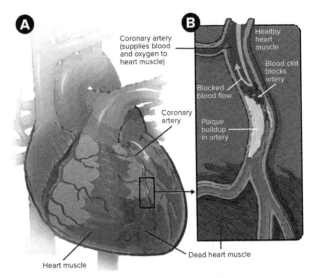

Figure 7. Blood can no longer flow to the body.

If the cerebral artery becomes restricted, blood flow to the brain is impacted. This can result in blood clots, also known as **aneurysms**, forming in the narrowed passages (Figure 6). If one ruptures or cuts off the flow entirely, it can result in a stroke. The restriction of the blood flow alone, even without a clot, can cause headaches, blurred vision, facial pain, and dementia (particular in the elderly).

Angina pectoris is what we call the pain people feel when experiencing symptoms of low blood flow to the heart. This could be a sensation of pain, pressure, fullness, or squeezing in the chest or discomfort in the neck, arm, shoulders, back, or jaw. Women often experience different pains than men because they more frequently develop disease in the smaller arteries that branch off of the coronary arteries. She could experience nausea, vomiting, sharp chest pain, abdominal pain, and a sensation of being out of breath.

Arrhythmias are when the heart beats in an irregular manner or beats unusually fast or slow. These can be life threatening. *Ventricular fibrillation* is a type of arrhythmia that causes an abnormal rhythm that must be corrected by electric shock (defibrillator) or the person will die. Other types of arrhythmias are not quite as serious but can lead to other issues, such as *atrial fibrillation*. This is an arrhythmia that can cause a rapid, irregular beat in the upper chambers of the heart. This can lead to the formation of clots, increasing the risk of stroke or heart attack (Figure 7).

Someone in the US has a **heart attack** (myocardial infarction) every 43 seconds. That's nearly 735,000 heart attacks each year. A heart attack occurs when a portion of the heart does not get enough blood. The longer the person stays in this state, the more damage to the organ.

According to the Centers for Disease Control, the five major symptoms of a heart attack are (Figure 8):

- Pain or discomfort in the neck, jaw, or back

- Feeling weak or light-headed, or as if you are going to faint

- Pain or discomfort in the chest

- Pain or discomfort in the shoulder or arms

- Being short of breath

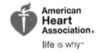

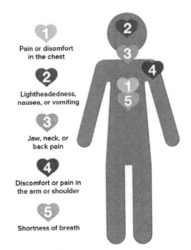

Figure 8. Warning signs for heart attack.

You may also feel unusually tired and experience nausea or vomiting. As mentioned, women are more than men to experience these other symptoms (see angina pectoris). If you suspect that you or someone you know could be having a heart attack, call 911. This would not be a situation to schedule an appointment with your doctor or attempt to drive yourself to the emergency room as this can be life threatening and time is critical (Figure 9).

If you survive the heart attack, your life will most certainly change significantly. At minimum, you will have to undergo a change in lifestyle, such as diet, exercise, and stress management. For some individuals, it could mean medications to prevent blood clots and frequent laboratory tests, lengthy hospitalization, and even risky surgery.

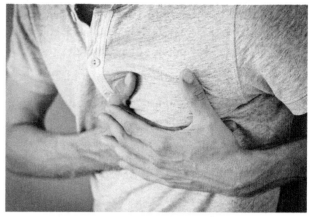

Figure 9. Any chest pain should be taken seriously.

Stroke

Stroke, or cerebrovascular accident (CVA), is the fifth leading cause of death in the US and affects 795,000 people each year. It is a significant source of disability for many Americans. There are two different types of strokes, an ischemic stroke and a hemorrhagic stroke.

An **ischemic stroke** can happen when the blood flow to the brain becomes blocked. Sometimes this blockage can be temporary, resulting in a transient ischemic attack (TIA). These are often called "mini-strokes" but warning stroke is a better term. People who suffer from TIAs are at high risk for a more severe blockage. A **hemorrhagic stroke** occurs when a blood vessel in the brain leaks or ruptures causing leaked blood to exert pressure on brain cells, damaging them (Figure 10).

Our brains need oxygen in order to do their job controlling our movements, emotions, memories, language, and nearly everything we do. Blood carries the oxygen to the brain. When it can't, the cells in that part of the brain begin to die or become permanently damaged, resulting in long-term disability and potentially, death. The nature of the disability will depend upon the part of the brain affected and what part of the body it controlled. Some stroke victims experience problems with speech, swallowing, a loss of control on one side of the body, or difficulty managing their emotions.

Strokes are one of the possible effects of heart diseases like coronary artery disease and atrial fibrillation. Essentially, any disease that can lead to an interruption in the normal flow of blood to the brain, whether it is through arterial plaque, leakage, or clotting, can lead to a stroke.

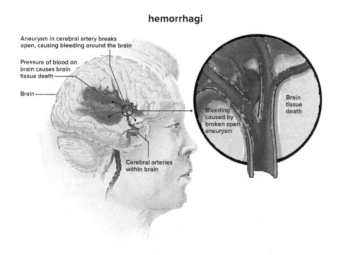

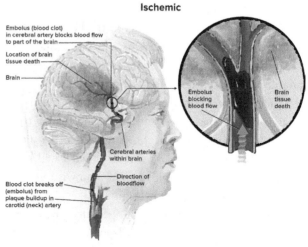

Figure 10. Stroke occurs when blood flow is blocked to the brain.

According to the National Institute of Neurological Disorders and Stroke (NINDS), some of the most common signs and symptoms of a stroke are:

- Sudden numbness in the face, arms, or legs

- Sudden confusion, and sudden difficulty speaking or understanding others

- Sudden difficulty seeing in one or both of your eyes

- Sudden difficulty with balance, walking, or coordination

- Sudden extreme headache with no apparent cause

F	Face: Ask the person to smile. Does on side of the face droop?
A	Arms: Ask the person to raise both arms. Does one arm drift downward?
S	Speech: Ask the person to repeat a simple phrase. Is their speech slurred or strange?
T	Time: If you see any of these signs, call 911 immediately.

Figure 11. Check these if someone might be having a stroke.

As with a heart attack, every minute is critical. If you or someone you know seems to be having a stroke, call 911.

Stroke Treatment

The NINDS states that generally there are three treatment stages for stroke: prevention, therapy immediately after the stroke, and post-stroke rehabilitation.

- *Therapies to prevent* a first or recurrent stroke are based on treating an individual's underlying risk factors for stroke, such as hypertension, atrial fibrillation, and diabetes.

- *Acute stroke therapies* try to stop a stroke while it is happening by quickly dissolving the blood clot causing an ischemic stroke or by stopping the bleeding of a hemorrhagic stroke.

- *Post-stroke rehabilitation* (physical, occupational, and speech therapy) helps individuals overcome disabilities that result from stroke damage. Medication or drug therapy is the most common treatment for antithrombotics and thrombolytics, which are intended to keep clots from forming and causing another stroke.

Recurrent stroke is frequent. About 25 percent of people who recover from their first stroke will have another within five years, so proper treatment is important to reduce the risk of reoccurrence.

Blood Pressure

Hypertension, otherwise known as sustained high blood pressure, is a form of cardiovascular disease in which the pressure of the blood in your body's vessels is higher than normal. This can lead to hardening of the arteries and weakening of the heart. Over time, high blood pressure can be dangerous to the body, causing such complications as aneurysms, chronic kidney disease, heart attack, cognitive changes, eye damage, heart failure, peripheral artery disease, and stroke.

The disease is common and known as "the silent killer" because one in five sufferers don't realize they have it. Often hypertension shows no noticeable symptoms, though occasionally a person affected will have nausea or vomiting. The only way to know is to check your blood pressure regularly (Figure 12).

This disease even impacts young adults. The results of studies are varied, but anywhere from 4–11% of adults in their mid-to-late twenties and early thirties have high

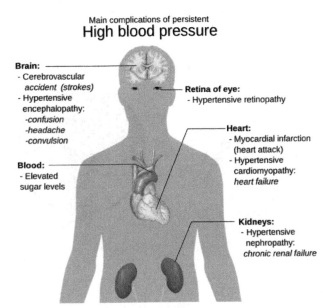

Figure 12. High blood pressure impacts several areas of the body.

blood pressure. Part of this may be because we now consider a "pre-hypertension stage" that wasn't previously recognized. This was added because blood pressures even in this stage can begin to impact the heart's function.

Hypertension has two types, primary and secondary. People with *primary hypertension* have no known cause for the disease. It can occur gradually over several years. *Secondary hypertension* stems from some other underlying condition, like a congenital defect in your blood vessels, kidney or thyroid problems, or the taking of medications that can cause the pressure to increase. Alcohol and drug abuse can also cause hypertension because they can damage the heart. Secondary hypertension can come on suddenly and even more dramatically than primary. Anything we do to cause blockage in our arteries can increase risk when it comes to hypertension.

Systolic vs. Diastolic

When we visit the doctor's office to have our blood pressure checked, the nurse reads off the number for us, 110 over 70 (110/70), and tells us everything is great. Great for what? Those numbers sound more like a speeding ticket than something related to your health. These are the systolic and diastolic readings (Figure 13).

- *Systolic* — The first or top number of the reading tells doctors how much pressure your blood is exerting against the walls of your arteries when your heart beats. Systole occurs when your ventricles contract and push blood out of the heart.

- *Diastolic* — The second or bottom number of the reading tells doctors how much pressure your blood is exerting against the walls of your arteries when your heart is resting (between beats). Diastole occurs when the ventricles relax, allowing blood to be pumped in.

So what is a healthy blood pressure and what would be considered high (see Chapter 3)? Your nurse was right. Your pressure was good — healthy numbers for adults of any age are a systolic reading below 120 and diastolic reading below 80. It is normal for blood pressures to change when you sleep, wake up, or are excited or nervous. It is also normal for your blood pressure to increase while you are active. However, once the activity stops, your blood pressure returns to your normal baseline range.

There are varying degrees of hypertension, ranging from prehypertension (numbers that are

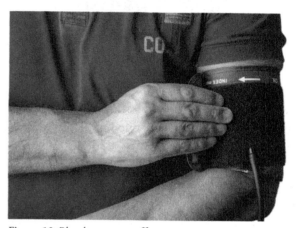

Figure 13. Blood pressure cuff.

slightly elevated and indicate hypertension could become a problem) to a hypertensive crisis requiring emergency medical care (Figure 14).

Blood pressure starts out low in infants and gradually rises as children grow into adults. A baby with a reading of 80/45 would be quite normal, but this would be cause for alarm in an adult. It's possible to have low blood pressure. **Hypotension** means a systolic reading

Blood Pressure Category	Systolic mm Hg (upper #)		Diastolic mm Hg (lower #)
Normal	less than 120	and	less than 80
Prehypertension	120 – 139	or	80 – 89
High Blood Pressure (Hypertension) Stage 1	140 – 159	or	90 – 99
High Blood Pressure (Hypertension) Stage 2	160 or higher	or	100 or higher
Hypertensive Crisis (Emergency care needed)	Higher than 180	or	Higher than 110

Figure 14. Blood pressure ranges based on systolic and diastolic pressure.

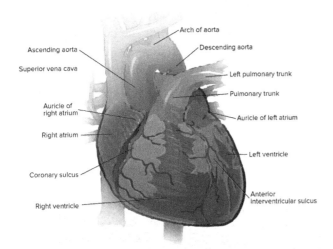

Figure 15. Anatomy of the heart.

below 90 and a diastolic below 60. This can occur during pregnancy, after a prolonged period of bed rest, from blood loss following trauma, or as the result of a severe infection or allergic reaction. It could also be the cause of something more chronic, such as a heart problem. Doctors typically become concerned about chronic hypotension when there are symptoms, such as nausea, dizziness, fatigue, clammy skin, and blurry vision.

Heart failure sounds as though the heart has stopped beating, but what it means is that the heart is no longer pumping enough blood to support the other organs in your body. Sometimes it affects only the right side of the heart, responsible for pumping blood to the lungs. A person may experience shortness of breath (particularly when lying flat), fatigue, and a cough that is worse when lying down. In most cases both sides of the heart are affected and sufferers will also experience shortness of breath and swelling of the ankles, legs, feet, liver, abdomen, and pain in the neck.

Electrocardiogram (ECG or EKG)	Electrodes are placed on the skin to detect the heart's electrical signals, which are recorded; the test can show problems with heart rate or rhythm and detect underlying damage to the heart.
Exercise Stress Test	An electrocardiogram is performed while the person is exercising on a treadmill or stationary bike; the test monitors the response to exercise and detects problems with the cardiovascular system during physical effort.
Coronary Angiography	A catheter is threaded through the artery, typically in the leg, and dye is injected into the arteries of the heart; special X-rays are then used to identify blockages. A similar procedure can be done to visualize the brain's blood vessels.
Blood Tests	In addition to checking cholesterol and glucose levels, blood samples can be analyzed for enzymes and proteins in the blood that indicate heart-muscle damage.
Chest X-ray	Ionizing radiation creates pictures of the heart, lungs, and blood vessels that can be used to determine the size and shape of the heart as well as to detect fluid buildup or damage.
Echocardiogram	A small device called a *transducer* transmits ultrasound waves into the chest, which are converted into computerized images of the heart; the test can show the heart's size, structure, and motion, as well as blood volume, speed. and direction of blood flow.
Nuclear Scan; Positron Emission Tomographic (PET) Scan	In both tests, small amounts if radioactive tracer materials are injected into the bloodstream; special imaging equipment monitors blood flow to the heart, as well as the heart's efficiency in pumping blood, and checks for heart-muscle damage.
Computed Tomography (CT) Scan	A special X-ray machine takes cross-sectional images that are used to create three-dimensional models of organs. Scans can be used to detect problems in the blood vessels in both the heart and the brain.
Magnetic Resonance Imaging (MRI)	A special scanner uses radio waves, magnets, and a computer to create images of organs and tissues; MRIs can evaluate the condition of the heart and blood vessels and detect the presence and size of aneurysms and malformed blood vessels that are potential causes of hemorrhagic stroke.
Electroencephalogram (EEG)	Electrodes are placed on the scalp, and the electrical activity of the brain is monitored for any indications of problems.

Figure 16. Tests for diagnosing and monitoring heart disease.

The primary causes of heart failure are diseases that damage the heart, such as coronary artery disease, hypertension, and diabetes. Heart failure can develop suddenly or over time. Approximately 5.7 million adults have heart failure in the US and of these about half will die within 5 years of being diagnosed.

There are many other heart diseases though not all of them are within our control. Some are congenital, meaning we are born with them, and some are acquired as a result of other illnesses.

With **cardiomyopathy**, for example, the heart becomes enlarged, rigid, or thick and in some cases the tissue is replaced with scar tissue. Cardiomyopathy can be inherited or acquired as the result of another disease or drug or alcohol abuse. As the disease progresses, the heart becomes less effective at pumping blood, leading to heart failure, arrhythmias, or heart valve problems. For most people, this is when they first begin experiencing symptoms.

Heart valve problems exist when one or more of the valves in your heart (tricuspid, mitral, pulmonary, or aortic) do not function properly. Each valve has a flap that opens and closes as the heart beats, responsible for distributing blood through the heart's chambers and through the body. A faulty or damaged valve may not open fully or may let blood back into the chamber when it is supposed to be pumping through (regurgitation), causing the heart to work harder.

Heart valve problems can be congenital, a condition of an aging heart, or damaged from an infection.

Many people live with valve problems a long time without noticing them, though others will need the valve replaced. Valve issues can lead to other heart diseases, like heart failure or stroke.

Some **heart murmurs** are actually an issue with a heart valve. A murmur is an atypical sound, like a whooshing noise, between heartbeats. They can occur when the blood flows more rapidly through the heart than normal, such as during exercise or pregnancy or during a child's growth spurt. The person may experience shortness of breath, bluish skin, a chronic cough, dizziness, or fainting. Many heart murmurs are innocent and cause no trouble to the person, but others are the result of a congenital defect or heart valve issue. Treatment, if necessary at all, depends upon what is causing the murmur.

Varicose veins are yet another indication that blood is not moving properly through the body. These are very common and usually harmless, occurring often during pregnancy, in people who stand for long periods of time, when we experience trauma to the leg, or when there is a lack of movement. Being overweight or obese increases your risk for varicose veins, though many are even hereditary.

When the valves in your veins are weakened or damaged, blood can begin to pool in the area, causing veins to swell. Some will swell just a little and be merely unappealing to look at. Others will swell to the point of pain, bulging, clotting, or ulceration on the skin. Painful veins may need to be surgically removed.

Cancer

Unfortunately for most of us, cancer is not an unfamiliar term. We've been forced to utter the "C" word more times than we would like. We've walked or ran in support of cures, donated money to research, given up a potentially hazardous food because of its association with the disease or, even worse, have known someone who has fought cancer. Cancer is the term we use for a number of diseases in which abnormal cells (sometimes in which the DNA has changed) divide uncontrollably and invade other parts of the body through our blood

and lymph systems. There are hundreds of different types of known cancers.

It seems like hardly a day goes by where we don't hear the word uttered. It's not surprising since cancers are the number two cause of death in the US, nearly 23% of deaths nationwide. The Agency for Healthcare research and Quality (AHRQ) estimates that the direct medical costs (total of all health care costs) for cancer in the US in 2014 were $87.8 billion.

How Cancer Develops

We begin life as a single cell. That cells divides and divides into more and more cells. Certain cells join

together to form parts of the body, like a toe or eye. Unlike us fully formed humans, these cells do not have to search for their soul mate. They have a set of instructions in their DNA telling them exactly which other cells to match up with to form the perfect union — or an ear. They know when to stop dividing and when to die. Some are meant to replicate as others die (such as skin cells) and others aren't (such as if we lose a toe).

When their DNA is affected, the cell becomes abnormal and no longer understands its instructions. Either they can divide and replicate too much within their area or they can spread to other parts of the body where they do not belong. Our immune system can handle only a few abnormal cells, but if they grow too rapidly, they begin to form lumps or growths called tumors.

Benign tumors are those that don't spread and usually don't pose a problem unless they get too large and in that way interfere with comfort or another part of the body. We consider them as non-cancerous. They are like the neutered house cat that eats too much. He stays home, bingeing on treats and getting chubby, but he doesn't bother anyone but his owner. These tumors can, however, become malignant over time in some cases.

Malignant tumors are invasive and considered as cancerous. They spread to other parts of the body (**metastasize**), destroy the surrounding tissue, and cause more tumors to grow. They are like the un-neutered tomcat that runs free in the neighborhood, tearing up kids' toys and making friends with other cats. Before you know it, the neighbors are angry and the neighborhood is filled

with kittens that can also run rampant if not kept in check (Figure 18).

Sometimes cancers are the result of exposure to an environmental factor known as a **carcinogen**, a substance capable of causing the abnormal cell division. We come into contact with many carcinogens voluntarily through our lifestyle, with or without our own knowledge. Smoking or chewing tobacco, poor nutrition (or the consumption of a carcinogenic food), and a lack of physical activity, for example, would relate to lifestyle carcinogens. Other carcinogens are the result of exposure to things like pollution, ultra-violet rays (skin cancer), workplace hazards (such as asbestos or coal dust), or radiation, just to name a few (Figure 19). More on this in a bit.

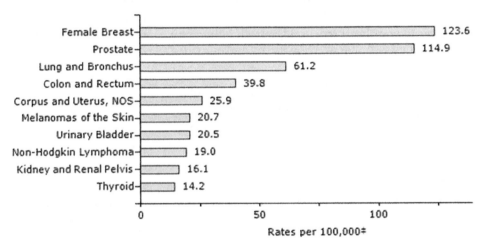

Figure 17. Common cancer sites on the body.

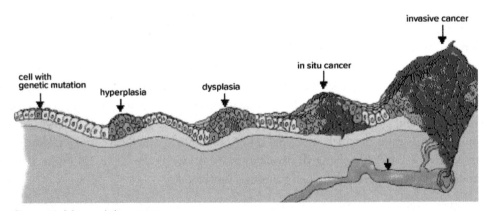

Figure 18. Metastasis in progress.

Types of Cancer

There are different forms of cancer, including carcinoma, sarcoma, lymphoma, and myeloma.

Carcinomas are one of the most common types of cancer. They occur in epithelial tissues, which are linings, such as the skin. Any part of your body with this type of tissue can be affected by carcinoma, such as the colon, breast, lung, or prostate, but we have many parts of the body lined with epithelial cells.

Sarcomas form in bones and in soft and connective tissues like blood vessels, muscles, tendons, and ligaments.

Lymphoma affects the lymph system, more specifically lymphocytes. These are our white blood cells, part of our immune system and are responsible for fighting disease.

Myeloma affects another type of immune cell, our plasma cells. The abnormal cells form tumors in bones any place in the body.

Cancers originating in the blood-forming tissues of our bone marrow are called **leukemia**. Rather than tumors forming, this cancer causes abnormal blood cells (white or red) to develop, accumulating in the blood and marrow and leaving little room for normal cells. Once this happens, the body has trouble getting enough oxygen to its cells, controlling bleeding, and fighting infection.

Cancer can happen at any age and to either gender. Some forms may strike a particular age or gender more often than another (Figure 20).

The symptoms of cancer vary greatly depending upon the type and location of the disease. Symptoms for breast cancer, for example, would include swelling of any part of the breast, dimpling, changes in shape, discharge, pain, or finding a lump in your breast. Symptoms of colon cancer might include changes in bowel movements (such as diarrhea), blood in the stool, and abdominal pain. The symptoms, to a large extent, are specific to the location of the disease though often fatigue accompanies illness.

For many cancers, symptoms do not present right away if at all, or are similar to the symptoms of common and less serious illnesses. Someone with colon cancer, for example, could easily assume they have the flu or irritable bowel syndrome. For that reason, it is important to have an annual physical, complete any tests recommended by your physician, and notify your physician if symptoms don't improve.

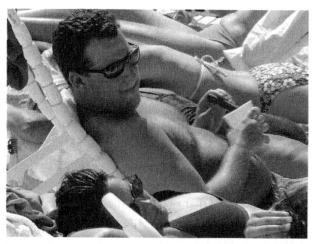

Figure 19. Excessive sun exposure can cause skin cancer.

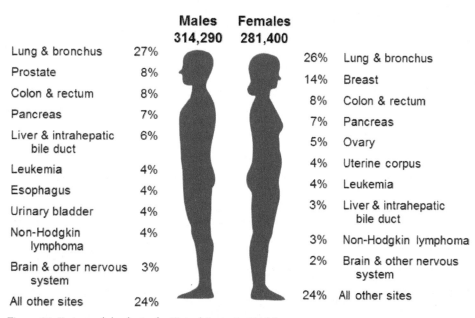

Estimated Cancer Deaths in the US in 2016

		Males 314,290	Females 281,400		
Lung & bronchus	27%			26%	Lung & bronchus
Prostate	8%			14%	Breast
Colon & rectum	8%			8%	Colon & rectum
Pancreas	7%			7%	Pancreas
Liver & intrahepatic bile duct	6%			5%	Ovary
Leukemia	4%			4%	Uterine corpus
Esophagus	4%			4%	Leukemia
Urinary bladder	4%			3%	Liver & intrahepatic bile duct
Non-Hodgkin lymphoma	4%			3%	Non-Hodgkin lymphoma
Brain & other nervous system	3%			2%	Brain & other nervous system
All other sites	24%			24%	All other sites

Figure 20. Estimated deaths in the United States in 2016 from cancers.

Cancer Detection and Diagnosis

Just as there are multiple cancers and multiple symptoms there are many ways of detecting and diagnosing the disease, including biopsy, imaging procedures, and lab tests. For many suspected cancers, your physician will begin with laboratory tests, such as blood and urine samples to determine the count of your white and red blood cells. This lets him or her know if your body may be attempting to fight off something.

Your physician will also look for **tumor markers**, usually particular proteins (or an increase in them) or possibly patterns of genes, which might indicate that

cancer could be developing within your body. These are essentially red flags to show further testing is needed. Imaging tests are also quite common. X-rays, ultrasounds, mammograms, and MRIs, among other types of procedures, help physicians see inside the body to determine if a tumor or other issue is present and how large or advanced the abnormal cells have become.

Biopsies are also quite common. A small sample of the abnormal growth is removed from the patient and tested to determine if it is benign or malignant, the type of cancer, and to plan the best treatment.

Early Screening

Last year your Aunt Phyllis was diagnosed with breast cancer. She underwent a few rounds of chemotherapy and a month of radiation. Her hair fell out and she spent several months not feeling so great, but everyone kept saying "Thank goodness they caught it in time!" You saw her after her third chemotherapy treatment and you didn't think there was anything good about it. She didn't look so great. Yet by the time it was all over and you had spent many hours in the clinic with her on her treatment days, and saw many people in different stages of the disease, you realized what it meant. She really was fortunate — she survived because a routine mammogram found the tumor in its early stage.

There are certain tests recommended to screen for certain types of cancer. What type of test you need often depends upon your age, gender, family history, and any illnesses or other risk factors you may have. The type of screening depends on the form of cancer the physician

Change in bowel or bladder habits

A sore that does not heal

Unusual bleeding or discharge

Thickening or lump in breast or elsewhere

Indigestion or difficulty in swallowing

Obvious change in wart or mole

Nagging cough or hoarseness

Figure 21. Use CAUTION to identify possible warning signs.

is looking for. It could be done with lab work, imaging, or something a bit more invasive like a colonoscopy. The following chart (Figure 22) can give you a basic guide of types of screenings and how often they're done.

Type of Screening	Gender	Age	Frequency
Mammogram	Female	40–44	Optional annual screenings
		45–54	Annually
		55 and up	Every 2 years
Colonoscopy for colon cancer	Male & Female	50 and up	Every 10 years
Stool sample for colon cancer	Male & Female	50 and up	1–3 years depending on type
Pap smear for cervical cancer	Female	21–65	Every 3 years or co-testing with HPV every. 5 yrs. for 30–65
Hpv test for cervical cancer	Female	30–65	Every 5 years
Chest ct scan for lung cancer	Either if smoking	55–74	Annually
Rectal exam & psa for prostate cancer	Men		Depends upon risk factors

Figure 22. Cancer screening tests.

Not all tests have set guidelines for completion. Imaging procedures pose their own risk, even though the radiation is often low-dose, as do other invasive procedures. Someone in good health with no family history may choose to screen less often to avoid unnecessary risk. Likewise, someone who is elderly and expected to live less than 10 years, or who is experiencing other illnesses, may not be a good candidate for these types of screenings. Often, blood work or stool samples will be done initially before more aggressive screening measures.

For some cancers, it is possible to do self-exams to detect problems. Monthly breast exams, for example, are recommended for women. If done routinely, a woman can become very aware of what her breast is like when normal and can often notice when something abnormal begins to form. Self-exams can also be a proactive approach for skin cancer. Checking your body for moles of an atypical shape, color, or that change shape can help you address the issue while it is still in the early stages.

A good beginning point is determining your risk. Know your family history of cancer, and risks related to your health and lifestyle, and ask your physician what screenings, both medically and through self-exam, should be done routinely.

Staging

Stage refers to the extent of your cancer, such as how large the tumor is, and if it has spread. Knowing the stage of your cancer helps your doctor understand how serious your cancer is and your chances of survival, as well as plan the best treatment for you. A cancer is always referred to by the stage it was given at diagnosis, even if it gets worse or spreads. New information about how a cancer has changed over time gets added on to the original stage. So, the stage doesn't change, even though the cancer might.

There are many staging systems. Some are used for many types of cancer. Others are specific to a particular type of cancer. Most staging systems include information about:

- Where the tumor is located in the body
- The cell type (such as, adenocarcinoma or squamous cell carcinoma)
- The size of the tumor
- Whether the cancer has spread to nearby lymph nodes
- Whether the cancer has spread to a different part of the body

Tumor grade, which refers to how abnormal the cancer cells look and how likely the tumor is to grow and spread.

Cancer Treatment

Research and treatment has come a long way over the years, giving many people a greater chance of surviving cancer. There are many methods of cancer treatment. The types that you have will depend on the type of cancer you have and how advanced it is. Some people with cancer will have only one treatment. But most people have a combination of treatments, such surgery to remove a part of the body or the cancer, along with chemotherapy and/or radiation therapy. You might also have immunotherapy, targeted therapy, or hormone therapy.

Chemotherapy is a form of intense treatment using drugs designed to stop the growth of cancer cells, either by killing the cells or by stopping them from dividing. Chemotherapy may be given by mouth, injection, or infusion, or on the skin, depending on the type and stage of the cancer being treated. It may be given alone or with other treatments, such as surgery, radiation therapy, or biologic therapy. Some patients may receive chemotherapy for several weeks or months, while others may try various forms of chemo over a period of years. Cancer is by no means easy to cure and many cells resist treatment.

The side effects can also become burdensome, particularly for patients already in a weakened state. These drugs do not only kill cancer cells. The drug does not differentiate between a rapidly growing cancer cell and a rapidly growing healthy one. Many of our cells are meant to die and regenerate often, such as those in our mouths, our hair, our intestines, our finger nails and so on. Patients often experience hair loss, nausea, mouth sores, and fingernail or tooth loss in addition to a great deal of fatigue when undergoing treatment. Chemo can be used alone or in combination with surgery or radiation, depending on the person's treatment plan.

Radiation is like a high-powered x-ray but without the pictures. We use radiation in lower doses to look for broken bones and dental cavities. Cancer treatment requires the use of high-energy radiation from x-rays, gamma rays, neutrons, protons, and other sources to kill cancer cells and shrink tumors. Radiation may come from a machine outside the body (external-beam radiation therapy), or it may come from radioactive material placed in the body near cancer cells (internal radiation therapy or brachytherapy). Systemic radiation therapy uses a radioactive substance that travels in the blood to tissues throughout the body.

The cancer cells die slowly and continue dying for a while after treatment is finished. Patients often need several doses given close together. For example, a patient may have to receive radiation 5 days each week for a month or more. As with chemo, there can be side effects as the healthy cells nearby the cancerous ones also become damaged. Fatigue, swelling, skin damage, and hair loss are just a few, though it does vary depending on the location of the cancer.

Immunotherapy is a type of biological therapy that uses substances to stimulate or suppress the immune system to help the body fight cancer, infection, and other diseases. Some types of immunotherapy only target certain cells of the immune system. Others affect the immune system in a general way.

Targeted therapy is a type of treatment that uses drugs or other substances to identify and attack specific types of cancer cells with less harm to normal cells. Some targeted therapies block the action of certain enzymes, proteins, or other molecules involved in the growth and spread of cancer cells. Other types of targeted therapies help the immune system kill cancer cells or deliver toxic substances directly to cancer cells and kill them. Targeted therapy may have fewer side effects than other types of cancer treatment.

Hormone therapy adds, blocks, or removes hormones. For certain conditions (such as diabetes or menopause), hormones are given to adjust low hormone levels. To slow or stop the growth of certain cancers (such as prostate and breast cancer), synthetic hormones or other drugs may be given to block the body's natural hormones. Sometimes surgery is needed to remove the gland that makes a certain hormone.

The effectiveness of these treatments varies with how early the cancer is detected, the overall health of the patient, and the type and aggressiveness of the cancer cells.

Diabetes

Diabetes has also become a familiar term to us over the past several years. You may have heard your older family members refer to it as "sugar diabetes," which makes it sound as though another type exists that doesn't relate to sugar. This is not the case. Diabetes develops when a person's blood glucose is too high and their bodies cannot make enough insulin to balance it out. Diabetes causes 3% of all deaths in the US, ranking at number 7 on the top causes of death. Its prevalence has also been expensive to the nation. The American Diabetes Association reports that annual costs for diabetes treatment in the US totals over $176 billion.

In order to produce energy, nearly all of the food we consume breaks down into glucose in our bodies. Insulin, a hormone secreted by the pancreas, aids this glucose in getting into our cells. In some people the pancreas does not make insulin at all or not enough to deal with the glucose, leaving too much of it in the blood. There are four different types of diabetes, Type 1, Type 2, gestational, and prediabetes.

Type 1 diabetes (juvenile onset), the body does not make insulin. The immune system attacks and destroys the cells in the pancreas that make it. It is usually diagnosed in children and young adults, although it can appear at any age. People with type 1 diabetes need to take insulin every day to stay alive.

Type 2 diabetes (usually occurs in adults), the body does not make insulin well. This is more common. A person can develop type 2 diabetes at any age, even during childhood. However, this type of diabetes occurs most often in middle-aged and older people.

Pregnant women can also get what's called **gestational** diabetes, which means that the body experiences a temporary problem producing enough insulin while the baby is still developing. This usually goes away after birth.

Prediabetes is a condition in which the blood sugar level is too high but not high enough to be considered diabetes. A person with prediabetes can have many of the same complications as diabetes and is at risk for diabetes if nothing within their body changes to lower the blood sugar.

Managing Diabetes

Healthy eating, physical activity, and insulin injections are the basic therapies for type 1 diabetes. The amount of insulin taken must be balanced with food intake and daily activities. Blood glucose levels must be closely monitored through frequent blood glucose testing (Figure 23).

Healthy eating, physical activity, and blood glucose testing are the basic therapies for type 2 diabetes. In addition, many people with type 2 diabetes require oral medication, insulin, or both to control their blood glucose levels.

Healthy eating with diabetes means following a meal plan that will help you manage your blood glucose, blood pressure, and cholesterol. Choose fruits and vegetables, beans, whole grains, chicken or turkey without the skin, fish, lean meats, and nonfat or low-fat milk and cheese. Drink water instead of sugar-sweetened beverages. Choose foods that are lower in calories, saturated fat, trans fat, sugar, and salt.

In addition, regular physical activity, as mentioned throughout this text, is important in managing your body's systems and keeping your body composition healthy. Work up to that recommended 150 minutes

Diabetes can take a large toll of the body. This abundance of sugar can cause serious damage to your eyes, kidneys, nerves, and heart. The impact to the nerves and to the circulatory system can make a person prone to skin sores that are difficult to heal and even lead to amputation of a limb. As if this isn't enough, the risk of stroke for a person with diabetes also increases.

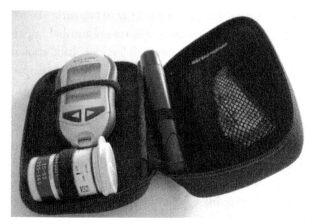

Figure 23. Common insulin testing kit.

of moderate or 75 minutes of vigorous-intensity exercise each week.

You can manage your diabetes and live a long and healthy life by taking care of yourself each day. Diabetes can affect almost every part of your body. Therefore, you will need to manage your blood glucose levels. Managing your blood glucose, as well as your blood pressure and cholesterol, can help prevent the health problems that can occur when you have diabetes, such as a heart attack or stroke.

Assessing and Lowering Individual Risk Factors for Chronic Diseases

Assessing your risk for chronic diseases in this chapter is a matter of comparing your current state to the recommendations for preventing these diseases. If any of your assessments show a need for improvement in a specific area, the other chapters in this book can help you create a targeted plan for improvement in that area of your life.

Risks for Heart Disease

Your risk for heart disease can be assessed by determining whether certain risk factors apply in your life.

You can potentially lower some of the risk by making healthy decisions in the controllable risk factors below.

Uncontrollable Risks

Not all risk is within our power of prevention. Several risk factors for heart disease are uncontrollable, including:

Heredity — Certain risks can be inherited genetic traits and make you predisposed to certain diseases, such as high blood pressure and cardiomyopathy. Hypertrophic cardiomyopathy, a condition in which the heart muscle is thickened, is thought to be the most common inherited or genetic heart disease. Several genetic disorders are associated with increased risk of premature heart attacks. A relatively common disorder is familial hypercholesterolemia, which causes high levels of "bad" cholesterol beginning at birth. About one out of 500 people in the United States inherit this condition (Figure 24).

Age — As you get older, your risk for atherosclerosis (hardening of the arteries) increases. Genetic or lifestyle factors cause plaque to build up in your arteries as you age. By the time you're middle-aged or older, enough plaque has built up to cause signs or symptoms. In men, the risk increases after age 45. In women, the risk increases after age 55.

Biological Sex — Heart disease is the number one killer for both sexes, though women have one risk factor that men don't — menopause. It is theorized that estrogen helps support heart health and as it declines, a woman's risk can increase.

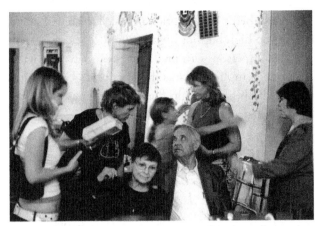

Figure 24. Family medical history is a good predictor for some chronic diseases.

Ethnicity — Although many of the risk factors correlate to socioeconomic class, even when studies adjust for these issues, some ethnicities still present with higher risks. Almost half of all African Americans have cardiovascular disease compared to one-third of whites. Hispanics and Latinos, though they have a higher risk for other diseases than whites, are 25% less likely to die of heart disease (though this could be due to under-reporting of the illness). Asian immigrants tend to have lower rates of heart disease, but their children raised in the US experience many of the same issues as whites, suggesting that environmental issues play a larger role.

Controllable Risks

Many risk factors that increase your likelihood of contracting heart disease are controllable, including:

Tobacco Use — The chemicals in tobacco cause buildup in the body's arteries, giving the blood a smaller passageway. It limits the flow of blood through the arteries forcing the heart to work harder, putting a strain on it and the rest of the body. If the buildup becomes too great, the artery can become totally blocked and the risk of heart attack is great. Smoking speeds up the accumulation of plaque from high cholesterol and robs your body of good cholesterol, putting you at even greater risk of forming dangerous blockage and clots. The nicotine in tobacco products also increases your heart rate and blood pressure. Even occasional smoking and second hand smoke increases your risk.

Smoking increases your risk of heart disease by 2 to 4 times compared to a non-smoker, according to the Centers for Disease Control. The CDC estimates

that 15.1% of people smoke and each day thousands of younger individuals take up the habit. The Midwest

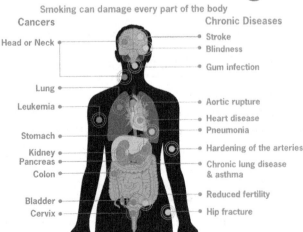

Figure 25. Smoking can contribute to many diseases.

shows the highest tobacco usage at 25.4%, the South at 24.2%, the Northeast 21.3%, and the West at 18%. People living in rural areas in particular have less access to health care services and so are more affected by this usage. Death rates attributed to tobacco use are lower in states with a lower population of smokers.

The CDC ranks smoking as the number one cause of preventable deaths in the US Approximately 90% of deaths from lung cancer result from smoking. Many people are aware of the high risks, but attempting to quit smoking or using tobacco can be difficult because of the addiction to nicotine. This chemical, found naturally in tobacco, is suspected by researchers to be as addictive as heroin and cocaine. People who attempt to quit often find the withdrawal symptoms difficult to manage. These include hunger, irritability, anger, anxiety, and cravings.

Yet more and more people find the will each day. Nearly 7 out of every 10 smokers report the desire to quit and half actually do make the move to do so. The CDC reports that the following tools have been helpful in those that have been successful:

- Consultation with health care provider

- Group or individual therapy/counseling or behavior therapy

- Treatments accessed by mobile phone

- Nicotine replacement products, either over-the-counter or prescription

- More information about quitting smoking can be found in Chapter 11.

The efforts are well worth it. When a person quits smoking, their risks begin to drop right away. Within one year, the improvements to health are dramatic, the risks are cut in half, and even individuals who have previously had a heart attack have a significantly lower risk of having another. Within five years, a former smoker has almost the same risk as a non-smoker. The younger you are when you quit, the greater you increase your potential life span. Someone who quits when they are 30 years of age can add at least 10 years to their life compared to a smoker. By age 60, that number decreases to three years.

Physical Activity — Most of us have heard the phrase "if you don't use it, you'll lose it." The key word in this sentence is *use*. As covered in previous chapters, many of the positive aspects of our health are lost through lack of usage. Muscles atrophy, tendons and ligaments become

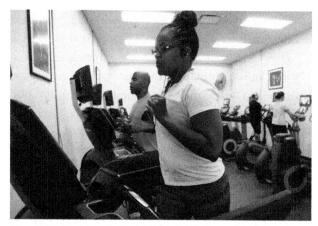

Figure 26. Regular physical activity can help prevent disease.

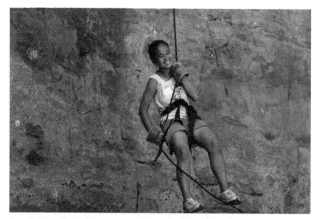

Figure 27. Staying active can lead to a long, full life.

inflexible, we lose agility and mobility when weight is gained, and our heart does not receive the aerobic benefits it needs to stay healthy (Figure 26).

Have you ever parked your car for a month or so without starting it? If you have, you likely found that you had a dead battery. Our heart functions in a similar way. It may not die as quickly, but it does experience the side effects of a sedentary lifestyle. Blood needs to pump in our bodies at times in the same way that a car's engine needs to rev. Physical activity improves circulation, improves cholesterol, improves the elasticity of arteries, helps control high blood pressure, diabetes and body weight. It helps us avoid so many of the risk factors that contribute to heart disease, such as overweight or obesity, high cholesterol, and hypertension, and keep our bodies functioning (Figure 27).

51% of US adults are not meeting the recommended guidelines for physical activity. The US Department of Health and Human Services recommends 150 minutes of moderate-intensity exercise, or 75 minutes of vigorous-intensity exercise each week to maintain a healthy fitness level and keep your heart functioning well.

High Cholesterol — The CDC describes cholesterol as a "waxy, fat-like substance" that our bodies use to make hormones, as well as digest fatty foods. Some of this our body makes, and some of it we ingest in the foods we eat. Cholesterol levels are primarily impacted by a few different factors — diet and physical activity.

We have different types of cholesterol in our bodies. The ones we hear about most often are the **low-density lipoproteins** (LDL) and **high-density lipoproteins** (HDL). Doctors consider LDL as the "bad" cholesterol or "less desirable cholesterol" because it does not flow as freely through the arteries and can lead to plaque buildup that results in heart disease and stroke. HDL, in contrast, absorbs cholesterol and helps it travel to the liver where it can be processed. Doctors test cholesterol levels with a fasting blood test to look at how much good and bad you have.

The science suggests that saturated fat encourages the liver to increase production of LDL and HDL. Trans fat can increase LDL and decrease HDL. The relationship is complicated, but most professionals recommend reducing saturated fat intake, particularly from animal sources. Experts are looking at inflammation as a marker for heart disease risk, but most guidelines (including the American Heart Association) continue to encourage people to be mindful of their saturated fat intake. The question isn't so much about how saturated fat impacts cholesterol levels, it's the degree to which that is dangerous for cardiovascular health. Researchers are considering what different factors may be affecting inflammation in the body to reduce heart disease risk. Physical activity, of course, plays a significant role. Research shows that exercise lowers LDL numbers and raises HDL. It also helps you lose weight, which is another contributing factor to risk. Being overweight increases cholesterol levels, largely due to a poor diet and lack of exercise. This allows bad cholesterol to build in your arteries, which leads to heart disease.

In the US, 71 million adults (33.5%) have high LDL numbers. An optimal LDL is below 100, though you aren't considered high until 160 or above, with 130 being borderline. HDL levels should be above 40. Doctors are now considering the relevance of your ratio of high to low density lipoproteins as a better predictor of your risk for cardiovascular disease. Divide your total cholesterol number by your HDL number. Ratios less than 3.5 to 1 are ideal.

Doctors check cholesterol levels through blood tests that measure LDL and HDL quantities, usually while the patient is fasting. Cholesterol should be checked every 4 to 6 years starting at age 20 unless the person has a problem with high LDL levels or have high risk factors for heart disease. Some physicians have begun testing children as young as 9, though there is some debate about whether this is necessary. Some studies suggest that genetic propensity toward high cholesterol can be determined early, as well as poor diet and exercise habits.

When doctors check cholesterol levels, they also check triglyceride levels. This gives them knowledge about how much fat is in your blood and adding to your risk of heart disease. **Triglycerides** are the storage centers for excess fat in our bodies. When our body needs energy, it uses these triglycerides to obtain it. If we never use it, our body keeps storing the fat as triglycerides indefinitely, which is why we become overweight.

A person can lower their cholesterol and triglycerides through a healthy diet, exercise, not smoking, and by maintaining a healthy weight. A diet aimed at lowering bad cholesterol is one low in saturated fats (though more research is needed), free of trans fat (a chemical form of fat engineered to lengthen food shelf life and shorten yours), and high in fruits, vegetables, fiber, whole grains, oats, and nuts (Figure 28). Individuals at high risk or with difficulty lowering their cholesterol numbers may need medications called statins, designed to help reduce blood cholesterol. These, however, can have side effects, which is why the preferred method is diet and exercise.

High Blood Pressure — As discussed earlier in the chapter, sustained high blood pressure (hypertension)

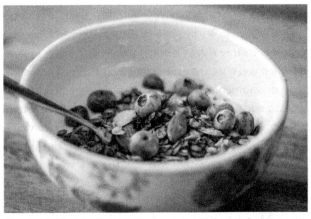

Figure 28. Healthy food choices improve the body's function.

means that the blood puts more pressure on the artery walls than normal. Whether it is primary or secondary hypertension, there are higher risks for certain individuals, such women over 45, blacks, and people with a family history of hypertension.

It's also important to consider that anything we do to either increase the pressure of our blood or make our heart pump harder will put us at greater risk. People who are overweight or obese, or are inactive, force their heart to pump harder to get oxygen and nutrients to the body, putting a strain on the vessels and the heart itself. Smoking or chewing tobacco also increases the risk because not only does nicotine temporarily increase your heart rate, the chemicals also build up in the artery walls and narrow the passage for the blood to travel and causing the heart to work harder. Over time, the arteries harden and lead to heart disease.

Stress can also play a negative role in our blood pressure levels (Figure 29). When we experience a stressful situation, our bodies can release fight or flight hormones that cause the heart to beat faster and the blood vessels to constrict. This is temporary but long-term stress can do damage. We also tend to pay less attention to other health aspects when stressed, such as our diet and exercise. See Chapter 8 for more information on stress.

About 75 million Americans suffer from hypertension at an annual cost to the nation of $46 billion each year. In fact, 1 in 3 adults have it. It's so common that many people aren't alarmed when they hear that they have high blood pressure. They begin taking the pills and continuing to live a normal life. Hypertension, however, should be a cause for concern. Seven out of every 10 people who have their first heart attack have hypertension, and 8 out of every 10 who have their first stroke. In addition to heart disease and stroke, your arteries in your kidneys and the vessels in your eyes can also be impacted by high blood pressure, as well as your ability to focus.

Your top number (systolic) should be below 120 and your bottom number (diastolic) below 80. A person with high blood pressure can lower it and their risks by eating a healthy diet, exercising, maintaining a healthy body composition, keeping cholesterol levels in a normal range, and controlling their stress level. Lowering your sodium intake can also help as salt can negatively affect pressure issues. Adults should have their blood pressure checked every two years if they have healthy blood pressure, and more frequently if their blood pressure is high.

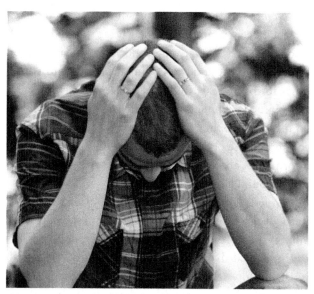

Figure 29. High blood pressure can stem from stress.

Overweight/Obesity — When your Body Mass Index (BMI) is above 30, you are considered obese, 25–29 is overweight. Over two in every three US adults are considered overweight or obese. As you can see by much of the material discussed in this text, many of the factors that cause someone to be overweight or obese, are the same factors that contribute to heart disease. Inactivity, a high fat diet (and high cholesterol levels), and visceral fat (abdominal fat) all contribute to stress on the heart and arteries. Visceral fat and poor cholesterol levels go hand-in-hand as a troubling tag-team to clog arteries and damage vital organs. Women tend to store fat on their hips and thighs, while men tend to store belly fat. Belly fat, which can be an indicator of visceral fat, is a greater risk. A healthy body composition remains your first line of defense. A fit man should have around 14–17% body fat, while a fit woman has between 21–24%. See Chapter 6 for more information.

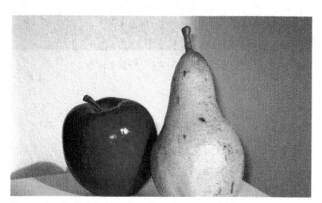

Figure 30. Body shapes tell us less about health than body composition.

Diabetes — The longer a person suffers from diabetes, the larger the impact to their heart. High levels of blood sugar can damage your blood vessels and the nerves that work with your heart, leading to atherosclerosis and other forms of heart disease. People with diabetes are also more likely to have issues with high cholesterol and high blood pressure. In fact, heart disease is the most common cause of death for people with diabetes. More information about how to lower your risk for diabetes can be found later in this chapter.

Psychological and Social Factors — These can also impact heart health in their connection to stress, personality type, chronic hostility and anger, suppressing psychological distress, depression and anxiety, social isolation, low socioeconomic status, and alcohol use (Figure 31). The common thread among most of these is stress. If you have difficulty managing anger, anxiety, depression, etc., your fight or flight hormones add stress to your body and you tend to have less concern for your health and lower motivation to manage it effectively. You may even drink more alcohol than recommended, which causes a temporary increase in heart rate. People with lower socioeconomic status tend to have more stress and, therefore, need to pay closer attention to how they manage it. See Chapter 8 for more information.

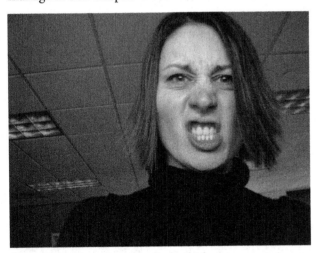

Figure 31. Persistant anger can lead to high stress.

Metabolic Syndrome — **Metabolic Syndrome** is a term the medical field uses for a group of risk factors or traits that contribute to heart disease and other health problems. These include many of the issues already discussed, such as obesity, high cholesterol and triglycerides, high blood pressure, and high blood sugar. When these are in check, your body is more likely to function as it should and your risk of heart disease is lower (Figure 32).

Metabolic Syndrome
Increased waist circumference or belly fat
High triglycerides
Elevated blood pressure
High blood sugar
A low HDL (good cholesterol)

Figure 32. Symptoms of metabolic syndrome.

Sleep Apnea — **Sleep apnea** is a common disorder in which you have one or more pauses in breathing or shallow breaths while you sleep. Untreated sleep apnea can increase your risk for high blood pressure, diabetes, and even a heart attack or stroke.

Alcohol Use — Heavy drinking can damage the heart muscle and worsen other CHD risk factors. Men should have no more than two drinks containing alcohol a day. Women should have no more than one drink containing alcohol a day.

Preeclampsia — This condition can occur during pregnancy. The two main signs of preeclampsia are a rise in blood pressure and excess protein in the urine. Preeclampsia is linked to an increased lifetime risk of heart disease, including CHD, heart attack, heart failure, and high blood pressure.

Risks for Cancer

Your risk of developing cancer can be assessed by determining whether certain risk factors apply in your life.

Uncontrollable Risks

Not all risk is within our power of prevention. Several risk factors for cancer are uncontrollable, including:

Heredity — There are certain inherited genetic mutations that result in an increase in some cancers, called Hereditary Cancer Syndrome (Figure 33).

Age — Natural aging is a significant risk factor in most cancers in general and also in certain types of cancer, such as breast, colon, and prostate. Half of all cancer diagnoses occurs in people with an average age of over 66.

Biological Sex — Hormones can also contribute to cancer growth, particularly in women. Menopausal women who undergo hormone replacement therapy for estrogen are at a higher risk for developing breast cancer. Cancer mortality rates, however, are higher among men than women.

Ethnicity — African American women have a higher incidence of aggressive breast cancers than other ethnicities while African American men have a higher rate of prostate cancer. Native Americans and Alaskan Natives have higher rates of kidney cancer. Asian and Pacific

Controllable Risks

Many risk factors that increase your likelihood of developing cancer are controllable. Make healthy decisions in the following areas to lower your risk (Figure 34).

Tobacco — Tobacco contains many chemicals above and beyond nicotine. When cigarettes are burned, these chemicals are released into the air and into the smoker's lungs. There is no such thing as a healthy cigarette, no matter how they are marketed. Tobacco use causes cancers in the lung, larynx, mouth, esophagus, throat, bladder, kidney, liver, stomach, pancreas, colon and rectum, and cervix. Smoking can also cause acute myeloid leukemia. For more information on quitting smoking, see Chapter 11.

Nutrition, Physical Activity, and Body Composition — Good nutrition habits are linked to preventing cancer by the American Cancer Society and several other governing associations. Good nutrition is about more than just calories and weight. It's about putting healthy, nutritional foods into your body that are more likely to help it than

You can potentially lower some of the risk by making healthy decisions in the controllable risk factors below.

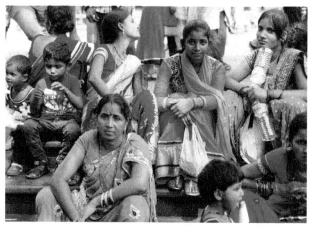

Figure 33. Heredity plays a role in your risk for chronic disease.

Islanders show a higher risk of liver cancer. Hispanic and African American women also see more risk of cervical cancers. It's uncertain why some ethnicities are more prone to certain forms of cancer aside from socioeconomic factors.

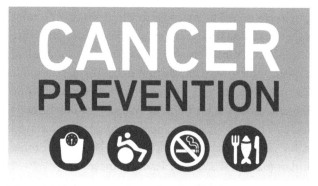

Figure 34. Prevent cancer by making healthy decisions.

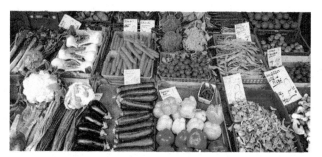

Figure 35. Vegetables are key in maintaining a healthy diet.

harm it. Healthy physical activity decreases the risks of colon, breast, and endometrial cancer according to the National Cancer Institute. It also keeps the organs and other systems of our body functioning properly and able to do their job effectively.

An unhealthy body composition, particularly obesity, can increase risks of breast, colon, rectum, endometrium, esophagus, kidney, pancreas, and bladder cancers. Good nutrition and physical activity if practiced regularly can lead to a healthy body composition. For more information on nutrition, physical activity, and body composition, see Chapters 2–7.

Alcohol Use — More than two drinks of alcohol a day can increase risk for cancers of the mouth, throat, esophagus, larynx, liver, and breast. It does this in a few different ways. One is that our bodies convert alcohol into a chemical called acetaldehyde, which damages DNA and hinders the body's cells from repairing the damage. Alcohol also impairs the body's ability to break down and absorb a variety of nutrients that may be associated with cancer risk, including vitamin A, nutrients in the vitamin B complex (such as folate), vitamin C, vitamin D, vitamin E, and carotenoids. In addition, it increases the risk of breast cancer by increasing blood levels of estrogen. For more information on alcohol use and abuse, see Chapter 11.

Infection — Approximately 16% of new cancer cases can be connected to infectious disease. Certain infectious agents such as viruses, bacteria, and parasites can cause chronic inflammation, which may increase your risk of cancer. Some viruses can disrupt signaling that normally keeps cell growth and proliferation in check. Also, some infections weaken the immune system, making the body less able to fight off other cancer-causing infections. And some viruses, bacteria, and parasites also cause chronic inflammation, which may lead to cancer.

Most of the viruses that are linked to an increased risk of cancer can be passed from one person to another through blood and/or other body fluids. Some examples include:

- Epstein-Barr Virus (EBV)
- Hepatitis B Virus and Hepatitis C Virus (HBV and HCV)
- Human Immunodeficiency Virus (HIV)
- Human Papillomaviruses (HPVs)
- Human T-Cell Leukemia/Lymphoma Virus Type 1 (HTLV-1)
- Kaposi Sarcoma-Associated Herpesvirus (KSHV)
- Merkel Cell Polyomavirus (MCPyV)
- Helicobacter pylori (H. pylori)
- Opisthorchis viverrini
- Schistosoma hematobium

You can lower your risk of infection from some infectious agents by getting vaccinated, not having unprotected sex, and not sharing hypodermic needles. For more information on infectious diseases, see Chapter 10.

Radiation — Environmental carcinogens (see earlier discussion in this chapter) can lead to cancer. Radiation from certain sources, like radon, x-rays, and gamma rays increase your risk of cancer by damaging DNA structure. The affected cells become abnormal and can become cancerous at a higher rate. Sunlight, sunlamps, and tanning booths give off ultraviolet (UV) radiation and should be avoided without protection. UV radiation damages skin cell's DNA, which may lead to skin cancer. For more information on radiation, see Chapter 12.

Stress — There is little evidence that stress directly causes cancer, but stress can impact your decision-making in the other risk factors above, leading to cancer indirectly. When a person becomes stressed they are less likely to focus on factors that don't immediately resolve issues and tend to put off healthy lifestyle changes in lieu of solving other concerns. This can become a difficult cycle since we are better able to manage stress when healthy and, certainly, a disease like cancer could add even more stress. For more information on stress management, see Chapter 8.

Chemicals and Toxic Environments — Exposure to chemicals in your environment can cause cancer, as well (environmental carcinogens). The highest risks are associated with radon radiation in basements, cigarette smoking, and pollution. The National Toxicology Project publishes a list of known human carcinogens every few years. For more information on environmental health, see Chapter 12.

Risks for Diabetes

Your risk of developing diabetes can be assessed by determining whether certain risk factors apply in your life. You can potentially lower some of the risk by making healthy decisions or managing certain risks in the controllable risk factors below.

Uncontrollable Risks

Heredity — Diabetes can run in families due to genetics. Type 1 diabetes can be inherited, autoimmune, or environmental. A predisposition to type 2 can also be inherited.

Age — Individuals 45 and older are more likely to develop type 2 diabetes. Research suggests that insulin resistance is more common due to muscle loss. As we age, fat can build in our muscles and liver, contributing to this resistance.

Biological sex — Men are at a greater risk for developing type 2 diabetes due to a higher incidence of visceral fat than women.

Ethnicity — American Indians and Alaskan Natives are at a higher risk at 15.9%, followed by blacks, Hispanics, Asian Americans, and whites.

Certain Health Conditions — including a history of gestational diabetes or having given birth to a baby over nine pounds, Polycystic ovary syndrome (PCOS), and *acanthosis nigricans* — dark, thick, and velvety skin around your neck or armpits.

Controllable Risks

Many risk factors that increase your likelihood of developing diabetes are controllable. Make healthy decisions in the following areas to lower your risk.

Overweight and obesity — A BMI over 25 increases your risk for diabetes.

Low HDL Cholesterol — HDL cholesterol is the "good" kind, so low levels of this or high levels of triglycerides can increase risks.

High Blood Pressure — High blood pressure, as mentioned above, is a result of lifestyle choices and can be lowered with improved nutrition and physical activity.

Physical Inactivity — Over and over, we have recommended fitness training to increase your physical activity, and lowering your risks for diabetes is yet another reason to strive for healthy physical fitness.

History of Heart Disease or Stroke — As above, some heart disease and stroke risk is preventable, so making healthier decisions overall can help you avoid multiple chronic diseases.

Depression — Clinical depression may not be preventable but it can be managed. See Chapter 8 for more information.

Online Resources for Lowering Risks

American Heart Association — Healthyforgood.heart.org
Centers for Disease Control — CDC.gov/cholesterol
The Franklin Institute — FI.edu/heart-engine-of-life
National Stroke Association — Stroke.org
American Diabetes Association — Diabetes.org

Conclusion

Your next steps should be to use the recommendations for each risk area to assess your own risk of developing a chronic disease. Using that information, you can create a plan for improving your wellness to lower those risks and live a healthier, longer life.

This chapter has looked closely at some of the life-threatening diseases that can be caused by poor health and fitness. We covered the causes, symptoms, and some treatments for disease, but most importantly, we explored several ways you can act now to avoid these diseases altogether. We all want to live longer, fuller lives, and understanding the consequences of unhealthy decisions can provide some of the motivation that may be lacking for you to make a change. Consider implementing lifestyle strategies that can reduce your risk for chronic disease, including habits in your diet, physical activity, stress, substance use, or other areas that may need attention.

Chapter 10
Infectious Disease

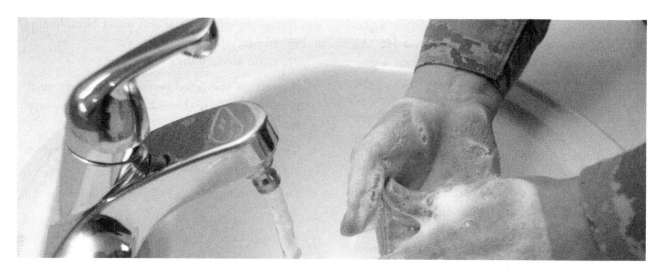

You and your friend are stopping for smoothies after an early-morning workout. You get some form of fruity concoction and she goes with some kale-filled, green, chunky mixture that looks intimidating. She's always trying to persuade you to join in her love of kale and makes yet another attempt, "Just taste it. It won't hurt you. It's good for you!" Little does she know that it's not your aversion to the leafy super-food that's causing you to hesitate. You are no longer distracted by the thought of drinking leaves but by the residue on her straw! She thinks she's offering you health — you see it as attempted assault. All you can think about are the millions of potential bacteria crawling around that tiny piece of plastic and respond with a polite "No thanks."

Your friend may have been completely healthy, but you have every right to be cautious. Infections are nothing to sneeze at. An infection is a disorder caused by the invasion of a disease-causing agent into your body. Dangers from infection surround us all the time, but most infectious diseases can be prevented with healthy strategies including engaging in good hygiene, protecting yourself against pathogens, and practicing safer sexual activity.

This chapter introduces the basics of infection and infectious diseases and how most of them can be prevented. It then turns to the dangers of sexually transmitted infections (STIs) and the importance of practicing safer sexual activity.

Infectious Diseases

No one gets through life without "catching a bug," not even your friend who consumes massive amounts of kale (though to be fair, she really is giving it a good shot). Infectious diseases accounted for over $120 billion in economic costs in 2014. As infectious diseases spread and new forms of them arise — and they do — the nation and its residents feel the burden physically and financially. Consider the common flu. Each year, on average, 5–20% of the US population gets the flu, tens of thousands are hospitalized and thousands die from flu-related illness. This costs an estimated $10.4 billion a year in direct medical expenses and an additional $16.3 billion in lost earnings annually.

We understand that diseases exist, and we know what it feels like to be sick, but what makes a disease infectious? Infectious diseases are caused by microorganisms. Microorganisms are tiny living things that are found everywhere — in air, soil, and water. You can get infected by touching, eating, drinking or breathing something that contains a germ. Microorganisms can also spread through animal and insect bites, kissing, and sexual contact.

The main kinds of microorganisms are:

- Bacteria — one-celled germs that multiply quickly and may release chemicals which can make you sick

- Viruses — capsules that contain genetic material and use your own cells to multiply

- Fungi — primitive plants, like mushrooms or mildew

- Protozoa — one-celled animals that use other living things for food and a place to live

- Helminths — intestinal worms transmitted through soil

These are all forms of **pathogens**. A pathogen is the first link in the chain of disease. Anything that causes disease is considered a pathogen.

Before going any further, it's important to remember that not all microbes are pathogens. Some bacteria, affectionately referred to as "good" bacteria, keep our bodies functioning properly. Some bacteria that live in our digestive tract, for example, aid in the digestion of food and help us process the things we eat. The microbes we focus on in this chapter are the ones we don't want in our bodies. Those are the ones we label pathogens.

Type	Description
Bacteria	Single celled organism that usually reproduce by splitting in two to create a pair of identical cells
Viruses	Multi-celled but can only reproduce inside a plant, animal, or person
Fungi	An organism that absorbs food from organic matter
Protozoa	One-celled creatures usually spread through water.
Parasitic worms	Causes intestinal and other infections

Figure 1. Five major types of pathogens.

Vaccines for Prevention	The primary method of controlling viral disease is by vaccination, which is used to prevent outbreaks by building immunity to a virus. Vaccines are prepared with live viruses, killed viruses, or molecular subunits of the virus.
Vaccines and Anti-Viral Drugs for Treatment	Vaccines can be used to treat an active viral infection. By giving the vaccine, immunity is boosted without adding more disease-causing virus. Another way of treating viral infections is the use of the antiviral drugs. These drugs have a limited success of curing viral disease, but can be used to control and reduce symptoms for a wide variety of viral diseases.

Figure 2. Treating viral infections.

Pathogens

We normally think of pathogens in hostile terms — as invaders that attack our bodies. But a pathogen or a parasite, like any other organism, is simply trying to live and procreate. Living at the expense of a host organism (in this case us) is a very attractive strategy, and it is possible that every living organism on Earth is subject to some type of infection or parasitism. A human host is a nutrient-rich, warm, and moist environment, which remains at a uniform temperature and constantly renews itself. It's not surprising that many microorganisms have evolved the ability to survive and reproduce in this desirable home.

Bacteria

Bacteria are living things that have only one cell. Under a microscope, they look like balls, rods, or spirals. They are so small that a line of 1,000 could fit across a pencil eraser. Most bacteria won't hurt you — less than 1 percent of the different types make people sick. Many are helpful. Some bacteria help to digest food, destroy disease-causing cells, and give the body needed vitamins. In fact, bacteria are used in making healthy foods like yogurt and cheese (you've seen the commercials). But infectious bacteria can make you ill. They reproduce quickly in your body and many give off chemicals called toxins or enzymes, which can damage tissue and give your immune system a run for its money.

Some of those that do cause disease can only replicate inside the cells of the human body and are called **obligate pathogens** (They feel obliged to be in your body — isn't that nice?). Others replicate in an environmental space such as water or soil and only cause disease if they happen to encounter a susceptible host. These are called **facultative pathogens**. Many bacteria are normally benign but have a latent ability to cause disease in someone with a compromised immune system. These are called **opportunistic pathogens**.

Some bacterial pathogens are fussy in their choice of host and will only infect a single species or a group of related species, whereas others are generalists. Shigella

Symptoms	Cold	Flu
Fever	Rare	High (100–102 F), can last 3–4 days.
Headache	Rare	Intense
General aches, pains	Slight	Usual, often severe
Fatigue, weakness	Mild	Intense, can last up to 2–3 weeks.
Extreme exhaustion	Never	Usual, starts early
Stuffy nose	Common	Sometimes
Sneezing	Usual	Sometimes
Sore throat	Common	Common
Cough	Mild to moderate	Common, can become severe.
Complications	Sinus, congestion or earache	Bronchitis, Pneumonia. You may need to go to a hospital.
Prevention	Wash your hands well and avoid sick people.	Flu vaccine once a year. Wash your hands well and avoid sick people. Antiviral drugs oseltamivir (Tamiflu) and zanamivir (Relenza)
Treatment	Over the counter products ease symptoms.	Over the counter products to ease symptoms. Prescription treatments: Oseltamivir (Tamiflu) or Zanamivir (Relenza) within 24-48 hours after symptoms start. Peramivir (Rapivab) for some cases; taken by IV.

Figure 3. Comparing the cold to the flu.

flexneri, for example, which causes epidemic dysentery (bloody diarrhea) in areas of the world lacking a clean water supply, will only infect humans and other primates. By contrast, the closely related bacterium Salmonella enterica, which is a common cause of food poisoning in humans, can also infect many other vertebrates, including chickens and turtles. A champion generalist is the opportunistic pathogen Pseudomonas aeruginosa, which is capable of causing disease in plants as well as animals. Other well-known bacteria that can harm us are Lyme disease, pneumonia, tuberculosis, E. coli, salmonella, listeria, meningitis, gonorrhea, chlamydia, and syphilis.

Viruses

Viruses are very tiny microorganisms. They contain just one or two molecules of RNA and DNA inside of a protein coating. Viruses cause some of the most familiar infectious diseases, such as the common cold, flu, and warts. They also cause more severe illnesses such as HIV/AIDS, smallpox, influenza, mononucleosis, measles, mumps, rabies, polio, hepatitis, and Ebola.

We often think of a virus as the runny nose and cough we get when catch the flu or the chicken pox. But what's actually happening in your body when you have a virus? Viruses are like a conquering clan. They invade living, normal cells and use those cells to multiply and reproduce. This can kill, damage, or change the cells and make you sick. Different viruses attack certain cells in your body such as your liver, respiratory system, or blood. When you get a virus, you may not always get sick from it. Your immune system may be able to fight it off.

For most viral infections, treatments can only help with symptoms while you wait for your immune system to fight off the virus. Antibiotics do not work for viral infections, though vaccines can help prevent you from getting many viral diseases, such as measles.

Fungus

If you have ever had athlete's foot or a yeast infection, you've had a **fungus**. A fungus is a primitive organism that may be single- or multi-celled, such as mushrooms, mold, and mildew. Fungi live in air, in soil, on plants, and in water. Some live in the human body, on the skin, as well as on many indoor surfaces. Common fungal infections are thrush, athlete's foot, meningitis, ringworm, and yeast infections.

Some fungi reproduce through tiny spores in the air. You can inhale the spores or they can land on you. As a result, fungal infections often start in the lungs or on the skin. Fungi are everywhere. There are approximately 1.5 million different species of fungi on Earth, but only about 300 of those are known to make people sick.

Anyone can get a fungal infection, even people who are otherwise healthy. Fungi are common in the environment, and people breathe in or come in contact with fungal spores every day without getting sick. However, in people with weak immune systems, these fungi are more likely to cause an infection.

Protozoa

Protozoa are microscopic, one-celled organisms that can be free-living or parasitic in nature. They are able to multiply in humans, which contributes to their survival and also permits serious infections to develop from just a single organism. Transmission of protozoa that live in a human's intestine to another human typically occurs through a fecal-oral route (for example, contaminated food or water or person-to-person contact). Protozoa that live in the blood or tissue of humans are transmitted to other humans by an arthropod vector (for example, through the bite of a mosquito or sand fly).

Examples include malaria, trichomoniasis (trich), toxoplasmosis, and naegleriasis. Some parasitic infections are rare, but deadly, like naegleriasis, which is contracted through warm, freshwater ponds or rivers and poorly chlorinated pools or hot tubs. Others, like toxoplasmosis, are much more common and contracted through poorly prepared foods and contact with cat feces.

Toxoplasmosis is considered to be a leading cause of death attributed to foodborne illness in the United States. More than 30 million men, women, and children in the US carry the toxoplasma parasite, but very few have symptoms because the immune system usually keeps the parasite from causing illness. However, women newly infected with Toxoplasma during pregnancy and anyone with a compromised immune system can experience severe consequences from it (this is why we frequently hear that pregnant women should not change kitty's litter box).

Helminths

Helminths are among the larger parasites. The word "helminth" comes from the Greek word for "worm." If this parasite — or its eggs — enters your body, it makes a home in your intestinal tract, lungs, liver, skin or brain, where it lives off your body's nutrients. These free-loading helminths include tapeworms and roundworms

Soil-transmitted helminths refer to the intestinal worms — such as whipworms, Ascaris, or hookworms — infecting humans through contaminated soil. This occurs mainly in areas with warm and moist climates where sanitation and hygiene are poor, including in temperate zones during warmer months. These STHs are considered Neglected Tropical Diseases (NTDs) because they inflict tremendous disability and suffering yet can be controlled or eliminated.

Soil-transmitted helminths live in the intestine and their eggs are passed in the feces of infected persons. If an infected person defecates outside (near bushes, in a garden, or field) or if the feces of an infected person are used as fertilizer, eggs are deposited on soil. Ascaris and hookworm eggs become infective as they mature in soil. People are infected with Ascaris and whipworm when eggs are ingested. This can happen when hands or fingers that have contaminated dirt on them are put in the mouth or by consuming vegetables and fruits that have not been carefully cooked, washed, or peeled. Hookworm eggs are not infective. They hatch in soil, releasing larvae (immature worms) that mature into a form that can penetrate the skin of humans. Hookworm infection is transmitted primarily by walking barefoot on contaminated soil. One kind of hookworm (Anclostoma duodenale) can also be transmitted through the ingestion of larvae.

People with light soil-transmitted helminth infections usually have no symptoms. Heavy infections can cause a range of health problems, including abdominal pain, diarrhea, blood and protein loss, rectal prolapse, and problems with physical and cognitive growth. These infections are treatable with medication prescribed by your health care provider.

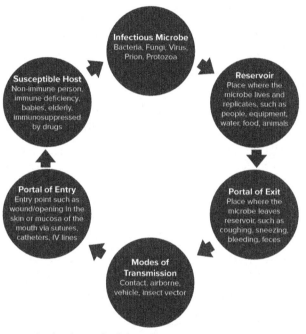

Figure 4. The chain of infection.

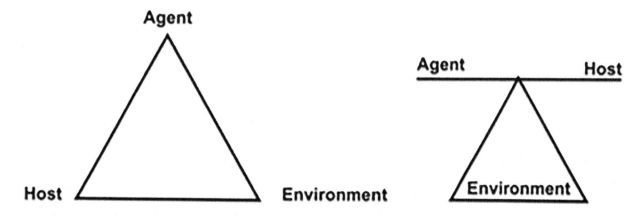

Figure 5. The epidemiologic triad.

Infection vs. Infectious Disease

There's a difference between infection and disease. The infection that occurs from the pathogen is often the first step. This is when the uninvited guest moves into its new home in your body and begins to take up residence, forming many new friends. Disease occurs when the cells in your body are damaged — as a result of the infection — and signs and symptoms of an illness appear. Your unwelcome houseguest hosts a large, messy party and trashes your house.

In response, your immune system gets busy. Your body calls in the police. A force of white blood cells, antibodies, and other mechanisms attempt to bust up the party and rid your body of whatever is causing the infection. For instance, in fighting off the common cold, your body might react with fever, coughing, and sneezing.

Chain of Infection

Each infection goes through a series of steps in this process. The traditional model (epidemiologic triad) holds that infectious diseases result when the agent (pathogen) leaves its reservoir or host (e.g. soil, air water) through a portal of exit (e.g. lungs, mouth), is conveyed by some mode of transmission (the droplets on your friend's smoothie straw), and enters through an appropriate portal of entry (your mouth, for example) to infect a susceptible host (you). This sequence is sometimes called the **chain of infection**. Each of the links must be present in a chronological order for an infection to develop.

Understanding how infectious diseases spread will help you protect yourself from contracting and spreading these illnesses to others. If you know how the chain works and where each connection is made, you can break the chain.

Reservoir

The reservoir of an infectious agent is the habitat in which the agent normally lives, grows, and multiplies. Reservoirs include humans, animals, and the environment. The reservoir may or may not be the source from which an agent is transferred to a host. For example, the reservoir of Clostridium botulinum is soil, but the source of most botulism infections is improperly canned food containing C. botulinum spores.

Many common infectious diseases have **human reservoirs**. Diseases that are transmitted from person to person without intermediaries include sexually transmitted diseases, measles, mumps, streptococcal infection, and many respiratory pathogens. Because humans were the only reservoir for the smallpox virus, for example, naturally occurring smallpox was eradicated after the last human case was identified and isolated.

Human reservoirs may or may not show the effects of illness. A carrier is a person who has the pathogen and is capable of transmitting it to others. Asymptomatic are otherwise healthy carriers are those who never experience symptoms despite being infected. **Incubatory** carriers are those who can transmit the agent during the incubation period before clinical illness begins. **Convalescent** carriers are those who have recovered from their illness but remain capable of transmitting to others. **Chronic** carriers are those who continue to harbor a pathogen such as hepatitis B virus or Salmonella Typhi (the causative agent of typhoid fever), for months or even years after their initial infection.

One notorious carrier is Mary Mallon, or Typhoid Mary, who was an asymptomatic chronic carrier of Salmonella Typhi. As a cook in New York City and New Jersey in the early 1900s, she unintentionally infected dozens of people until she was placed in isolation on an island in the East River, where she died 23 years later. It sounds odd now that a person would be isolated in such a way. However, Mary, not understanding the chain of infection, continued to work as a cook (infecting more people) even after being instructed to find a new profession. This lead authorities to step in and permanently remove her from the chain.

Carriers commonly transmit disease because they do not realize they are infected, and consequently take no special precautions to prevent transmission. Symptomatic persons who are aware of their illness, on the other hand, may be less likely to transmit infection because they are either too sick to be out and about, take precautions to reduce transmission, or receive treatment that limits the disease.

Humans are also subject to diseases that have **animal reservoirs**. Many of these diseases are transmitted from animal to animal, with humans as incidental hosts. The term "zoonosis" refers to an infectious disease that is transmissible under natural conditions from vertebrate animals to humans. Long recognized zoonotic diseases include brucellosis (cows and pigs), anthrax (sheep), plague (rodents), trichinellosis/trichinosis (swine), tularemia (rabbits), and rabies (bats, raccoons, dogs, and other mammals). Zoonoses newly emergent in North America include West Nile encephalitis (birds), and monkeypox (prairie dogs). Many newly recognized infectious diseases in humans, including HIV/AIDS, Ebola infection, and SARS, are thought to have emerged from animal hosts, although those hosts have not yet been identified.

Plants, soil, and water in the environment are also reservoirs (**environmental reservoirs**) for some infectious agents. Many fungal agents, such as those that cause histoplasmosis, live and multiply in the soil. Outbreaks of Legionnaire's disease are often traced to water supplies in cooling towers and evaporative condensers, reservoirs for the pathogen Legionella pneumophila.

Portal of Exit

The portal of exit is the path by which a pathogen leaves its host. It usually corresponds to the site where the pathogen is localized. For example, the pathogens for influenza viruses and tuberculosis exit the respiratory tract, cholera in feces, scabies in scabies skin lesions, and conjunctivitis (pink eye) through the eye. Some blood borne agents can exit by crossing the placenta from mother to fetus (rubella, syphilis, toxoplasmosis), while others exit through cuts or needles in the skin (hepatitis B) or blood-sucking arthropods (malaria).

An infectious agent may be transmitted from its natural reservoir to a susceptible host in different ways, both direct and indirect.

Direct Transmission

In direct transmission, an infectious agent is transferred from a reservoir to a susceptible host by **direct contact** or **droplet spread**. Direct contact occurs through skin-to-skin contact, kissing, and sexual intercourse. Direct contact also refers to contact with soil or vegetation harboring infectious organisms. Infectious mononucleosis ("mono" or "kissing disease") and gonorrhea, for example, are spread from person to person by direct contact. Hookworm is spread by direct contact with contaminated soil.

Droplet spread refers to spray with relatively large, short-range aerosols produced by sneezing, coughing, or even talking (such as that disheartening spray when someone neglects to cover their sneeze). Droplet spread is classified as direct because transmission is by direct spray over a few feet, before the droplets fall to the ground. Pertussis and meningococcal infections are examples of diseases transmitted from an infectious person to a susceptible host by droplet spread.

Indirect Transmission

Indirect transmission refers to the transfer of an infectious agent from a reservoir to a host by suspended air particles, inanimate objects (vehicles), or animate intermediaries (vectors).

Airborne transmission occurs when infectious agents are carried by dust or droplet nuclei (tiny, dried residue of droplets) suspended in air. Airborne dust includes material that has settled on surfaces and re-circulated by air currents as well as infectious particles blown from the soil by the wind. In contrast to droplets that fall to the ground within a few feet, droplet nuclei may remain suspended in the air for long periods of time and may be blown over great distances. Measles, for example, has occurred in children who came into a physician's office after a child with measles had left, because the measles virus remained suspended in the air. Viruses that cause the common cold can spread through either direct or indirect transmission.

Vehicles that may indirectly transmit an infectious agent include food, water, biologic products (blood), and fomites (inanimate objects such as handkerchiefs, bedding, or surgical scalpels). A vehicle may passively carry a pathogen, as food or water may carry the hepatitis A virus. The vehicle may also provide an environment in which the agent grows, multiplies, or produces toxin, as improperly canned foods provide an environment that supports production of botulinum toxin by Clostridium botulinum.

Vectors such as mosquitoes, fleas, and ticks may carry an infectious agent through purely mechanical means or may support growth or changes in the agent. Examples of mechanical transmission are flies carrying Shigella (which leads to a stomach infection) on their appendages, mosquitos carrying Malaria and Zika, ticks carrying Lyme disease, and fleas carrying Yersinia pestis (the agent of plague) in their gut.

Portal of Entry

The **portal of entry** refers to the manner in which a pathogen enters a susceptible host. The portal of entry must provide access to tissues in which the pathogen can multiply or a toxin can act. Often, infectious agents use the same portal to enter a new host that they used to exit the source host. For example, influenza virus exits the respiratory tract of the source host and enters the respiratory tract of the new host. In contrast, many pathogens that cause gastroenteritis follow a so-called "fecal-oral" route because they exit the source host in feces, are carried on inadequately washed hands to a vehicle such as food, water, or utensil, and enter a new host through the mouth. Other portals of entry include the skin (hookworm), mucous membranes (syphilis), and blood (hepatitis B, HIV).

Host

The final link in the chain of infection is a susceptible **host** (this could be you). Susceptibility of a host depends on genetic or constitutional factors, specific immunity, and nonspecific factors that affect an individual's ability to resist infection or to limit their reaction to it. An individual's *genetic makeup* may either increase or decrease susceptibility. For example, persons with sickle cell trait seem to be at least partially protected from a particular type of malaria.

Specific immunity refers to protective antibodies that are directed against a specific agent. Such antibodies may develop in response to infection, vaccine, or toxoid (toxin that has been deactivated but retains its capacity to stimulate production of toxin antibodies) or may be acquired by transfer from mother to fetus or by injection of antitoxin. *Nonspecific* factors that defend against infection include the skin, mucous membranes, gastric acidity, cilia in the respiratory tract, the cough reflex, and immune response.

Our immune system is critical in the process of fighting infection. Its strength and abilities can make or break our body's ability to stand up to these tiny invaders. Most humans are not easily infected. People with compromised immune systems are more susceptible to disease and can have a more difficult time getting healthy again. Factors that may increase susceptibility to infection by disrupting host defenses include malnutrition, alcoholism, and disease or therapy that impairs the immune response. Those who are weak, sick, malnourished, have cancer or are diabetic have increased susceptibility to chronic or persistent infections. Individuals who have a suppressed immune system are particularly susceptible to opportunistic infections.

Colonization

Infection begins when an organism successfully enters the body, grows, and multiplies. This is referred to as **colonization**. Think for a moment about what a colony is and what it means to colonize. The first Americans were part of a colony. They came from foreign lands to a new country and established a new home. They built houses, had children, and "colonized" America. Sometimes this was painless, as it is with some pathogens. Other times this was accomplished at the expense of the present inhabitants (in this case, your cells and tissues). Sometimes the colonists stayed at their original port of entry (say Plymouth Rock, for example) and other times they travelled great distances to set up home. While a few organisms can grow at the initial site of entry, many migrate and cause systemic infection in different organs. Some pathogens grow within our cells while others grow freely in bodily fluids.

Types of Infection

Many times, we are exposed to a pathogen but do not become ill. Disease can arise if the host's protective immune mechanisms aren't up to the task or are compromised and the organism inflicts damage on the host. Not all infectious agents cause disease in all hosts. For example, less than 5% of individuals infected with polio develop the disease. On the other hand, some infectious agents are highly virulent. The pathogens causing mad cow disease and Creutzfeldt–Jakob disease invariably kills all animals and people that are infected.

Just as the first colonists arriving in America came from many different lands, there are many different types of pathogens looking for a new home. It stands to reason that they will all react differently to their new environment, even if some have similarities. We categorize infections by how quickly they settle in, how they treat their new home, and how long they stay.

Acute

An **acute infection** has a rapid onset and relatively brief period of symptoms, often resolving within days, though it could be six months depending upon the pathogen and your general health. Bouts of the flu, sinus infections, and even Ebola are good examples. The disease itself could be sudden, severe, and fairly miserable — even fatal in some people — but you won't live with it long-term.

Often an acute infection may cause little or no clinical symptoms, what is called an "inapparent" infection. The poliovirus that affected so many people years ago is a good example. Over 90% of people infected were without symptoms. During an inapparent infection, the pathogens reproduce enough in the host to call upon your antibodies, but not enough to cause disease. This may seem preferable, but it can be problematic because the disease can spread easily this way. During the polio epidemic in the US, the quarantine of paralyzed patients did not stop the spread of the disease because most of the infected individuals had no symptoms and continued on with their lives, spreading the disease to others.

Acute infections begin with an **incubation** period. This is the time it takes after a person is infected until he becomes ill. Sometimes the incubation is short (e.g., a day or so for the flu), while other times it is quite long (e.g, 2 weeks for chickenpox and many years for HIV). In

Illness (Pathogen)	Symptoms	Home Treatment	When to Seek Medical Care
Common cold (Over 200 different viruses)	Runny nose, nasal congestion, mild cough, sore throat, low-grade fever, sneezing	Usually resolves on its own; fluid, rest, and over-the-counter medications to treat symptoms; avoid alcohol and tobacco	Worsening symptoms after third day, difficulty breathing, stiff neck
Influenza (Influenza A or B virus)	Sudden-onset fever, extreme fatigue, head-ache, body aches, cough	Usually resolves on its own; same home treatment as for colds; prescription anti-virals available	Difficulty breathing, severe head-ache or stiff neck, confusion, fever lasting more than 3 days; new, localized pain in ear, chest, sinuses; people at high risk for complications should contact a health care provider if they develop flu symptoms
Bronchitis (different viruses or bacteria)	Cough that may start out dry and later produce mucus; sore throat, fever	Usually resolves on its own; same home treatment as colds	Shortness of breath, high fever, shaking chills (signs of pneumonia); wheezing and cough that last more than 2 weeks; people at high risk for complications should check with a health care provider
Mononucleosis (Epstein-Barr virus)	High fever, swollen glands, severe sore throat, fatigue; nausea, vomiting, and loss of appetite can occur	Usually resolves on its own; rest, fluids; avoid contact sports until symptoms resolve due to risk of spleen rupture	Fever lasting more than 3 days; symptoms lasting longer than 7-10 days; severe abdominal pain (possibly indicating ruptured spleen)

Figure 6. Common illnesses and their symptoms and treatment.

some cases, a person is contagious during the incubation period, while in others the person is not contagious until the illness begins. The amount of time a person remains contagious depends on the infection and the person.

In such cases, a **prodrome** isn't apparent. A prodome is an early sign or symptom (or set of signs and symptoms), which often indicate the onset of a disease before specific symptoms develop. Prodromes may be non-specific symptoms or, in a few instances, may clearly indicate a particular disease, such as the tingling that occurs just before getting a cold sore, or the feeling you get when it seems like you are "fighting a bug," just before getting the full symptoms.

Acute viral infections are responsible for epidemics of disease involving millions of individuals each year, such as influenza and measles. When a vaccine doesn't exist for the virus or is unavailable, these infections can be difficult to control. Often, between the incubation period and the time a person feels symptoms (prodromes), they've already spread it to someone else. This is an even larger problem in crowded areas, like college campuses and health care facilities.

After the symptoms begin to fade we enter a stage of **convalescence**, where we start regaining energy and acute symptoms subside. The time it takes for this to occur depends on the infection severity and the overall health of the individual. Yet with some infections, we could be convalescent carriers, spreading the disease despite our own improvement.

Chronic Infection

In contrast to acute infections, a **chronic infection** lasts for long periods, and can occur when the primary infection is not cleared by the immune system. Varicella-zoster virus (chicken pox), measles virus, hepatitis, and HIV-1 are examples. Whether an infection becomes chronic depends on a combination of factors, such as the nature of the pathogen and the immune system of the host.

Infections can go through periods where the virus lays dormant (or latent) then returns under the right circumstances, like the virus that causes chicken pox. If we get chicken pox when we are young, it can resurface again later in our lives in the form of shingles. That's because it is a **latent infection**. This type of infection is hidden or inactive. As opposed to active infections, where a virus or bacterium is actively replicating and potentially causing symptoms, latent infections are essentially static. While an infection is latent, it may hide from the immune system and/or be difficult to treat with drugs and other therapies. The reason why people don't have cold sores on their mouths all their lives is because the herpes virus that causes cold sores (HSV-1) goes dormant, hiding out in the nervous system.

Illness (Pathogen)	Symptoms	Home Treatment	When to Seek Medical Care
Meningitis (several different viruses or bacteria)	High fever, stiff and painful neck, headache; vomiting, sleepiness, confusion, seizures	Requires medical evaluation; if determined to be a viral infection, home treatment to relieve symptoms is appropriate	Immediately; bacterial meningitis requires treatment with antibiotics to avoid serious or deadly complications
Strep throat (streptococcus bacteria)	Sudden-onset sore throat and fever swollen glands; red and white pus on tonsils; absence of cold symptoms	A visit to health care provider is appropriate; saltwater gargles, throat lozenges, over-the-counter medications to treat symptoms	Treated with antibiotics to reduce duration of symptoms and risk of complications
Bacterial skin infection (staphylococcus aureus or streptococcus)	Skin sore or rash; red, swollen, warm, and painful areas of skin; if infection spreads, general symptoms of fever, chills, swollen glands	A visit to health care provider is appropriate; warm compresses; keep infected area clean and dry; topical antibiotics if advised by health care provider	Usually treated with antibiotics; be alert to worsening symptoms or infection to the face
Urinary tract infection (different bacteria)	Cloudy, bloody, or strong smelling urine; frequent urination; pain or burning with urination; low fever; pain in lower abdomen	Requires medical evaluation; drink plenty of water; in women, drinking cranberry juice has been shown to help prevent but not treat urinary tract infections	Usually treated with antibiotics; be alert to worsening symptoms, which may indicate that the infection has spread to the kidneys

Figure 7. When to seek medical care for infections.

Many sexually transmitted diseases go through periods of latency, where individuals are asymptomatic and the infection is lying dormant in their bodies. Herpes and HIV are good examples. One of the reasons that STIs are a hidden epidemic. People can spread the disease if the dormant infection reactivates before symptoms appear.

People with chronic infections are considered carriers. They serve as reservoirs of the infectious virus and will likely always carry it around. In populations with a high proportion of carriers, the disease is said to be endemic, such as HIV is in certain parts of Africa.

Immune System

Your **immune system** is a complex network of cells, tissues, and organs that work together to defend against germs. It helps your body to recognize these "foreign" invaders. Then its job is to keep them out, or if it can't, to find and destroy them.

An example of this principle is found in **immune-compromised** people, including those with genetic immune disorders, immune-debilitating infections like HIV, and even pregnant women, who are susceptible to a range of microbes that typically do not cause infection in healthy individuals.

The immune system can distinguish between normal, healthy cells and unhealthy cells by recognizing a variety of "danger" cues called danger-associated molecular patterns (DAMPs). Cells may be unhealthy because of infection or because of cellular damage caused by non-infectious agents like sunburn or cancer. Infectious microbes, such as viruses and bacteria, release another set of signals recognized by the immune system called pathogen-associated molecular patterns (PAMPs).

When the immune system first recognizes these signals, it responds to address the problem. If an immune response cannot be activated when there is sufficient need, problems arise, like infection. On the other hand, when an immune response is activated without a real threat or is not turned off once the danger passes, different problems arise, such as allergic reactions and autoimmune disease.

The immune system is quite complex and stays very busy. There are numerous cell types that either circulate throughout the body or reside in a particular tissue. Our white blood cells, for example, are made by bone marrow and help the body fight infection and other diseases. There are lots of types of white blood cells and other cells that contribute to our immune system. Each cell type plays a unique role, with different ways of recognizing problems, communicating with other cells, and performing their functions.

All immune cells come from precursors in the bone marrow and develop into mature cells through a series of changes that can occur in different parts of the body. Our skin, for example, is usually the first line of defense against germs. Skin cells produce and secrete important antimicrobial proteins, and immune cells can be found in specific layers of the skin. Another important helper is our bloodstream. Immune cells constantly circulate throughout the bloodstream, patrolling for problems.

Mucosal tissue also pitches in to help defend the body against infection. Mucosal surfaces are prime entry points for pathogens, and specialized immune hubs are strategically located in mucosal tissues like the respiratory tract and gut. For instance, Peyer's patches are important areas in he small intestine where immune cells can access samples from the gastrointestinal tract.

The Lymphatic System

Perhaps the biggest player in the game of defense is our **lymphatic system**. The lymphatic system is a network of vessels and tissues composed of lymph, an extracellular fluid, and lymphoid organs, such as lymph nodes. The lymphatic system is a conduit for travel and communication between tissues and the bloodstream. Immune cells are carried through the lymphatic system and converge in lymph nodes, which are found throughout the body.

Lymph nodes are a communication hub where immune cells sample information brought in from the body. For instance, if adaptive immune cells in the lymph node recognize pieces of a microbe brought in from a distant area, they will activate, replicate, and leave the lymph node to circulate and address the pathogen. Thus, doctors may check patients for swollen lymph nodes, which may indicate an active immune response.

The lymph system gets help from other players, such as the thymus and spleen. The thymus is an organ in the chest behind the breastbone. T lymphocytes grow and multiply in the thymus. The spleen is an organ located behind the stomach. While it is not directly connected to the lymphatic system, it is important for processing information from the bloodstream. Immune cells are enriched in specific areas of the spleen, and upon recognizing blood-borne pathogens, they will activate and respond accordingly.

White blood cells patrol the body. When they come across an antigen, they produce an antibody. An **antigen** is a foreign substance (the invading microbe or pathogen) that causes a response in the immune system. Antigens are proteins that are found on the surface of the pathogen. They are unique to that pathogen. Antigens can be bacterium, viruses, etc. There's a different antigen for every cold that you've ever had.

When an antigen enters the body, the immune system produces **antibodies** against it. It is like a battle with the police (antibody) fighting off the intruders (antigen). Lymphocytes (a type of white blood cell) recognizes the antigen as being uninvited and produces antibodies that are specific to that antigen. The antibodies gang up on and destroy the antigen.

White blood cells can also produce chemicals called antitoxins, which destroy the toxins (poisons) some bacteria produce when they have invaded the body. Tetanus, diphtheria and scarlet fever are all diseases where the bacteria secrete toxins.

Once a person has had a disease they don't normally catch it again because the body produces memory cells that are specific to that antigen. Once someone has trashed your home, you aren't likely to invite them back. The memory cells remember the microbe that caused the disease and rapidly make the correct antibody if the body is exposed to infection again. The pathogen is quickly destroyed, preventing symptoms of the disease from occurring.

Preventing Infections

To prevent infection, good hygiene, practicing safer sex, and getting vaccinated are key. It takes a large amount of individual and teamwork to effectively prevent and control infections. Below, you will find examples of specific practices that are ongoing and that you can do to help minimize your exposure to pathogens.

Public Health

Disease knows no borders. In today's interconnected world, a disease threat anywhere can become a health threat in the US We know that disease exploits even the smallest gap to spread and grow. With the ease and speed of global travel, along with rapidly expanding commerce and trade, the need to shut down the expressways available to infectious disease into the US and within its borders is more important today than ever before.

The Centers for Disease Control has the large job of looking not only at what happens here in the US but also what happens abroad. The most effective way to protect Americans from known and unknown health threats is to stop those that occur overseas before they spread to our shores. CDC's global activities protect Americans from major health threats such as Ebola, Zika, and pandemic influenza. Importantly, CDC helps other countries build capacity to prevent, detect, and respond to their health threats through our work.

CDC works with an array of partners, including the World Health Organization. WHO convenes its 194 member nations, including the US, to direct and coordinate global health strategies, tactics, and priorities. CDC works in more than 60 countries, with staff from the US, but with even more staff from the respective countries to carry on the work, working with ministries of health and other partners on the front lines where outbreaks occur. This work protects Americans because it strengthens countries to respond to disease threats as close to their source as possible, and not spread.

CDC also works globally to eradicate the world of vaccine-preventable diseases such as polio. The US Government's commitment for over two decades to eradicate the second human disease ever after smallpox, ensures that children in the US will never repeat history when people with polio had to be in iron lungs to breathe and children had to spend their summer indoors in fear of being paralyzed for life

How We Can Protect Ourselves

Within the US we have many challenges when it comes to controlling the spread of infection. Much of it comes through the process of education. Knowledge of common infection control practices and vaccinations are the primary way that citizens can help keep themselves and others healthy.

Getting Vaccinated

For a few weeks after birth, babies have some protection from germs that cause diseases. This protection is passed from their mother through the placenta before birth, and through antibodies in breastmilk. After a short period, this natural protection goes away.

Vaccines help protect against many diseases that used to be much more common. Examples include tetanus, diphtheria, mumps, measles, pertussis (whooping cough), meningitis, and polio. Many of these infections can cause serious or life-threatening illnesses and may lead to life-long health problems. Because of vaccines, many of these illnesses are now rare.

Vaccines are our most effective and cost-saving tools for disease prevention. For each annual group of children in the US receiving the recommended 13 vaccines, approximately 42,000 lives are saved, 20 million cases of disease are prevented, $13.6 billion in direct costs are saved, and $68.9 billion in direct plus indirect (societal) costs are saved.

How Vaccines Work

Vaccines (immunizations) are used to boost your immune system and prevent serious, life-threatening diseases. Vaccines "teach" your body how to defend itself when germs, such as viruses or bacteria, invade it:

- They expose you to a very small, very safe amount of viruses or bacteria that have been weakened or killed.

- Your immune system then learns to recognize and attack the infection if you are exposed to it later in life.

- As a result, you will not become ill, or you may have a milder infection. This is a natural way to deal with infectious diseases.

Four types of vaccines are currently available:

- **Live virus vaccines** use the weakened (attenuated) form of the virus. The measles, mumps, and rubella (MMR) vaccine and the varicella (chickenpox) vaccine are examples.

- **Killed (inactivated) vaccines** are made from a protein or other small pieces taken from a virus or bacteria. The flu vaccine is an example.

- **Toxoid vaccines** contain a toxin or chemical made by the bacteria or virus. They make you immune to the harmful effects of the infection, instead of to the infection itself. Examples are the diphtheria and tetanus vaccines.

- **Biosynthetic vaccines** contain manmade substances that are very similar to pieces of the virus or bacteria. The Hib (*Haemophilus influenzae* type B) conjugate vaccine is an example.

Safety of Vaccines

Some people worry that vaccines are not safe and may be harmful, especially for children. They may ask their health care provider to wait or even choose not to have the vaccine. Overwhelming scientific consensus, including The American Academy of Pediatrics, the CDC, and the Institute of Medicine, concludes that vaccines are not dangerous, but even if they were, their benefits far outweigh their risks.

Vaccines, such as the measles, mumps, rubella, chickenpox, and nasal spray flu vaccines contain live, but weakened viruses. Unless a person's immune system is weakened, it is unlikely that a vaccine will give the person the infection. People with weakened immune systems should not receive these live vaccines. These live vaccines may be dangerous to the fetus of a pregnant woman. To avoid harm to the baby, pregnant women should not receive any of these vaccines. Your health care provider can tell you the right time to get these vaccines.

Thimerosal is a preservative that was found in most vaccines in the past. People feared that the preservative could cause autism. But now:

- Only one third of flu shots still have thimerosal.

- No other vaccines commonly used for children or adults contain thimerosal.

- Research done over many years has not shown any link between thimerosal and autism or other medical problems.

- Allergic reactions are rare and are usually to some other (component) of the vaccine.

Staying Up-to-Date on Vaccinations

Even if you were vaccinated at a younger age, the protection from some vaccines can wear off or the viruses or bacteria that the vaccines protect against change so your resistance is not as strong. As you get older, you may also be at risk for vaccine-preventable diseases due to your age, job, hobbies, travel, or health conditions.

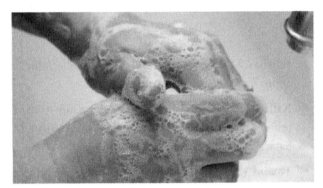

Figure 8. Washing hands helps prevent infection.

The CDC recommends that all adults get the following vaccines:

- Influenza vaccine every year to protect against seasonal flu

- Td vaccine every 10 years to protect against tetanus

- Tdap vaccine once instead of Td vaccine to protect against tetanus and diphtheria plus pertussis (whooping cough) and during each pregnancy for women

- Other vaccines you need as an adult are determined by factors such as age, lifestyle, job, health condition and vaccines you have had in the past. Vaccines you need may include those that protect against: shingles, human papillomavirus (which can cause certain cancers), pneumococcal disease, meningococcal disease, hepatitis A and B, chickenpox (varicella), measles, mumps, and rubella.

Practice Good Infection Control Habits

There are a number of additional strategies that can help you avoid infection.

- **Wash your hands frequently** — Use soap and water that is as hot as you can stand. Thoroughly lather your hands and make sure to wash under your fingernails, if possible.

- **Stay home if you are sick** — Easier said than done, sometimes, but going out and contacting other people when you are sick can spread disease. In some instances, you may be legally required to stay home. Someone working with food, for example, is required by the state of Oregon to stay home if they have diarrhea, for example.

- **Use single-use tissues, and dispose of them immediately after use** — Once you have used a tissue, it becomes a vector for spreading disease. Also, it's gross to leave tissues lying around.

- **Wash your hands after coughing, sneezing, or using a tissue** — If you cough or sneeze into your hands, they become coated in infectious materials and anything you touch becomes a vector for spreading disease.

- **Do not touch your eyes, nose, or mouth** — If you are in public and touch door handles, shake hands, etc., you may contact contagions. Your eyes, nose, and mouth all have mucous membranes, which are thin enough to make it easy for pathogens to pass into your system.

- **Do not share cups, glasses, dishes, or cutlery** — Your smoothie-sharing friend may be offended, but people can be contagious before and after being visibly sick, making their cups and cutlery vectors for infection.

- **Be careful how you cover your sneeze or cough** — We are taught to cough and sneeze into our hands, which is a good thing — it keeps pathogens from spreading through the air in droplets. However, a better practice is to sneeze or cough into your shoulder or elbow, which comes into contact with fewer surfaces than your hands.

Sexually Transmitted Infections (STIs)

STIs are among the most common infections in the US with over 20 million new cases each year. Half of these cases are 15–24 year-olds. STIs can be dangerous when left untreated. In most cases, they can be prevented by practicing "safer" sex. The "safest" sex practice is not having sex with other people (abstinence). But there are a number of other ways to have safer sex, such as having sex within a mutually monogamous relationship and using barriers, like condoms, the correct way, consistently, with each new sex act.

STIs are more common than people think. For example, HPV is so common that nearly all sexually active men and women contract the virus at some point in their lives. The CDC estimates that there are over 20 million new STI cases each year, and that annual costs of treatment for STIs is over $16 billion.

Sexually transmitted infections are diseases that get transmitted via sexual contact between partners. Most STIs are transmitted via fluid exchanges during oral, anal, and vaginal sex, but some diseases can be transmitted via skin-to-skin contact. Many STIs do not exhibit symptoms and people may spread them unknowingly to their partners. Some exhibit symptoms that make transmission easier, even for other STIs, because of open sores or breaks in the skin.

Some STIs are treatable, if detected early, while others are chronic, incurable, and even life-threatening (e.g. HIV and herpes). Engaging in risk-aware, "safer sex" practices significantly reduce the chances of infection. Treatable sexually transmitted infections carry an unfortunate social stigma, which can cause people to become depressed or too embarrassed to talk to a doctor.

STI	Estimated Annual Incidence	Estimated Prevalence*	Outlook if Diagnosed
Trichomoniasis	1.1 million	n/a	Curable with antibiotics
HPV infection	14 million	20 million	Vaccine-preventable; incurable but often resolves on its own; can cause cancer
Chlamydia	2.8 million	1.9 million	Curable with antibiotics
Genital herpes	750,000	45 million	Chronic and incurable; treatments can reduce symptoms and outbreaks
Gonorrhea	820,000	n/a	Curable with antibiotics
Syphilis	55,000	n/a	Curable with antibiotics
HIV infection	41,000	1.2 million	Chronic and potentially fatal; treatable but incurable
Hepatitis B	19,000	1.25 million	Vaccine-preventable; incurable but often resolves on its own; can cause fatal liver disease

*Because viral STIs can be persistent and incurable, the number of currently infected people capable of transmitting the infections (prevalence) greatly exceeds the annual number of new cases (incidence).

Figure 9. Common STI incidence in the United States.

It is important to regularly test for infection if you are sexually active (even if married) and seek treatment as soon as an infection is discovered.

Despite being a relatively small portion of the sexually active population, young people between the ages of 15 and 24 accounted for the highest rates of chlamydia and gonorrhea in 2014 and almost two thirds of all reported cases. Additionally, previous estimates suggest that young people in this age group acquire half of the estimated 20 million new STIs diagnosed each year.

There are several reasons for this. Young people:

- Often underestimate their risk;

- Are more likely to participate in risky sexual behavior;

- Are more likely to have their sexual activity affected by alcohol or substance abuse

- Are more prone to peer and media influences.

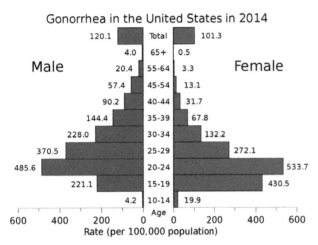 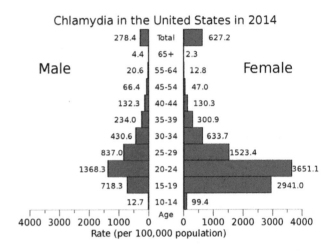

Figure 10. Gonorrhea and.Chlamydia cases in the United States.

Gender and STIs

Some people are at greater risk than others for acquiring an STI. It is easier for men to transmit STIs to women than the other way around, and people limited to "abstinence only" education have a higher infection rate than people who have had a more comprehensive education. The old saying holds true — knowledge is power, or in this case, protection. Studies suggest that women who learn abstinence-only and promise to wait for sex until marriage and young women who haven't made the same pledge become sexually active at roughly the same rates, but the women who haven't learned

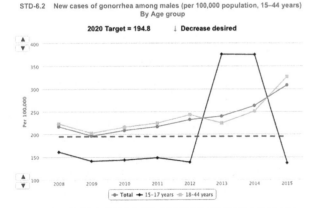 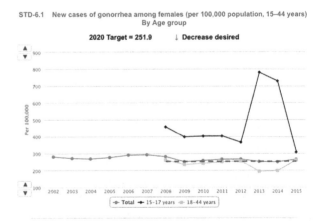

Figure 11. Healthy People 2020 goals for STI incidence.

how to have safer sex, per CDC recommendations, via comprehensive sex education, contract STIs, like HPV, at a higher rate than their peers and are also more likely to become pregnant earlier.

Women experience a different type of risk when it comes to STIs. Their bodies are different and do not show the same signs and symptoms and the impact can be more severe. According to the CDC:

- **A woman's anatomy can place her at a unique risk for STI, compared to a man** — The lining of the vagina is thinner and more delicate than the skin on a penis, so it's easier for bacteria and viruses to penetrate. The vagina is a good environment (moist) for bacteria to grow.

- **Women are less likely to have symptoms of common STIs — such as chlamydia and gonorrhea — compared to men** — If symptoms do occur, they can go away even though the infection may remain.

- **Women are more likely to confuse symptoms of an STI for something else** — Women often have normal discharge or think that burning/itching is related to a yeast infection. Men usually notice symptoms like discharge because it is unusual.

- **Women may not see symptoms as easily as men** — Genital ulcers (like from herpes or syphilis) can occur in the vagina and may not be easily visible, while men may be more likely to notice sores on their penis

- **STIs can lead to serious health complications and affect a woman's future reproductive plans** — Untreated STIs can lead to pelvic inflammatory disease, which can result in infertility and ectopic pregnancy. Chlamydia (one of the most common STIs) results in few complications in men.

- **Women who are pregnant can pass STDs to their babies** — Genital herpes, syphilis and HIV can be passed to babies during pregnancy and at delivery. The harmful effects of STDs in babies may include stillbirth (a baby that is born dead), low birth weight (less than five pounds), brain damage, blindness and deafness.

- **Human papillomavirus (HPV) is the most common sexually transmitted infection in women, and is the main cause of cervical cancer** — While HPV is also very common in men, most do not develop any serious health problems.

Each year untreated STDs cause infertility in at least 24,000 women in the US, and untreated syphilis in pregnant women results in infant death in up to 40 percent of cases. The fact that many women go untreated, unknowingly, presents an increased risk of transmission for both genders. The good news is that regular pap screenings can catch many infections before they progress and HPV now has a vaccine for both men and women to reduce the risk of contracting cancer.

Diagnosis and Treatment of Common STIs

This section provides information on the top seven most common STIs in the US, including a description of symptoms, how they are diagnosed, and how they are treated. Some of these sections are more complex than others, just as some STIs are more complex than others. They are listed below in descending order of total new infections each year.

Human Papillomavirus (HPV)

Human papillomavirus (HPV), commonly known as genital or anal warts, is the most common STI in the United States (Figure 12). There are approximately 20 million current cases of HPV and 6 million new cases each year. It is easily transmitted via vaginal, oral, or anal intercourse, but is also transmitted skin-to-skin, which reduces the effectiveness of condoms somewhat (still — mostly protected is always better than unprotected!). HPV can be passed

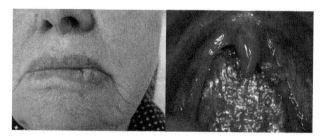

Figure 12. HPV symptoms on face and throat.

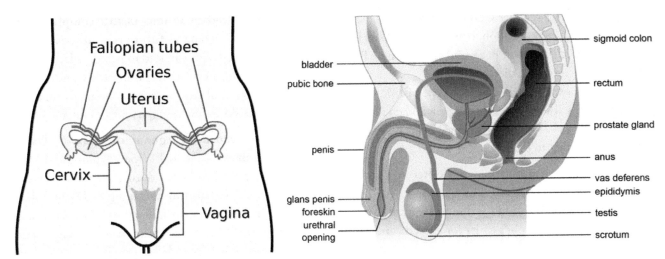

Figure 13. Female and male sexual anatomy.

even when an infected person has no signs or symptoms.

HPV often goes away on its own and does not cause any health problems. In other cases, the individual develops warts or even cancer, not necessarily in that order. The strains of HPV that are connected to cancer are different than the strains that cause warts. HPV could lead to cancer without first producing warts as a symptom. These cancers include cervical, vulva, penis, anus, and even cancer in the back of the throat or base of the tongue and tonsils (propharyngeal cancer). Cancer often takes years, even decades, to develop after a person gets HPV.

When there are genital warts they may appear as a small bump or group of bumps in the genital area. They can be small or large, raised or flat, or shaped like a cauliflower and can appear anywhere in or around the genitals. A healthcare provider can usually diagnose warts by looking at the genital area (Figure 13).

Test or Test Combination	Strategy	Frequency (Years)	Age When Screening Strategy Begins		
			18 years	25 years	18–24 via Miller 25+ via strategy
Pap only	Pap	1 (age 18–20) and 3 (age 21+)	X (screening Strategy (SS) 1)		
	Pap	1	X (SS 2)		
	Pap	2	X (SS 3)		
HPV testing only	HPV	3	X (SS 4)	X (SS 5)	X (SS 6)
	HPV	5	X (SS 7)	X (SS 9)	X (SS 9)
Co-testing	Pap + HPV	2	X (SS 10)	X (SS 11)	X (SS 12)
	Pap + HPV	3	X (SS 13)	X (SS 14)	X (SS 15)
	Pap + HPV	5	X (SS 16)	X (SS 17)	X (SS 18)
Triage (Pap followed by HPV)	Pap with HPV triage	1	X (SS 19)	X (SS 20)	X (SS 21)
Triage (HPV followed by Pap)	HPV with Pap triage	3	X (SS 22)	X (SS 23)	X (SS 24)
	HPV with Pap triage	5	X (SS 25)	X (SS 26)	X (SS 27)

Figure 14. HPV testing.

Diagnosis and Treatment

Most people with HPV do not know they are infected and never develop symptoms or health problems from it. Some people find out they have HPV when they develop visible genital warts. Others may only find out once they've developed more serious problems. Women, who are at higher risk of developing cancer from HPV than men, may find out they have HPV when they get an abnormal Pap test result (during cervical cancer screening). Women should get their first Pap test within three years of becoming sexually active (Figure 14). DNA tests conducted on cells from your cervix can recognize the DNA of the high-risk varieties of HPV that have been linked to genital cancers. There is no other test that detects someone's "HPV status."

There is no treatment for the virus itself. However, there are treatments for the health problems that HPV can cause. Fortunately, we have recently developed a vaccine for the HPV virus, which is the most effective preventative measure available. This vaccine protects against the types of HPV that cause about 70% of cervical cancers and 90% of genital warts cases.

Who Should Get Vaccinated?

The HPV vaccine is safe and effective when given in the recommended age groups. CDC recommends that all boys and girls age 11 to 12 get two doses of HPV vaccine to protect against cancers caused by HPV. Males can receive the vaccine through age 21 and females through age 26 if they did not get vaccinated when they were younger. This applies to any gender whether heterosexual, gay, or bisexual. It is also recommended for men and women with compromised immune systems (including those living with HIV/AIDS) up to age 26 (Figure 15).

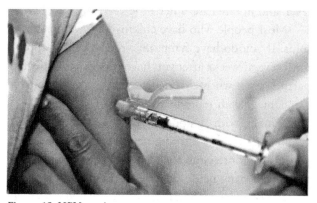

Figure 15. HPV vaccine.

Chlamydia

Chlamydia (caused by the bacteria Chlamydia trachomatis) is a common STI that can infect both men and women. There are more than 1.5 million reported cases of chlamydia in the US It is transmitted through vaginal, anal, or oral sex. Women can contract it in the cervix, rectum, or throat, men in the urethra (inside the penis), rectum, or throat.

Women can potentially experience long-term effects from the infection. It can cause pelvic inflammatory disease and lead to permanent damage to a woman's

Women	Sexually active women under 25 years of age. Sexually active women aged 25 years and older if at increased risk. Retest approximately 3 months after treatment
Pregnant Women	All pregnant women under 25 years of age. Pregnant women, aged 25 and older if at increased risk. Retest during the 3rd trimester for women under 25 years of age or at risk. Pregnant women with chlamydial infection should have a test-of-cure 3-4 weeks after treatment and be retested within 3 months
Men	Consider screening young men in high prevalence clinical settings or in populations with high burden of infection (e.g. MSM)
Men Who Have Sex with Men (MSM)	At least annually for sexually active MSM at sites of contact (urethra, rectum) regardless of condom use. Every 3 to 6 months if at increased risk
Persons with HIV	For sexually active individuals, screen at first HIV evaluation, and at least annually thereafter. More frequent screening for might be appropriate depending on individual risk behaviors and the local epidemiology

Figure 16. Who should get tested for Chlamydia?

reproductive system, making it difficult or impossible for her to get pregnant later on. If you are pregnant and have chlamydia, you can pass the infection to your baby during delivery, leading to pneumonia, lung infections, and eye infections that can lead to blindness in newborns. Chlamydia can also cause a potentially fatal ectopic pregnancy (pregnancy that occurs outside the womb) or make it more likely to deliver your baby too early. Health care providers often screen for chlamydia during pregnancy check-ups.

Men do not experience long-term effects as often as women, but if the infection is left untreated they can sustain scarring of the urethra and infection in the epididymis (the tube that carries sperm). This can lead to pain, fever, and in rare cases infertility.

Most people who have chlamydia have no symptoms. If you do have symptoms, they may not appear until several weeks after you have sex with an infected partner. Even when chlamydia causes no symptoms, it can damage your reproductive system.

Women with symptoms may notice an abnormal vaginal discharge; a burning sensation when urinating; pain during intercourse; and in advanced cases lower abdominal pain, nausea, and fever (Figure 17).

Symptoms in men can include a discharge from their penis; difficulty urinating, including pain or a burning sensation; redness, swelling, or itching at the opening of

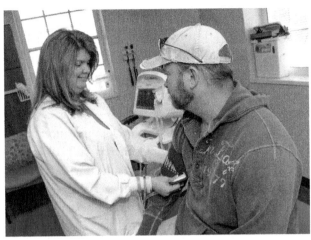

Figure 17. Talk with your healthcare provider about STIs.

the urethra (tip), and pain and swelling in one or both testicles (although this is less common).

Men and women can also get infected with chlamydia in their rectum. This happens either by having receptive anal sex, or by spread from another infected site (such as the vagina). While these infections often cause no symptoms, they can cause rectal pain, discharge, and bleeding.

Since chlamydia is transmitted via oral, anal, or vaginal sex, using barriers, like condoms, correctly during these activities is the only way for a sexually active people to reduce risk. Chlamydia can be cured with antibiotics provided by your health care provider.

Diagnosis and Treatment

Chlamydia is treated with antibiotics provided by your health care provider. Repeat infection with chlamydia or a gonorrhea infection occurring at the same time

is common. You should be tested again about three months after you're treated, even if your sex partner(s) was treated.

Gonorrhea

There are nearly 400,000 cases of **gonorrhea** reported in the US, the most common population being young adults aged 15–24. It is transmitted through vaginal, oral, or anal sex, leading to infections in the genital tract, mouth, or anus.

Gonorrhea does not always cause symptoms. In men, gonorrhea can cause pain when urinating and discharge from the penis. If untreated, it can cause swelling of the testicles and problems with the prostate.

In women, the early symptoms of gonorrhea (if present at all) often are mild. Later, it can cause bleeding between periods, pain when urinating (often mistaken

for a bladder infection), and increased discharge from the vagina. If untreated, it can lead to pelvic inflammatory disease, which causes problems with pregnancy and infertility. As with many STIs, gonorrhea can be passed to a child from an infected mother during birth, and can cause infections in the eyes, blood, and joints of newborns. This is rare, but serious.

Rectal infections in both men and women can also go unnoticed. When present, symptoms include anal itching, soreness, bleeding, or discharge and pain during bowel movements.

Diagnosis and Treatment

Your health care provider will diagnose gonorrhea with lab tests and treat with antibiotics. However, treating gonorrhea is becoming more difficult because drug-resistant strains are increasing. Correct usage of latex condoms greatly reduces, but does not eliminate, the risk of catching or spreading gonorrhea.

Untreated gonorrhea can cause serious and permanent health problems in both women and men. Rarely, untreated gonorrhea can spread to your blood or joints, which can be life threatening.

In women, untreated gonorrhea can cause pelvic inflammatory disease (PID), scar tissue blocking the fallopian tubes, ectopic pregnancy, infertility, and long-term pelvic or abdominal pain. In men, gonorrhea can cause a painful condition in the tubes attached to the testicles. In rare cases, this may cause a man to be sterile, or prevent him from being able to father a child.

Gonorrhea is treated with antibiotics prescribed by your health care provider. As with many commonly occurring bacteria, it is becoming harder to treat some gonorrhea, as drug-resistant strains are increasing. If your symptoms continue for more than a few days after receiving treatment, you should return to a healthcare provider to be checked.

Syphilis

Syphilis is caused by the bacteria known as Treponema pallidum and can cause serious health problems if it is not treated. You can get syphilis by direct contact with a syphilis sore during vaginal, anal, or oral sex. You can find sores on or around the penis, vagina, or anus, or in the rectum, on the lips, or in the mouth.

In 2015, there were 23,872 reported cases of primary and secondary syphilis in the US, with men representing the vast majority of cases, at 21,547. In Oregon, the rate of primary and secondary syphilis was 2.5 per 100,000 in 2011 and 8.7 per 100,000 in 2015. Oregon now ranks 9th in rates of primary and secondary stage syphilis among 50 states.

Syphilis is divided into stages — primary, secondary, latent, and tertiary. These stages can be overlapping and there are different signs and symptoms associated with each stage.

Primary Stage

During the first (primary) stage of syphilis, you may notice a single sore or multiple sores. The sore is the location where syphilis entered your body. Sores are usually (but not always) firm, round, and painless. Because the sore is painless, it can easily go unnoticed. The sore usually lasts 3 to 6 weeks and heals regardless of whether or not you receive treatment. Even after the sore goes away, you must still receive treatment. This will stop your infection from moving to the secondary stage.

Secondary Stage

During the secondary stage, two to ten weeks after infection, you may have skin rashes and/or mucous membrane lesions. Mucous membrane lesions are sores in your mouth, vagina, or anus. This stage usually starts with a rash on one or more areas of your body. The rash can show up when your primary sore is healing or several weeks after the sore has healed. It can look like rough, red, or reddish-brown spots on the palms of your hands and/or the bottoms of your feet. The rash usually won't itch and it is sometimes so faint that you won't notice it.

Other symptoms you may have can include fever, swollen lymph glands, sore throat, patchy hair loss, headaches, weight loss, muscle aches, and fatigue (feeling very tired). The symptoms from this stage will go away whether or not you receive treatment. Without the right treatment, your infection will move to the latent and possibly tertiary stages of syphilis.

Latent Stage

The latent stage of syphilis is a period of time when there are no visible signs or symptoms of syphilis. If you do not receive treatment, you can continue to have syphilis in your body for years without any signs or symptoms, making the risk of transmission greater.

Tertiary Stage

Most people with untreated syphilis do not develop tertiary syphilis. However, when it does happen it can affect many different organ systems. These include the heart and blood vessels, and the brain and nervous system. Tertiary syphilis is very serious and would occur 10–30 years after your infection began. In tertiary syphilis, the disease damages your internal organs and can result in death.

Complications

Like most STIs, f you are pregnant and have syphilis, you can give the infection to your unborn baby (Figure 18). This can lead to a low birth weight baby and also make it more likely you will miscarry, deliver your baby too early, or deliver a stillborn baby. Health care providers typically screen for syphilis during the first trimester of pregnancy because the impact to the child can be severe and potentially fatal, and because it can be treated in time if found early. An infected baby may be born without signs or symptoms of disease. However, if not treated immediately, the baby may develop serious problems within a few weeks. Untreated babies can have health problems and birth defects or developmental delays such as cataracts, deafness, or seizures.

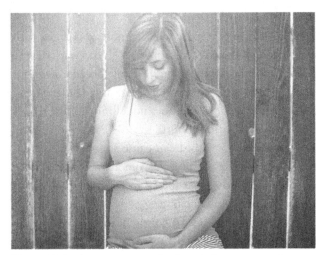

Figure 18. Pregnant women and unborn infants can experience severe complications from untreated STIs.

Without treatment, syphilis can spread to the brain and nervous system (neurosyphilis) or to the eye (ocular syphilis). This can happen during any of the stages described above. Symptoms include severe headache, poor muscle coordination, partial paralysis, numbness, dementia, and changes in your vision, including blindness.

Pregnant Women	All pregnant women at the first prenatal visit. Retest early in the third trimester and at delivery if at high risk.
Men Who Have Sex with Men (MSM)	At least annually for sexually active MSM at sites of contact (urethra, rectum, pharynx) regardless of condom use. Every 3 to 6 months if at increased risk.
Persons with HIV	For sexually active individuals, screen at first HIV evaluation, and at least annually thereafter. More frequent screening for might be appropriate depending on individual risk behaviors and the local epidemiology.

Figure 19. Who should get tested for Syphilis?

Diagnosis and Treatment

Most of the time, a blood test is used to test for syphilis. Some healthcare providers will diagnose syphilis by testing fluid from a syphilis sore. Syphilis can be cured with the right antibiotics from your healthcare provider. However, treatment might not undo any damage that the infection has already done, which is why it is important to get tested if you think you may have been exposed.

Herpes

Herpes simplex virus (HSV) is transmitted through skin-to-skin contact. There are varying forms of the herpes virus — herpes simplex virus type 1 (HSV 1) and herpes simplex virus type 2 (HSV 2) — and various effects. These viruses form either oral or genital herpes.

Oral herpes (such as cold sores or fever blisters on or around the mouth) is usually caused by HSV-1. Most people are infected with HSV-1 during childhood from non-sexual contact. For example, people can get infected from a kiss from a relative or friend with oral herpes. More than half of the population in the US has HSV-1, even if they don't show any signs or symptoms. HSV-1 can also be spread from the mouth to the genitals through oral sex. This is why some cases of genital herpes are caused by HSV-1.

Genital herpes (usually caused by HSV 2) shows itself as sores, usually appearing as one or more blisters on or around the genitals, rectum, or mouth — most often at the site of infection. It may start with a tingling feeling, then red bumps, and then blisters or red sores. The blisters break and leave painful sores that may take weeks to heal. These symptoms are sometimes called "having an outbreak." The first time someone has an outbreak they may also have flu-like symptoms such as fever, body aches, or swollen glands.

Repeat outbreaks of genital herpes are common, especially during the first year after infection, though they are usually shorter and less severe than the first outbreak. Although the infection can stay in the body for the rest of your life, the number of outbreaks tends to decrease over a period of years.

You should be examined by your doctor if you or your partner notice symptoms, such as an unusual sore, a smelly discharge, burning when urinating, or, for women specifically, bleeding between periods. Most people who have herpes have no, or very mild symptoms. It is important to know that even without signs of the disease, it can still spread to sexual partners.

Often times, your healthcare provider can diagnose genital herpes by simply looking at your symptoms. Providers can also take a sample from the sore(s) and test it.

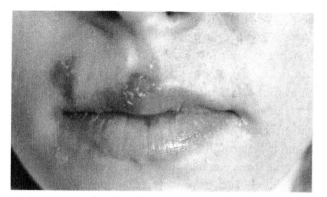

Figure 20. A herpes outbreak.

	Prevalence (%)
Total	**16.2%**
Age Group (Years)	
14–19	1.4%
20–29	10.5%
30–39	19.6%
40–49	26.1%
Reported Number of Lifetime Sex Partners	
1	3.9%
2–4	14.0%
5–9	16.3%
>10	26.7%

*Over 80 percent of those whose blood test was positive for HSV 2 had never received a diagnosis of genital herpes.

Figure 21. Herpes risks rise with age and number of partners.

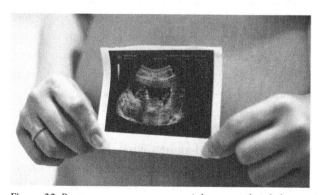

Figure 22. Pregnant women can transmit herpes to their baby.

Living with Herpes

There is no cure for herpes. Herpes is a chronic infection, but there are medicines that can shorten outbreaks and reduce the chance that you will pass the infection on to your sex partner(s).

The sores produced with genital herpes can be quite painful and can be severe in people with suppressed immune systems. If you touch your sores or the fluids from the sores, you may transfer herpes to another part of your body, such as your eyes, so immediate and thorough hand-washing is imperative If sores are touched to prevent the spread of infection.

Some people who get genital herpes have concerns about how it will impact their overall health, sex life, and relationships. It is best for you to talk to a healthcare provider about those concerns, but it also is important to recognize that while herpes is not curable, it can be managed. Since a genital herpes diagnosis may affect how you will feel about current or future sexual relationships, it is important to understand how to talk to sexual partners about STIs.

Herpes symptoms can occur in both male and female genital areas that are covered by a latex condom. However, outbreaks can also occur in areas that are not covered by a condom so condoms may not fully protect you from getting herpes.

HSV can be transmitted during delivery, so pregnant women are usually monitored towards the end of pregnancy, and a C-section may be performed. Research suggests that women who contract herpes during latter part of pregnancy are at a higher risk of transmitting to their baby. It can also be transmitted in utero and can cause premature birth and miscarriage.

HIV and AIDS

HIV stands for human immunodeficiency virus. It is the virus that can lead to acquired immunodeficiency syndrome, or AIDS, if not treated. Unlike some other viruses, the human body can't get rid of HIV completely, even with treatment.

When we first began hearing about **HIV** and **AIDS** as a nation back in the 1980s, we knew little about how the disease was transmitted and viewed the disease as a certain death sentence. Today, we are much more educated and better at preventing the spread of the virus and offering treatments to those affected. Yet it still remains a significant threat in certain populations (in the US 82% of the people affected are gay or bisexual). There were over 6,000 deaths in 2014 attributed directly to HIV and it was the 8th leading cause of death for those aged 25–34 and 9th for those aged 35–44.

No effective cure currently exists, but with proper medical care, HIV can be controlled. The medicine used to treat HIV is called antiretroviral therapy or ART. If taken the right way, every day, this medicine can dramatically prolong the lives of many people infected with HIV, keep them healthy, slow or prevent the advancement of the disease to AIDS, and greatly lower their chance of infecting others. Before the introduction of ART in the mid-1990s, people with HIV could progress to AIDS in just a few years. Today, someone diagnosed with HIV and treated before the disease is far advanced can live nearly as long as someone who does not have HIV.

An estimated 1.1 million people in the United States were living with HIV at the end of 2014, the most recent year for which this information is available. Of those people, about 15%, or 1 in 7, did not know they were infected. There are a disproportionate number of people affected who are African American (45%), sex workers, or living in prison.

In 2014, there were an estimated 37,600 new HIV infections — down from 45,700 in 2008. HIV disease continues to be a serious health issue for parts of the world. Worldwide, there were about 2.1 million new cases of HIV in 2015. About 36.7 million people are living with HIV around the world, and as of June 2016, 17 million people living with HIV were receiving ART.

Sub-Saharan Africa, which bears the heaviest burden of HIV/AIDS worldwide, accounts for 65% of all new HIV infections. Other regions significantly affected by HIV/AIDS include Asia and the Pacific, Latin America and the Caribbean, and Eastern Europe and Central Asia. Women represent half of adult AIDS cases worldwide. In Oregon, 7,254 men and women are currently living with HIV/AIDS, as of 2016, with 447 cases in Marion County. An estimated 1.1 million people died from AIDS-related illnesses in 2015.

Though we know more about the illness, and have methods of treatment, HIV can still be intimidating. HIV attacks the body's immune system, specifically the CD4 cells (T cells), which help the immune system fight off infections. Untreated, HIV reduces the number of CD4 cells in the body, making the person more likely to get other infections or infection-related cancers. Over time, HIV can destroy so many of these cells that the body can't fight off infections and disease. These opportunistic infections or cancers take advantage of a very weak immune system and signal that the person has AIDS, the last stage of HIV infection.

Without treatment, HIV advances in stages, overwhelming your immune system and getting worse over time. The three stages of HIV infection are: (1) acute HIV infection, (2) clinical latency, and (3) AIDS (acquired immunodeficiency syndrome).

State 1 — Acute HIV Infection Stage

Within two to four weeks after infection, many, but not all, people develop flu-like symptoms, often described as "the worst flu ever." Symptoms can include fever, swollen glands, sore throat, rash, muscle and joint aches and pains, and headache. This is called "acute retroviral syndrome" (ARS) or "primary HIV infection," and it's the body's natural response to the HIV infection. People who think that they may have been infected recent-

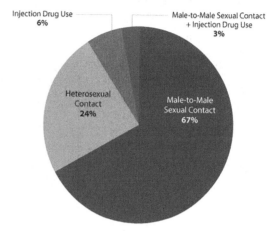

New HIV Diagnoses by Transmission Category
(2014, n=44,073)

Injection Drug Use 6%

Male-to-Male Sexual Contact + Injection Drug Use 3%

Heterosexual Contact 24%

Male-to-Male Sexual Contact 67%

Figure 23. Some activities have a higher likelihood of causing HIV transmission.

ly and are in the acute stage of HIV infection should seek medical care right away. Starting treatment at this stage can have significant benefits to your health.

During this early period of infection, large amounts of virus are being produced in your body. The virus uses

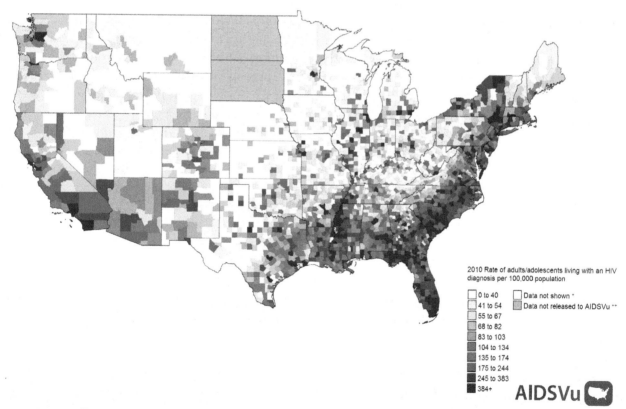

2010 Rate of adults/adolescents living with an HIV diagnosis per 100,000 population

0 to 40	Data not shown *
41 to 54	Data not released to AIDSVu **
55 to 67	
68 to 82	
83 to 103	
104 to 134	
135 to 174	
175 to 244	
245 to 383	
384+	

AIDSVu

Figure 24. AIDS affects parts of the country differently.

CD4 cells to replicate and destroys them in the process. Because of this, your CD4 cells can fall rapidly. Eventually your immune response will begin to bring the level of virus in your body back down to a level called a viral set point, which is a relatively stable level of virus in your body. At this point, your CD4 count begins to increase, but it may not return to pre-infection levels. It may be particularly beneficial to your health to begin ART during this stage.

During the acute HIV infection stage, you are at very high risk of transmitting HIV to your sexual or needle-sharing

partners because the levels of HIV in your blood stream are extremely high. For this reason, it is very important to take steps to reduce your risk of transmission.

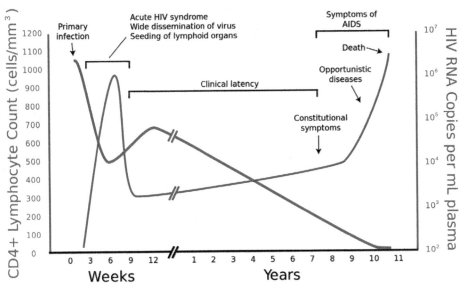

Figure 25. How HIV infection progresses.

Stage 2 — Clinical Latency

After the acute stage of HIV infection, the disease moves into a stage called the **clinical latency stage**, a period where a virus is living or developing in a person without producing symptoms. During the clinical latency stage, people who are infected with HIV experience no symptoms, or only mild ones. (This stage is sometimes called "asymptomatic HIV infection" or "chronic HIV infection.")

During the clinical latency stage, the HIV virus continues to reproduce at very low levels, even if it cannot be detected with standard laboratory tests. If you take ART, you may live with clinical latency for decades and never progress to AIDS because treatment helps keep the virus in check.

People in this symptom-free stage are still able to transmit HIV to others, The risk of transmission is greatly reduced by HIV transmission. In studies looking at the effects of HIV treatment on transmission, no new HIV infections have been linked to someone with very low or undetectable (suppressed) viral load.

For people who are not on ART, the clinical latency stage lasts an average of 10 years, but some people may progress through this stage faster. As the disease progressions, eventually your viral load will begin to rise and your CD4 count will begin to decline. As this happens, you may begin to have constitutional symptoms of HIV as the virus levels increase in your body before you develop AIDS.

Stage 3 — AIDS

This is the stage of HIV infection that occurs when your immune system is badly damaged and you become vulnerable to opportunistic infections. Common symptoms of AIDS include chills, fever, sweats, swollen lymph glands, weakness, and weight loss. People with AIDS can have a high viral load and be very infectious.

When the number of your CD4 cells falls below 200 cells per cubic millimeter of blood (200 cells/mm3), you are considered to have progressed to AIDS. (In someone

with a healthy immune system, CD4 counts are between 500 and 1,600 cells/mm3.) You are also considered to have progressed to AIDS if you develop one or more opportunistic illnesses — such as certain forms of pneumonia, toxoplasmosis, and Kaposi's carcoma — regardless of your CD4 count.

Without treatment, people who progress to AIDS typically survive about 3 years. Once you have a dangerous opportunistic illness, life-expectancy without treatment falls to about 1 year. ART can be helpful for people who have AIDS when diagnosed and can be lifesaving. Treatment is likely to benefit people with HIV no matter when it is started, but people who start ART soon after they get HIV experience more benefits from treatment than do people who start treatment after they have developed AIDS.

In the United States, most people with HIV do not develop AIDS because effective ART stops disease progression. People with HIV who are diagnosed early can have a life span that is about the same as someone like them who does not HIV.

People living with HIV may progress through these stages at different rates, depending on a variety of factors, including their genetic makeup, how healthy they were before they were infected, how much virus they were exposed to and its genetic characteristics, how soon after infection they are diagnosed and linked to care and treatment, whether they see their healthcare provider regularly and take their HIV medications as directed, and different health-related choices they make, such as decisions to eat a healthful diet, exercise, and not smoke. Someone who is HIV-positive, receiving treatment, and in optimal health — meaning they don't do drugs and are free of other infections — may live to be in their late 70s.

Transmission

Only certain body fluids — blood, semen, pre-seminal fluid, rectal fluids, vaginal fluids, and breast milk — from a person who has HIV can transmit HIV. These fluids must come in contact with a mucous membrane or damaged tissue or be directly injected into the bloodstream (from a needle or syringe) for transmission to occur. Mucous membranes are found inside the rectum, vagina, penis, and mouth.

In the United States, HIV is spread mainly by:

- Sharing needles or syringes, rinse water, or other equipment (works) used to prepare drugs for injection with someone who has HIV. HIV can live in a used needle for up to 42 days depending on temperature and other factors.

- Having anal or vaginal sex with someone who has HIV without using a condom or taking medicines to prevent or treat HIV

- For the HIV-negative partner, receptive anal sex (bottoming) is the highest-risk sexual behavior, but you can also get HIV from insertive anal sex (topping). Either partner can get HIV through vaginal sex, though it is less risky than receptive anal sex.

Less commonly, HIV may be spread:

- From mother to child during pregnancy, birth, or breastfeeding. Although the risk can be high if a mother is living with HIV and not taking medicine, recommendations to test all pregnant women for HIV and start HIV treatment immediately have lowered the number of babies who are born with HIV.

- By being stuck with an HIV-contaminated needle or other sharp object. This is a risk mainly for health care workers.

In extremely rare cases, HIV has been transmitted by:

- Oral sex — putting the mouth on the penis, vagina, or anus. In general, there's little to no risk of getting HIV from oral sex. But transmission of HIV, though extremely rare, is theoretically possible if an HIV-positive man ejaculates in his partner's mouth during oral sex.

- Receiving blood transfusions, blood products, or organ/tissue transplants that are contaminated with HIV. This was more common in the early years of HIV, but now the risk is extremely small because of rigorous testing of the US blood supply and donated organs and tissues.

- Contact between broken skin, wounds, or mucous membranes and HIV-infected blood or blood-contaminated body fluids.

HIV is *not* transmitted:

- By hugging, shaking hands, sharing toilets, sharing dishes, or closed-mouth or "social" kissing with someone who is HIV-positive

- Through saliva, tears, or sweat that is not mixed with the blood of an HIV-positive person

- By mosquitoes, ticks or other blood-sucking insects

- Through the air

HIV Diagnosis

The only way to know for sure whether you have HIV is to get tested. CDC recommends that everyone between the ages of 13 and 64 get tested for HIV at least once as part of routine healthcare (Figure 26). Knowing your HIV status gives you powerful information to help you take steps to keep you and your partner healthy.

There are three broad types of tests available: antibody tests, combination or fourth-generation tests, and nucleic acid tests (NAT). HIV tests may be performed on blood, oral fluid, or urine. Most HIV tests, including most rapid tests and home tests, are antibody tests. Antibodies are produced by your immune system when you're exposed to viruses like HIV or bacteria. HIV antibody tests look for these antibodies to HIV in your blood or oral fluid. In general, antibody tests that use blood can detect HIV slightly sooner after infection than tests done with oral fluid.

It can take 21–84 days for an HIV-positive person's body to make enough antibodies for an antibody test to detect HIV infection. This is called the window period. Approximately 97% of people will develop detectable antibodies during this window period. If you get a negative HIV antibody test result during the window period, you should be re-tested three months after your possible exposure to HIV.

- With a rapid antibody screening test, results are ready in 30 minutes or less.

- The OraQuick HIV Test, which involves taking an oral swab, provides fast results. You have to swab your mouth for an oral fluid sample and use a kit to test it. Results are available in 20 minutes.

- The Home Access HIV-1 Test System involves pricking your finger to collect a blood sample, sending the sample by mail to a licensed laboratory, and then calling in for results as early as the next business day.

If you use any type of antibody test and have a positive result, you will need to take a follow-up test, typically through your healthcare provider, to confirm your results. Most labs will retest your sample for accuracy.

- A combination, or fourth-generation, test looks for both HIV antibodies and antigens. Combination screening tests are now recommended for testing done in labs and are becoming more common in the United States.

- A nucleic acid test (NAT) looks for HIV in the blood. It looks for the virus and not the antibodies to the virus. The test can give either a positive/negative result or an actual amount of virus present in the blood (known as a viral load test). This test is very expensive and not routinely used for screening individuals unless they recently had a high-risk exposure or a possible exposure with early symptoms of HIV infection.

Individuals should talk to their healthcare provider to see what type of HIV test is right for them and get in touch right away if a result comes back positive. Thanks to better treatments, people with HIV are now living longer — and with a better quality of life — than ever before. If you are living with HIV, it's important to make choices that keep you healthy and protect others.

Women	All women aged 13-64 years (opt-out) All women who seek evaluation and treatment for STDs
Pregnant Women	All pregnant women should be screened at first prenatal visit (opt-out) Retest in the third trimester if at high risk
Men	All men aged 13-64 (opt-out) All men who seek evaluation and treatment for STDs
Men Who Have Sex with Men (MSM)	At least annually for sexually active MSM if HIV status is unknown or negative and the patient himself or his sex partner(s) have had more than one sex partner since most recent HIV test

Figure 26. Who should get tested for HIV?

HIV Treatment

HIV is a type of virus called a retrovirus, and the drugs used to treat it are called antiretrovirals (ARV). These drugs are always given in combination with other ARVs. This combination therapy is called antiretroviral therapy (ART). HIV medicines prevent the virus from multiplying (making copies of itself), which reduces the amount of HIV in the body. Having less in the body gives the immune system a chance to recover. Even though there is still some HIV in the body, the immune system is strong enough to fight off infections and certain HIV-related cancers. By reducing the amount, HIV medicines also reduce the risk of HIV transmission. ART can keep you healthy for many years.

HIV and Pregnancy

Perinatal HIV transmission, also known as mother-to-child transmission, can happen at any time during pregnancy, labor, delivery, and breastfeeding. Approximately 8,500 women living with HIV give birth annually. CDC recommends that all women who are pregnant or planning to get pregnant take an HIV test as early as possible before and during every pregnancy. This is because the earlier HIV is diagnosed and treated, the more effective HIV medicines, called antiretroviral treatment (ART), will be at preventing transmission and improving the health outcomes of both mother and child.

Advances in HIV research, prevention, and treatment have made it possible for many women living with HIV to give birth without transmitting the virus to their babies. The annual number of HIV infections through perinatal transmission have declined by more than 90% since the early 1990s. Today, if a woman takes HIV medicines as prescribed throughout pregnancy, labor and delivery, and provides HIV medicines to her baby for 4–6 weeks, the risk of transmitting HIV can be 1% or less.

In some cases, a Cesarean delivery can also prevent HIV transmission. After delivery, a mother can prevent transmitting HIV to her baby by not breastfeeding and not pre-chewing her baby's food. For babies living with

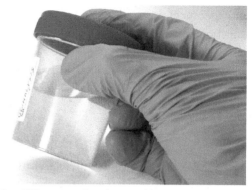

Figure 27. Most STI tests are done by urinalysis.

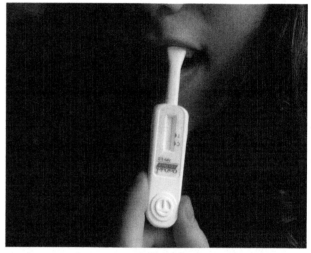

Figure 28. Oral tests are available for HIV.

HIV, starting treatment early is important because the disease can progress more rapidly in children than adults. Providing ART early can help children with perinatal HIV live longer, healthier lives.

It is important that all women who are pregnant or trying to get pregnant encourage their partners to also get tested for HIV. Women who are HIV-negative but have an HIV-positive partner should talk to their doctor about taking HIV medicines daily, called pre-exposure prophylaxis (PrEP), to protect themselves while trying to get pregnant, and to protect themselves and their baby during pregnancy and while breastfeeding.

Looking Toward a Solution

There is currently no vaccine available that will prevent HIV infection or treat those who have it. However, scientists are working to develop one. Building on the findings of an earlier study that found for the first

time, albeit modestly, that a vaccine could prevent HIV infection in 2016, an NIH-supported clinical trial was launched to test a modified HIV vaccine. This current vaccine trial, called HVTN 702, is testing whether an experimental vaccine regimen safely prevents HIV infection among South African adults.

The long-term goal is to develop a safe and effective vaccine that protects people worldwide from getting infected with HIV. However, even if a vaccine only protects some people who get vaccinated, or even if it provides less than total protection by reducing the risk of infection, it could still have a major impact on the rates of transmission and help control the pandemic, particularly for populations at high risk of HIV infection.

Viral Hepatitis

Hepatitis A, Hepatitis B, and Hepatitis C are diseases of the liver caused by three different viruses. Although each can cause similar symptoms, they have different modes of transmission and can affect the liver differently. Hepatitis A appears only as an acute or newly occurring infection and does not become chronic. People with Hepatitis A usually improve without treatment. Hepatitis B and Hepatitis C can also begin as acute infections, but in some people, the virus remains in the body, resulting in chronic disease and long-term liver problems. There are vaccines to prevent Hepatitis A and B. However, there is not one for Hepatitis C. If a person has had one type of viral hepatitis in the past, it is still possible to get the other types.

In 2015, a total of 48 states submitted reports of acute hepatitis B virus (HBV) infection, 40 submitted reports of acute hepatitis C virus (HCV) infection, 40 submitted reports of chronic HBV infection, and 40 submitted reports of chronic HCV infection.

Hepatitis A is caused by the hepatitis A virus (HAV). Hepatitis A is highly contagious. It is usually transmitted by the fecal-oral route, either through person-to-person contact or consumption of contaminated food or water. HAV does not result in chronic infection. More than 80% of adults with Hepatitis A have symptoms, but the majority of children do not have symptoms or have an unrecognized infection. Antibodies produced in response to HAV last for life and protect against reinfection.

Hepatitis B is a liver infection caused by the Hepatitis B virus (HBV). HBV is transmitted when blood, semen, vaginal fluid, or another body fluid from a person infected with the virus enters the body of someone who is not infected. This can happen through sharing needles, syringes, or other drug-injection equipment, through sexual contact, or from mother to baby at birth. This virus is more easily transmitted than HIV, so even sharing razors or toothbrushes with someone infected is considered risky.

For some people, HBV is an acute, or short-term, illness but for others, it can become a long-term, chronic infection. Risk for chronic infection is related to age at infection: approximately 90% of infected infants become chronically infected, compared with 2–6% of adults. Chronic HBV can lead to serious health issues, like cirrhosis or liver cancer (Figure 29).

Hepatitis C is a blood-borne infection caused by the Hepatitis C virus (HCV). Most people become infected with HCV by sharing needles or other equipment to inject drugs. For some people, HCV is a short-term illness but for 70–85% of people who become infected, it becomes a long-term, chronic, potentially fatal infection. The majority of infected persons might not be aware of their infection because they are not clinically ill. There is no vaccine for Hepatitis C. The best way to prevent

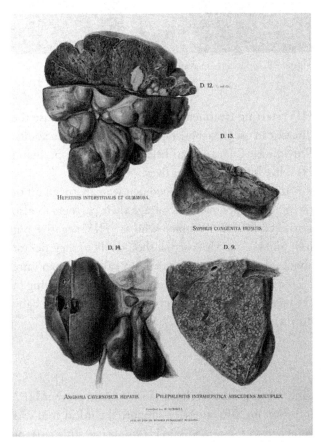

Figure 29. Many STIs affect the shape and function of the liver.

Hepatitis C is by avoiding behaviors that can spread the disease, especially injecting drugs.

Many people with hepatitis do not have symptoms and do not know they are infected. If symptoms occur with an acute infection, they can appear anytime from 2 weeks to 6 months after exposure. Symptoms of chronic viral hepatitis can take decades to develop. Acute symptoms of hepatitis that show up in 1–6 months can include: fever, fatigue, loss of appetite, nausea, vomiting, abdominal pain, dark urine, grey-colored stools, joint pain, and jaundice.

Diagnosis, Treatment, and Prevention

Hepatitis is diagnosed via blood test. There is no medication available for acute hepatitis. It is best addressed through supportive care. In chronic cases of hepatitis, regular monitoring for signs of liver disease progression is required. Some patients are treated with antiviral drugs.

The best way to prevent Hepatitis A and B is by getting vaccinated. Because of how easily transmitted hepatitis B is, vaccination against HBV is routinely given to infants as a preventative measure.

Pelvic Inflammatory Disease

Pelvic inflammatory disease is an infection of a woman's reproductive organs primarily caused by untreated chlamydia and gonorrhea. This can occur when bacteria from the vagina or cervix travel to your womb, fallopian tubes, or ovaries.

Bacteria can also enter your body during a medical procedure such as:

- Childbirth
- Endometrial biopsy (removing a small piece of your womb lining to test for cancer)
- Getting an intrauterine device (IUD)
- Miscarriage
- Abortion

In the United States, nearly 1 million women have PID each year. About 1 in 8 sexually active girls will have PID before age 20.

You are more likely to get PID if you:

- Have an STI and do not get treated
- Have more than one sex partner
- Have a sex partner who has sex partners other than you
- Have had PID before
- Are sexually active and are age 25 or younger
- Douche
- Use an intrauterine device (IUD) for birth control. However, the small increased risk is mostly limited to the first three weeks after the IUD is placed inside the uterus by a doctor.

Women	Women born between 1945-1965. Other women If risk factors are present. Women at increased risk
Pregnant Women	Women born between 1945-1965. Other pregnant women If risk factors are present. Test for HBsAg at first prenatal visit of each pregnancy regardless of prior testing; retest at delivery if at high risk
Men	Men at increased risk
Men Who Have Sex with Men (MSM)	MSM born between 1945-1965. Other MSM if risk factors are present. Annual HCV testing in MSM with HIV infection. All MSM should be tested for HBsAg
Persons with HIV	Serologic testing at initial evaluation. Annual HCV testing in MSM with HIV infection. Test for HBsAg and anti-HBc and/or anti-HBs.

Figure 30. Who should get tested for Hepatitis?

Diagnosis and Treatment

There are no tests for PID. A diagnosis is usually based on a combination of your medical history, physical exam, and other test results. You may not realize you have PID because your symptoms may be mild, or you may not experience any symptoms. However, if you do have symptoms, you may notice:

- Pain in your lower abdomen

- Fever

- An unusual discharge with a bad odor from your vagina

- Pain and/or bleeding when you have sex

- Burning sensation when you urinate

- Bleeding between periods

Screening for chlamydia and gonorrhea, and getting treatment for these infections if present, can help prevent PID in addition to safer sex practices.

If PID is diagnosed early, it can be treated. However, treatment won't undo any damage that has already happened to your reproductive system. The longer you wait to get treated, the more likely it is that you will have complications from PID, such as scar tissue blocking the fallopian tubes, ectopic pregnancy, infertility, and long-term pelvic or abdominal pain.

Safer Sex

The transmission of STIs can be prevented by practicing safer sexual activity. "Safer" sex means exactly that: you are less likely to receive or transmit an STI if you educate yourself on risk factors, communicate with partners, and get tested regularly when you are sexually active.

The Only "Safe" Sex

Abstinence is the safest way to avoid STIs. If you aren't having sex with other people, then you aren't at risk for STIs, right? Abstinence is the idea that you wait to have any kind of sex with another person until you are in a committed, monogamous relationship. Once you are in a mutually monogamous relationship (i.e. both partners remain dedicated to monogamy), your risk levels are much lower. This is especially true if neither partner has been very active sexually prior to this relationship.

Formal abstinence education is often misleading and people who haven't learned about risks will sometimes narrowly define "sex" as "vaginal intercourse" in order to preserve "virginity." This approach causes young people who become sexually active to engage in high-risk sex activities, like unprotected anal intercourse, which is a direct cause for the high rate of infection in places where abstinence-only sex education is taught.

Condoms and Barriers

Condoms have been around for a very long time. They are basically a sealed sheath that covers the penis and were originally used to prevent pregnancy, though now we use them to control the spread of infection. Although the materials used to make condoms have been pretty creative over the years, modern condoms are primarily made from latex, polyurethane, polyisoprene, nitrile, or gut (like sausage casings). The latter variety only protects against pregnancy and are not safe for use against STIs.

Correctly using male condoms and other barriers like female condoms and dental dams, every time, can reduce (though not eliminate) the risk of sexually transmitted diseases (STIs), including HIV and viral hepatitis. They can also provide protection against other diseases that may be transmitted through sex like Zika and Ebola. Using male and female condoms correctly, every time, can also help prevent pregnancy. However, male and female condoms should not be used at the same time as it could cause breakage to either.

Male condoms fit over the penis and usually have a reservoir at the tip to catch ejaculate. Female condoms look like a tube with an opening at one end and are inserted into the vagina. Dental dams are latex sheets that are placed over women's genitals for safer oral sex.

Correctly Using Male Condoms

Male condoms are the most readily available barrier method and one of the easiest to use. Correct use is key. Condom failure is almost always due to user error.

First make sure you haven't been carrying around a condom in your wallet for months. Heat, wear and tear, and age are all factors that can cause condom failure — condoms have expiration dates! Always use a fresh condom with each new sex act (even if there was no orgasm).

When opening the condom, do not use anything sharp. Most condom packages are easy to open. After opening it, look to see which way it is going to roll. Pinch the tip of the condom and place it at the tip of the penis. Once it's placed, you can roll the condom all the way down to the base of the penis. If you don't roll the condom all the way down to the base, you are receiving no protection from the condom.

When you are done using the condom, remove the condom by pulling from the tip and either tie a knot in it (like a balloon) or wrap it in some tissue and throw it away. Remember, never attempt to reuse a condom.

You may have to use lubricant with condoms, because friction has a "drying" effect. If so, use water or silicone-based lubricants. Petroleum or oil-based lubricants break down the latex and increase likelihood of breakage. If a condom ever breaks, stop sexual activity immediately and put on a new condom.

The FC2 "Female" (frequently referred to as "internal") condom offers many advantages for people who want to ensure protection from pregnancy or sexually transmitted infection. The internal condom is a strong, thin, and flexible nitrile sheath inserted into the vagina (up to 4 hours) prior to sex. It has a flexible inner ring for easy insertion and is absolutely latex-free. It is pre-lubricated with a slick silicone-based lubricant, but additional lubricant can be used as well.

Latex condoms are easy to acquire at grocery and drug stores. Although rare, latex allergies may make regular condoms unusable. Reported data suggest that the average prevalence of latex allergy worldwide remains 9.7%, 7.2%, and 4.3% among healthcare workers, susceptible patients, and general population. High contact with latex products, like gloves in a medical setting, seems to increase the likelihood of a latex allergy.

There are also "traditional" style condoms designed to fit over a penis that are made from polyurethane, polyisoprene, and synthetic resins. These are latex-free and some

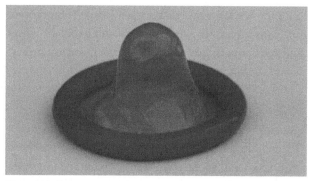

Figure 31. A common protection against STIs is the male condom.

people like them for the relative thinness of the material along with the higher level of heat transfer, which combine to create a more "natural" feeling. These materials are less flexible than latex, so correct sizing is important. Some examples of latex free condom varieties are:

- SKYN, SKYN Extra Lubricated, SKYN Extra Studded (polyisoprene)

- Durex (Avanti Bare) RealFeel (polyisoprene)

- Unique Pull (synthetic resin)

- Trojan Supra (polyurethane)

Used correctly with every new sex act, condoms have a success rate close to 100 percent in most cases for protecting against infection and avoiding pregnancy. For preventing pregnancy, they have the additional benefit over hormonal birth control of providing protection against STIs.

Condoms have some other benefits as well. They come in a wide variety of shapes, textures, thicknesses, and styles, making them something that can "spice things up" a little. Men who want to last longer can experiment with different condom thicknesses until they find something that gives them the effect they want.

Some people complain that they don't like the "feeling" of wearing a condom, or that putting one on "kills the mood." Both of these are easy problems to fix. A drop or two of lubricant in the tip of the condom before putting it on makes it feel almost like there is no condom. The "mood killer" probably has more to do with where the condom is located, than the act of putting it on. Put the condom in an easily accessible location to reduce how much time it takes to get the condom and put it on.

Most resistance to condom use is purely psychological — if you feel like they are a hassle, or that condoms aren't sexy, that's exactly what they will be. If you think condoms are sexy and easy-to-use (while they protect you from infection), you will have no problem using condoms correctly and effectively. Also, if you are embarrassed about buying condoms at your local grocery store, there are plenty of alternate ways to get them online via sites like Lucky Bloke (luckybloke.com), which also offer advice on finding the right fit.

Safer Sex Overview

Reducing the chance of contracting or transmitting STI include limiting your number of sexual partners, communicating about your health, and practicing safer sexual activities. It's a simple statistical likelihood that you are more likely to contract an STI the more partners you have. If you are sexually active with multiple partners, it's important to communicate and protect yourself (and them).

Communication means talking about health concerns, sharing information, and setting boundaries. It's important to be upfront and honest about your sexual activity with your partner(s), so everyone can make informed decisions. For example, if one person isn't being monogamous, and they are sexually active with someone who thinks the relationship IS monogamous, that's unethical. One person in the equation isn't able to make informed decisions about his or her sexual health.

If you already have, or end up contracting an STI, it's your ethical (and in some states, legal) obligation to inform partner(s) so that they can quickly seek treatment and/or decide whether they are comfortable with the risk of contracting an STI. For example, herpes (HSV-2) is transmittable during a flare up, but otherwise isn't a problem. It's even less of a problem when a person with HSV-2 is using treatments that control outbreaks. Therefore, someone who is aware that it's a relatively low risk to date someone with herpes might choose to do so.

Communicating safe sex boundaries is important as well. If you tell a man that you require he wear a condom during sex, and he balks, makes excuses, or refuses, then you know that he isn't a safe sexual partner. Or you may discover that you have different safer sex expectations. He may prefer condoms for any kind of genital contact and require oral barriers in addition to condoms for vaginal or anal sex. Figuring out where your boundaries are beforehand is an important first step to having a useful conversation about safer sex.

No Age Limit to Safer Sex

Even though most new STIs are in younger people, older adults are just as susceptible to infections. Safer sex has no age limit. In a recent AARP survey of singles 45 and older in 2009, only one in five reported using condoms every time — 32% of women and 12% of men.

While STIs are by far most common among those under 30, those in their 50s are still at risk. Syphilis, for example, is the most prevalent STI in people 45 and older, though the percentages are low.

Older singles also neglect condoms because they're less likely to have sex involving the main route of STI transmission — vaginal intercourse. Interest in sex often fades with age. Erectile medications are not as effective as we see on television, and menopausal changes can take the fun out of intercourse as it becomes uncomfortable or impossible. As a result, AARP reports that older couples adapt to sex without intercourse — hand massage, oral sex, and sex toys.

As we've learned, however, many STIs can infection the mouth and throat. Most other STIs, however, are rarely transmissible orally. Public-health authorities insist they need to continue condom use. As people continue to live longer and more actively, older adults' STI rates have risen. Since 2005, their risk of syphilis has jumped 67% and chlamydia 40%. No wonder health experts recommend consistent condom use for anyone who dates, at least until they are in a monogamous relationship and have been tested for STIs.

These actions increase your risk of contracting an STI:

- Having unprotected sex. Vaginal or anal penetration by an infected partner who isn't wearing a latex condom significantly increases the risk of getting an STI. Improper or inconsistent use of condoms can also increase your risk. Oral sex may be less risky, but infections can still be transmitted without a latex condom or dental dam. Dental dams — thin, square pieces of rubber made with latex or silicone — prevent skin-to-skin contact.

- Having sexual contact with multiple partners. The more people you have sexual contact with, the greater your risk. This is true for concurrent partners as well as monogamous consecutive relationships.

- Having a history of STIs. Having one STI makes it much easier for another STI to take hold.

- Anyone forced to have sexual intercourse or sexual activity. Dealing with rape or assault can be difficult, but it's important to be seen as soon as possible. Screening, treatment and emotional support can be offered.

- Abusing alcohol or using recreational drugs. Substance abuse can inhibit your judgment, making you more willing to participate in risky behaviors.

- Injecting drugs. Needle sharing spreads many serious infections, including HIV, hepatitis B and hepatitis C.

- Being young. Half of STIs occur in people between the ages of 15 and 24.

Men who request prescriptions for drugs to treat erectile dysfunction. Men who ask their doctors for prescriptions for certain drugs — such as sildenafil (Viagra), tadalafil (Cialis) and vardenafil (Levitra) — have higher rates of STIs. Be sure you are up to date on safe sex practices if you ask your doctor for one of these medications.

Are There Any Sexual Activities I Should Avoid?

The short answer is no. Different sexual activities have different levels of risk, and this question is really only one that can be answered by consenting partners who have taken the time to educate themselves and determine what their boundaries are. If the activity is too far outside your comfort zone in terms of risk, it's something you can choose to avoid. As noted above, unprotected anal sex presents the highest level of risk for transmitting STIs, whereas activities like kissing or mutual masturbation present the least amount of risk.

The discovery of treatment-resistant gonorrhea elevates the risk of unprotected penile oral sex, which was previously considered moderate- to low-risk activity. Some S&M practices that include the possibility of blood are extremely high-risk and require the same precautions one would expect in a medical setting.

Screening

Getting regularly tested and screened for STIs is a major part of preventing the spread of infection. Testing after each new partner is considered good practice and people in monogamous relationships should consider being tested at least once a year.

STI screening requires blood and urine samples and results come back within a couple of days. Some tests, like herpes, may require special request as HSV-2 screenings aren't necessarily a part of the regular screening process.

Early diagnosis is vital for avoiding the more serious complications of sexually transmitted infections. Not only are most infections preventable via safer sex practices, many are relatively harmless when detected quickly. It's kind of a no-brainer when we put it that way.

Resources for Diagnosis and Treatment of STIs

If you have medical insurance, it usually covers STI screening. You can also try any of these resources in the Salem area:

- Yakima Valley Farm Workers Clinic Salud Medical Center, 1175 Mt Hood Ave, Woodburn, OR 97071 503-982-2000

- Oregon Health Division Marion County Health Department, 3180 Center St NE Rm 200, Salem, OR 97301 503-588-5342

- Planned Parenthood Columbia Willamette Salem Center, 3825 Wolverine St NE, Salem, OR 97305 888-875-7820

Planned Parenthood is an excellent resource for comprehensive sexual health services for women and men. They offer a sliding scale for testing services and low-cost or free STI prevention measures, like condoms.

Conclusion

Your next steps should be to become more aware of risk factors for infection in your life. If you find that risks are high in certain areas, practice more caution and take action to combat the spread of infectious diseases in that area. Your chances of contracting and transmitting an STI depend on your individual decisions about safe sex. If you are sexually active, make sure you communicate with each of your partners about your concerns. Protect yourself and your partner from potential infection by practicing safe sex.

Chapter 11
Substances

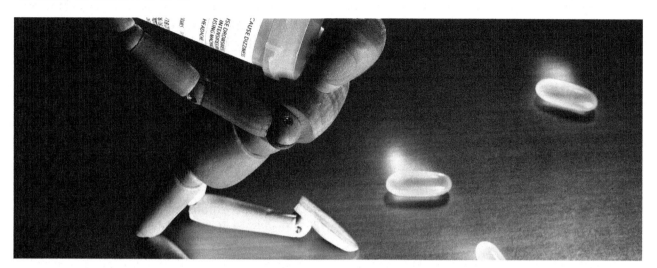

Last night you came home late to find your roommate passed out on the floor in the prone position with his foot resting in the remnants of what looks to have been a pepperoni pizza. He'd been out with friends and had clearly drank more than he should have. In fact, he reeked of alcohol, had a half-eaten slice in his hand, and when you tried to wake him he mumbled something about calling his ex-girlfriend (never a good idea). You decided to let him sleep it off right where he was. Fearing he would die the cliché rock-star death and choke on his own vomit, you roll him over on his side and put pillows behind his back. It's not your first rodeo even if it is only your first term in school. Along with adjusting to classes, homework, and independent life, you've also learned the realities of substance use.

Any substance (other than food) that causes a physiological or chemical change in the body when ingested is considered a drug. Some drugs are used medicinally, but some are used recreationally. You probably use the antihistamine in your bathroom medicinally, while the alcohol your roommate consumed was most definitely recreational. We use the term "substance" collectively to refer to alcohol, tobacco, and any drugs (medicinal or recreational) that are used in a non-therapeutic manner.

Substance misuse and abuse can have a negative impact on wellness, particularly when the use of these substances results in addiction or dependence. Substance abuse and addiction, including problems with prescription drugs, cost Americans more than $700 billion a year in increased health care costs, crime, and lost productivity. Alcohol, illicit, and prescription drugs contribute to 90,000 deaths every year in the US, plus an additional 480,000 linked to tobacco.

This chapter defines what substances are and how they can impact your health. It then introduces the concepts of substance abuse and addiction, focusing on the inherent dangers of substance use that leads to addiction. Then, this chapter examines several different drugs that have addictive properties, addressing the prevalence of addiction and abuse, the short- and long-term effects of each drug, and recovery and treatment options for addiction.

Defining Substance Abuse, Drugs, and Addiction

Not all drug use is harmful. Prescription and over-the-counter medicines are typically **drugs**, but they are not a problem unless they are misused or abused. When used correctly, following the directions or the pharmacist's instructions, drugs can help with any number of psychological and physiological ailments. However, all drugs, whether medicinal or recreational, have the potential to be abused.

Medicinal and Recreational Substances

The differences between medical and recreational substances can be confusing sometimes, especially as laws and attitudes change. The simplest difference between the two, however, is that one type of drug is usually prescribed by a doctor or qualified health professional for specific medicinal purposes, such as temporary pain relief after surgery or to control a cough. The other type has no clear medical use.

Your friend may take Ritalin for his ADD — for him it's medicinal. But if you take one to stay awake, you are using it recreationally. You have no diagnosis to support its use. You may think you *need* the energy, but a doctor would most likely disagree with your approach. Drinking alcohol, for example, is only done for recreational purposes. We hear periodically that a glass of wine or beer a day is healthy, but there are a lot of variables as for whom it's healthy and under what circumstances. It would be a stretch to call it medicinal.

The same applies to marijuana. Your friend praises this plant like it's an organic super-food, a cure-all for every ailment — unfortunately, he spent more time "healing" himself than studying last term and failed his math class for the second time. You can tell yourself that anything is medicinal, but when it impacts your life in a negative way, it is not medicine and you aren't being honest with yourself. A medicinal drug is prescribed to solve problems with your health or improve it. Anything that shifts your priorities away from a productive, healthy life is not medicinal.

Misuse and Abuse

The line between misuse and abuse can be a bit thin at times, but they are not the same. Many of us have misused a substance at one time or another, probably unintentionally. Not all of us have crossed the line from misuse to abuse.

Drug Misuse

Your cousin, Dave, recently had his wisdom teeth removed. The oral surgeon gave him Oxycodone "just in case" the pain could not be resolved with the extra-strength ibuprofen he also prescribed. The procedure had gone well, no complications, and Dave took the ibuprofen for a few days with only a little discomfort. He didn't need the Oxycodone — this time. He decided to save it, just in case. After all, it's not easy to get pain killers this strong and he'd heard that people would lie, cheat, and steal to get their hands on it. A few weeks later he had a rotten headache that he couldn't shake and the bottle of Oxycodone came out of his sock drawer.

Drug misuse is a broad term. It often involves prescription drugs being used in ways other than they were intended, such as for non-medical reasons, taking a drug that was not prescribed for you, or taking it at a higher dosage than recommended. Examples of drug misuse include taking Vicodin for a headache or Xanax for nausea. This kind of misuse can be a result of people self-diagnosing a problem, or discovering that a prescription drug has side effects that help with something other than its purpose. This is dangerous.

Misuse can happen with any drugs, even those that we purchase over-the-counter. Using cold medicine like a sleeping pill, taking four acetaminophens at a time instead of two because "you're tall," or chasing a few ibuprofens with a beer in anticipation of the headache you plan to have — none of these examples sound like the instructions on the bottle. Drugs come with warnings for a reason — mixing drugs or using them for some other purpose than intended can have dire consequences. The most commonly misused drugs are prescription drugs like opioids (painkillers), depressants (e.g. sleeping pills, anti-anxiety medications), and stimulants (e.g. ADD medications). These can be misused for many reasons, particularly among teens:

- After marijuana and alcohol, prescription drugs are the most commonly misused substances by Americans age 14 and older.

- Teens misuse prescription drugs for a number of reasons, such as to get high, to stop pain, or because they think it will help them with schoolwork.

- Many teens get prescription drugs they misuse from friends and relatives, sometimes without the person knowing.

- Boys and girls tend to misuse some types of prescription drugs for different reasons. For example, boys are more likely to misuse prescription stimulants to get high, while girls tend to misuse them to stay alert or to lose weight.

Prescription drug misuse has become a large public health problem, because misuse can lead to addiction, and even overdose deaths. Following the directions printed on the bottle or provided by a pharmacist and only using a drug for its intended purpose can save lives. Being aware of the active ingredients and possible drug interactions is vital to making sure the drugs are safe and effective.

Substance Abuse

People use substances for many different reasons. It becomes **substance abuse** when they use substances that are illegal or use legal substances inappropriately. For example, when a person takes drugs for the express purpose of producing pleasure, alleviating stress, and altering or avoiding reality it's considered abuse. The drug is used to experience euphoria, relaxation, or otherwise "getting high."

Drugs and other substances capable of such mood-altering feats impact wellness because they often substitute a synthetic, temporary solution for the long-term, natural effects of other wellness-increasing activities. This is why many people will continue to use the substance, regaining that high or low they desire. Substance abuse is a harmful pattern of drug use that persists, continually or intermittently, despite negative consequences. Those negative consequences include both the harmful effects experienced by the user and those impacting others (e.g. victims of drunk driving accidents).

Substance abuse is a serious public health problem that affects almost every community and family in some way. Each year drug abuse causes millions of serious illnesses or injuries among Americans. Issues such as drugged driving, violence, stress, child abuse, homelessness, crime, harm to unborn babies, and job loss are just a few of the ways substance abuse can impact you and those around you. Some of the drugs commonly abused include methamphetamine, anabolic steroids, cocaine, heroin, marijuana, inhalants, opioids (like Oxycodone), and club drugs (like Ecstasy).

Psychoactive Drugs

Psychoactive drugs are what we typically think of when we consider substance abuse. Drugs in the **psychoactive** category act on the central nervous system, causing intoxication. This alters the brain's normal, everyday activity, causing changes in mood, awareness, and behavior. They disrupt the communication between neurons (brain cells), so abusing them can have serious short- and long-term effects on the brain.

Psychoactive drugs include four groups of drugs: depressants (e.g. alcohol, sleeping pills), stimulants (nicotine, ecstasy), opioids (heroin, pain medications), and hallucinogens (LSD). The term psychoactive drug might immediately make you think of **hallucinogens**, like LSD and mushrooms, which change your brain and behavior in extreme ways. Hallucinogens, or "psychedelic" drugs (like we envision from the 1960s), significantly alter the user's perception of reality, causing hallucinations that can be visual, auditory, or even emotional — hallucinations that seem very real. They are also an illicit, or illegal, drug.

But not all psychoactive drugs are illegal. Caffeine is a **stimulant** found in coffee and energy drinks. Ritalin and Adderall, both used by prescription for attention deficit disorder are some of the most commonly abused drugs. Stimulants increase alertness, attention, and energy, as well as elevate blood pressure, heart rate, and respiration.

Historically, stimulants were used to treat asthma and other respiratory problems, obesity, neurological disorders, and a variety of other ailments (such as Attention Deficit Disorder). Stimulants increase wakefulness, motivation, and aspects of cognition, learning, and memory. Some people take these drugs in the absence of medical need in an effort to enhance mental performance.

Opioids like Vicodin, Oxycodone, or morphine are often prescribed by doctors. These medications act on opioid receptors (found on the nerve cells) in both the spinal cord and brain to reduce the intensity of pain-signal perception. They also affect brain areas that control emotion, which can further diminish the effects of painful stimuli.

Depresssants, like alcohol, Xanax, and Valium are also legal when used responsibly. These include tranquilizers, sedatives, and hypnotics — substances that can slow brain activity. This property makes them useful for treating anxiety and sleep disorders. It also makes them commonly misused or abused by individuals looking to relax.

Abusing prescribed psychoactive drugs *is* illegal though, and can be as dangerous as abusing cocaine or heroin. That is one reason why they come with warning labels telling people not to drive or operate heavy machinery. Your brain may not think or respond rationally when under the influence of these substances. Even an excess of caffeine and nicotine (from heavy tobacco use) can have significant mood-altering effects (Figure 1).

This alteration in the brain is called **intoxication**. This is, essentially, a type of poisoning though most individuals seek it for the high or low feeling they sustain. It causes a marked reduction in your physical and mental capacities that people often find enjoyable. If you consider other uses for the word "intoxicating," you'll find that often we attach the term to enjoyable things with which we like to be overwhelmed, such as comforting aromas or pleasant settings. However, any intoxication we receive from drugs is short-lived and generally followed by unpleasant side effects.

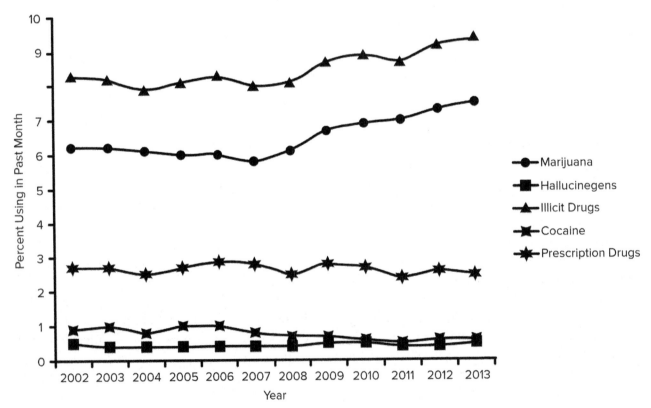

Past–Month Use of Selected illicit Drugs

Figure 1. How many people use drugs in the United States?

Psychoactive Drugs Impact Public Health

Our nation pays a high price in dollars and lives for these misused and abused substances. Abuse of tobacco, alcohol, and illicit drugs exacts more than $740 billion annually in costs related to crime, lost work productivity, and health care. In illness and injury alone, smoking costs approximately 168 billion, alcohol 27 billion, illicit drugs 11 billion, and prescription opioids 26 billion.

Many people die each year from overdose and other injuries sustained due to substance usage. Opioid-related deaths in the US have quadrupled since 1999 and are not at approximately 33,000 annually, 18,000 for prescription opioids alone. That could be because as many as one in four people who receive long-term prescription opioids for non-cancer pain struggle with addiction. There has been a growing trend of 'pill mills' and 'doctor shopping' to feed this addiction. In the US, the non-medical use of these drugs by 12 million people made them the second most common form of illicit drug use after cannabis in 2010 (Figure 2).

Drug Abuse Impacts Mental Health

Chronic use of some drugs can lead to both short- and long-term changes in the brain, which can lead to mental health issues including paranoia, depression, anxiety, aggression, hallucinations, and the impairment of cognitive function. It is not uncommon for people with substance addictions to have a diagnosis of mental illness as well. Compared with the general population, people addicted to drugs are roughly twice as likely to suffer from mood and anxiety disorders, with the reverse also true.

In 2015, an estimated 43.4 million (17.9 percent) adults ages 18 and older experienced some form of mental illness (other than a developmental or substance use disorder). Of these, 8.1 million had both a substance use disorder and another mental illness. Although substance use disorders commonly occur with other mental illnesses, it's often unclear whether one helped cause the other or if common underlying risk factors contribute to both disorders.

Type	Health Care	Overall	Year Estimate Based On
Tobacco	$168 Billion	$300 Billion	2010
Alcohol	$27 Billion	$249 Billion	2010
Illicit Drugs	$11 Billion	$193 Billion	2007
Prescription Opioids	$26 Billion	$78.5 Billion	2013

Figure 2. Drug use and abuse accounts for healthcare treatment that costs billions of dollars each year.

Dependence and Addiction

Drug **dependence** develops when the neurons adapt to the repeated drug exposure and only function normally in the presence of the drug. When the drug is withdrawn, several physiologic reactions occur. These can be mild (e.g., for caffeine) or even life threatening (e.g., for alcohol). This is known as the withdrawal syndrome. In the case of heroin, for example, withdrawal can be very serious and the abuser will use the drug again to avoid the withdrawal syndrome.

Drug **addiction** is defined as a chronic, relapsing brain disease that is characterized by compulsive drug seeking and use, despite harmful consequences. It is characterized by an inability to stop using a drug; failure to meet work, social, or family obligations; and, sometimes (depending on the drug), tolerance and withdrawal. It is considered a brain disease because drugs change the brain — they change its structure and how it works. These brain changes can be long-lasting, and can lead to the harmful behaviors seen in people who abuse drugs.

Physical dependence can happen with the chronic use of many drugs — including many prescription drugs, even if taken as instructed. Thus, physical dependence in and of itself does not constitute addiction, but it often accompanies addiction. This distinction can be difficult to discern, particularly with prescribed pain medications, for which the need for increasing dosages can represent tolerance or a worsening underlying problem, as opposed to the beginning of abuse or addiction.

Addiction Development

According to the National Institute on Drug Abuse (NIDA), our brains are wired to ensure that we will repeat life-sustaining activities by associating those activities with pleasure or reward. Whenever this reward circuit is activated, the brain notes that something important is happening that needs to be remembered, and teaches us to do it again and again without thinking about it. Because abusing drugs stimulates the same circuit, we learn to abuse drugs in the same way.

The NIDA explains that for the brain, the difference between normal rewards and drug rewards can be described as the difference between someone whispering into your ear and someone shouting into a microphone. Just as we turn down the volume on a radio that is too loud, the brain adjusts to the overwhelming surges in dopamine (and other neurotransmitters) by producing less dopamine or by reducing the number of receptors that can receive signals. As a result, dopamine's impact on the reward circuit of the brain of someone who abuses drugs can become abnormally low, and that person's ability to experience *any* pleasure is reduced.

This is why a person who abuses drugs eventually feels flat, lifeless, and depressed, and is unable to enjoy things that were previously pleasurable. Now, the person needs to keep taking drugs again and again just to try and bring his or her dopamine function back up to normal — which only makes the problem worse, like a vicious cycle. Also, the person will often need to take larger amounts of the drug to produce the familiar dopamine high — an effect known as **tolerance**.

The initial decision to take drugs is typically voluntary. However, with continued use, a person's ability to exert self-control can become seriously impaired. This impairment in self-control is the hallmark of addiction. Brain imaging studies of people with addiction show physical changes in areas of the brain that are critical to judgment, decision making, learning and memory, and behavior control. Scientists believe that these changes alter the way the brain works and may help explain the compulsive and destructive behaviors of addiction.

Many people don't understand why or how other people become addicted to drugs. They may mistakenly think that those who use drugs lack moral principles or willpower and that they could stop their drug use simply by choosing to. In reality, drug addiction is a complex disease, and quitting usually takes more than good intentions or a strong will. Drugs change the brain in ways that make quitting hard, even for those who want to. can help people recover from drug addiction and lead productive lives.

Risk Factors for Addiction

As with any other disease, vulnerability to addiction differs from person to person, and no single factor determines whether a person will become addicted to drugs. No one factor can predict if a person will become addicted to drugs. In general, the more risk factors a person has, the greater the chance that taking drugs will lead to abuse and addiction. Protective factors, on the other hand, reduce a person's risk of developing addiction.

Risk and protective factors may be influenced by:

Biology — The genes that people are born with account for about half of a person's risk for addiction. Gender, ethnicity, and the presence of other mental disorders may also influence risk for drug use and addiction.

Environment — A person's environment includes many different influences, from family and friends to economic status and general quality of life. Factors such as peer pressure, physical and sexual abuse, early exposure to drugs, stress, and parental guidance can greatly affect a person's likelihood of drug use and addiction.

Development — Genetic and environmental factors interact with critical developmental stages in a person's life to affect addiction risk. Although taking drugs at any age can lead to addiction, the earlier that drug use begins, the more likely it will progress to addiction. This is particularly problematic for teens. Because areas in their brains that control decision-making, judgment, and self-control are still developing, teens may be especially prone to risky behaviors, including trying drugs.

Method of Administration — Smoking a drug or injecting it into a vein increases its addictive potential. Both smoked and injected drugs enter the brain within seconds, producing a powerful rush of pleasure. However, this intense "high" can fade within a few minutes, taking the abuser down to lower, more normal levels. Scientists believe this starkly felt contrast drives some people to repeated drug taking in an attempt to recapture the fleeting pleasurable state.

Long-Term Effects on the Brain

The NIDA suggests that the same sort of mechanisms involved in the development of tolerance can eventually lead to profound changes in neurons and brain circuits, with the potential to severely compromise the long-term health of the brain (Figure 3). For example, glutamate is another neurotransmitter that influences the reward circuit and the ability to learn. When the optimal concentration of glutamate is altered by drug abuse, the brain attempts to compensate for this change, which can cause impairment in cognitive function.

Similarly, long-term drug abuse can trigger adaptations in habit or non-conscious memory systems. Conditioning is one example of this type of learning, in which cues in a person's daily routine or environment become associated with the drug experience and can trigger uncontrollable cravings whenever the person is exposed to these cues, even if the drug itself is not available. This learned "reflex" is extremely durable and can affect a person who once used drugs even after many years of abstinence.

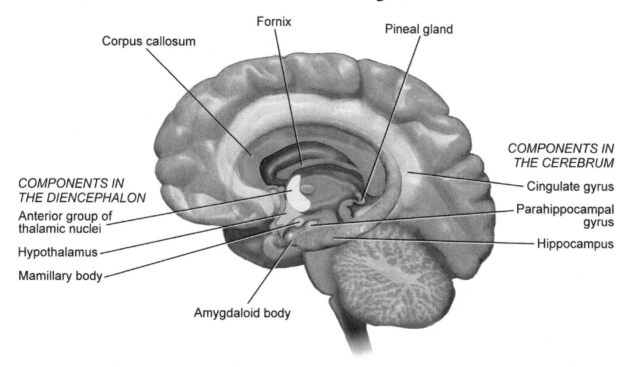

Figure 3. Drug use has long-term effects on the brain.

Process Addictions

Though this chapter is about substance abuse primarily, it is important to note that we can become addicted to many things, such as gambling, gaming, Internet usage, work, exercise, sex, and so on. These are called **process addictions**, or behavioral addictions. Anything capable of stimulating us can be addictive. Whenever a habit becomes an obligation — the person must complete it fulfill a need, it becomes an addiction. How many times have you watched a friend stay up all night gaming with an excuse that their online community needed them? How many times have you become anxious because you didn't have your phone? These seem minor initially, but over time they can become significant.

Addiction is a lot like other diseases, such as heart disease. Both disrupt the normal, healthy functioning of the underlying organ, have serious harmful consequences, and are preventable and treatable, but if left untreated, can last a lifetime.

Signs of Drug Dependency or Addiction

Drug dependency and addiction have some common symptoms. You may notice increased drug-seeking behaviors or irritability, anxiety, depression, and restlessness, particularly when the drug is not available. When dependence is severe, some drugs, like alcohol, have potentially lethal withdrawal symptoms that require a person trying to break their dependence to seek medical intervention.

Other symptoms or behaviors include, among others:

- Feeling that you have to use the drug regularly — whether daily or several times throughout the day

- Having intense urges for the drug

- Needing more and more of the drug to get the same effect

- Making sure that you maintain a supply of the drug

- Spending money on the drug, even when you can't afford it

- Not meeting obligations and work responsibilities, or cutting back on social or recreational activities because of drug use

- Doing things to get the drug that you normally wouldn't do, such as stealing or prostitution

- Driving or doing other risky activities when you're under the influence of the drug

- Focusing more and more time and energy on getting and using the drug

- Trying to quit and failing

- Experiencing withdrawal symptoms when you attempt to stop taking the drug

Drug Addiction Treatment

As with most other chronic diseases, such as diabetes, asthma, or heart disease, treatment for drug addiction generally isn't a cure. However, addiction is treatable and can be successfully managed. People who are recovering from an addiction will be at risk for relapse for years and possibly for their whole lives. Research shows that combining addiction treatment medicines with behavioral therapy ensures the best chance of success for most patients. Treatment approaches tailored to each patient's drug use patterns and any co-occurring medical, mental, and social problems can lead to continued recovery.

Treatment involves many steps, depending upon the nature of the drug and the level of addiction. This could include detoxification (ridding the body of the drug), behavioral therapy and counseling, assessment of any co-existing mental illness, and long-term monitoring. Sometimes drugs need to be used as well to help ease withdrawal symptoms.

Methadone, for example, is often used to treat heroin addiction because it provides a similar effect on the body as the opiate (though legal) and allows treatment centers to wean the person off the illicit drug.

More good news is that drug use and addiction are preventable. Results from NIDA-funded research have shown that prevention programs involving families, schools, communities, and the media are effective for preventing or reducing drug use and addiction. Although personal events and cultural factors affect drug use trends, when young people view drug use as harmful, they tend to decrease their drug taking. Therefore, education and outreach are key in helping people understand the possible risks of drug use. Teachers, parents, and health care providers have crucial roles in educating young people and preventing drug use and addiction.

Addiction and Dependence Stigma

Like many mental health issues, addiction is hard for people who don't experience addiction to understand. A person with addiction is hard to predict, will do and say hurtful things, and are compelled by their addiction to make decisions that harm themselves and others. Treatment is labor-intensive and can take a long time, which can be frustrating for close friends or the family of someone with addiction. It can take a depth of patience to help an addict that many people just don't have.

Many people worry over whether addiction is a disease or a result of choices. Technically, it's a complicated combination of both. Addiction often occurs amidst a perfect storm of genetic predisposition (disease) and environmental factors. The compulsive behavior of a person with addiction tells us that they have limited control of their actions and their choices are more in line with the kind of choices a person with bipolar disorder or acute social anxiety might make. To make different choices, a person suffering from bipolar disorder needs lifelong treatment and can expect to suffer episodes despite treatment, which appears similar to what we see among people suffering from addiction.

Common Addictive Substances and Treatments

People most often think of "hard" illegal drugs like meth and heroin when they think of addictive substances. As we've covered so far there are a wide variety of them, many of which are legal for over the counter medical and recreational use.

Alcohol

People drink to socialize, celebrate, and relax. Alcohol often has a strong effect on people — and throughout history, we've struggled to understand and manage alcohol's power. Why does alcohol cause us to act and feel differently? How much is too much? Why do some people become addicted while others do not? (Figure 4)

Here's what we know. Alcohol's effects vary from person to person, depending on a variety of factors, such as how much and how often you drink, your age, your biological gender, your health, and your family history. While drinking alcohol is itself not necessarily a problem — drinking too much can cause a range of consequences, and increase your risk for a variety of problems.

Ethyl Alcohol (ethanol) is the alcohol found in alcoholic drinks such as beer or whiskey. It is made from the fermentation or chemical breakdown of sugars by yeasts. Alcohol is made from plants and grains such as corn, wheat, and barley, or from grapes (for wine). Ethanol can be produced by milling the grains and then fermenting them with yeast (wine is similar but requires the grapes

to be stored under the right conditions). During the fermentation process, the starches of the grains (or the sugar in the grapes) are turned into alcohol.

Alcoholic drinks come in two types: fermented and distilled. Examples of fermented drinks include beer, malt liquor, wine, cider, mead, etc. Beer and cider have a lower alcohol content by volume (usually below 10%) than wine and mead (which can get up to 20% in the case of fortified wines and some meads). Distilled alcohols basically take fermented alcohol and refine it by a process called distillation, which uses heat to remove water from the original source to create a drink with higher alcohol percentage (usually 40% or more). This percentage is taken when the alcohol is at 60 degrees Fahrenheit and multiplied by two, which is called "proof." Examples of distilled alcohol are vodka, whiskey, tequila, and rum.

How Your Body Processes Alcohol

As soon as you take a drink it enters the stomach and small intestine. Here small blood vessels carry it to the bloodstream. Approximately 20% of alcohol is absorbed through the stomach and most of the remaining 80%

Age	Lifetime Abstainer	Former Regular	Current Regular
16–44	22.3%	3.3%	56.6%
45–64	16.7%	7.6%	51.8%
65–74	21.8%	10.4%	41.6%
75 and over	30.9%	12.3%	29.6%

Figure 4. Alcohol use is common throughout life.

through the small intestine. Enzymes in the liver then break down the alcohol.

Understanding the rate of metabolism is critical to understanding the effects of alcohol. For the average person, the liver processes one ounce of liquor (or one standard drink) in one hour. Consume any more than this, and your system becomes saturated. The additional alcohol will accumulate in the blood and body tissues until it can be metabolized. This is why doing shots, and playing drinking games like beer pong, can result in high **blood alcohol concentrations** (BAC) that last for several hours, making your behavior potentially risky. Driving with a blood alcohol concentration of .08% or more, for example, is considered dangerous and illegal (Figure 5).

Factors Affecting Your BAC

Not everyone metabolizes alcohol the same. There are different factors that affect the way our body processes alcohol that have a direct impact on our BAC, such as:

Age — The amount of water in your body goes down with age, which affects your body's metabolism process. You also have lower muscle mass. Muscle absorbs alcohol.

Biological sex — Women absorb and metabolize alcohol differently from men. They have higher BAC's after consuming the same amount of alcohol as men. The difference in BAC's has been attributed to women's smaller amount of body water, lower muscle mass, and lower activity of the alcohol-metabolizing enzyme ADH (alcohol dehydrogenase) in the stomach, causing a larger proportion of the ingested alcohol to reach the blood.

Weight — In general, people who weigh less have less water in their bodies and are able to drink less.

Physical fitness level — The health of your liver, your hydration level, and the amount of fat in your body affect alcohol metabolism. If you're in better physical health, your body metabolizes it more efficiently.

Amount of food consumed before drinking — Drinking alcohol after a meal that includes fat, protein, and carbohydrates allows the body to absorb the alcohol about three times more slowly than when alcohol is consumed on an empty stomach.

How quickly the alcohol was consumed — The faster you drink, the higher your BAC.

Use of drugs or prescription medicines — Certain medications can speed up the feeling of intoxication or can

Number of Drinks		Body Weight in Pounds								Driving Condition
		100	120	140	160	180	200	220	240	
0	Male	.00	.00	.00	.00	.00	.00	.00	.00	Only Safe Driving Limit
	Female	.00	.00	.00	.00	.00	.00	.00	.00	
1	Male	.06	.05	.04	.04	.03	.03	.03	.02	Driving Skills Impaired
	Female	.07	.06	.05	.04	.04	.03	.03	.03	
2	Male	.12	.10	.09	.07	.07	.06	.05	.05	
	Female	.13	.11	.09	.08	.07	.07	.06	.06	
3	Male	.18	.15	.13	.11	.10	.09	.08	.07	
	Female	.20	.17	.14	.12	.11	.10	.09	.08	Legally Intoxicated
4	Male	.24	.20	.17	.15	.13	.12	.11	.10	
	Female	.26	.22	.19	.17	.15	.13	.12	.11	
5	Male	.30	.25	.21	.19	.17	.15	.14	.12	
	Female	.33	.28	.24	.21	.18	.17	.15	.14	

Subtract .01% for each 40 minutes of drinking.
1 drink = 1.5 oz. 80 proof liquor, 12 oz. 5% beer, or 5 oz. 12% wine.
Fewer than 5 persons out of 100 will exceed these values.

Figure 5. Blood alcohol concentrations by number of drinks, weight, and sex.

BAC Level	Effects
0.02	Light to moderate drinkers begin to feel relaxed.
0.04	Most drinkers begin to feel relaxed.
0.06	Judgment is impaired. Legally drunk in some states.
0.08	Judgment is further impaired. More likely to do things that you would not do when sober. Legally drunk in all states.
0.10	Reaction time and muscle control are impaired. A person drinking at this level is 10x more likely to cause a fatal car crash. Normal social drinkers rarely reach this level.
0.12	Vomiting for most people.
0.15	Balance and movement are substantially imaired. Difficulty walking or talking. Heavy drinkers with substantial tolerance may learn to look sober at this level. One half pint of whiskey is circulating in the blood stream. 25x more likely to cause a fatal car crash.
0.20	Blackout and memory loss. A person driving at this level is 100x more likely to cause a fatal car crash.
0.30	Loss of consciousness and passing out. Being ble to remain concious at this level indicates a tolerance that is a serious risk factor for health problems.
0.40–0.60	FATAL: Causes paralysis to brain area that controls breathing and heart rate. This can happen when someone drinks a lot, passes out and the alcohol in the stomach continues to be absorbed into the blood stream. Drinking contests are frequent cause of lethal overdose.

Figure 6. BAC concentrations and their effects.

have dangerous affects when mixed with alcohol.

Knowing how much alcohol constitutes a "standard" drink can help you determine how much you are drinking and understand the risks. One standard drink contains about 0.6 fluid ounces or 14 grams of pure alcohol (Figure 7). In more familiar terms, the following amounts constitute one standard drink:

- 12 fluid ounces of beer (about 5% alcohol)

- 8 to 9 fluid ounces of malt liquor (about 7% alcohol)

- 5 fluid ounces of table wine (about 12% alcohol)

- 1.5 fluid ounces of 80-proof distilled spirits (40% alcohol)

Regular Beer (5% alc/vol)	Malt Liquor (7% alc/vol)	Table Wine (12% alc/vol)	80–proof Distilled Spirits (40% alc/vol)
12 fl oz = 1 16 fl oz = 1 ⅓ 22 fl oz = 2 40 fl oz = 3 ⅓	12 fl oz = 1.5 16 fl oz = 2 22 fl oz = 2.5 40 fl oz = 4.5	750 ml (a regular wine bottle) = 5	a shot (1.5-oz glass/50-ml bottle=1) a mixed drink or cocktail = 1 or more 200 ml (a "half pint") = 4.5 375 ml (a "pint" or "half bottle") = 8.5 750 ml (a "fifth") = 17

Figure 7. Common alcohol containers and how many "drinks" they represent.

Consequences of Drinking Too Much

Alcohol's immediate effects can appear within about ten minutes. Your BAC increases as you drink. The higher your BAC, the more impaired you become by alcohol's effects. These effects can be **short-term**, including reduced inhibitions, slurred speech, confusion, motor impairment, blacking out, and risky or violent behav-iors. It can lead us to overeat (get the munchies), get into arguments, drunk-dial former love interests, and say things we don't mean and do things we wouldn't normally do.

One of the first consequences we think of when we think about the effects of alcohol is the notorious hangover! A **hangover** is largely the result of dehydration. Alcohol consumption leads to increased urination, which leads to less water in the body. This makes your mouth dry and your headache. Alcohol also causes your blood sugar to fall, which can result in that weak, tired, shaky feeling. Some alcohols also contain other chemicals that can lead to headaches and irritate your stomach lining. Some champagne, for example, has arsenic to make them bubble. Even some of the chemicals that naturally form during the fermentation process can contribute to that miserable feeling of having socks on your teeth and a pounding in your brain. This is typically resolved within a day with water intake, sleep, and over-the-counter painkillers.

But there are other consequences that can be quite serious and can occur from even one night of heavy drinking. These can be the direct physical result of a high BAC or the indirect result of a decreased mental capacity. These include alcohol poisoning, coma, unintended pregnancy, sexual abuse, breathing problems, and death, including suicide and homicide. Car crashes and other accidents, often fatal, are quite common. Alcohol related crashes alone account for over 10,000 deaths each year.

People who drink too much over a long period of time may experience **long-term effects** that can significantly impact their health, such as:

Alcohol use disorder (AUD) — This is a chronic relapsing brain disease characterized by compulsive alcohol use, loss of control over alcohol intake, and a negative emotional state when not using. AUD may result in Wernicke-Korsakoff syndrome, a brain disorder due to thiamine (vitamin B1) deficiency. Lack of vitamin B1 is common in people with alcohol use disorder.

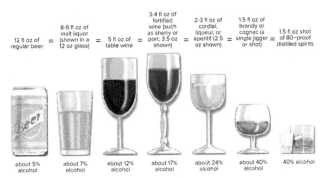

Figure 8. Common serving sizes of different alcohols.

Heart disease — Drinking a high amount over a long time or too much on a single occasion can damage the heart, causing problems including cardiomyopathy, arrhythmias, stroke, and high blood pressure.

Liver damage — Heavy drinking takes a toll on the liver, and can lead to a variety of problems and liver inflammations, including steatosis (fatty liver), alcoholic hepatitis, fibrosis (thickening or scarring), and cirrhosis.

Pancreas damage — Alcohol causes the pancreas to produce toxic substances that can eventually lead to pancreatitis, a dangerous inflammation and swelling of the blood vessels in the pancreas that prevents proper digestion.

Cancer — Drinking too much alcohol can increase your risk of developing certain cancers, including cancers of the mouth, esophagus, throat, liver, and breast.

Compromised immune system — Excessive alcohol use can weaken your immune system, making your body a much easier target for disease. Chronic drinkers are more liable to contract diseases like pneumonia and tuberculosis than people who do not drink too much. Drinking a lot on a single occasion slows your body's ability to ward off infections — even up to 24 hours after getting drunk.

Alcohol and Public Health

Excessive alcohol use led to approximately 88,000 deaths and 2.5 million years of potential life lost each year in the United States from 2006–2010, shortening the lives of those who died by an average of 30 years. Further, excessive drinking was responsible for one in ten deaths among working-age adults aged 20–64 years. The economic costs of excessive alcohol consumption in 2010 were estimated at $249 billion, or $2.05 a drink.

But when does drinking become excessive? When do we cross the line from fun, responsible drinking toward something dangerous and unhealthy?

For women, **low-risk drinking** is defined as no more than three drinks on any single day and no more than seven drinks per week. For men, it is defined as no more than four drinks on any single day and no more than 14 drinks per week. Research shows that only about 2 in 100 people who drink within these limits have AUD.

Excessive alcohol consumption includes binge drinking, heavy drinking, and any drinking by pregnant women or people younger than age 21.

Binge Drinking

Binge drinking is the most common, costly, and deadly pattern of excessive alcohol use in the United States. Three-quarters of the total cost of alcohol misuse in the US is related to binge drinking. The National Institute on Alcohol Abuse and Alcoholism defines binge drinking as a pattern of drinking that brings a person's blood alcohol concentration (BAC) to 0.08% or above. This typically happens when men consume five or more drinks or women consume four or more drinks in about two hours. However, most people who binge drink are not alcohol dependent.

Of the $249 billion price tag to the US in terms of losses in workplace productivity, health care expenditures, criminal justice costs, and other expenses binge drinking was responsible for 77% of these costs, or $191 billion. The health and safety risks mentioned earlier can all arise from binge drinking. When done on a regular basis, those long-term effects can set in, even for younger individuals like college students (Figure 9).

Binge drinking is a major public health problem. One in six US adults binge drink about four times a month, consuming about eight drinks per binge. Binge drinking is most common among younger adults aged 18–34 years, but is reported into higher ages. Binge drinking is twice as prevalent among men than women. Binge drinking is more common among people with household incomes of $75,000 or more than among people with lower incomes. People with lower incomes binge drink in lower numbers, but those that do binge more often and consume more drinks. Over 90% of US adults who drink excessively report binge drinking in the past 30 days. Most people younger than age 21 who drink report binge drinking, usually on multiple occasions.

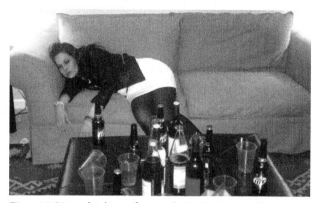

Figure 9. Binge-drinking often results in "passing out."

Heavy Drinking

Heavy drinking is defined as consuming eight or more drinks per week for women and fifteen or more for men. Too much combined with too often makes it too risky. It makes a difference both *how much* you drink on any day and *how often* you have a "heavy drinking day," that is, more than four drinks on any day for men or more than three drinks for women.

In short, the more drinks on any day and the more heavy drinking days over time, the greater the risk — not only for an alcohol use disorder, but also for other health and personal problems. About one in four people who exceed these limits already has an alcohol use disorder, and the rest are at greater risk for developing these and the other problems previously mentioned.

Consequences of College Drinking

College students and heavy alcohol use have coexisted for many years. When was the last time that you watched a movie about college life that didn't highlight at least some elements of the party life? There aren't many, and if they exist, they aren't very realistic. Your friend passed out on the floor of your apartment? That happens more often than we care to admit. College students are known for excessive drinking, particularly those at four-year universities.

Drinking at college has become a ritual that students often see as an integral part of their higher education experience (Figure 10). In fact, it has become so commonplace that we tend to normalize it, make light of it, which underscores the severity of the issue. Many students come to college with established drinking habits, and the college environment can exacerbate the problem. According to a national survey, almost 60 percent of college students ages 18–22 drank alcohol during any given month, and almost two in three of them engaged in binge drinking during that same timeframe.

Factors Affecting Student Drinking

Although the majority of students come to college already having some experience with alcohol, certain aspects of college life, such as unstructured time, the widespread availability of alcohol, inconsistent enforcement of underage drinking laws, and limited interactions with parents and other adults, can intensify the problem. In fact, college students have higher binge-drinking rates and a higher incidence of driving under the influence of alcohol than their non-college peers. The dangers of college drinking include:

Death — About 1,825 college students between 18–24 die from alcohol-related, unintentional injuries, including motor vehicle crashes.

Assault — About 696,000 students between 18–24 are assaulted by another student who has been drinking.

Sexual Assault — About 97,000 students between 18–24 report experiencing alcohol-related sexual assault or date rape.

Academic Problems — About one in four college students report academic consequences from drinking, including missing class, falling behind in class, doing poorly on exams or papers, and receiving lower grades overall, particularly those who binged.

Alcohol Use Disorder (AUD) — About 20% of college students meet the criteria for AUD.

Other Consequences — These include suicide attempts, health problems, injuries, unsafe sex, and driving under the influence of alcohol, as well as vandalism, property damage, and involvement with the police.

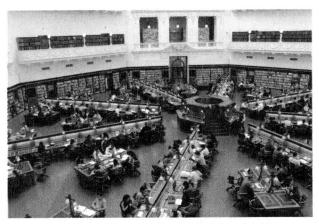

Figure 10. College campuses are known for binge-drinking.

Alcohol Poisoning

Some people getting a kick out of watching people get drunk. Some think it's even funnier when they pass out. But there is nothing funny about the aspiration of vomit leading to asphyxiation or the poisoning of the respiratory center in the brain, both of which can result in death.

Do you know about the dangers of an alcohol overdose — also referred to as **alcohol poisoning**? When should you seek professional help for a friend? Sadly enough, too many college students say they wish they had sought medical treatment for someone they thought was just drunk. Many end up feeling responsible for alcohol-related tragedies that could have easily been prevented.

Common myths about sobering up include drinking black coffee, taking a cold bath or shower, sleeping it off, or walking it off. These are just myths, and they don't work. The only thing that reverses the effects of alcohol is time — something you may not have if you are suffering from an alcohol overdose. And many different factors affect the level of intoxication of an individual, so it's difficult to gauge exactly how much is too much.

Alcohol depresses nerves that control involuntary actions, such as breathing and the gag reflex (which prevents choking). A fatal dose of alcohol will eventually stop these functions.

It is common for someone who drank excessive alcohol to vomit since alcohol is an irritant to the stomach. There is then the danger of choking on vomit, which could cause death by asphyxiation in a person who is not conscious.

You should also know that a person's BAC can continue to rise even while he or she is passed out. Even after a person stops drinking, alcohol in the stomach and intestine continues to enter the bloodstream and circulate throughout the body. It is dangerous to assume the person will be fine by sleeping it off. Critical signs of alcohol poisoning include:

- Mental confusion, stupor, coma, or person cannot be roused

- Vomiting

- Seizures

- Slow breathing (fewer than eight breaths per minute)

- Irregular breathing (ten seconds or more between breaths)

- Hypothermia (low body temperature), bluish skin color, paleness

If you suspect an alcohol overdose (poisoning), call 911. Do not try to handle it on your own. An alcohol overdose can lead to irreversible brain damage. Rapid binge drinking (which often happens on a bet or a dare) is especially dangerous because the victim can ingest a fatal dose before even becoming unconscious (Figure 11).

Some people should never drink alcohol, even if their usage is considered low-risk. Low-risk does not mean no risk (Figure 12). According to the US Dietary Guidelines, the following groups of people should not drink at all:

- Anyone under age 21

- People of any age who are unable to restrict their drinking to moderate levels

- Women who may become pregnant or who are pregnant

- People who plan to drive, operate machinery, or take part in other activities that require attention, skill, or coordination

- People taking prescription or over-the-counter medications that can interact with alcohol.

Women and Alcohol Use

An estimated 5.3 million women in the United States drink in a way that threatens their health, safety, and general well-being. We discussed earlier about the physiological differences between men and women and how they impact the metabolism of alcohol (Figure 13). Between the lower muscle mass, differences in enzymes, and lower body water (lower body weight), women generally can (or should) consume less alcohol. Due to this, a woman's brain and other organs are exposed to more alcohol and to more of the toxic byproducts that result when the body breaks down and eliminates alcohol. This makes them more at risk for motor vehicle crashes, other injuries, high blood pressure, liver damage, cardiovascular disease, brain injury, stroke, violence, suicide, and certain types of cancer.

Research suggests that as little as one drink per day can slightly raise the risk of breast cancer in some women, especially those who are postmenopausal or have a family history of breast cancer. It is not possible, however, to

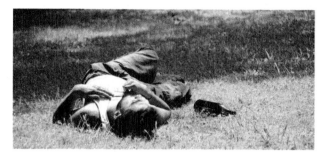

Figure 11. Passing out from drinking is always dangerous.

Low-risk drinking limits	**Men**	**Women**
On any single **DAY**	No more than 4 ▾▾▾▾ drinks on any **day**	No more than 3 ▾▾▾ drinks on any **day**
	AND	*AND*
On any single **WEEK**	No more than 14 ▾▾▾▾▾▾▾▾▾▾▾▾▾▾ drinks on any **week**	No more than 7 ▾▾▾▾▾▾▾ drinks on any **week**
To stay low risk, keep within **both** the single-day **and** weekly limits.		

Figure 12. Low-risk drinking has strict limits.

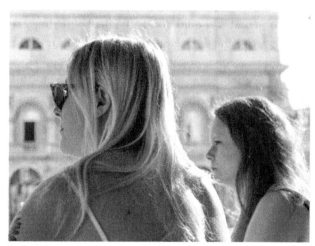

Figure 13. Women who are or may become pregnant should not drink at all.

predict how alcohol will affect the risk for breast cancer in any one woman.

It's important to highlight that drinking makes young women more vulnerable to sexual assault and unsafe and unplanned sex. On college campuses, assaults, unwanted sexual advances, and unplanned and unsafe sex are all more likely among students who drink heavily on occasion — for men, five drinks in a row, for women, four. In general, when a woman drinks to excess she is more likely to be a target of violence or sexual assault.

Alcohol Use and Pregnancy

There is no known safe amount of alcohol use during pregnancy or while trying to get pregnant. There is also no safe time during pregnancy to drink. All types of alcohol are equally harmful, including all wines and beer. When a pregnant woman drinks alcohol (Figure 14), so does her baby.

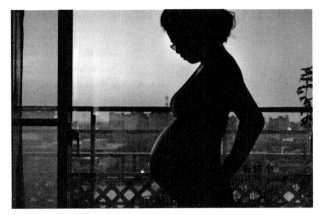

Figure 14. FASDs are very serious.

Women also should not drink alcohol if they are sexually active and do not use effective birth control. This is because a woman might get pregnant and expose her baby to alcohol before she knows she is pregnant. This recommendation is from the CDC, and it may sound extreme but this recommendation is due to the seriousness of fetal alcohol spectrum disorders. Nearly half of all pregnancies in the United States are unplanned. Most women will not know they are pregnant for up to four to six weeks from the time of conception.

Alcohol in the mother's blood passes to the baby through the umbilical cord. Drinking alcohol during pregnancy can cause miscarriage, stillbirth, and a range of lifelong physical, behavioral, and intellectual disabilities. These disabilities are known as **fetal alcohol spectrum disorders** (FASDs). Children with FASDs might have the following characteristics and behaviors:

- Abnormal facial features, such as a smooth ridge between the nose and upper lip (this ridge is called the philtrum)
- Small head size
- Shorter-than-average height
- Low body weight
- Poor coordination
- Hyperactive behavior
- Difficulty with attention
- Poor memory
- Difficulty in school (especially with math)
- Learning disabilities
- Speech and language delays
- Intellectual disability or low IQ
- Poor reasoning and judgment skills
- Sleep and sucking problems as a baby
- Vision or hearing problems
- Problems with the heart, kidney, or bones

FASD is most likely to occur in infants whose mothers drank heavily (three or more drinks per occasion or more than seven drinks per week) and continued to drink heavily throughout pregnancy. It can also occur even with lesser amounts — even moderate usage of one drink per day. There is no safe time or safe level to drink alcohol during pregnancy. Alcohol can cause problems for the developing baby throughout pregnancy, including before a woman knows she is pregnant. If you find out you are pregnant and have been drinking, it is important to stop immediately, see your healthcare provider, and begin prenatal care.

Alcohol and Driving

Drunk driving laws make it illegal nationwide to drive with a BAC at or above 0.08%. For people under 21, "zero tolerance" laws make it illegal to drive with any measurable amount of alcohol in their system.

Every day, 28 people in the United States die in motor vehicle crashes that involve an alcohol-impaired driver.

This is one death every 51 minutes. The annual cost of alcohol-related crashes totals more than $44 billion.

Consuming alcohol prior to driving greatly increases the risk of car accidents, highway injuries, and vehicular deaths. The greater the amount of alcohol consumed, the more likely a person is to be involved in an accident.

When alcohol is consumed, many of the skills that safe driving requires — such as judgment, concentration, comprehension, coordination, visual acuity, and reaction time — become impaired.

How can you avoid driving while intoxicated? It's simple. Your options are to:

- Stay put — Leave your location when you are sober.

- Have a designated driver — One friend should assume the responsibility of getting everyone home safely.

- Call a taxi

- Walk if the environment is safe and/or you are with a group of people

Alcohol and Sexual Activity

We discussed the increased risks for women, but any gender can be impacted by the combination of sex and alcohol. We frequently hear about sexual assault, particularly on college campuses and there are many factors to consider for everyone involved. When sex and alcohol are combined there is an increased risk that you could:

- Make unwanted or unintended sexual advances toward someone

- Participate in unwanted or unintended sex

- Experience sexual assault

- Be accused of sexual assault, even if you thought it was consensual

- Have unprotected sex, leading to pregnancy, and/or an STI

- Have sex with multiple partners

There are certain things you aren't legally allowed to do while you are drinking, such as get a tattoo, drive, or get married. There is a good reason for this — you're impaired and unable to make a rational decision on an important issue. Add sex to the list. If someone is drinking, they are not capable of making the decision about whether or not to engage in sexual activity, safely if at all — end of discussion. If they agree to it while intoxicated, they aren't really agreeing and if you are also intoxicated your ability to interpret their intentions is also compromised.

While women are at greater risk in these situations, the dangers and adverse outcomes are not limited to one gender. Any person of any gender or sexual preference is vulnerable when sex and alcohol are mixed.

Alcohol Abuse and Alcoholism

Problem drinking that becomes severe is given the medical diagnosis of **alcohol use disorder**, or AUD. AUD is a chronic relapsing brain disease characterized by compulsive alcohol use, loss of control over alcohol intake, and a negative emotional state when not using.

An estimated 16 million people in the United States have AUD. In 2015 alone, approximately 6.2%, or 15.1 million adults in the United States ages 18 and older had AUD. This includes 9.8 million men and 5.3 million women. Adolescents can be diagnosed with AUD as well, and in 2015, an estimated 623,000 adolescents ages 12–17 had AUD.

Anyone meeting any two of the eleven criteria (listed below) during the same 12-month period receives a diagnosis of AUD. The severity of AUD — mild, moderate, or severe — is based on the number of criteria met. To assess whether you or loved one may have AUD, here are some questions to ask. In the past year, have you:

- Had times when you ended up drinking more, or longer than you intended?

- More than once wanted to cut down or stop drinking, or tried to, but couldn't?

- Spent a lot of time drinking? Or being sick or getting over the aftereffects?

- Experienced craving — a strong need, or urge, to drink?

- Found that drinking — or being sick from drinking — often interfered with taking care of your home or family? Or caused job troubles? Or school problems?

- Continued to drink even though it was causing trouble with your family or friends?

- Given up or cut back on activities that were important or interesting to you, or gave you pleasure, in order to drink?

- More than once gotten into situations while or after drinking that increased your chances of getting hurt (such as driving, swimming, using machinery, walking in a dangerous area, or having unsafe sex)?

- Continued to drink even though it was making you feel depressed or anxious or adding to another health problem? Or after having had a memory blackout?

- Had to drink much more than you once did to get the effect you want? Or found that your usual number of drinks had much less effect than before?

- Found that when the effects of alcohol were wearing off, you had withdrawal symptoms, such as trouble sleeping, shakiness, irritability, anxiety, depression, restlessness, nausea, or sweating? Or sensed things that were not there?

If you have any of these symptoms, your drinking may already be a cause for concern. The more symptoms you have, the more urgent the need for change. A health professional can conduct a formal assessment of your symptoms to see if AUD is present.

However severe the problem may seem, most people with AUD can benefit from treatment. Unfortunately, less than ten percent of them receive any treatment. Ultimately, receiving treatment can improve an individual's chances of success in overcoming AUD.

Treatment for Alcohol Abuse

Many people struggle with controlling their drinking at some time in their lives. Approximately 17 million adults ages 18 and older have an alcohol use disorder (AUD) and 1 in 10 children live in a home with a parent who has a drinking problem.

The good news is that no matter how severe the problem may seem, most people with an alcohol use disorder can benefit from some form of treatment. Research suggests that about one-third of people who are treated for alcohol problems have no further symptoms 1 year later. Many others substantially reduce their drinking and report fewer alcohol-related problems.

When asked how alcohol problems are treated, people commonly think of 12-step programs or 28-day inpatient rehab, but may have difficulty naming other options. In fact, there are a variety of treatment methods currently available, thanks to significant advances in the field over the past 60 years.

Ultimately, there is no one-size-fits-all solution, and what may work for one person may not be a good fit for someone else. Simply understanding the different options can be an important first step.

Behavioral treatments are aimed at changing drinking behavior through counseling. They are led by health professionals and supported by studies showing they can be beneficial.

Three medications are currently approved in the US to help people stop or reduce their drinking and prevent relapse. They are prescribed by a health care provider and may be used alone or in combination with counseling.

Mutual-support groups like Alcoholics Anonymous (AA) and other 12-step programs provide peer support for people quitting or cutting back on their drinking. Combined with treatment led by health professionals, mutual-support groups can offer a valuable added layer of support. Due to the anonymous nature of mutual-support groups, it is difficult for researchers to determine their success rates compared with those led by health professionals.

Overcoming an alcohol use disorder is an ongoing process, one that can include setbacks. Because an alcohol use disorder can be a chronic relapsing disease, persistence is key. It is rare that someone would go to treatment once and then never drink again. More often, people must repeatedly try to quit or cut back, experience recurrences, learn from them, and then keep trying. For many, continued follow-up with a treatment provider is critical to overcoming problem drinking, as are mental health services for those suffering from coexisting mental illness.

Relapse is common among people who overcome alcohol problems. People with drinking problems are most likely to relapse during periods of stress or when exposed to people or places associated with past drinking. Just as some people with diabetes or asthma may have flare-ups of their disease, a relapse to drinking can be seen as a temporary set-back to full recovery and not a complete failure.

Seeking professional help can prevent relapse — behavioral therapies can help people develop skills to avoid and overcome triggers, such as stress, that might lead to drinking. Most people benefit from regular checkups with a treatment provider. Medications also can deter drinking during times when individuals may be at greater risk of relapse (e.g., divorce, death of a family member).

Alcohol Treatment Resources

- Al-Anon & Al-Ateen: Phone: (503) 370-7363

- Bridgeway Recovery Services: 3325 Harold Dr NE, Salem, OR 97305 Phone: (503) 363-2021

- Willamette Valley Intergroup: 687 Cottage St NE, Salem, OR 97301 Phone: (800) 615-3851

- Chemeketa Community College Advising and Counseling: Phone: 503.399.5120

- Center for Substance Abuse Treatment: samhsa.gov/about-us/who-we-are/offices-centers/csat 1-800-662-HELP (4357)

- Narconon: narconon.org/drug-rehab/alcoholic-family.html Phone: 1-888-391-7310

Tobacco and Nicotine

Tobacco use is the leading cause of preventable disease and death in the United States, accounting for more than 480,000 deaths every year, or one of every five deaths. In 2015, about 15 of every 100 US adults aged 18 years or older (15.1%) currently smoked cigarettes. This means an estimated 36.5 million adults in the United States currently smoke cigarettes (Figure 15). It's not hard to imagine then why more than 16 million Americans live with a smoking-related disease. Smoking causes many different cancers as well as chronic lung diseases, such as emphysema and bronchitis, heart disease, pregnancy-related problems, and many other serious health problems.

Tobacco is a leafy plant grown around the world. Four countries — China, Brazil, India, and the United States — produce approximately two-thirds of the world's tobacco. Tobacco is currently grown in 16 US states. The largest tobacco-producing states are Kentucky and North Carolina. They account for 71% of all tobacco grown in the United States.

Dried tobacco leaves can be:

- Shredded and smoked in cigarettes, cigars, and pipes

- Ground into snuff, which is sniffed through the nose

- Cured and made into chewing tobacco

- Moistened, ground or shredded into dip, which is placed in the mouth between the lip and gum

Tobacco is an addictive substance because it contains the chemical **nicotine**. Like heroin or cocaine, nicotine is a highly addictive substance that changes the way your brain works and causes you to crave more and more of it to achieve the same effect. This addiction to nicotine is what makes it so difficult to quit smoking and other tobacco.

Each day, more than 3,200 people under 18 smoke their first cigarette, and approximately 2,100 youth and young adults become daily smokers. Nine out of ten smokers start before the age of 18, and 98% start smoking by age 26. One in five adults and teenagers smoke. Men (16.7%) smoke more than women (13.6%). From 1964 to 2014, the proportion of adult smokers declined from 42.0% to 18.0%. People with no high school diploma are among the highest population of smokers, while people with graduate degrees are among the lowest. The prevalence of smoking declines as the level of education increases. Adults aged 25–44 smoke the most, followed closely by adults aged 45–64. American Indians and Alaskan Natives are more likely to smoke (21.9%) compared to whites and blacks (approximately 16%), Hispanics (10%), and Asians (7%). People in the Midwest are most likely to smoke (18.7%), followed by the South (15.3%), Northeast (13.5%), and West (12.7%). People living below the federal poverty level are among the highest population of smokers.

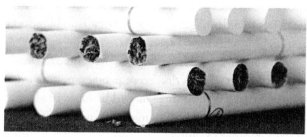

Figure 15. Cigarettes are a common source of nicotine.

Tobacco smoke contains a deadly mix of more than 7,000 chemicals. Hundreds are toxic. About 70 are known carcinogens, including some that you've likely heard related to forms of pollution. When you smoke, you inhale some of the same pollutants that come from the exhaust of your car!

There are approximately 93 harmful and potentially harmful chemicals in cigarettes. These include nicotine, cadmium, lead, ammonia, carbon monoxide, arsenic, chromium, hydrogen cyanide, mercury, and formaldehyde. And these are just the chemicals that may sound familiar to you. Formaldehyde is commonly used by morticians as a preservative in the process of preparing bodies for burial — not something we should be looking to put in our bodies while we are still living.

Some tobacco products also contain additives used to enhance flavor. Menthol is a flavor additive widely used in consumer and medicinal products. However, its use in tobacco products is not currently regulated. It has a minty taste and aroma, and may have cooling or painkilling properties — which can reduce the irritation and harshness of smoking when used in cigarettes and may allow a person to breathe in more deeply. Studies suggest that it also reinforces smoking behaviors by making the side effects less bothersome and the process more rewarding.

The cocktail of both naturally occurring and added chemicals make for a perfect storm of potential carcinogens. **Carbon Monoxide** (CO), for example, is a pollutant we've long associated with driving. In fact, our nation has worked hard to cut down on this form of pollution in our environment. Did you know that cigarettes contain CO? Breathing CO can cause headaches, dizziness, vomiting, and nausea. If CO levels are high enough, you may become unconscious or die. Exposure to moderate and high levels of CO over long periods of time has also been linked with increased risk of heart disease. People who survive severe CO poisoning may suffer long-term health problems. CO interferes with the body's ability to absorb oxygen, which strains the heart and can cause suffocation. Someone who smokes a pack a day can have a 3% to 6% carboxyhemoglobin (COHb) level in the blood. If they smoke two packs a day, the number is 6% to 10%. At three packs a day, it climbs as high as 20% COHb blood level.

Many of the chemicals are dangerous and problematic, but the big culprit that keeps people coming back for more, doing serious damage to their bodies, is nicotine.

Nicotine

About 5% (by weight) of the tobacco plant is **nicotine**, a naturally occurring liquid alkaloid. An alkaloid is an organic compound made out of carbon, hydrogen, nitrogen, and sometimes oxygen, and it can have potent effects on the human body.

When you use tobacco products, nicotine is quickly absorbed into your bloodstream. Within ten seconds of entering your body, the nicotine reaches your brain. It causes the brain to release adrenaline, creating a buzz of pleasure and energy.

The buzz fades quickly though, and leaves you feeling tired, a little down, and wanting the buzz again. This feeling is what makes you light up the next cigarette. Since your body is able to build up a high tolerance to nicotine, you'll need to smoke more and more cigarettes in order to get the nicotine's pleasurable effects and prevent withdrawal symptoms.

This up and down cycle repeats over and over, leading to addiction. Addiction keeps people smoking even when they want to quit. Breaking addiction is harder for some people than others. Many people need more than one try in order to quit.

Cigarette makers know that nicotine addiction helps sell their products. Cigarettes today deliver more nicotine more quickly than ever before. Tobacco companies also use additives and chemicals to make them more addictive.

Nicotine addiction happens quickly making it harder and harder to quit. It is also easy to relapse, especially if your social group contains a lot of others who smoke. Relapse is common, especially when a person is experiencing a lot of stress. People also tend to have certain triggers that often cause them to crave the tobacco. These can be emotional, physical, social, or pattern triggers.

When you stop smoking or cutback your tobacco use, your body begins to withdrawal. You may experience anxiety, irritability, headache, hunger, and cravings for cigarettes and other sources of nicotine. This does make it hard to quit. However, nicotine withdrawal is short-lived and symptoms pass in time, usually less than a week. Withdrawal is the most uncomfortable part of quitting, but the real challenge is beating long-term cravings and staying away from tobacco.

Other Nicotine Delivery Systems

Pipes and **cigars** are very similar to cigarettes, except that people usually don't inhale. This means all the harmful chemicals in cigarettes are only lingering in the mouth. Avid pipe and cigar smokers can expect to have damage in discoloration to their teeth, bad breath, and are at a high risk for developing oral cancer. They also still take in second-hand smoke.

Chewing tobacco — otherwise known as dip, chew, and snuff — contains more nicotine than cigarettes. These give you a more concentrated delivery system, one you can partake in nearly everywhere — no designated smoking area. You may not be as invasive to others in public as someone who smokes, but these products still pack an unhealthy punch.

- Holding an average-sized dip in your mouth for 30 minutes can give you as much nicotine as smoking three cigarettes.

- Using two cans of snuff a week gives you as much nicotine as someone who smokes one and a half packs of cigarettes a day.

Oral, esophageal, and pancreatic cancer are common among people who chew. Other regular problems include uncontrolled drooling and stained clothing, not to mentioned discolored teeth, bad breath, and dental issues. And to make matters worse, almost no one will want to kiss you!

Cloves, or kretek, smoking is associated with an increased risk for acute lung injury (i.e., lung damage that can include a range of characteristics, such as decreased oxygen, fluid in the lungs, leakage from capillaries, and inflammation), especially among susceptible individuals with asthma or respiratory infections. Regular kretek smokers have 13 to 20 times the risk for abnormal lung function (e.g., airflow obstruction or reduced oxygen absorption) compared with nonsmokers.

Electronic cigarettes (e-cigarettes), or vaporizers (Figure 16), are battery-operated products designed to turn nicotine and other chemicals into a vapor that you inhale. These products are often made to look like cigarettes, cigars, pipes, or pens. Many people use e-cigarettes

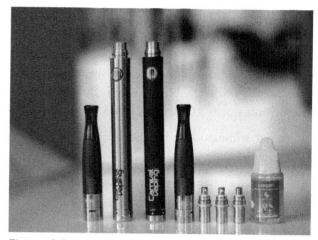

Figure 16. E-cigarettes or vaporizers are a relatively new and popular nicotine delivery system.

because they assume they are healthier than traditional ones. Others use them as a way of tapering their cigarette usage because they allow the person to still inhale nicotine. Currently, there are no e-cigarettes approved by FDA for therapeutic uses so they cannot be recommended as a cessation aid.

E-Cigarettes may contain ingredients that are known to be toxic to humans. Because clinical studies about the safety of e-cigarettes have not been submitted to the US Food and Drug Administration (FDA), you have no way of knowing if they are safe, which chemicals they contain, or how much nicotine you are inhaling.

Additionally, these products may be attractive to kids. They are attracted to anything that looks like an electronic device and with the different styles and shiny exterior, these devices have an added "cool" factor that traditional cigarettes don't. Since many adults use them as a transitional tool when they are trying to quit smoking, young people may be under the impression that they aren't harmful. However, they still contain nicotine and we don't yet know the side effects of the vaping process. Using e-cigarettes may also lead kids to try other tobacco products — including conventional cigarettes.

We may not know a lot about their long-term use, but we do know that e-cigarettes don't put carbon monoxide into the air because there is no flame ignition to produce smoke.

Effects of Tobacco on the Body

Smoking harms nearly every organ of the body. Some of these harmful effects are immediate and can become chronic (see below). One of the obvious short-term effects of smoking is the smell — whoever just smoked a cigarette is usually the worst-smelling person in the room. It permeates your clothing, hair, breath, fingernails, home, car, and anything it comes into contact with. Once the immediate smell dissipates, the stale smell sets in and really becomes foul. But odor is the least of your worries. Other short-term effects include:

- Initial stimulation, then reduction in activity of brain and nervous system

- Increased alertness and concentration

- Feelings of mild euphoria

- Feelings of relaxation

- Increased blood pressure and heart rate

- Decreased blood flow to fingers and toes

- Decreased skin temperature

- Decreased appetite

- Dizziness

- Nausea, abdominal cramps and vomiting

- Headache

- Coughing due to smoke irritation

The sheer quantity of potential long-term effects of smoking should be enough to make people never light their first cigarette, and cause people who already smoke to quit. Nearly every vital organ and system in your body is impacted from cigarette smoke (Figure 17) and other forms of tobacco, including:

Ears — Smoking reduces the oxygen supply to the cochlea, a snail-shaped organ in the inner ear. This may result in permanent damage to the cochlea and mild to moderate hearing loss.

Eyes — Smoking causes physical changes in the eyes that can threaten your eyesight. Nicotine from cigarettes restricts the production of a chemical necessary for you to be able to see at night. Smoking also increases your risk of developing cataracts and macular degeneration (both can lead to blindness).

Mouth — Smoking takes a toll on your mouth. Smokers have more oral health problems than non-smokers, like mouth sores, ulcers, and gum disease. You are more likely to have cavities and lose your teeth at a younger age. You are also more likely to get cancers of the mouth and throat.

Face — Smoking can cause your skin to be dry and lose elasticity, leading to wrinkles and stretch marks. Your skin tone may become dull and grayish.

Heart — Carbon monoxide from inhaled cigarette smoke contributes to a lack of oxygen, making the heart work harder. It also makes your blood thick and sticky, and increases your cholesterol levels, further straining the heart and increasing your risk of blood clots, heart disease, and heart attacks.

Lungs — Smoking causes inflammation in the small airways and tissues of your lungs. Continued inflammation builds up scar tissue, which leads to physical changes to your lungs and airways that can make breathing hard. It can also lead to serious and potentially fatal lung diseases, such as emphysema, frequent respiratory infections, and of course lung cancer.

Belly — People who smoke have bigger bellies and less muscle than non-smokers. They are more likely to develop type 2 diabetes, even if they don't smoke every day. Smoking also makes it harder to control diabetes once you already have it.

Female hormones — Smoking lowers a female's level of estrogen, making it harder for them to become pregnant or have a healthy baby. Smoking can also lead to early menopause, which increases your risk of developing certain diseases (like heart disease).

Male sexual performance — Smoking increases the risk of erectile dysfunction in men — the inability to get or keep and erection. Toxins from cigarette smoke can also damage the genetic material in sperm, which can cause infertility or genetic defects.

Healing Systems — When you smoke, the number of white blood cells (the cells that defend your body from infections) stays high. A high white blood cell count is like a signal from your body, letting you know you've been injured. White blood cell counts that stay elevated for a long time are linked with an increased risk of heart attacks, strokes, and cancer.

Cigarette smoke contains high levels of tar and other chemicals, which can make your immune system less effective at fighting off infections. This means you're more likely to get sick. Continued weakening of the immune system can make you more vulnerable to autoimmune diseases like rheumatoid arthritis and multiple sclerosis. It also decreases your body's ability to fight off cancer!

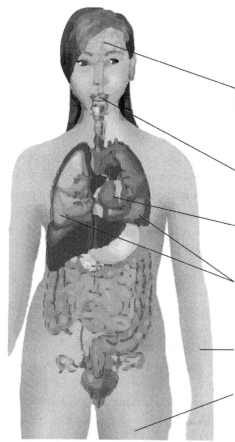

How tobacco affects your body

Brain

Nicotine, the drug that makes tobacco addictive, goes to your brain. It makes you feel good when you are smoking, but it can make you anxious, nervous, moody, and depressed after you smoke. Using tobacco also can cause headaches and dizziness.

Mouth

Tobacco stains your teeth and gives you bad breath. Tobacco ruins some of your taste buds, so you won't be able to taste your foods as well.

Heart

Smoking incrases your heart rate and blood pressure. If you try to do activities like exercise or play sports, your heart rate has to work harder to keep up.

Lungs

Smokers have trouble breathing because smoking damages the lungs. If you have asthma, you can have more frequent and more serious attacks. Smoking causes a lot of coughing with phlegm (mucus) and lung cancer.

Skin

Smoking causes dry, yellow skin and wrinkles. the smell sticks to your skin too.

Muscles

Less blood and oxygen flow to your muscles, which causes them to hurt more when you exercise or play sports.

Figure 17. Tobacco has short- and long-term effects on the body.

People who smoke also have difficulty healing. Nutrients, minerals, and oxygen are all supplied to the tissue through the blood stream. Nicotine causes blood vessels to tighten, which decreases levels of nutrients supplied to wounds. As a result, wounds take longer to heal. Slow wound healing increases the risk of infection after an injury or surgery and painful skin ulcers can develop, causing the tissue to slowly die.

Muscles and Bones — When you smoke, less blood and oxygen flow to your muscles, making it harder to build muscle. The lack of oxygen also makes muscles tire more easily, giving you more muscle aches and pains than non-smokers.

Ingredients in cigarette smoke also disrupt the natural cycle of bone health. Your body is less able to form healthy new bone tissue, and it breaks down existing bone tissue more rapidly. Over time, smoking leads to a thinning of bone tissue and loss of bone density, increasing your risk of bone fractures.

Unique Effects for Women

Risks from tobacco use that are unique to women include a higher risk of breast cancer, lung cancer, osteoporosis, thyroid-related diseases, and menstrual problems. They also can experience problems with:

Decreased bone density — Women who have gone through menopause and who smoke have lower bone density. This means they have a higher chance of breaking a hip than women who do not smoke.

Rheumatoid arthritis — Women who smoke are more likely to get rheumatoid arthritis (RA), an inflammatory, chronic disease causing swelling and pain in their joints.

Cataracts — Women who smoke are more likely to get cataracts that affect their vision. Cataracts are an eye disease where the lens of the eye is cloudy or foggy.

Depression — It is important for women to know about the link between smoking and depression because women are more likely than men to be diagnosed with depression.

Menopause — Women who smoke are more likely than non-smokers to go through menopause at a younger age, and they may have worse symptoms of menopause.

Smoking while Pregnant

Women who smoke may have a harder time getting pregnant. Smoking during pregnancy causes premature birth, low birth weight, certain birth defects, and ectopic pregnancy in which the fertilized egg implants somewhere in the abdomen other than the womb. Smoking during pregnancy also causes complications with the placenta, the organ through which nutrients pass from mother to fetus. These complications include placenta previa and placental abruption, conditions that jeopardize the life and health of both mother and child.

After birth, studies show there is an increased risk of SIDS (sudden infant death syndrome, also called "crib death") in babies born to women smokers, along with an increased risk of asthma, colic, and obesity for the child. Even emotional and behavioral problems in children can occur when the mother smokes while pregnant. These risks can be reduced if the woman quits within the first four months of pregnancy.

Women who are pregnant or who are planning a pregnancy should not smoke. It's important to encourage women to quit smoking before or early in pregnancy, when the most health benefits can be achieved, but cessation in all stages, even in late pregnancy, benefits maternal and fetal health.

Secondhand Smoke

So, why does it matter if you quit smoking? You're only hurting yourself, right? Among the more than 7,000 chemicals that have been identified in **secondhand** tobacco smoke, at least 250 are known to be harmful or cancerous, for example, hydrogen cyanide, carbon monoxide, ammonia, arsenic, benzene, butadiene (a hazardous gas), beryllium (a toxic metal), cadmium, chromium, ethylene oxide, nickel, polonium-210, vinyl chloride, formaldehyde, Benzo[a]pyrene, and toluene.

Secondhand smoke (also called **environmental tobacco smoke**, involuntary smoke, and passive smoke) is the combination of **sidestream** smoke (the smoke given off by a burning tobacco product) and **mainstream** smoke (the smoke exhaled by a smoker). In the US, the source of most secondhand smoke is from cigarettes, followed by pipes, cigars, and other tobacco products.

The amount of smoke created by a tobacco product depends on the amount of tobacco available for burning.

The amount of secondhand smoke emitted by smoking one large cigar is similar to that emitted by smoking an entire pack of cigarettes.

Inhaling secondhand smoke causes lung cancer in nonsmoking adults. Approximately 3,000 lung cancer deaths occur each year among adult nonsmokers in the United States as a result of exposure to secondhand smoke. The US Surgeon General estimates that living with someone who smokes increases a nonsmoker's chances of developing lung cancer by 20–30%.

There is no safe level of exposure to secondhand smoke. Even low levels of secondhand smoke can be harmful. The only way to fully protect nonsmokers from secondhand smoke is to completely eliminate smoking in indoor spaces. Separating smoking from nonsmoking areas, cleaning the air, and ventilating buildings cannot completely eliminate exposure to secondhand smoke.

Environmental Smoke's Effects on Children

Secondhand smoke causes numerous health problems in infants and children, including more frequent and severe asthma attacks, respiratory infections, ear infections, bronchitis, pneumonia, and sudden infant death syndrome (SIDS). It's so risky that smoking with children in the car (where they cannot even hope to distance themselves from the source) is illegal in some states (Figure 18). The impact can be significant, even fatal.

Parents can help protect their children from secondhand smoke by taking some simple precautions, such as not allowing anyone to smoke in or near your home, and definitely not in your car, even with the window down.

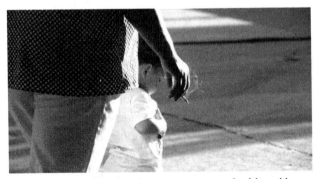

Figure 18. Secondhand smoke causes numerous health problems in infants and children.

Make sure your child's day care center and school are tobacco-free campuses. And choose restaurants and other venues of entertainment that do not allow smoking. "No smoking" sections do not protect you and your family from secondhand smoke. Sometimes you are still only a table away — the barrier is really an imaginary line.

Reducing Environmental Smoke

Secondhand smoke can travel into buildings and drift hundreds of feet from a smoker, while still threatening the health of anyone who inhales it. In Oregon, we don't have many areas where smoking is allowed, but we do face challenges periodically. In outdoor event venues, there are frequently no restrictions. Drive right across the border into Washington and you may find yourself sitting through an uncomfortable outdoor concert. Here are a few things you can do to avoid smoke:

- Vote for legislation that bans public smoking

- Avoid businesses and venues that allow smoking. Let those businesses know that you are choosing not to frequent them as a consumer and why.

- Educate your children and set a good example. Don't rely on the school system to do this for you — they will learn first from you!

- Encourage your friends and family members to quit and be supportive. If you have children and do not want them around the smoke, be honest with your loved ones about why.

The news isn't all bad. Among all current US adult cigarette smokers in 2015, nearly seven out of every ten (68.0%) reported that they wanted to quit completely. In fact, since 2002 the number of former smokers has been greater than the number of current smokers. According to a 2015 study, 55.4% of adult cigarette smokers reported stopping cigarettes for more than one day in an attempt to quit smoking.

The Benefits of Quitting Smoking

Unlike the slow process of trying to reduce your body fat percentage, the minute you quit smoking, you begin to reap the benefits! After you quit, your body begins to heal within 20 minutes of your last cigarette. The nicotine leaves your body within three days. As your body starts to repair itself, you may feel worse instead of better, temporarily. Withdrawal can be difficult, but it's a sign that your body is healing.

There are plenty of long-term rewards, too. Quitting smoking can add years to your life. Smokers who quit before age 40 reduce their chance of dying early from smoking-related diseases by about 90%. Those who quit by age 45–54 reduce their chance of dying early by about 60%. You can take control of your health by quitting and staying smoke free. Over time, you'll greatly lower your risk of death from lung cancer and other diseases such as heart disease, stroke, chronic bronchitis, emphysema, and at least 13 other kinds of cancer.

When you quit, you'll also protect your loved ones from dangerous secondhand smoke. You'll set a good example and show your family that a life without cigarettes is possible. See Chapter 1, Figure 30.

Ways to Quit Smoking

According to the CDC, most former smokers quit without using one of the treatments that scientific research has shown can work. However, the following treatments are proven to be effective for smokers who want help to quit.

Nicotine Replacement Therapy (NRT)

Nicotine replacement therapy (NRT) is the most commonly used type of medication to help you quit smoking. NRT reduces withdrawal feelings by giving you a small controlled amount of nicotine-but none of the other dangerous chemicals found in cigarettes. This small amount of nicotine helps satisfy your craving for nicotine and reduces the urge to smoke.

Doctors and other medical experts think NRT is the one of the most helpful tools smokers can use to quit. Some smokers have mild to moderate side effects. However, research shows that NRT is safe and effective. NRT can be an important part of almost every smoker's strategy to quit. NRT products are sold over-the-counter (nicotine patch, gum, or lozenge) or by prescription (nicotine patch, inhaler, or nasal spray).

NRT Type	How to Get Them	How to Use Them
Patch	Over the counter	Place on the skin. Gives a small and steady amount of nicotine
Gum	Over the counter	Chew to release nicotine. Chew until you get a tingling feeling, then place between cheek and gums
Lozenge	Over the counter	Place in the mouth like hard candy. Releases nicotine as it slowly dissolves in the mouth
Inhaler	Prescription	Cartridge attached to a mouthpiece. Inhaling through the mouthpiece gives a specific amount of nicotine
Nasal Spray	Prescription	Pump bottle containing nicotine. Put into nose and spray

Figure 19. Nicotine replacement therapy types and availability.

NRT and other medications like bupropion SR (Zyban®) and varenicline tartrate (Chantix®) can't do all the work. It can help with withdrawal and cravings. But it won't completely take away the urge to smoke. Even if you use NRT to help you stop smoking, quitting can still be hard. Combining NRT with other strategies can improve your chances of quitting and staying quit. To give yourself the best chance for success, explore other quit methods you can combine with medication.

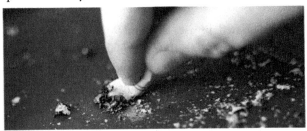

Figure 20. Cigarette smoke impacts more than just the smoker's health.

Community-Based Options

Community support is a major factor for whether or not a person will quit. Quitting is less likely, for example, if you are in an intimate relationship with someone who doesn't also want to quit. Other smokers, even good friends, are not reliable tools to help you quit. Anyone who has ever smoked knows how easy it is to get another smoker to give them a cigarette.

Smoking Prevention Policy

Tobacco control programs aim to reduce disease, disability, and death related to tobacco use. A comprehensive approach — one that includes educational, clinical, regulatory, economic, and social strategies — has been established as the best way to eliminate the negative health and economic effects of tobacco use.

Counseling and medication are both effective for treating tobacco dependence, and using them together is more effective than using either one alone. The American Lung Association also offers the following tips that can help you along the way:

It's never too late to quit — Earlier in life is better but quitting at any age will improve your quality of life.

Learn from past mistakes — If you've tried to quit before, consider what worked well and what didn't and adapt your approach.

You don't have to quit alone — Enlist support from friends and family or join a support group.

Use medication — Be sure to follow the directions. They don't work well if you aren't using them properly or long enough.

Every person can quit — It's just a matter of finding the right combination of approaches that work for you.

However, having a strong social support system can double your chances of quitting. Seeking counseling and support groups is a good start. You can also join groups, bringing you in contact with people who are less likely to smoke.

Federal laws, like the Family Smoking Prevention and Tobacco Control Act (Tobacco Control Act) are usually enforced through executive branch agencies, such as the Food and Drug Administration (FDA).

Laws can also be enacted at the state and local level to protect public health and make tobacco products less affordable, less accessible, and less attractive. For example, states may pass smoke-free indoor air laws and cigarette price increases, which have been proven to reduce cigarette use, prevent youth from starting to smoke, and encourage people to try to quit. The purpose of laws to eliminate smoking includes economic reasons, too.

Oregon's Anti-Smoking Policies

In August 2017, Oregon became the fifth state to raise the tobacco age to 21, along with California, Hawaii, Maine and New Jersey. The new law includes an increase on fines for vendors who sell nicotine products to people under 21 (Figure 21).

The Oregon Indoor Clean Air Act (ICAA), also known as the Smokefree Workplace Law, prohibits smoking in the workplace and within ten feet of all entrances, exits, accessibility ramps that lead to and from an entrance or exit, windows and air-intake vents.

Under Oregon's Smokefree Workplace Law, smoking is prohibited in public places and workplaces (Figure 22), with few exceptions. Public place means any enclosed area open to the public. Place of employment means an enclosed area that is under the control of a public or private employer and that employees frequent during the course of employment. Oregonians may not use e-cigarettes and other inhalant delivery systems in workplaces, restaurants bars and other indoor public places.

The Family Smoking Prevention and Tobacco Control Act (FSPTCA), also known as the Tobacco Control Act, gives the Food and Drug Administration (FDA) the authority to regulate the manufacture, distribution, and marketing of tobacco products to protect public health. The Tobacco Control Act gave the FDA immediate authority to regulate cigarettes, cigarette tobacco, roll-your-own tobacco, and smokeless tobacco.

For other kinds of tobacco products, the statute authorizes the FDA to issue regulations "deeming" them to be subject to such authorities. Consistent with the statute, once a tobacco product is deemed, the FDA may put in place "restrictions on the sale and distribution of a tobacco product," including age-related access restrictions as well as advertising and promotion restrictions,

The total economic cost of smoking is more than $300 billion a year, including nearly $170 billion in direct medical care for adults, and more than $156 billion in lost productivity due to premature death and exposure to secondhand smoke

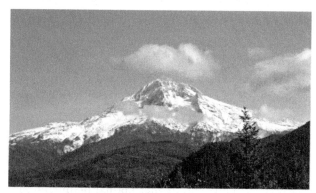

Figure 21. Clean air in Oregon.

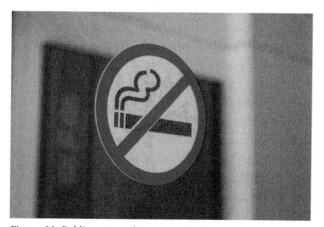

Figure 22. Public anti-smoking campaign.

if the FDA determines the restrictions are appropriate for the protection of the public health.

This act is important because it has effectively taken control away from tobacco companies, who have shown a universal willingness to mislead the public on the universally negative effects of tobacco use, and is proven to be a major factor in the reduction of smoking and tobacco use throughout the US.

Marijuana

Marijuana is a green, brown, or gray mixture of dried, shredded leaves, stems, seeds, and flowers of the hemp, or *Cannabis sativa*, plant. It goes by many different names — pot, herb, weed, grass — and stronger forms include sinsemilla (sin-seh-me-yah), hashish (*hash* for short), and hash oil. It can be rolled up and smoked like a cigarette or cigar or smoked in a pipe. Sometimes people mix it in food (edibles) or inhale it using a vaporizer.

All forms of marijuana are psychoactive, changing how the brain works. Marijuana contains more than 400 chemicals, including **THC** (delta-9-tetrahydrocannabinol). Since THC is the main active chemical in marijuana, the amount of THC in marijuana determines its potency, or strength, and therefore its effects. The THC content of marijuana has been increasing over the past few decades.

Cannabinoids

The active ingredient of marijuana, and the thing people seek from it are cannabinoids. There are two, specifically, that produce significant physio/psychological effects — THC and CBD.

Delta-9 tetrahydrocannabinol (THC)

THC's chemical structure is similar to the brain chemical anandamide. Similarity in structure allows the body to recognize THC and to alter normal brain communication.

Endogenous cannabinoids, such as anandamide, function as neurotransmitters because they send chemical messages between nerve cells (neurons) throughout the nervous system. They affect brain areas that influence pleasure, memory, thinking, concentration, movement, coordination, and sensory and time perception. Because of this similarity, THC is able to attach to molecules called cannabinoid receptors on neurons in these brain areas and activate them, disrupting various mental and physical functions and causing the effects described earlier. The neural communication network that uses these cannabinoid neurotransmitters, known as the endocannabinoid system, plays a critical role in the nervous system's normal functioning, so interfering with it can have profound effects.

For example, THC is able to alter the functioning of the hippocampus and orbitofrontal cortex, brain areas that enable a person to form new memories and shift his or her attentional focus. As a result, using marijuana causes impaired thinking and interferes with a person's ability to learn and perform complicated tasks. THC also disrupts functioning of the cerebellum and basal ganglia, brain areas that regulate balance, posture, coordination, and reaction time. This is the reason people who have used marijuana may not be able to drive safely and may have problems playing sports or engaging in other physical activities.

People who have taken large doses of the drug may experience an acute psychosis, which includes hallucinations, delusions, and a loss of the sense of personal identity.

THC, acting through cannabinoid receptors, also activates the brain's reward system, which includes regions that govern the response to healthy pleasurable behaviors such as sex and eating. Like most other drugs that people misuse, THC stimulates neurons in the reward system to release the signaling chemical dopamine at levels higher than typically observed in response to natural stimuli. This flood of dopamine contributes to the pleasurable "high" that those use who recreational marijuana seek.

Organs in the body have fatty tissues that quickly absorb the THC in marijuana. In general, standard urine tests can detect traces of THC several days after use. In heavy marijuana users, however, urine tests can sometimes detect THC traces for weeks after use stops.

A Rise in Marijuana's THC Levels

The amount of THC in marijuana has been increasing steadily over the past few decades. For a person who is new to marijuana use, this may mean exposure to higher THC levels with a greater chance of a harmful reaction. Higher THC levels may explain the rise in emergency room visits involving marijuana use.

The popularity of edibles also increases the chance of harmful reactions. Edibles take longer to digest and produce a high. Therefore, people may consume more to feel the effects faster, leading to dangerous results. Higher THC levels may mean a greater risk for addiction if people are regularly exposing themselves to high doses.

Cannabidiols (CBD)

Rigorous clinical studies are still needed to evaluate the clinical potential of CBD for specific conditions. However, pre-clinical research (including both cell culture and animal models) has shown CBD to have a range of effects that may be therapeutically useful, including anti-seizure, antioxidant, neuroprotective, anti-inflammatory, analgesic, anti-tumor, anti-psychotic, and anti-anxiety properties.

Effects of Marijuana on the Body

Some people feel nothing at all when they smoke marijuana. Others may feel relaxed or "high." Some experience sudden feelings of anxiety and paranoid thoughts (even more likely with stronger varieties of marijuana). In the **short-term**, marijuana can cause:

- Problems with learning and memory

- Distorted perception (sights, sounds, time, touch)

- Poor coordination

- Increased heart rate

Regular use of marijuana has also been linked to depression, anxiety, and a loss of drive or motivation, which means a loss of interest even in previously enjoyable activities. Its effects can be unpredictable (Figure 23), especially when mixed with other drugs.

We know a lot about where marijuana acts in the brain and how it affects specific sites called cannabinoid receptors. These receptors are found in brain regions that influence learning and memory, appetite, coordination, and pleasure. That's why marijuana produces the effects it does. Research suggests that the effects on memory, learning, and intelligence can be long-term and even

Marijuana During Pregnancy

Women who are pregnant should not smoke or consume marijuana. Marijuana use during pregnancy is linked to lower birth weight and increased risk of both brain and behavioral problems in babies. If a pregnant woman uses marijuana, the drug may affect certain developing parts of the fetus's brain. Resulting chal-

Bodily effects of
Cannabis

Eyes:
- Reddening
- Decreased intra-ocular pressure

Mouth:
- Dryness

Skin:
- Sensation of heat or cold

Heart:
- Increased heart rate

Muscles:
- Relaxation

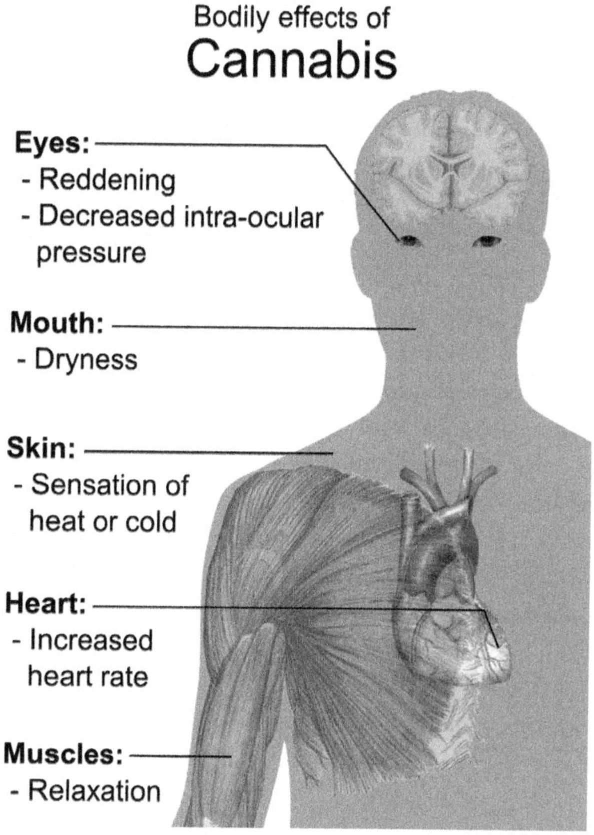

Figure 23. Cannabis use affects several parts of the body.

permanent in people who begin using marijuana regularly as teens. Lost mental abilities might not fully return even if a person quits using marijuana as an adult

Someone who smokes marijuana regularly may have many of the same breathing and lung problems that tobacco smokers do, such as a daily cough and a greater risk of lung infections like pneumonia. As with tobacco smoke, marijuana smoke has a toxic mixture of gases and tiny particles that can harm the lungs. Although we don't yet know if marijuana causes lung cancer, many people who smoke marijuana also smoke cigarettes, which do cause cancer — and smoking marijuana can make it harder to quit cigarette smoking.

lenges for the child may include problems with attention, memory, and problem-solving. Some research also suggests that moderate amounts of THC are excreted into the breast milk of nursing mothers. With regular use, THC can reach amounts in breast milk that could affect the baby's developing brain.

Marijuana in the US

In the United States, marijuana is the most commonly used illicit drug. In 2013, 7.5% of the US population over 12 years old (19.8 million people) reported using marijuana during the preceding month. In 2014, a total of 2.5 million persons over 12 years had used marijuana for the first time during the preceding 12 months, an average of approximately 7,000 new users each day. During 2002–2014, the prevalence of marijuana use during the past month, past year, and daily or almost daily increased among persons over 18 years, but not among those between 12–17 years old.

The increase in adult usage is likely due to the drug's legalization in some states. In other words, it's still illegal for people under 21, so their numbers have not increased, while it has for legal adults. Among persons over 12 years old, studies also showed that their perception that the drug carried risk decreased — again, possibly due to relaxing laws on the substance.

In 2016, 9.4% of 8th graders reported marijuana use in the past year and 5.4% in the past month (current use). Among 10th graders, 23.9% had used marijuana in the past year and 14% in the past month. Rates of use among 12th graders were higher still — 35.6% had used marijuana during the year prior to the survey and 22.5 percent used in the past month. 6% said they used marijuana daily or near-daily.

Medical emergencies possibly related to marijuana use have also increased. The Drug Abuse Warning Network (DAWN), a system for monitoring the health impact of drugs, estimated that in 2011, there were nearly 456,000 drug-related emergency department visits in the United States in which marijuana use was mentioned in the medical record (a 21% increase over 2009). About two-thirds of patients were male and 13% were between the ages of 12 and 17. It is unknown whether this increase is due to increased use, increased potency of marijuana (amount of THC it contains), or other factors. It should be noted, however, that mentions of marijuana in medical records do not necessarily indicate that these emergencies were directly related to marijuana intoxication.

Medical Marijuana and Therapeutic Theories

Marijuana has been a point of controversy for some time now. You could say that we have a love-hate relationship with it as a country. Many people fully support the idea that it has therapeutic value, while others focus on the negative effects and federal status as an illicit drug and theories that it can be a "gateway" to more harmful substances.

Despite this, some states have approved "medical marijuana" to ease symptoms of various health problems. The term medical marijuana refers to using the whole, unprocessed marijuana plant or its basic extracts to treat symptoms of illness and other conditions. The US Food and Drug Administration (FDA) has not approved the marijuana plant (Figure 24) as a medicine. However, there have been scientific studies of cannabinoids, the chemicals in marijuana. This has led to two FDA-approved medicines.

They contain THC, the active ingredient in marijuana. They treat nausea caused by chemotherapy and increase appetite in patients who have severe weight loss from HIV/AIDS. Scientists are doing more research with marijuana and its ingredients to treat many diseases and conditions.

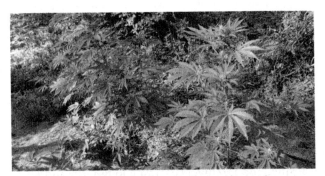

Figure 24. Marijuana grows in nature, but is still unsafe.

Anti-Seizure Theories

A number of studies over the last two decades or more have reported that CBD has anti-seizure activity. In addition, there have been a number of case studies and anecdotal reports suggesting that CBD may be effective in treating children with drug-resistant epilepsy. However, there have only been a few small, randomized clinical trials examining the efficacy of CBD as a treatment for epilepsy with significant flaws in both method and statistical analysis.

Neuroprotective and Anti-Inflammatory Theories

CBD has also been shown to have neuroprotective properties in cell cultures as well as in animal models of several neurodegenerative diseases, including Alzheimer's, stroke, glutamate toxicity, multiple sclerosis (MS), Parkinson's disease, and neurodegeneration caused by alcohol abuse.

Analgesic Theories

There have been multiple clinical trials demonstrating the efficacy of nabiximols on nerve pain, rheumatoid arthritis, and cancer pain. Research is inconclusive as to whether both THC and CBD have an impact or whether it is CBD alone.

Anti-Tumor Theories

In addition to the research on the use of cannabinoids in comfort treatments for cancer — reducing pain and nausea and in increasing appetite — there are also several pre-clinical reports showing anti-tumor effects of CBD in cell culture and in animal models. Reduced cell viability, increased cancer cell death, decreased tumor growth, and inhibition of metastasis may be due to the antioxidant and anti-inflammatory effects of CBD.

Anti-Psychotic Theories

Marijuana can produce acute psychotic episodes at high doses, and several studies have linked marijuana use to increased risk for chronic psychosis in individuals with specific genetic risk factors. Research suggests that these effects are prompted by THC, and it has been suggested that CBD may mitigate these effects.

Anti-Anxiety Theories

CBD has shown therapeutic efficacy in a range of animal models of anxiety and stress, reducing both behavioral and physiological (e.g., heart rate) measures of stress and anxiety. In addition, CBD has been shown to be effective in small human laboratory and clinical trials. CBD reduced anxiety in patients with social anxiety subjected to a stressful public speaking task. In a laboratory protocol designed to model post-traumatic stress disorders, CBD improved the ability to forget traumatic memories. Again, more research is needed.

Sometimes people will say marijuana is "harmless," pointing to the idea that it is "natural" and that the active ingredient comes from a plant. This is faulty reasoning — cocaine and heroin also come from plants. Marijuana can be harmful if misused, like any medicine. Also, the primary method of ingesting marijuana is through smoking, which isn't safe.

Marijuana Addiction

Marijuana use can lead to the development of problem use, known as a **marijuana use disorder**, which takes the form of addiction in severe cases. Recent data suggests that 30 percent of those who use marijuana may have some degree of marijuana use disorder. People who begin using marijuana before the age of 18 are four to seven times more likely to develop a marijuana use disorder than adults.

Marijuana use disorders are often associated with dependence — in which a person feels withdrawal symptoms when not taking the drug. People who use marijuana frequently often report irritability, mood and sleep difficulties, decreased appetite, cravings, restlessness, and/or various forms of physical discomfort that peak within the first week after quitting and last up to 2 weeks. Marijuana dependence occurs when the brain adapts to large amounts of the drug by reducing production of and sensitivity to its own endocannabinoid neurotransmitters.

Marijuana use disorder becomes addiction when the person cannot stop using the drug even though it interferes with many aspects of his or her life. In 2015, about 4.0 million people in the United States met the diagnostic criteria for a marijuana use disorder, and 138,000 people voluntarily sought treatment for their marijuana use.

Dangers of Smoking

Like tobacco smoke, marijuana smoke is an irritant to the throat and lungs and can cause a heavy cough during use. It also contains levels of volatile chemicals and tar that are similar to tobacco smoke, raising concerns about risk for cancer and lung disease.

Marijuana smoking is associated with large airway inflammation, increased airway resistance, and lung hyperinflation, and those who smoke marijuana regularly report more symptoms of chronic bronchitis than those who do not smoke. One study found that people who frequently smoke marijuana had more outpatient medical visits for respiratory problems than those who do not smoke. Smoking marijuana may also reduce the respiratory system's immune response, increasing the likelihood of the person acquiring respiratory infections, including pneumonia.

Whether smoking marijuana causes lung cancer, as cigarette smoking does, remains an open question.

Marijuana smoke contains carcinogenic combustion products. Because of how it is typically smoked (deeper inhale, held for longer), marijuana smoking leads to four times the deposition of tar compared to cigarette smoking. Studies are still inconclusive.

One complexity in comparing the lung-health risks of marijuana and tobacco concerns the very different ways the two substances are used. While people who smoke marijuana often inhale more deeply and hold the smoke in their lungs for a longer duration than is typical with cigarettes, marijuana's effects last longer, so people who use marijuana may smoke less frequently than those who smoke cigarettes. Additionally, the fact that many people use both marijuana and tobacco makes determining marijuana's precise contribution to lung cancer risk, if any, difficult to establish.

A Gateway Drug?

Long-term studies of drug use patterns indicate that most high school students who use other illegal drugs have tried marijuana first. However, many young people who use marijuana do not go on to use other drugs. To explain why some do, here are a few theories:

- Exposure to marijuana may affect the brain, particularly during development, which continues into users' early twenties. Effects may include changes to the brain that make other drugs more appealing. For example, animal research suggests that early exposure to marijuana makes opioid drugs (like Vicodin® or heroin) more pleasurable.

- Someone who is using marijuana is likely to be in contact with other users and sellers of other drugs, increasing the risk of being encouraged or tempted to try them.

- People at high risk of using drugs may use marijuana first because it is easy to get (like cigarettes and alcohol).

Legalization of Marijuana

Twenty-nine states (including Oregon) and the District of Columbia have legalized marijuana for medical and recreational purposes. It is still a schedule I drug at the federal level, which makes it a potential federal felony offense to possess and sell pot. There are a lot of reasons behind these state legislations — changing social attitudes, prisons overflowing with nonviolent drug offenders, and the potential state income taxing marijuana represents.

Whether this legalization will continue to other states and even a federal level remains to be seen. It also remains to be seen whether we will benefit from this legalization as a nation or begin seeing a host of problems related to marijuana usage.

Marijuana Use After Medical Legalization
for adults age 21 and older, 2004 to 2011

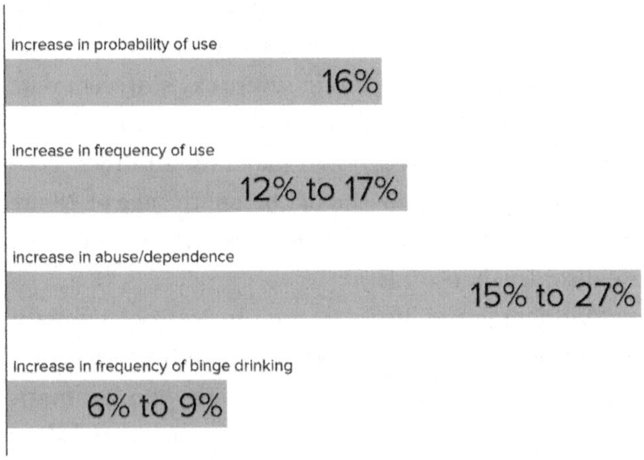

increase in probability of use

16%

increase in frequency of use

12% to 17%

increase in abuse/dependence

15% to 27%

increase in frequency of binge drinking

6% to 9%

Figure 25. Marijuana use has grown since it became legalized for medical and recreational use.

Marijuana's Impact on Mental Illness

Several studies have linked marijuana use to increased risk for psychiatric disorders, including psychosis (schizophrenia), depression, anxiety, and substance use disorders, but whether and to what extent it actually causes these conditions is not always easy to determine. The amount of drug used, the age at first use, and genetic vulnerability have all been shown to influence this relationship. Studies are still inconclusive.

Recent research has suggested that people who use marijuana and carry a specific variant of the AKT1 gene, which codes for an enzyme that affects dopamine signaling in the striatum, are at increased risk of developing psychosis. The striatum is an area of the brain that becomes activated and flooded with dopamine when certain stimuli are present. One study found that the risk of psychosis among those with this variant was seven times higher for those who used marijuana daily compared with those who used it infrequently or used none at all.

Narcotics, Opioids, Painkillers, and Prescriptions

Narcotic medications (Figure 26) have psychoactive (mind-altering) properties and, because of that, are sometimes abused — that is, taken for reasons or in ways or amounts not intended by a doctor, or taken by someone other than the person for whom they are prescribed. In fact, prescription and over-the-counter (OTC) drugs are, after marijuana (and alcohol), the most commonly abused substances by Americans 14 and older.

The classes of prescription drugs most commonly abused are: opioid pain relievers (Figure 27), such as Vicodin or Oxycodone; stimulants for treating Attention Deficit Hyperactivity Disorder (ADHD), such as Adderall, Concerta, or Ritalin; and central nervous system (CNS) depressants for relieving anxiety, such as Valium or Xanax. The most commonly abused OTC drugs are cough and cold remedies containing dextromethorphan.

Prescription Drugs Abuse

You've been studying for days for finals. You only have two exams to go but are finding yourself completely exhausted. Your roommate offers you some Ritalin that she borrowed from a friend, claiming it will give you energy and improve your attention span. In desperation, you give it a try. This is a common example of how prescription drugs are misused and potentially abused.

Prescription and OTC drugs may be abused in one or more of the following ways:

- Taking a medication that has been prescribed for somebody else. Unaware of the dangers of sharing medications, people often unknowingly contribute to this form of abuse by sharing their unused pain relievers with their family members.

People often think that prescription and OTC drugs are safer than illicit drugs. But they can be as addictive and dangerous and put users at risk for other adverse health effects, including overdose — especially when taken along with other drugs or alcohol. Before prescribing drugs, a health care provider considers a patient's health conditions, current and prior drug use, and other medicines to assess the risks and benefits for a patient.

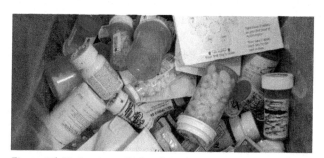

Figure 26. Various prescription drugs.

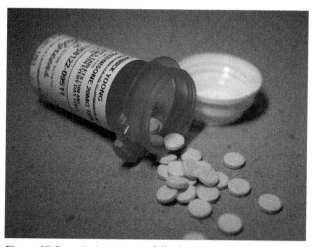

Figure 27. Prescriptions are carefully designed to treat medical conditions and should never be misused.

- Taking a drug in a higher quantity or in another manner than prescribed. Most prescription drugs are dispensed orally in tablets, but abusers sometimes crush the tablets and snort or inject the powder to hasten the effect.

- Taking a drug for another purpose than prescribed. Many of the drugs mentioned can produce pleasurable effects at sufficient quantities, so taking them for the purpose of getting high is one of the main reasons people abuse them.

- ADHD drugs like Adderall and Ritalin are also often abused by students seeking to improve their academic performance. However, although they may boost alertness, there is little evidence they improve cognitive functioning for those without a medical condition.

Effects of Prescription Drugs on the Brain

Taken as intended, prescription and OTC drugs safely treat specific mental or physical symptoms. But when taken in different quantities or when such symptoms aren't present, they may affect the brain in ways very similar to illicit drugs.

For example, stimulants such as Ritalin achieve their effects by acting on the same neurotransmitter systems as cocaine. Opioid pain relievers such as Oxycodone attach to the same cell receptors targeted by illegal opioids like heroin. Prescription depressants produce sedating or calming effects in the same manner as the club drugs GHB and Rohypnol. And when taken in very high doses, dextromethorphan acts on the same cell receptors as PCP or ketamine, producing similar out-of-body experiences.

When abused, all of these classes of drugs directly or indirectly cause a pleasurable increase in the amount of dopamine in the brain's reward pathway. Repeatedly seeking to experience that feeling can lead to addiction.

Opioids and Brain Damage

Opioids can produce drowsiness, cause constipation, and — depending upon the amount taken — depress breathing. The latter effect makes opioids particularly dangerous, especially when they are snorted or injected or combined with other drugs or alcohol.

While the relationship between opioid overdose and depressed respiration (slowed breathing) has been confirmed, researchers are also studying the long-term effects on brain function. Depressed respiration can affect the amount of oxygen that reaches the brain, a condition called hypoxia. Hypoxia can have short- and long-term psychological and neurological effects, including coma and permanent brain damage.

Researchers are also investigating the long-term effects of opioid addiction on the brain. Studies have suggested some deterioration of the brain's white matter due to heroin use, which may affect decision-making abilities, the ability to regulate behavior, and responses to stressful situations.

Prescription Opioid Overdose Epidemic

More people die from overdoses of prescription opioids than from all other drugs combined, including heroin and cocaine. More than 2 million people in the United States suffer from substance use disorders related to prescription opioid pain relievers. The terrible consequences of this trend include overdose deaths, which have more than quadrupled in the past decade and a half. The causes are complex, but they include over-prescription of pain medications. In 2013, 207 million prescriptions were written for prescription opioid pain medications.

CNS depressants slow down brain activity and can cause sleepiness and loss of coordination. Continued use can lead to physical dependence and withdrawal symptoms if discontinuing use.

Dextromethorphan can cause impaired motor function, numbness, nausea or vomiting, and increased heart rate and blood pressure. On rare occasions, hypoxic brain damage — caused by severe respiratory depression and a lack of oxygen to the brain — has occurred due to the combination of dextromethorphan with decongestants often found in the medication.

All of these drugs have the potential for addiction, and this risk is amplified when they are abused. Also, as with other drugs, abuse of prescription and OTC drugs can alter a person's judgment and decision making, leading to dangerous behaviors such as unsafe sex and drugged driving.

Prescription Drug Abuse in the US

Prescription drug abuse-related emergency department visits and treatment admissions have risen significantly in recent years. Other negative outcomes that may result from prescription drug misuse and abuse include overdose and death, falls and fractures in older adults, and, for some, initiating injection drug use with resulting risk for infections such as hepatitis C and HIV. According to results from a 2014 study, 12.7% of new illicit drug users began with prescription pain relievers. It is estimated that the abuse of opioid analgesics costs the US $72 billion in medical costs annually.

What makes this such a problem is that prescription opioid and painkiller abuse often starts as a legitimate prescription for painkillers. The potential for addiction to drugs like Oxycodone, for example, has practically become common knowledge and it can affect anyone. The idea that all drug addicts became so because they "chose" a way of life through partying just doesn't hold water. This could be an uncle who hurt his back on the job, your mother, grandparents, or siblings — a little bad luck may result in a treatment that turns someone you know into someone you don't.

Improving the way opioids are prescribed through clinical practice guidelines can ensure patients have access to safer, more effective chronic pain treatment while reducing the number of people who misuse, abuse, or overdose from these drugs.

CDC developed and published the CDC Guideline for Prescribing Opioids for Chronic Pain to provide recommendations for the prescribing of opioid pain medication for patients 18 and older in primary care settings. Recommendations focus on the use of opioids in treating chronic pain (pain lasting longer than 3 months or past the time of normal tissue healing) outside of active cancer treatment, palliative care, and end-of-life care.

Classifications

Commonly abused classes of prescription drugs include opioids (for pain), central nervous system (CNS) depressants (for anxiety and sleep disorders), and stimulants (for ADHD and narcolepsy).

- Opioids include Fentanyl (Duragesic®), Hydrocodone (Vicodin®), Oxycodone (OxyContin®), Oxymorphone (Opana®), Propoxyphene (Darvon®), Hydromorphone (Dilaudid®), Meperidine (Demerol®), and Diphenoxylate (Lomotil®).

- CNS depressants include Pentobarbital sodium (Nembutal®), Diazepam (Valium®), and Alprazolam (Xanax®).

- Stimulants include: Dextroamphetamine (Dexedrine®), Methylphenidate (Ritalin® and Concerta®), and Amphetamines (Adderall®).

Opioids are not the only problem when it comes to their misuse or abuse — studies suggest that many opioid abusers often later develop problem usage of heroin. When talking about opioid abuse and deaths, we often discuss heroin at the same time.

Drug overdose deaths involving prescription opioid pain relievers have increased dramatically since 1999 (Figure 28). Combined federal and state efforts have been made to curb this epidemic. In 2011, the White House released an interagency strategy for Responding to America's Prescription Drug Crisis. Enacting this strategy, federal agencies have worked with states to educate providers, pharmacists, patients, parents, and youth about the dangers of prescription drug abuse and the need for proper prescribing, dispensing, use, and disposal.

Improvements have been seen in some regions of the country in the form of decreasing availability of prescription opioid drugs and a decline in overdose deaths in states with the most aggressive policies. However, since 2007, overdose deaths related to heroin have started to increase. The Centers for Disease Control and Prevention counted 10,574 heroin overdose deaths in 2014, which represents more than a fivefold increase of the heroin death rate from 2002 to 2014.

In an effort to combat the intertwined problems of prescription opioid misuse and heroin use, in March of 2015 the Secretary of Health and Human Services announced the Secretary's Opioid Initiative, which aims to reduce addiction and mortality related to opioid drug abuse by (HHS takes strong steps, 2015):

- Reforming opioid prescribing practices

- Expanding access to the overdose-reversal drug naloxone

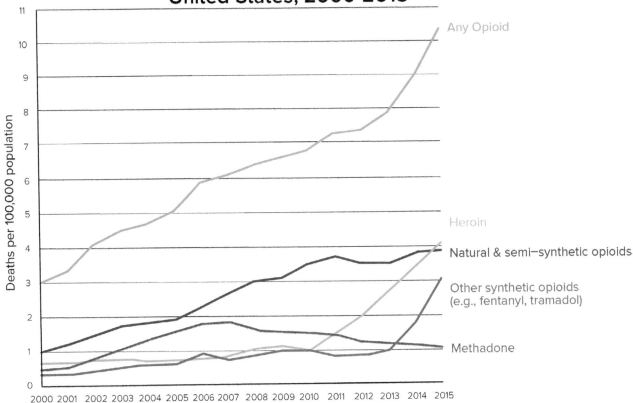

Source: CDC/NCHS, National Vital Statistics System, Mortality. CDC WONDER, Atlanta, GA: US Department of Health and Human Services, CDC; 2016. https://wonder.CDC.gov/.

Figure 28. Opioid overdose is becoming increasingly common.

- Expanding access to medication-assisted treatment for opioid use disorder

The relationship between prescription opioid abuse and increases in heroin use in the US is under scrutiny. These substances are all part of the same opioid drug category and overlap in important ways. Currently available research demonstrates:

- Prescription opioid use is a risk factor for heroin use.

- Heroin use is rare in prescription drug users.

- Prescription opioids and heroin have similar effects, different risk factors.

- A subset of people who abuse prescription opioids may progress to heroin use.

- Increased drug availability is associated with increased use and overdose.

- Heroin use is driven by its low cost and high availability.

- Emphasis is needed on both prevention and treatment.

Treatment

Medications, including buprenorphine (Suboxone®, Subutex®), methadone, and extended release naltrexone (Vivitrol®), are effective for the treatment of opioid use disorders. Buprenorphine and methadone are "essential medicines" according to the World Health Organization. Medications should be combined with behavioral counseling for a "whole patient" approach, known as Medication Assisted Treatment (MAT).

MAT Decreases opioid use, opioid-related overdose deaths, criminal activity, and infectious disease transmission. After buprenorphine became available in Baltimore, heroin overdose deaths decreased by 37%.

MAT Increases social functioning and retention in treatment. Patients treated with medication were more likely to remain in therapy compared to patients receiving treatment that did not include medication.

Treatment of opioid-dependent pregnant women with methadone or buprenorphine improves outcomes for their babies. MAT reduces symptoms of neonatal abstinence syndrome and length of hospital stay.

Less than 1/2 of privately-funded substance use disorder treatment programs offer MAT and only 1/3 of patients with opioid dependence at these programs actually receive it.

- The proportion of opioid treatment admissions with treatment plans that included receiving med-

Additional Information

If you or someone you care about has an opioid use disorder, ask your doctor about available MAT options and about naloxone, an opioid antagonist that can

ications fell from 35 percent in 2002 to 28 percent in 2012.

- Nearly all US states do not have sufficient treatment capacity to provide MAT to all patients with an opioid use disorder.

Methadone and buprenorphine do not just substitute one addiction for another. When someone is treated for an opioid addiction, the dosage of medication used does not get them high — it helps reduce opioid cravings and withdrawal. These medications restore balance to the brain circuits affected by addiction, allowing the patient's brain to heal while working toward recovery.

reverse an opioid overdose. Many states allow you to get naloxone from a pharmacist without bringing in a prescription from a physician.

Club Drugs

Club drugs are a group of psychoactive drugs that tend to be abused by teens and young adults at bars, nightclubs, concerts, and parties. Rohypnol, ketamine, cocaine, and LSD, as well as MDMA (Ecstasy) and methamphetamine are some of the drugs included in this group. They all have slightly different origins and effects. Some are natural, like cocaine, and others have synthetic versions.

These drugs are popular because they are relatively inexpensive to obtain, come in a variety of forms (making them easy to circulate), and their properties are believed to enhance the club experience. These drugs most often provide a burst of energy and heightened sensitivity to sights and sounds. This heightened awareness also tends to apply to the users sense of arousal.

Club Drug Addiction Treatment

With most drugs, regardless of their nature, there are traditional methods for treatment. Most involve:

- Detoxification (the process by which the body rids itself of a drug)
- Behavioral therapy
- Medication (for opioid, tobacco, or alcohol addiction)
- Evaluation and treatment for co-occurring mental health issues such as depression and anxiety
- Contingency management, or motivational incentives — providing rewards to patients who remain substance free

- Therapeutic communities — drug-free residences in which people in recovery from substance use disorders help each other to understand and change their behaviors
- Long-term follow-up to prevent relapse

A range of care with a tailored treatment program and follow-up options can be crucial to success. Treatment should include both medical and mental health services as needed. Follow-up care may include community- or family-based recovery support systems.

Club Drugs	Effects	Short-Term Dangers	Long-Term Dangers
MDMA (Ecstasy)	Stimulant and hallucinogen: increased energy, pleasure, emotional warmth, distorted sensory and time perception, euphoria	Increased risk of unwanted sexual activity, chills, involuntary teeth clenching, nausea, muscle cramps, blurred vision, sweating, overdose	Anxiety, irritability, sleep problems, aggressiveness, liver failure, heart failure, kidney failure, addiction
Rohypnol (Roofies)	Sedative: extreme fatigue, memory loss	Lethal if mixed with alcohol or other depressants	Impaired attention span, decreased learning ability, memory loss, coma, death
Ketamine (K)	Anesthetic: dissociation, distorted perception of sight and sound, detachment, hallucinations, delirium, amnesia	Impaired motor function, high blood pressure, potentially fatal respiratory problems, painlessness causing traumatic injury to go untreated	Severe injury from refusing treatment (e.g., walking on a broken leg), thickened bladder and urinary tracts, severe abdominal pain, kidney failure
Cocaine	Stimulant and anesthetic: dopamine floods, extreme happiness, energy, hypersensitivity	Constricted blood vessels, irritability, extreme paranoia, nausea, increased heart rate, restlessness, muscle tremors, bizarre, violent, and unpredictable behavior, overdose	Lose of smell, frequent nosebleeds, difficulty swallowing, addiction
LSD (Acid, DMT, Mushrooms)	Hallucinogen: altered sensory perception, increased heart rate, nausea, intense emotion, changed perception of time	Increased blood pressure, loss of appetite, dry mouth, uncoordinated movement, excessive sweating, panic, paranoia, psychosis, poisoning, seizures, coma	Persistent psychosis, visual disturbances, disorganized thinking, paranoia, mood changes
Methamphetamine	Stimulant, dopamine floods, euphoria, increased wakefulness, excitement, decreased appetite	Rapid breathing and heart rate, increased body temperature, poisoning, overdose	Nerve damage, dopamine irregularity, sleep problems, anxiety, weight loss, dental problems, excessive itching, paranoia, hallucinations, loss of memory, addiction

Figure 29. Club drugs' effects and dangers.

Caffeine

None of us are strangers to caffeine use. We often consider it a common and necessary drug for daily functioning. Didn't sleep well? Have a cup of coffee (Figure 30). Hanging out with friends? Let's get coffee. Energy drinks are on the rise as sleep is on the decrease, particularly for college students. But what is it about caffeine that feeds our love and need for this drug?

Caffeine is a bitter substance that occurs naturally in more than 60 plants including coffee beans, tea leaves, kola nuts (used to flavor colas), and cacao pods (used to make chocolate).

There is also synthetic (man-made) caffeine, which is added to some medicines, foods, and drinks. For example,

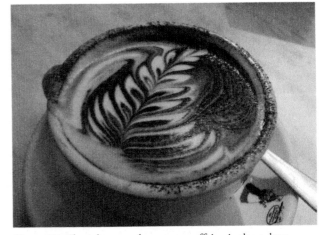

Figure 30. Though not as dangerous, caffeine is also a drug.

some pain relievers, cold medicines, and over-the-counter medicines for alertness contain synthetic caffeine. So do energy drinks and "energy-boosting" gums and snacks.

Most people consume caffeine from drinks. The amounts of caffeine in different drinks can vary a lot (Figure 31), but it is generally:

- An 8-ounce cup of coffee: 95–200mg

- A 12-ounce can of cola: 35–45mg

- An 8-ounce energy drink: 70–100mg

- An 8-ounce cup of tea: 14–60mg

Caffeine's Effects on the Body

Caffeine has many effects on your body's metabolism. It stimulates your central nervous system, making you feel more awake and giving you that boost of energy. It also acts like a diuretic, helping salt (and other bodily fluids) move through your system.

Not all of its effects are comfortable. It increases acid in the stomach leading to heartburn or a sour belly. That jolt of energy you got? This increases your blood pressure. Within one hour of eating or drinking caffeine, it reaches its peak level in your blood. You may continue to feel the effects of caffeine for four to six hours.

Side Effects from Too Much Caffeine

For most people, it is not harmful to consume up to 400mg of caffeine a day. If you do eat or drink too much caffeine, it can cause health problems, such as restlessness and shakiness, insomnia, headaches, dizziness, dehydration, anxiety, and dependency.

How many times have you gotten a headache from *not* drinking caffeine? Probably plenty, even if you didn't realize it. Your body gets used to its daily fix. We don't often consider it as a drug from which we will withdrawal, but we do! If we go without it, we become more tired than usual, irritable, and even nauseous.

Energy Drinks

Energy drinks are beverages that have added caffeine. The amount of caffeine in energy drinks can vary widely, and sometimes the labels on the drinks do not give you the actual amount of caffeine in them. Energy drinks may also contain sugars, vitamins, herbs, and supplements.

Companies that make energy drinks claim that the drinks can increase alertness and improve physical and mental performance. This has helped make the drinks popular with American teens and young adults. There's limited data showing that energy drinks might

Beverage/Food	Serving Size	Caffeine
Tea	8 oz. (240 ml)	15-70 mg
Decaffeinated Tea	8 oz. (240 ml)	less than 12 mg
Roobios Tea	8 oz. (240 ml)	0 mg
Herbal Tea or Tisane	8 oz. (240 ml)	0 mg
Coffee	8 oz. (240 ml)	27-200 mg
Decaffeinated Coffee	8 oz. (240 ml)	2-12 mg
Espresso	1 oz. (30 ml)	29-120 mg
Decaffeinated Espresso	1 oz. (30 ml)	8 mg
Chocolate (Dark)	1 oz.	20 mg
Chocolate (Milk)	1 oz.	6 mg
Pepsi MAX	12 oz.	69 mg
Mountain Dew	12 oz.	54 mg
Cocoa–Cola Classic	12 oz.	34 mg
7–Up and Root Beers	12 oz.	0 mg
Rockstar Energy Drink	16 oz.	160 mg
Red Bull Energy Drink	8.4 oz.	80 mg

Figure 31. Amount of caffeine in common drinks.

temporarily improve alertness and physical endurance. There is not enough evidence to show that they enhance strength or power. But what we do know is that energy drinks can be dangerous because they have large amounts of caffeine. And since they have lots of sugar, they can contribute to weight gain and worsen diabetes.

Sometimes young people mix their energy drinks with alcohol. It is dangerous to combine alcohol and caffeine. Caffeine can interfere with your ability to recognize how drunk you are, which can lead you to drink more. This also makes you more likely to make bad decisions.

Some people either cannot tolerate caffeine or are at high risk for other reasons. Pregnant women, for example, are advised to limit caffeine usage to 200 mg a day. It is a stimulant and can be passed to the child with negative effects (including while breastfeeding).

People with anxiety, heart disease, high blood pressure, ulcers, migraines, and sleep disorders should also avoid it. Consider the reactions of caffeine on the body. If this is likely to interfere with an existing problem, you should keep consumption limited. For example, if you are already prone to headaches, and caffeine causes headaches, its usage would exacerbate the problem.

Caffeine's Impact on Sports Performance

Despite considerable research in this area, the role of caffeine as a performance enhancing drug is still controversial. Some of the data are conflicting, which is in part due to how the experimental studies were designed and what methods were used. However, there is general agreement in a few areas:

- Caffeine may benefit short term, high intensity exercise (e.g., sprinting)

- Caffeine can enhance performance in endurance sports.

Glycogen is the principal fuel for muscles and exhaustion occurs when it is depleted. A secondary fuel, which is much more abundant, is fat. As long as there is still glycogen available, working muscles can utilize fat. Caffeine mobilizes fat stores and encourages working muscles to use fat as a fuel.

This delays the depletion of muscle glycogen and allows for a prolongation of exercise. The critical time period in glycogen sparing appears to occur during the first 15 minutes of exercise, where caffeine has been shown to decrease glycogen utilization by as much as 50%. Glycogen saved at the beginning is thus available during the later stages of exercise. Although the exact method by which caffeine does this is still unclear, caffeine caused sparing in all of the human studies where muscle glycogen levels were measured. The effect on performance, which was observed in most experimental studies, was that subjects were able to exercise longer until exhaustion occurred.

Caffeine Overdose

The death of an Ohio high school senior caused by an overdose of powdered caffeine has prompted the FDA to issue a safety advisory about caffeine powders. Bulk bags of pure caffeine powder are readily available online, and these products may be attractive to young people looking for added caffeine stimulation or for help losing weight, but they are extremely dangerous. Just a teaspoon of pure caffeine powder is equivalent to about 25 cups of coffee — a lethal amount. Besides death, severe caffeine overdose can cause fast and erratic heartbeat, seizures, vomiting, diarrhea, and disorientation — symptoms much more extreme than those of drinking too much coffee or tea or consuming too many sodas or energy drinks.

Although caffeine is generally safe at the dosages contained in popular beverages, caffeine powder is so potent that safe amounts cannot be measured with ordinary kitchen measuring tools, making it very easy to overdose on them even when users are aware of their potency. The FDA thus recommends that consumers avoid caffeine powder altogether, and wishes to alert parents to the existence of these products and their hazards.

Cutting Back on Caffeine

If you know you've been overdoing it or are experiencing negative side effects from too much caffeine, it's probably time to cut back or eliminate it from your daily routine. Here are a few tips to help you do that:

Taper your usage — Don't go "cold turkey" unless you have instructions from your physician to immediately stop using it. Wean yourself off of it, consuming a bit less each day. This will help you avoid the really unpleasant side effects of withdrawal.

Keep tabs — Caffeine is in many substances, such as drinks and foods and medications that we may not be aware of. Keep track of where your caffeine is coming from.

Go decaf — Decaffeinated drinks can help give you the same level of emotional comfort without the risk (Coffee is a comfort food for many people).

Conclusion

Your next steps should be to avoid substance abuse in all forms. If you drink alcohol, drink responsibly. If you consume caffeinated beverages, make sure that you aren't drinking an amount that harms your health. It's also worth examining your behaviors to notice any behavioral addictions that may be developing. Educating yourself and others about the risks associated with drug use is often the most effective deterrent to using drugs.

If you or someone you know has a substance abuse problem, getting help requires behavioral change. Review the stages of change theoretical model in Chapter 1 and look for information on addiction treatment in your area.

Chapter 12
Environmental Health

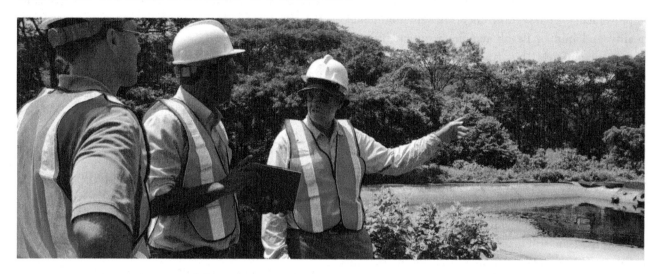

You've considered yourself a friend to the environment for years! You're from Oregon — of course you know everything there is to know about protecting Mother Earth and all of her natural resources. You recycle like a champ (Reduce, Reuse, Recycle — right?), drive an electric car, and wear your Earth Day shirt on any day you choose. But did you know that it wasn't just the safety of the planet you were protecting?

Environmental health refers to the ways all aspects of natural and man-made environment impact human health. It covers everything from your home, workplace, and neighborhood, to the places you might go fishing, hunting, and camping. Environmental health is about the water you drink, the air you breathe, and the soil in which you grow your food. Environmental health is at risk because of increased human population, but it can be improved by better managing the pollutants that people expel into the world.

This chapter defines environmental health and its importance to wellness. It then describes population growth and the concerns associated with unmanageable pollution levels. Finally, this chapter defines several types of pollution and makes suggestions to decrease your own pollution to contribute to better environmental health.

Environmental Health and Wellness

The environment plays a crucial role in people's physical, mental, and social well-being. Despite significant improvements, major differences in environmental quality and human health remain between different states and nations. This can make it challenging to make improvements and control damage to the areas we live, work, eat, and breathe.

Have you ever seen a photo taken from space of the smog over China? Or the amount of garbage piled on the shores of a developing country? Maybe even noticed that when you drove away from the west coast, you no longer had a place to recycle your plastic bottle? That's because not every country or state has the infrastructure required to protect the environment in the same way we do here.

But there are still many ways we can approach this problem. The complex relationships between environmental factors and human health, taking into account multiple pathways and interactions, should be seen in a broader spatial, socio-economic, and cultural context.

Environmental health refers to protection against environmental factors that may adversely impact human health or the ecological balances essential to long-term human health and environmental quality, whether in the natural or man-made environment. Humans interact with the environment constantly. These interactions affect quality of life, years of healthy life lived, and health disparities. The World Health Organization (WHO) defines **environment**, as it relates to health, as "all the physical, chemical, and biological factors external to a person, and all the related behaviors." Environmental health consists of preventing or controlling disease, injury, and disability related to the interactions between people and their environment.

The Healthy People 2020 Environmental Health objectives focus on six themes, each of which highlights an element of environmental health:

- Outdoor air quality
- Surface and groundwater quality
- Toxic substances and hazardous wastes
- Homes and communities
- Infrastructure and surveillance
- Global environmental health

Creating healthy environments can be complex and relies on continuing research to better understand the effects of exposure to environmental hazards on people's health.

Maintaining a healthy environment is central to increasing our quality of life and years of healthy life. Globally, 23% of all deaths and 26% of deaths among children under age five are due to preventable environmental factors. Environmental factors are diverse and far reaching. They include:

- Exposure to hazardous substances in the air, water, soil, and food
- Natural and technological disasters
- Climate change
- Occupational hazards
- The built environment

Poor environmental quality has its greatest impact on people whose health status is already at risk. Therefore, environmental health must address the societal and environmental factors that increase the likelihood of exposure and disease.

The degradation of the environment, through air pollution, noise, chemicals, poor quality water and loss of natural areas, combined with lifestyle changes, may be contributing to substantial increases in rates of obesity, diabetes, diseases of the cardiovascular and nervous systems and cancer — all of which are major public health problems for the US population. Reproductive and mental health problems are also on the rise. Asthma, allergies, and some types of cancer related to environmental pressures are of particular concern for children.

The six Health People 2020 themes for Environmental health draw attention to separate elements of the environment and their links to health.

Environmental health is a dynamic and evolving field. While not all complex environmental issues can be predicted, some known emerging issues in the field include:

Climate change — This is projected to impact sea level, patterns of infectious disease, air quality, and the severity of natural disasters such as floods, droughts, and storms.

Outdoor Air Quality	Poor air quality is linked to premature death, cancer, and long-term damage to respiratory and cardiovascular systems. Progress has been made to reduce unhealthy air emissions, but in 2008, approximately 127 million people lived in US counties that exceeded national air quality standards. Decreasing air pollution is an important step in creating a healthy environment.
Surface and Groundwater	Surface and groundwater quality concerns apply to both drinking water and recreational waters. Contamination by infectious agents or chemicals can cause mild to severe illness. Protecting water sources and minimizing exposure to contaminated water sources are important parts of environmental health.
Toxic Substances and Hazardous Wastes	The health effects of toxic substances and hazardous wastes are not yet fully understood. Research to better understand how these exposures may impact health is ongoing. Meanwhile, efforts to reduce exposures continue. Reducing exposure to toxic substances and hazardous wastes is fundamental to environmental health.
Homes and Communities	People spend most of their time at home, work, or school. Some of these environments may expose people to indoor air pollution, inadequate heating and sanitation, structural problems, electrical and fire hazards, or lead-based paint hazards. These hazards can impact health and safety. Maintaining healthy homes and communities is essential to environmental health.
Infrastructure and Surveillance	Preventing exposure to environmental hazards relies on many partners, including state and local health departments. Personnel, surveillance systems, and education are important resources for investigating and responding to disease, monitoring for hazards, and educating the public. Additional methods and greater capacity to measure and respond to environmental hazards are needed.
Global Environmental Health	Water quality is an important global challenge. Diseases can be reduced by improving water quality and sanitation and increasing access to adequate water and sanitation facilities.

Figure 1. Environmental health factors.

Disaster Preparedness — for the environmental impact of natural disasters as well as disasters of human origin includes planning for human health needs and the impact on public infrastructure, such as water and roadways.

Nanotechnology — The potential impact of nanotechnology is significant and offers possible improvements to disease prevention, detection and treatment along with electronics, clean energy, manufacturing, and environmental risk assessment.

The Built Environment — Features of the built environment appear to impact human health — influencing behaviors, physical activity patterns, social networks, and access to resources.

Several major environmental health issues exist on a global scale, while others are relatively local in scope. Some issues are important in both, such as air quality. First, let's look at how some global trends in population growth, biodiversity, food supply, land degradation, water pollution, and energy consumption impact any discussion of environmental health. These are the major issues that affect us all, and must be taken into account when describing environmental health.

Population Growth

Population growth and density are important factors to environmental health because each person has an impact on the global environment. They produce waste that needs to be removed, increase the need for farmlands (which are limited), and increase the number of pollutants in the air and water. One way you can see this is in action is by visiting a major city and looking around. What does the air look like or smell like? How much garbage do you see lying around? What kind of infrastructure (like the Big Pipe project in Portland,

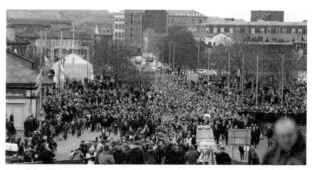
Figure 2. Populations around the world are growing.

OR) is needed to keep sewage out of nearby waterways? These signs are all representative of problems we face when the population grows (Figure 2).

The current world population of 7.3 billion is expected to reach 8.5 billion by 2030, 9.7 billion in 2050 and 11.2 billion in 2100, according to a new UN DESA report, "World Population Prospects: The 2015 Revision."

Most of the projected increase in the world's population can be attributed to a short list of high-fertility countries, mainly in Africa, or countries with already large populations. During 2015–2050, half of the world's population growth is expected to be concentrated in nine countries: India, Nigeria, Pakistan, Democratic Republic of the Congo, Ethiopia, United Republic of Tanzania, United States of America (USA), Indonesia and Uganda, listed according to the size of their contribution to the total growth (Figure 3).

Earth's Carrying Capacity

Human population cannot continue to grow indefinitely without it having a negative impact. We have limits to the life-sustaining resources earth can provide us. In other words, there is a **carrying capacity** for human life on our planet. The carrying capacity is the maximum number of a particular species an environment can support indefinitely. Every species on Earth has a carrying capacity, including humans. However, it is very difficult for ecologists to calculate human carrying capacity. We are a complex species. From culture to culture and nation to nation, we do not reproduce, consume resources, and interact with our living environment uniformly. Carrying capacity estimates involve making predictions about future trends in population, resource availability, technological advances, and economic development.

We project what is going to happen with the population and attempt to determine our carrying capacity in part by estimating the fertility rates of women in different countries, in order to try and prepare for what kind

Global Trends

Globally, the TFR has dropped from 4.45 in 1970 to around 2.5 in 2014. If the rate keeps falling, the world population will eventually stop growing and may actually start shrinking towards the end of the 21st century.

A country's population is stable when TFR is equal to replacement rates. These vary by country but globally work out to around 2.1 children per woman. The

Country	2016 Est. Total Fertility Rate (Children Born/Woman)
Niger	6.62
Chad	4.45
Somalia	5.89
Congo	4.53
India	2.45
Mexico	2.25
United States	1.87
Australia	1.77
Canada	1.6
China	1.6
Russia	1.61
Germany	1.44
Japan	1.41

Figure 3. Fertility rates in countries around the world.

of population burden is yet to come and how each country is probably going to have to deal with this growth.

Total fertility rate (**TFR**) compares figures for the average number of children that would be born per woman if all women lived to the end of their childbearing years and bore children according to a given fertility rate at each age. TFR is a more direct measure of the level of fertility than the crude birth rate, since it refers to potential births per woman. The highest total birth rate in the world, as of 2016, belongs to Niger, with almost seven births per woman, and the lowest is in Singapore which averaged a little less than one birth per woman. The United States' average for 2016 was 1.82 births per woman.

Tracking TFR is important for a number of reasons. From an environmental health standpoint, a rapid increase in population means we need to increase infrastructure to deal with major issues like sewage processing, which is vital for preventing catastrophic pandemics of sewage-related infectious disease.

replacement rate is slightly higher than two is not only do women need to replace themselves and the father but also to factor in children who die before reaching adulthood and women who die before the end of their childbearing years.

With that in mind, many countries in the world are now below replacement level, including China, Russia, Brazil, all of Europe (except France, Ireland, and Turkey), Japan, Canada, and Australia, among others. This means that without immigration all these countries will see long term population decreases (Figure 4).

Human population growth is having such a profound effect on the environment and geology of earth that some geologists have proposed we call the current epoch the Anthropocene to reflect these impacts. Our current geological age could be measured more by what we've contributed to the planet as humans than at any other point in history. Rather than nature doing its job to move, shift, and adapt, we've forced changes that would not have otherwise occurred.

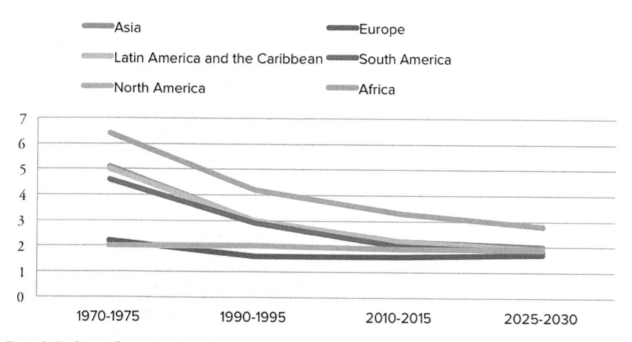

Figure 4. Fertility rates by continent through time.

Biodiversity

Biodiversity is the variety of life forms on our planet and within specific ecosystems. Scientists have tracked the loss of biodiversity on Earth for decades. Our planet has always experienced declines and even the extinction of entire species. Our physical, geological, and biological data show us that his is true. So, why are we worried if this is a natural part of our life and existence on this planet?

Much of these changes and losses come from natural environmental change. It happens slowly, giving different species time to adapt to or transition to new environments. For example, many humans are no longer born with wisdom teeth. Our bodies have slowly, over many centuries, learned that we do not need them. At first, much of the species loss in the twentieth century was attributed to these typical changes in biodiversity that occur in living ecosystems.

Scientists that study biodiversity now believe that we are seeing more than usual fluctuations and adaptations. What we are now seeing is that much of the extinct, such as with mammals, birds, and amphibians, is related to human activity. Our actions are causing certain species to decline — potentially die off.

There is no doubt that humans have had a negative impact on biodiversity (Figure 5), particularly since the industrial revolution. We fish too much, hunt too much, and build massive subdivisions that remove the habitats of many animals. Our agriculture and pollutants have forced pesticides, herbicides, and other toxic substances into the natural world. It is estimated that there are over 5,000 vertebrates, over 2,000 invertebrates, and an excess of 8,000 plants on the list of threatened species. The number of documented extinctions since 1500 AD is now 784 species and it is estimated that extinction rates are now 50 to 500 times higher than previous estimated rates.

The popularity of seafood has lead to overfishing, which is a problem compounded by toxic chemicals and fecal waste entering oceans, raising nitrogen levels, and creating huge "dead zones" that don't support most types of sea life. Popular types of edible fish are becoming increasingly rare and expensive. Combine this with the very manmade problem of plastic in our oceans (ever heard of the Great Pacific Garbage Patch?), and our sea life could continue to see a marked decline.

Other industrial farming techniques, such as the "intensive" farming methods used to meet the demand for meat, produces 9% of the greenhouse gasses in the US and an astronomical amount of fecal waste. A pig farm with 2,400 swine, for example, produces as much waste as 24,000 people.

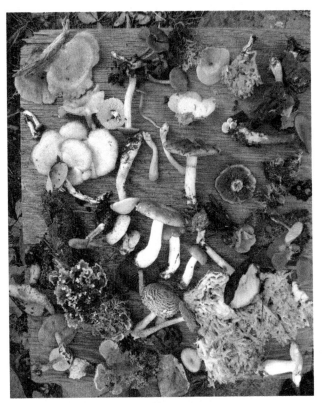

Figure 5. Biodiversity in agriculture.

Food Supply

As food demand increases, we have to become more and more industrialized with our food production (Figure 6). We've developed intensive farming techniques, artificial fertilization methods to replace nutrients stripped from the soil, and are converting important biospheres into grazing land.

The demand for meat, which increases globally as more people enter the middle class in developing nations, creates the most environmental health problems, because there are limited uses for the vast quantities of waste produced by livestock, which often finds its way into the water supply, and livestock also needs a massive amount of water to drink and for growing feed.

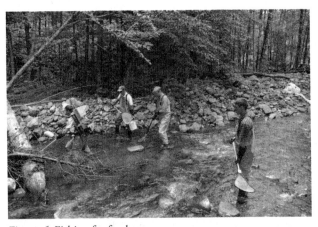

Figure 6. Fishing for food.

Land Degradation

Land degradation is the decline in the quality of the land, largely due to human activities. It can be considered in terms of the loss of actual or potential productivity or utility. This can occur through natural factors, such as the way water causes soil erosion, or through the way we care for the land.

Land degradation has been a major global issue during the last century and will likely remain high on the international agenda. The importance of land degradation among global issues is enhanced because of its impact on world food security and quality of the environment. High population density is not necessarily related to land degradation — it is what a population does to the land that determines the extent of degradation. People can be a major asset in reversing a trend towards degradation. However, they need to be healthy and politically and economically motivated to care for the land, as subsistence agriculture, poverty, and illiteracy can be important causes of land and environmental degradation.

Land degradation often leads to desertification, which is the process of fertile irrigated land transforming into dry dead desert with loss of fertility and vegetation.

According to the World Health Organization, weather extremes — particularly drought — and human activities that pollute or degrade land (including over-cultivation, overgrazing and deforestation) convert arable land into desert. As ecosystems change and deserts expand, food production diminishes, water sources dry up and populations are pressured to move to more hospitable areas.

Water Pollution

Water pollution is any contamination of water with chemicals or other foreign substances that are detrimental to human, plant, or animal health. These pollutants include fertilizers and pesticides from agricultural runoff; sewage and food processing waste; lead, mercury, and other heavy metals; chemical wastes from industrial discharges; and chemical contamination from hazardous waste sites. Worldwide, nearly 2 billion people drink contaminated water that could be harmful to their health.

Energy Consumption

The outlook for energy use worldwide continues to show rising levels of demand over the next three decades. Countries where demand is drive by strong economic growth, like China and India, account for more than half of the world's total projected increase in energy consumption. The US Energy Information Administration projects that world energy consumption will grow by 48% by the year 2040.

Concerns about energy security, effects of fossil fuel emissions on the environment, and sustained, long-term high world oil prices support expanded use of nonfossil renewable energy sources and nuclear power. Renewables and nuclear power are the world's fastest-growing energy sources over the projection period. Renewable energy is expected to increase by an average 2.6% per year through 2040, nuclear power by 2.3% per year (Figure 7).

Even though nonfossil fuels are expected to grow faster than fossil fuels (petroleum and other liquid fuels, natural gas, and coal), fossil fuels will still likely account for more than three-quarters of world energy consumption through 2040. Natural gas, which has a lower carbon intensity than coal

and petroleum, is the fastest-growing fossil fuel in the outlook, with global natural gas consumption increasing by 1.9% per year.

Although liquid fuels — mostly petroleum-based — remain the largest energy source, the liquids' share of world marketed energy consumption is projected to fall from recent the 33% to 30% in 2040. As oil prices rise in the long term, many energy users adopt more energy-efficient technologies and switch away from liquid fuels when feasible.

Coal is the world's slowest-growing energy source, expected to rise by only 0.6% per year through 2040. Throughout the projection period, the top three coal-consuming countries are China, the United States, and India,

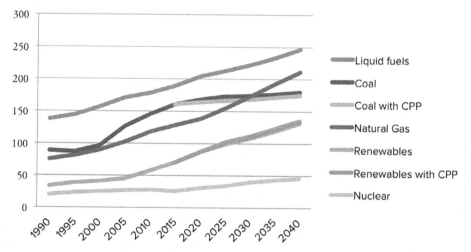

Figure 7. Energy consumption predictions.

which together account for more than 70% of world coal consumption. China alone currently accounts for almost half of the world's total coal consumption, but a slowing economy and plans to implement policies to address air pollution and reduce carbon dioxide emissions mean that coal use in China will begin to decline in the later years of the projection period. Coal use in India is expected to continue to rise and surpasses US coal consumption after 2030.

Though we are making some progress toward renewable energies that are less damaging to the air, soil, and wildlife, all forms of energy have some environmental impact. Most energy sources still require land use and water use at minimum, in addition to any waste produced in the process. Moving toward clean energy is important, but humans will continue to leave a footprint, no matter how clean, for many years to come.

Pollution: The Greatest Threat to Environmental Health

The rest of this chapter expands on the largest threats to environmental health. All of these threats can be described as pollution of some kind. There are a variety of pollutants people produce that can be reduced on a personal and systemic level. Taking personal responsibility and reducing pollution in our immediate vicinity (e.g. neighborhood, town, county, and state) has far-reaching results. The trash you recycle each day, the water you conserve while brushing your teeth, and the days you bike to work instead of drive all have a cumulative positive impact.

Air Quality and Pollution

Most of us fear the thought of not being able to breathe. Just imagining it can make us feel short of breath and even a bit panicked. But when it comes to the quality of our air, we don't often think of it as a shortage — more often see it as an aesthetic issue. The fact is that we need clean air to breathe, which is why **air pollution** is a growing concern.

Air pollution is a mixture of natural and man-made substances in the air we breathe. People who live near major sources of air pollutants develop respiratory illnesses at an alarming rate. Even being in traffic causes your respiratory system to work at a lower efficiency as

carbon monoxide basically cuts in front of oxygen in the line to get into your bloodstream.

The Clean Air Act requires the Environmental Protection Agency (EPA) to set National Ambient Air Quality Standards (NAAQS) for maximum allowable concentrations of six "criteria" pollutants in outdoor air. The six pollutants are carbon monoxide, lead, ground-level ozone, nitrogen dioxide, particulate matter, and sulfur dioxide. The standards are set at a level that protects public health with an adequate margin of safety. These pollutants are found all over the US They can harm your health, the environment, and even cause property damage.

The Six Criteria Air Pollutants

Ground level ozone, or "bad" ozone is not emitted directly into the air, but is created by chemical reactions between oxides of nitrogen (NOx) and volatile organic compounds (VOC) in the presence of sunlight. Emissions from industrial facilities and electric utilities, motor vehicle exhaust, gasoline vapors, and chemical solvents are some of the major sources of NOx and VOC. Breathing ozone can trigger a variety of health problems, particularly for children, the elderly, and people of all ages who have lung diseases such as asthma. Ground level ozone can also have harmful effects on sensitive vegetation and ecosystems.

Carbon monoxide (CO) is a colorless, odorless gas that can be harmful when inhaled in large amounts. CO is released when something is burned. The greatest sources of CO to outdoor air are cars, trucks, and other vehicles or machinery that burn fossil fuels. A variety of items in your home such as unvented kerosene and gas space heaters, leaking chimneys and furnaces, and gas stoves also release CO and can affect air quality indoors.

Breathing air with a high concentration of CO reduces the amount of oxygen that can be transported in the blood stream to critical organs like the heart and brain. At very high levels, which are possible indoors or in other enclosed environments, CO can cause dizziness, confusion, unconsciousness and death.

Very high levels of CO are not likely to occur outdoors. However, when CO levels are elevated outdoors, they can be of particular concern for people with some types of heart disease. These people already have a reduced ability for getting oxygenated blood to their hearts in situations where the heart needs more oxygen than usual. They are especially vulnerable to the effects of CO when exercising or under increased stress. In these situations, short-term exposure to elevated CO may result in reduced oxygen to the heart accompanied by chest pain also known as angina.

The EPA's NAAQS for **sulfur dioxide** (SO2) are designed to protect against exposure to the entire group of sulfur oxides (SOx). SO2 is the component of greatest concern and is used as the indicator for the larger group of gaseous sulfur oxides. Other gaseous SOx (such as SO3) are found in the atmosphere at concentrations much lower than SO2.

The largest source of SO2 in the atmosphere is the burning of fossil fuels by power plants and other industrial facilities. Smaller sources of SO2 emissions include: industrial processes such as extracting metal from ore; natural sources such as volcanoes; and locomotives, ships and other vehicles and heavy equipment that burn fuel with a high sulfur content. Emissions that lead to high concentrations of SO2 generally also lead to the formation of other SOx. These chemicals can react with other compounds in the atmosphere to form small particles. These particles contribute to particulate matter (PM) pollution (particles may penetrate deeply into sensitive parts of the lungs and cause additional health problems).

Short-term exposures to SO2 can harm the human respiratory system and make breathing difficult. Children, the elderly, and those who suffer from asthma are particularly sensitive to effects of SO2.

PM, or **particulate matter** (also called particle pollution), is the term for a mixture of solid particles and liquid droplets found in the air. Some particles, such as dust, dirt, soot, or smoke, are large or dark enough to be seen with the naked eye. Others are so small they can only be detected using an electron microscope. They range in size from 10 micrometers to 2.5 or smaller. To give you an idea of how small that is, one strain of human hair is 70 micrometers in diameter. We can inhale PM without realizing it's happening.

These particles come in many sizes and shapes and can be made up of hundreds of different chemicals. Some are emitted directly from a source, such as construction sites, unpaved roads, fields, smokestacks or fires. Most particles form in the atmosphere as a result of complex reactions of chemicals such as sulfur dioxide and nitrogen oxides, which are pollutants emitted from power plants, industries and automobiles.

Inhaled PM can cause serious health problems. Particles less than 10 micrometers in diameter pose the greatest problems, because they can get deep into your lungs, and some may even get into your bloodstream. Fine particles (PM2.5) are the main cause of reduced visibility (haze) in parts of the United States, including many of our national parks and wilderness areas.

Sources of **lead** emissions vary from one area to another. At the national level, major sources of lead in the air are ore and metals processing and piston-engine aircraft operating on leaded aviation fuel. Other sources are waste incinerators, utilities, and lead-acid battery manufacturers. The highest air concentrations of lead are usually found near lead smelters.

As a result of EPA's regulatory efforts, including the removal of lead from motor vehicle gasoline, levels of lead in the air decreased by 98 percent between 1980 and 2014.

Lead is persistent in the environment and can be added to soils and sediments through deposits from sources of lead air pollution. Other sources of lead to ecosystems include direct discharge of waste streams to water bodies and mining. Elevated lead in the environment can result in decreased growth and reproductive rates in plants and animals, and neurological effects in vertebrates.

Once taken into the body, lead distributes throughout the body in the blood and is accumulated in the bones. Depending on the level of exposure, lead can adversely affect the nervous system, kidney function, immune system, reproductive and developmental systems and the cardiovascular system. Lead exposure also affects the oxygen carrying capacity of the blood. The lead effects most commonly encountered in current populations are neurological effects in children and cardiovascular effects (e.g., high blood pressure and heart disease) in adults. Infants and young children are especially sensitive to even low levels of lead, which may contribute to behavioral problems, learning deficits, and lowered IQ.

As of 2017, there are approximately 4 million houses or buildings that have children living in them who are potentially being exposed to lead. Nearly half a million US children ages 1 to 5 have blood lead levels at or above 5 micrograms per deciliter (µg/dL), which is currently the reference level at which CDC recommends public health actions be taken. Even blood lead exposure levels as low as 2 micrograms per deciliter (µg/dL) can affect a child's cognitive function. Since no safe blood lead level has been identified for children, any exposure should be taken seriously. However, since lead exposure often occurs with no obvious signs or symptoms, it often remains unrecognized.

Nitrogen Dioxide (NO2) is one of a group of highly reactive gases known as oxides of nitrogen or nitrogen oxides (NOx). NO2 primarily gets in the air from the burning of fuel from cars, trucks and buses, power plants, and off-road equipment. NO2 along with other NOx reacts with other chemicals in the air to form both particulate matter and ozone. Both of these are also harmful when inhaled due to effects on the respiratory system.

It sounds bad enough, but it gets worse. NO2 and other NOx interact with water, oxygen, and other chemicals in the atmosphere to form acid rain. Acid rain harms sensitive ecosystems such as lakes and forests. The nitrate particles that result from NOx make the air hazy and difficult to see though. Picture those days in downtown Portland in the summer when we haven't had enough rain. Mt. Hood, usually our biggest selling point as a scenic destination, can be difficult to see.

And yet, as we attempt to stand and stare in awe of our majestic mountain, we may be breathing in the same thing obstructing our view (fortunately, we don't experience this type of air quality very often here). Breathing air with a high concentration of NO2 can irritate airways in the human respiratory system. Such exposures over short periods can aggravate respiratory diseases, particularly asthma, leading to respiratory symptoms (such as coughing, wheezing or difficulty breathing), hospital admissions and visits to emergency rooms. Longer exposures to elevated concentrations of NO2 may contribute to the development of asthma and potentially increase susceptibility to respiratory infections. People with asthma, as well as children and the elderly are generally at greater risk for the health effects of NO2.

Air Quality Index

As discussed in Chapter 2, the **Air Quality Index** (AQI) is a measurement for reporting daily air quality (Figure 8). It tells you how clean or polluted your air is, and what associated health effects might be a concern for you. The AQI focuses on health effects you may experience within a few hours or days after breathing polluted air. EPA calculates the AQI for five of the six major air pollutants with the exception of lead. Ground-level ozone and airborne particles are the two pollutants that pose the greatest threat to human health in this country.

Think of the AQI as a yardstick that runs from 0 to 500. The higher the AQI value, the greater the level of air pollution and the greater the health concern. For

Air Quality Index Levels	Numerical Value	Color	Meaning
Good	0 to 50	Green	Air quality is considered satisfactory, and air pollution poses little or no risk.
Moderate	51 to 100	Yellow	Air quality is acceptable; however, for some pollutants there may be a moderate health concern for a very small number of people who are unusually sensitive to air pollution.
Unhealthy for Sensitive Groups	101 to 150	Orange	Members of sensitive groups may experience health effects. The general public is not likely to be affected.
Unhealthy	151 to 200	Red	Everyone may begin to experience health effects; members of sensitive groups may experience more serious health effects.
Very Unhealthy	201 to 300	Purple	Health alert: everyone may experience more serious health effects.
Hazardous	301 to 500	Maroon	Health warnings of emergency conditions. The entire population is more likely to be affected.

Figure 8. AQI helps indicate dangerous conditions.

example, an AQI value of 50 represents good air quality with little potential to affect public health, while an AQI value over 300 represents hazardous air quality.

An AQI value of 100 generally corresponds to the national air quality standard for the pollutant, which is the level EPA has set to protect public health. AQI values below 100 are generally thought of as satisfactory. When AQI values are above 100, air quality is considered to be unhealthy, at least for certain sensitive groups of people, then for everyone as AQI values get higher.

Indoor Air Quality

It seems like a safe assumption that once inside the doors of your home, you would be safe from pollution. Yet this is not the case. **Indoor Air Quality** (IAQ) refers to the air quality within and around buildings and structures, especially as it relates to the health and comfort of building occupants. Understanding and controlling common pollutants indoors can help reduce your risk of indoor health concerns.

There are many ways for us to experience pollutants like carbon monoxide, nitrogen and sulfur dioxide, lead, and other chemicals at home. This is in addition to cigarette smoke, animal dander, mold, and many other elements that can cause discomfort and health hazards. Our water supply, ventilation systems and air ducts, fireplaces, and the general location of our homes can put us at greater risk.

Some health effects may show up shortly after a single exposure or repeated exposures to a pollutant. These include irritation of the eyes, nose, and throat, headaches, dizziness, and fatigue. Such immediate effects are usually short-term and treatable. Sometimes the treatment is simply eliminating the person's exposure to the source of the pollution, if it can be identified. Soon after exposure to some indoor air pollutants, symptoms of some diseases such as asthma may show up, be aggravated, or worsened.

Detecting Indoor Pollutants

Some health effects can be useful indicators of an indoor air quality problem, especially if they appear after a person moves to a new residence, remodels or refurnishes a home, or treats a home with pesticides. If you think that you have symptoms that may be related to your home environment, discuss them with your

The purpose of the AQI is to help you understand what local air quality means to your health. Under the Clean Air Act, the EPA sets limits on certain air pollutants, including on how much can be in the air anywhere in the United States. It also gives the EPA the authority to limit emissions of air pollutants coming from sources like chemical plants, utilities, and steel mills. Individual states or tribes may have stronger air pollution laws, but they may not have weaker pollution limits than those set by the EPA.

The likelihood of immediate reactions to indoor air pollutants depends on several factors including age and preexisting medical conditions. In some cases, whether a person reacts to a pollutant depends on individual sensitivity, which varies tremendously from person to person. Some people can become sensitized to biological or chemical pollutants after repeated or high level exposures.

Certain immediate effects are similar to those from colds or other viral diseases, so it is often difficult to determine if the symptoms are a result of exposure to indoor air pollution. For this reason, it is important to pay attention to the time and place symptoms occur. If the symptoms fade or go away when a person is away from the area, for example, an effort should be made to identify indoor air sources that may be possible causes. Some effects may be made worse by an inadequate supply of outdoor air coming indoors or from the heating, cooling or humidity conditions prevalent indoors.

Other health effects from may show up either years after exposure has occurred or only after long or repeated periods of exposure. These effects, which include some respiratory diseases, heart disease and cancer, can be severely debilitating or fatal. It is prudent to try to improve the indoor air quality in your home even if symptoms are not noticeable.

doctor or your local health department to see if they could be caused by indoor air pollution. You may also want to consult a board-certified allergist or an occupational medicine specialist for answers to your questions.

Another way to judge whether your home has or could develop indoor air problems is to identify potential sources of indoor air pollution. Although the presence of such sources does not necessarily mean that you have an indoor air quality problem, being aware of the type and number of potential sources is an important step toward assessing the air quality in your home.

A third way to decide whether your home may have poor indoor air quality is to look at your lifestyle and activities. Human activities, such as smoking cigarettes or open fires, can be significant sources of indoor air pollution. Finally, look for signs of problems with the ventilation in your home. Signs that can indicate your home may not have enough ventilation include:

- smelly or stuffy air

- moisture condensation on windows or walls

- dirty central heating and air cooling equipment

- and areas where books, shoes, or other items become moldy

To detect odors in your home, step outside for a few minutes, and then upon reentering your home, note whether odors are noticeable.

Measuring Radon Levels

Radon (Figure 9) forms when uranium in water, rocks, and soil begins to break down, releasing radon gas into the dirt beneath your home. This can seep in through cracks in walls, gaps in floors, space around pipes, fire-places and furnaces, water (usually well water), and even blow in through open windows.

In the United States, an estimated 21,000 people die from radon-related lung cancer every year. It is the second

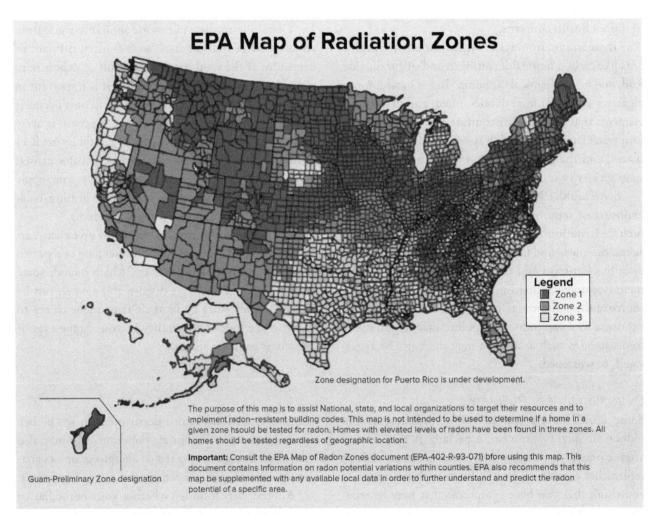

Figure 9. Radiation zones help shape policy around radon.

leading cause of lung cancer next to tobacco smoke and the primary cause for non-smokers.

The federal government recommends that you measure the level of radon in your home. Without measurements there is no way to tell whether radon is present because it is a colorless, odorless, radioactive gas.

Weatherizing Your Home

Winter rolls around and you begin to think of ways to keep the cold out and the heat in. In the summer, as temperatures rise, you go through the same process of trying to keep your inside cool and protected from the heat. While weatherization for temperature is underway, steps should also be taken to minimize pollution from sources inside the home. In addition, you should be alert to the emergence of signs of inadequate ventilation, such as stuffy air, moisture condensation on cold surfaces, or mold and mildew growth. Additional weatherization measures should not be undertaken until these problems have been corrected.

Inexpensive devices are available for measuring radon. EPA provides guidance as to risks associated with different levels of exposure and when the public should consider corrective action. There are specific mitigation techniques that have proven effective in reducing levels of radon in the home.

Weatherization generally does not cause indoor air problems by adding new pollutants to the air. (There are a few exceptions, such as caulking, that can sometimes emit pollutants.) However, measures such as installing storm windows, weather stripping, caulking, and blown-in wall insulation can reduce the amount of outdoor air infiltrating into a home. Consequently, after weatherization, concentrations of indoor air pollutants from sources inside the home, such as radon, can increase. This is why being alert to signs of trouble and checking the radon levels of your home is important.

Acid Deposition (Acid Rain)

Acid rain, or acid deposition, is a broad term that includes any form of precipitation with acidic components, such as sulfuric or nitric acid that fall to the ground from the atmosphere in wet or dry forms. This can include rain, snow, fog, hail or even dust that is acidic.

Acid rain results when sulfur dioxide (SO2) and nitrogen oxides (NOX) are emitted into the atmosphere and transported by wind and air currents. The SO2 and NOX react with water, oxygen and other chemicals to form sulfuric and nitric acids. These then mix with water and other materials before falling to the ground.

Wet deposition is what we most commonly think of as acid rain. The sulfuric and nitric acids formed in the atmosphere fall to the ground mixed with rain, snow, fog, or hail.

Acidic particles and gases can also deposit from the atmosphere in the absence of moisture as dry deposition. The acidic particles and gases may deposit to surfaces (water bodies, vegetation, buildings) quickly or may form larger particles that can be harmful to human health. When the accumulated acids are washed off a surface by the next rain, this acidic water flows over and through

the ground, and can harm plants and wildlife, such as insects and fish.

The amount of acidity in the atmosphere that deposits to earth through dry deposition depends on the amount of rainfall an area receives. For example, in desert areas the ratio of dry to wet deposition is higher than an area that receives several inches of rain each year.

When acid deposition is washed into lakes and streams, it can cause some to turn acidic (Figure 10). This sounds like it would burn our skin. But walking in acid rain, or even swimming in a lake affected by acid rain, is no more dangerous to humans than walking in normal rain or swimming in non-acidic lakes. For humans, it's the particles in the air that matter.

Acid rain has many ecological effects, but its impact on lakes, streams, wetlands, and other aquatic environments is the greatest. It increased acid levels in the water and causes them to absorb the aluminum that makes its way from soil into lakes and streams. Our water systems contain many creatures not suited to this acidic environment. It becomes toxic to crayfish, clams, fish, and other aquatic animals.

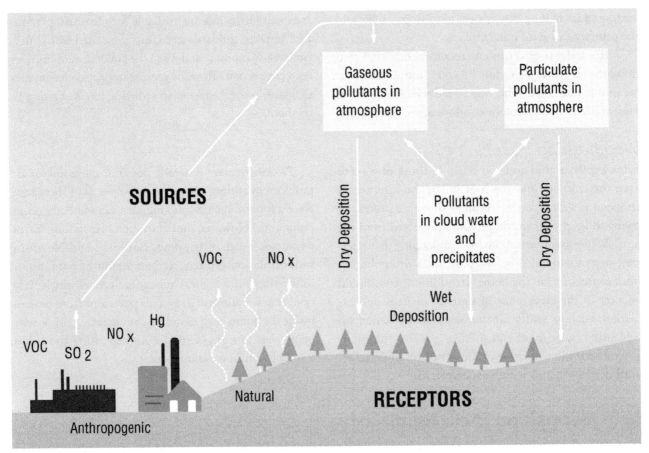

Figure 10. How acid rain forms.

Measuring Acid Rain

Acid rain is measured by its acidity and alkalinity using a pH scale for which 7.0 is neutral. The lower a substance's pH (less than 7), the more acidic it is. The higher a substance's pH (greater than 7), the more alkaline it is. Normal rain has a pH of about 5.6 — it is slightly acidic because carbon dioxide (CO_2) dissolves into it forming weak carbonic acid. Acid rain usually has a pH between 4.2 and 4.4.

Preventing Acid Rain

Reducing the amount of acid rain means first reducing the amount of sulfur dioxide in the air. Can we do it? Scientists believe so and are at work coming up with new methods, ways to let science and technology help us solve the problem. For example, scientists are working to develop a coal that contains less sulfur or a method to "wash" the coal to remove some of the sulfur. Forms of alternative energy and technology also provide hope in the form of:

Fossil fuel reduction — The use of renewable energy, such as wind and solar power

Cleaner cars — Manufacturers have been improving methods for reducing emissions for many years now with good success. Some are now looking toward cleaner fuels and power sources as well, such as bio-fuels, natural gas, hydrogen, and electricity.

The Ozone Layer

The **ozone layer** is an important atmospheric layer in the stratosphere that protects the Earth's surface (and everything on it) from harmful solar radiation. It's like the Earth's sunscreen. Plants, animals, humans — we all need protection from the sun. In areas of human population where ozone depletion has been more severe, instances of deadly skin cancers, like malignant melanoma, are much higher than normal (Figure 11). This is because ozone layer depletion increases the amount of Ultraviolet B rays (UVB) that reaches the Earth's surface. UVB has been linked to the development of cataracts, a clouding of the eye's lens.

Atmospheric ozone has two effects on the temperature balance of the Earth. It absorbs solar ultraviolet radiation, which heats the stratosphere. It also absorbs infrared radiation emitted by the Earth's surface, effectively trapping heat in the troposphere. Therefore, the climate impact of changes in ozone concentrations varies with the altitude at which these ozone changes occur.

The major ozone losses that have been observed in the lower stratosphere due to the human-produced chlorine- and bromine-containing gases have a cooling effect on the Earth's surface. On the other hand, the ozone increases that are estimated to have occurred in the troposphere (the lowest region) because of surface-pollution gases have a warming effect on the Earth's surface, thereby contributing to the "greenhouse" effect.

Carbon dioxide concentrations are significant contributors to this problem. However, chlorofluorocarbons (CFCs), chemicals found mainly in spray aerosols, are the primary culprits in ozone layer breakdown. When CFCs reach the upper atmosphere, they are exposed to ultraviolet rays. This causes them to break down into substances that include chlorine. The chlorine reacts with the oxygen atoms in ozone and rips apart the ozone molecule. According to the EPA, one atom of chlorine can destroy more than a hundred thousand ozone molecules. In areas where the sun shines for significant parts of the day, such as the Antarctic, the ozone layer is very thin. This is what we like to call a "hole in the ozone layer."

Industrialized countries like the US and Europe are responsible for about 90 percent of CFCs currently in the atmosphere. These countries banned CFCs by 1996, and the amount of chlorine in the atmosphere is falling now. Scientists estimate it will take another 50 years for chlorine levels to return to their natural levels.

Continued declines in ozone depleting substance emissions are expected to result in a near complete recovery of the ozone layer near the middle of the twenty-first century. These substances take a long time to be removed through natural processes, but we are seeing improvement.

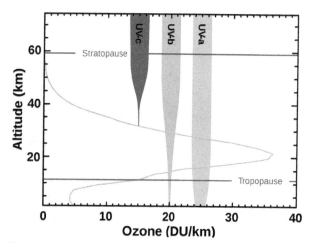

Figure 11. Ozone Altitude UV graph.

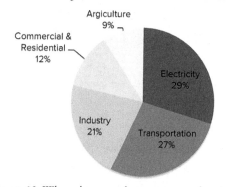

Figure 12. Where does greenhouse gas come from?

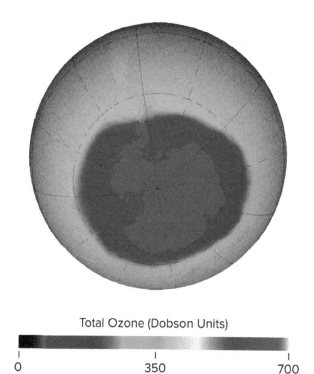

Figure 13. The ozone layer hole over the south pole.

Total Emissions in 2015 by Sector

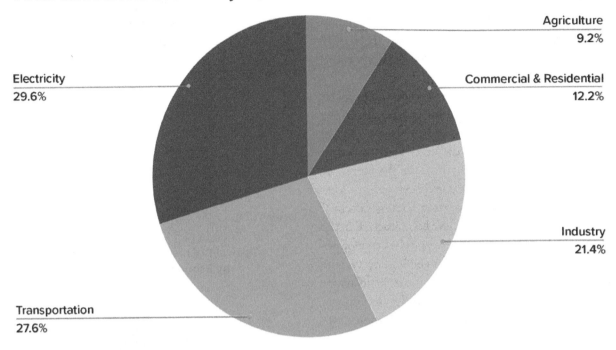

Figure 14. CO_2 emissions from different sources.

Climate Change

Climate change is occurring as we speak. The US and the world are warming, global sea level is rising, and some types of extreme weather events are becoming more frequent and more severe. These changes have already resulted in a wide range of impacts across every region of the country and many sectors of the economy. This change has the potential to affect human health in a number of ways, according to the World Health Organization. The changing seasonal nature of our environment through the global warming process, for example, could encourage certain infectious diseases, disturb food-producing ecosystems, and increase the frequency of extreme weather events, such as hurricanes.

Earth-orbiting satellites and other technological advances have enabled scientists to see the big picture, collecting many different types of information about our planet and its climate on a global scale. This body of data, collected over many years, reveals the signals of a changing climate.

The heat-trapping nature of carbon dioxide and other gases (the result of pollutants) was demonstrated in the mid-19th century. Their ability to affect the transfer of infrared energy through the atmosphere is the scientific

basis of many instruments flown by NASA. There is no question that increased levels of greenhouse gases must cause the Earth to warm in response (Figure 14).

The current warming trend is of particular significance because most of it is extremely likely (greater than 95% probability) to be the result of human activity since the mid-20th century and proceeding at a rate that is unprecedented.

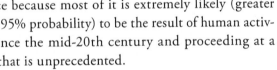

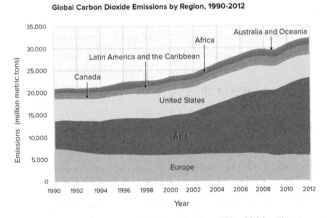

This figure shows carbon dioxide emissions from 1990 to 2012 for different regions of the world. These totals do not include emissions or sinks related to land–use change or forestry. Inclusion of land–use change and forestry would increase the apparent emissions from some regions while decreasing the emissions from others.

Figure 15. Where does CO_2 come from?

The planet's average surface temperature has risen about 2.0 degrees Fahrenheit (1.1 degrees Celsius) since the late nineteenth century, a change driven largely by increased carbon dioxide and other human-made emissions into the atmosphere. Most of the warming occurred in the past 35 years, with 16 of the 17 warmest years on record occurring since 2001. Not only was 2016 the warmest year on record, but eight of the 12 months that make up the year — from January through September, with the exception of June — were the warmest on record for those respective months.

U.S. GHG Emissions Flow Chart
Sector/IPCC Reporting category

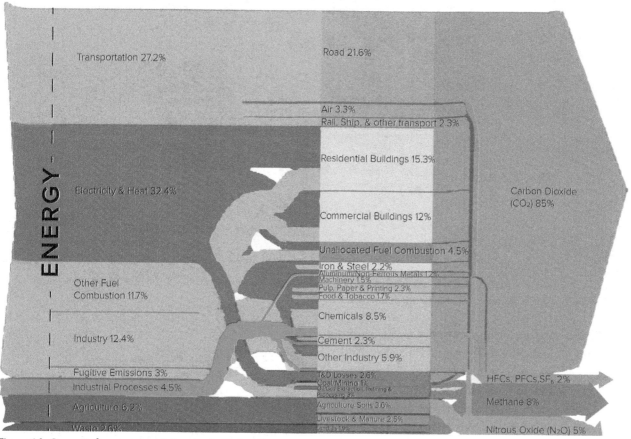

Figure 16. Sources of ozone gas emissions in the United States.

Effects of Climate Change

Global climate change has already had observable effects on the environment. Glaciers have shrunk, ice on rivers and lakes is breaking up earlier, plant and animal ranges have shifted and trees are flowering sooner. Effects that scientists had predicted are now occurring — loss of sea ice, accelerated sea level rise, and longer, more intense heat waves. We've already seen a number of alarming short-term effects of global warming (Figure 17), which will develop into harmful long-term effects if left untreated.

Global sea level rose about eight inches in the last century and it is increasing at a stronger rate. The oceans have absorbed much of the increased heat, with the top 700 meters (about 2,300 feet) of ocean showing warming of 0.302 degrees Fahrenheit since 1969.

The Greenland and Antarctic ice sheets have decreased in mass. Data from NASA's equipment shows Greenland lost 150 to 250 cubic kilometers of ice per year between 2002 and 2006, while Antarctica lost about 152 cubic kilometers between 2002 and 2005.

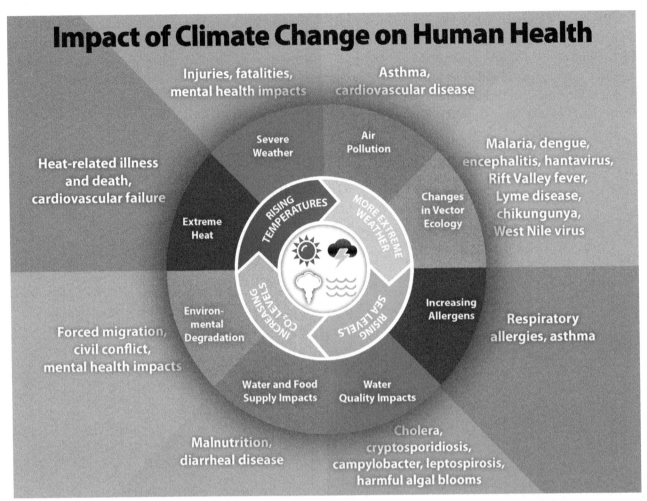

Figure 17. Climate change impacts human health in several ways.

Glaciers are retreating almost everywhere around the world — including in the Alps, Himalayas, Andes, Rockies, Alaska and Africa. Annual glacial melt is an important source of fresh water for drinking and agriculture. Without this melt, droughts are longer and more frequent. Satellite observations reveal that the amount of spring snow cover in the Northern Hemisphere has decreased over the past five decades and that the snow is melting earlier (Figure 18), which could have a similar impact over the long run.

Long-Term Impact

If we continue to ignore the problem, we can expect the situation to get much worse. Scientists have high confidence that global temperatures will continue to rise for decades to come, largely due to greenhouse gases produced by human activities. The Intergovernmental Panel on Climate Change (IPCC), which includes

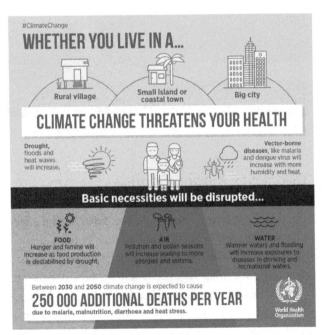

Figure 18. How climate change impacts you.

more than 1,300 scientists from the United States and other countries, forecasts a temperature rise of 2.5 to 10 degrees Fahrenheit over the next century.

Global climate is projected to continue to change over this century and beyond. The magnitude of climate change beyond the next few decades depends primarily on the amount of heat-trapping gases emitted globally, and how sensitive the Earth's climate is to those emissions. Because human-induced warming is superimposed on a naturally varying climate, the temperature rise has

not been, and will not be, uniform or smooth across the country or over time.

However, the damages are likely to be significant. We can expect to see:

- More severe droughts and more frequent heat waves
- More intense and frequent hurricanes
- Continued rising of sea level globally along with increased flooding in many regions.

Impact on Human Health

When you live in an inhospitable environment, you can experience negative effects. It may sound cliché, but the Earth really is our home. Climate change is no exception. The World Health Organization suggests:

- Climate change affects the social and environmental determinants of health — clean air, safe drinking water, sufficient food, and secure shelter.
- Between 2030 and 2050, climate change is expected to cause approximately 250,000 additional

deaths per year, from malnutrition, malaria, diarrhea, and heat stress.

- The direct damage costs to health (i.e. excluding costs in health-determining sectors such as agriculture and water and sanitation), is estimated to be between $2–4 billion/year by 2030.
- Areas with weak health infrastructure — mostly in developing countries — will be the least able to cope without assistance to prepare and respond.

Solutions to Air Pollution and Reducing the Threat of Global Warming

Climate change is one of the most complex issues facing us today. It involves many dimensions — science, economics, society, politics and moral and ethical questions. It is a global problem, felt on local scales that will be around for decades and centuries to come. Carbon dioxide, the heat-trapping greenhouse gas that has driven recent global warming, lingers in the atmosphere for hundreds of years, and the planet (especially the oceans) takes a while to respond to warming. So even if we stopped emitting all greenhouse gases today, global warming and climate change will continue to affect future generations. In this way, humanity is "committed" to some level of climate change.

How much climate change? NASA indicates that will be determined by how our emissions continue and also exactly how our climate system responds to those emissions. Despite increasing awareness of climate change, our emissions of greenhouse gases continue on a relentless rise. In 2013, the daily level of carbon dioxide in the atmosphere surpassed 400 parts per million for the first time in human history. The last time levels were that high was about three to five million years ago, during

the Pliocene era.

Because we are already committed to some level of climate change, responding to climate change involves a two-pronged approach:

- Reducing emissions of and stabilizing the levels of heat-trapping greenhouse gases in the atmosphere ("mitigation")
- Adapting to the climate change already in the play ("adaptation")

Mitigation involves reducing the flow of heat-trapping greenhouse gases into the atmosphere, either by reducing sources of these gases (for example, the burning of fossil fuels for electricity, heat, or transport) or enhancing the "sinks" that accumulate and store these gases (such as the oceans, forests, and soil). The goal of mitigation is to avoid significant human interference with the climate system, and stabilize levels to allow ecosystems to naturally adapt before food production is threatened.

Adaptation involves adjusting to actual or expected future climate. The goal is to reduce our vulnerability to the harmful effects of climate change (like sea-level encroachment, more intense extreme weather events, or food insecurity). It also encompasses making the most of any potential beneficial opportunities associated with climate change (for example, longer growing seasons or increased yields in some regions).

Mitigation of air pollution is a significant step. In the US, we have the EPA, which sets standards that no state can drop below (and every state is welcome to exceed), and we have agreements and treaties with other nations to help curb emissions. These global agreements are important to the goal of reducing pollutants because chemical and particulate matter in the air does not respect borders — a factory on the east coast of the US polluting the air around it is also polluting the air of nations on the other side of the Atlantic. These agreements have the following goals:

- Slowing depletion of the ozone layer
- Making changes in energy, transportation, and industrial practices
- Ending rapid deforestation (the destruction of animal and plant habitats for human use)
- Practicing sustainable development

Sustainable Development

In 2015, the United Nations and world leaders joined together to establish 17 sustainable development goals as part of their commitment to the protection of our planet and prosperity of its inhabitants. Their goals are focused on the climate change, as well as fighting poverty and inequalities around the world.

The concept of sustainability revolves around using renewable resources and conserving the ones we have. That means choosing products and methods that don't contribute to the problem. For the U.N. it means larger issues, such as a focus on how urban areas manage their infrastructure and transportation systems, the creation of

Things You Can Do from Your Couch	Save electricity — Plug appliances into a power strip and turn them off completely when not in use, including your computer. Save paper — Stop automated paper statements from utilities and banks and pay your bills online. No paper, no need for forest destruction. Don't print — See something online you need to remember? Jot it down in a notebook or a digital post-it note and spare the paper. Turn off the lights — Your TV or computer screen provides a cosy glow, so turn off other lights if you don't need them.
Things You Can Do from Home	Air dry — Let your hair and clothes dry naturally instead of running a machine. If you do wash your clothes, make sure the load is full. Take short showers — Bathtubs require gallons more water than a 5-10 minute shower. Eat less meat, poultry, and fish — More resources are used to provide meat than plants. Avoid pre-heating the oven. Unless you need a precise baking temperature, start heating your food right when you turn on the oven. Replace old appliances with energy efficient models and light bulbs
Things You Can Do Outside Your House	Shop local — Supporting neighbourhood businesses keeps people employed and helps prevent trucks from driving far distances. Shop Smart — plan meals, use shopping lists and avoid impulse buys. Don't succumb to marketing tricks that lead you to buy more food than you need, particularly for perishable items. Though these may be less expensive per ounce, they can be more expensive overall if much of that food is discarded. Buy Funny Fruit — many fruits and vegetables are thrown out because their size, shape, or color are not "right". Buying these perfectly good funny fruit, at the farmer's market or elsewhere, utilizes food that might otherwise go to waste. Eat sustainably — At restaurants ask if they serve sustainable seafood? Let your favorite businesses know that ocean-friendly seafood is a priority.

Figure 19. What you can do to lower your carbon footprint.

jobs that do not strain the land and its resources, increasing green spaces, and working toward cleaner energies.

Locally and at home, the concepts are the same. What can we do to lessen traffic and emissions? What can we do to preserve resources like water? How can we reduce waste and the harmful gasses that arise from it? The United Nations offers a list of tips as to how you can help as an individual (Figure 19). These include methods of conserving water, paper, electricity, and food as well as being smart with how much you purchase. For us, much of the issues come down to waste. We waste everything. We leave lights on in empty rooms, buy more food than we need, and throw away massive amounts of trash. Our waste means more production — of clothing, food, electricity, fuel, you name it! The more we manufacture and transport, the more resources used and the more greenhouse gases are emitted. Think about whether your actions lead to sustainability.

Another way individuals can make an impact is to start thinking about the internal and external spaces they encounter on a regular basis and to what types of pollution they may expose themselves to regularly. For example, what is the air quality inside your home (Figure 20)? In your workplace? What steps are necessary to improve this quality? Another thing to think about is how much time you spend outdoors and what you do while there. In

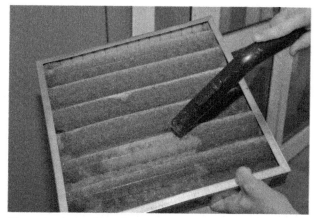

Figure 20. Air quality at home.

Oregon, for example, most of us enjoy hunting, fishing, and hundreds of other outdoor activities. A person who is an avid hunter, or who enjoys fishing, has a vested interest in the quality of the water and land because contaminants have a nasty habit of making it into the flesh of the animals we eat.

If all you want to do is go camping and enjoy the scenery, making yourself aware of what kinds of pollution negatively affects the experience is a good idea. What sorts of litter do you see on the trail? How clean is the air? Even people who aren't that interested in the wilderness can ask the same questions about their own neighborhoods.

How to Reduce and Reuse	Benefits of Reducing and Reusing
Buy used. You can find everything from clothes to building materials at specialized reuse centers and consignment shops. Often, used items are less expensive and just as good as new.	Prevents pollution caused by reducing the need to harvest new raw materials
Look for products that use less packaging. When manufacturers make their products with less packaging, they use less raw material. This reduces waste and costs. These extra savings can be passed along to the consumer. Buying in bulk, for example, can reduce packaging and save money.	Saves energy
Buy reusable over disposable items. Look for items that can be reused; the little things can add up. For example, you can bring your own silverware and cup to work, rather than using disposable items.	Reduces greenhouse gas emissions that contribute to global climate change
Maintain and repair products, like clothing, tires and appliances, so that they won't have to be thrown out and replaced as frequently.	Helps sustain the environment for future generations
Borrow, rent or share items that are used infrequently, like party decorations, tools or furniture.	Reduces the amount of waste that will need to be recycled or sent to landfills and incinerators
	Allows products to be used to their fullest extent

Figure 21. How and why to reduce and reuse.

After thinking about it, you will find that you can make minor changes to your habits that end up having positive environmental and health effects. You can choose not to drive to locations that are less than a couple of miles away, for example, which will cut down on auto emissions while giving you necessary exercise.

The list goes on, but you get the idea: a whole lot of people can do things that aren't really an inconvenience and make real, lasting changes (Figure 21).

Learn more about buying greener products at:
www.epa.gov/greenerproducts
For more tips on sustainability visit:
www.un.org/sustainabledevelopment/takeaction

Water Quality and Pollution

When the water in our rivers, lakes, and oceans becomes polluted, it can endanger wildlife, make our drinking water unsafe, and threaten the waters where we swim and fish. Safe and readily available water is more important for public health than we realize, going far beyond the faucet in our homes. We use it for food production, drinking, showering, cleaning, recreation, and any number of things. Think about how many times each day you access water in some way.

The United States enjoys one of the World's most reliable and safest supplies of drinking water. Congress passed the Safe Drinking Water Act (SDWA) in 1974 to protect public health by regulating public water systems. This requires EPA to establish and enforce standards that public drinking water systems must follow.

Over 151,000 public water systems provide drinking water to most Americans. Customers that are served by a public water system can contact their local water supplier and ask for information on contaminants in their drinking water, and are encouraged to request a copy of their Consumer Confidence Report. This report lists the levels of contaminants that have been detected in the water, including those by EPA, and whether the system meets state and EPA drinking water standards.

About 10 percent of people in the United States rely on water from private wells. Private wells are not regulated under the SDWA. People who use private wells need to take precautions to ensure their drinking water is safe.

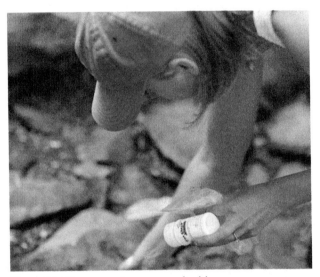

Figure 22. Clean water impacts your health.

The Great Pacific Garbage Patch

Later in the chapter you will learn about land pollution. Unfortunately, much of our land pollution now resides in the ocean, lodged in gyres — circular currents driven by the Earth's rotation. There are many gyres in our oceans, but the most famous (or notorious) is the Great Pacific Garbage Patch. This gyre holds an inestimable amount of trash, much of it plastic. Plastic does not biodegrade — ever. It only breaks down into smaller pieces of plastic (microplastics) that animals feed on, consuming toxins and deadly objects that they cannot rid from their systems. Ocean trash is a large threat to our eco-systems. To control this form of water pollution, we must first control land pollution.

Groundwater and Surface Water

The nation's freshwater supply, shaped by rainfall, snowmelt, runoff, and infiltration, is distributed unevenly across the landscape, throughout the seasons, and from year to year. In many areas, concerns are growing about the adequacy of the available ground and surface water supply and the quality of the water to support intended uses.

Groundwater is water lives and moves in the spaces in soil, sand, or cracks in the rocks known as **aquifers**. It supplies drinking water for 51% of the US population and 99% in rural areas. The largest portion of it is used to irrigate crops. Surface water is exactly that, water collected on the surface. This is water we can see in our lakes, streams, rivers, and reservoirs. Approximately 80% of all the water used in the US comes from surface water, to drink, irrigate crops, and support our power systems.

Groundwater may become surface water if it seeps into streams, lakes, and oceans.

Aquifers are typically made up of gravel, sand, sandstone, or fractured rock, like limestone (Figure 23). Water can move through these materials because they have large connected spaces that make them permeable. The pace at which groundwater travels depends upon the size of the spaces in the aquifers. When people dig wells for their homes, they dig into an aquifer to retrieve groundwater.

Aquifers and wells

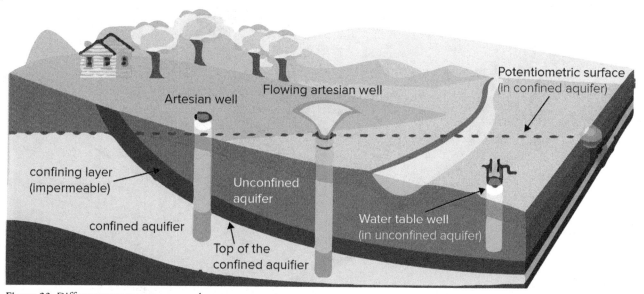

Figure 23. Different ways to access groundwater.

Threats to Groundwater

In areas where material above the aquifer is permeable, pollutants can easily sink into our groundwater supplies. Groundwater can be polluted by landfills, storage tanks, septic tanks, leaky underground gas tanks, factories, livestock farms, and from overuse of fertilizers and pesticides. This is referred to as **point source pollution**, which means that we can identify the source of the problem. If groundwater becomes polluted, it will no longer be safe to drink (Figure 24).

Nonpoint source pollution generally results from land runoff, precipitation, atmospheric deposition, drainage, seepage or hydrologic modification (alteration of stream flow by human activities). NPS pollution is caused by rainfall or snowmelt moving over and through the ground. As the runoff moves, it picks up and carries away natural and human-made pollutants (gasoline, oil, road salt, livestock waste, etc.), finally depositing them into lakes, rivers, wetlands, coastal waters, and ground waters (Figure 25).

Groundwater contamination is nearly always the result of human activity. In areas where population density is high and human use of the land is intensive, groundwater is especially vulnerable. Virtually any activity whereby chemicals or wastes may be released to the environment, either intentionally or accidentally, has the potential to pollute groundwater.

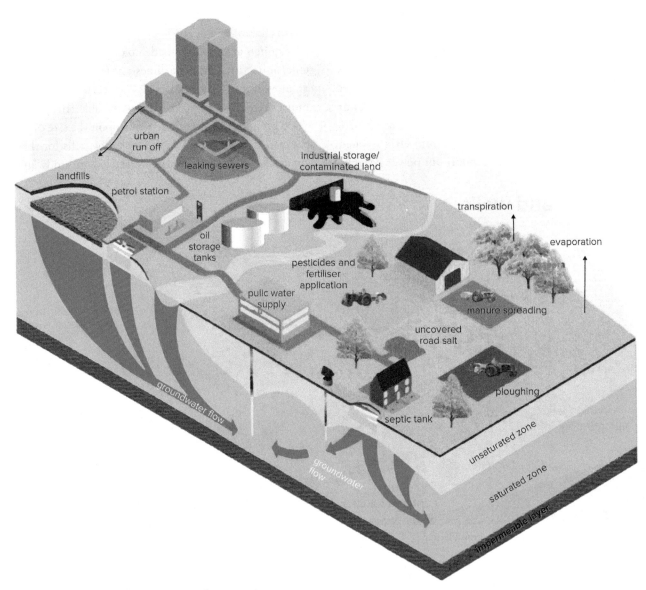

Figure 24. Hazards to clean water come from several sources.

Dangers of Contaminated Groundwater

Contamination of ground water can result in poor drinking water quality, loss of water supply, degraded surface water systems, high cleanup costs, high costs for alternative water supplies, and/or potential health problems. The consequences of contaminated ground water or degraded surface water are often serious. For example, estuaries that have been impacted by high nitrogen from ground water sources have lost critical shellfish habitats.

In terms of water supply, in some instances, ground water contamination is so severe that the water supply must be abandoned as a source of drinking water. In other cases, the ground water can be cleaned up and used again, if the contamination is not too severe and if the municipality is willing to spend a good deal of money. Follow-up water quality monitoring is often required

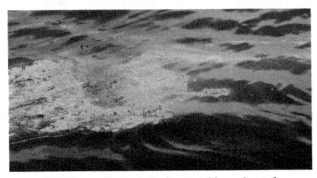

Figure 25. Water pollution isn't always visible on the surface.

for many years. Because ground water generally moves slowly, contamination often remains undetected for long periods of time. This makes cleanup of a contaminated water supply difficult, if not impossible. If a cleanup is undertaken, it can cost thousands to millions of dollars.

A number of microorganisms and thousands of synthetic chemicals have the potential to contaminate ground water. Drinking water containing bacteria and viruses can result in illnesses such as hepatitis, cholera, or giardiasis (infection of the small intestine). Methemoglobinemia or "blue baby syndrome," an illness affecting infants, can be caused by drinking water that is high in nitrates. **Benzene**, a component of gasoline, is a known human carcinogen. The serious health effects of lead are well known — learning disabilities in children; nerve, kidney, and liver problems along with pregnancy risks. Concentrations in drinking water of these and other substances are regulated by federal and state laws. Hundreds of other chemicals, however, are not yet regulated, and many of their health effects are unknown or not well understood.

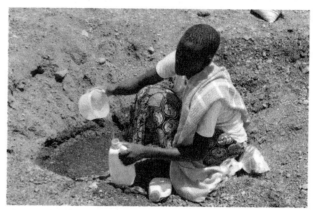

Figure 26. Clean water is not readily available everywhere.

Overuse

Where surface water, such as lakes and rivers, are scarce or inaccessible, groundwater supplies many of the hydrologic needs of people everywhere. In the United States, aside from being the main source of drinking water it provides over 50 billion gallons per day for agricultural needs. **Groundwater depletion**, a term often defined as long-term water-level declines caused by sustained groundwater pumping, is a key issue associated with groundwater use. Many areas of the United States are experiencing groundwater depletion.

The water stored in the ground can be compared to money kept in a bank account. If you withdraw money at a faster rate than you deposit new money you will eventually start having account-supply problems.

Pumping water out of the ground faster than it is replenished over the long-term causes similar problems. The volume of groundwater in storage is decreasing in many areas of the United States in response to pumping. Groundwater depletion is primarily caused by sustained groundwater pumping. Some of the negative effects of groundwater depletion:

- Drying up of wells
- Reduction of water in streams and lakes
- Deterioration of water quality
- Increased pumping costs
- Land subsidence (collapse of soil)

Is My Tap Water Safe to Drink?

Some people think tap water is always unsafe, and prefer to drink bottled water. The problem with that approach is that people are often wrong about the quality of their tap water and bottling water is often expensive and wasteful.

EPA standards require tap water to be safe to drink at the tap and this is usually the case. Unfortunately, unethical practices in Flint, Michigan and the failure of Portland Public Schools to update their plumbing have cast doubts on the safety of tap water. Luckily, it is easy to conduct a test to check water safety.

There are a couple of factors that may lead to valid questions about the quality of your tap water. One factor is the age of the infrastructure through which the water travels and whether there are contaminants in the water. For example, an older home may be on a system that is newer, but the pipes leading from the water main to the house may be lead. As we've already learned there is no safe amount of lead, which means checking for lead at the tap.

If the lead test is clear, the water is safe to drink. You can usually request a test kit from your water provider. If you are still worried, you can buy a water filter. Water filters can improve flavor and, when used properly, keep potential contaminants, like lead, out of the water (Figure 27).

The United States has one of the safest drinking water supplies in the world, at least in comparison to other countries. We are picky about our pollutants and have the knowledge and resources to deal with them when they are known. That doesn't mean that it doesn't happen, as we've seen. Ask your water department to provide you with a list of chemicals in your water and the levels at which they exist.

Here in Oregon, we pride ourselves on our clean water systems. In fact, we can barely get to work when it snows because of the regulations limiting salt and other chemicals on our roadways. Many water bureaus have increased regulations above and beyond the EPA checkpoints.

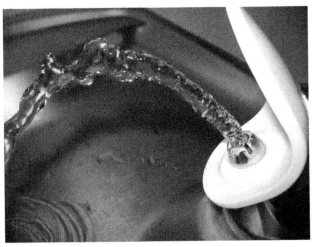

Figure 27. Public fountains are typically filtered for contaminants.

Protecting Groundwater

The following tips can help you establish a routine that works to protect our water supplies:

- Carefully follow instructions for the use, storage, and disposal of household chemicals.

- Check your vehicles for leaks. Leaks often go unnoticed and can contribute to groundwater contamination.

- Avoid overtreating your garden or lawn with fertilizers and other chemicals. Consider less toxic or natural alternatives.

- Water wisely. Avoid overwatering, especially after applying fertilizers and pesticides.

- Landscape with native plants. Natives are adapted to our local soils and climate and require less fertilizer, pesticides, and water.

- Never pour household chemicals or used motor oil down storm drains.

- Recycle or dispose of batteries properly to keep heavy metals out of the environment.

- Check underground storage tanks for leaks. Many older homes have underground heating oil tanks.

- Report chemical spills and illegal dumping. Call Oregon Emergency Response System at 1.800.452.0311 and Bureau of Environmental Services at 503.823.7180.

- Clean up pet waste.

Water Use Issues

A major issue with water pollution is that individuals use too much water, contributing to waste and extra energy being spent on recycling water unnecessarily. When water goes into the sewer system, it winds up at a treatment plant, where it is processed until it is safe to reintroduce the water into the water supply. This process is expensive and consumes a lot of energy, which is why it is important to use water frugally. Another concern is that we currently use potable water in our toilets, to water our lawns, and for a variety of other purposes that can produce water waste.

Reducing the Threat of Water Pollution

The EPA advocates a program they call P2 — Pollution prevention. This is any practice that reduces, eliminates, or prevents pollution at its source. P2, also known as "source reduction," is the ounce-of-prevention approach to waste management. Reducing the amount of pollution produced means less waste to control, treat, or dispose of. Less pollution means less hazards posed to public health and the environment, including our water supplies.

Pollution prevention approaches can be applied to all potential and actual pollution-generating activities, including those found in the energy, agriculture, federal, consumer, and industrial sectors. Prevention practices are essential for preserving wetlands, groundwater sources, and other critical ecosystems — areas in which we especially want to stop pollution before it begins.

In the energy sector, pollution prevention can reduce environmental damages from extraction, processing, transport and combustion of fuels. Pollution prevention approaches include increasing efficiency in energy use and the use of environmentally benign fuel sources.

In the agricultural sector, pollution prevention approaches include reducing the use of water and chemical inputs; adoption of less environmentally harmful pesticides or cultivation of crop strains with natural resistance to pests; and protection of sensitive areas.

In the industrial sector, examples of P2 practices include modifying a production process to produce less waste; using non-toxic or less toxic chemicals as cleaners, degreasers, and other maintenance chemicals; implementing water and energy conservation practices, and reusing materials such as drums and pallets rather than disposing of them as waste.

In homes and schools examples of P2 practices include using reusable water bottles instead of throw-aways; automatically turning off lights when not in use; repairing leaky faucets and hoses; switching to "green" cleaners.

Pollution prevention reduces both financial costs (waste management and cleanup) and environmental costs (health problems and environmental damage). Pollution prevention protects the environment by conserving and protecting natural resources while strengthening economic growth through more efficient production in industry and less need for households, businesses and communities to handle waste.

Global Protection

There are agencies that work on a global level to protect our water supplies. These include the Convention on the Protection and Use of Transboundary Watercourses and International Lakes (Water Convention), the World Health Organization/UNECE, and the Global Environmental Facility (GEF). These agencies and others work together to implement systems, lobby for new regulation, coordinate research, protect public health, and implement better systems aimed at cooperation among nations and agencies.

Area	Pollution Prevention Tips
Bathroom	Install a toilet dam or plastic bottle in your toilet tank. Install a water-efficient showerhead (2.5 gallons or less per minute). Take short showers and draw less water for baths. When you buy a new toilet, purchase a low flow model. Check your toilet for "silent" leaks by placing a little food coloring in the tank and seeing if it leaks into the bowl. Turn off water while brushing teeth and shaving.
Kitchen or Laundry	Compost your food scraps rather than using a garbage disposal in your sink. Keep a gallon of drinking water in the refrigerator rather than running the tap for cold water. Run your washing machine with a full load of clothes. Wash with warm water instead of hot, rinse with cold water instead of warm. Wash with cold water when you can. (When possible) hang your wash out to dry.
Outdoors	Install a drip-irrigation water system for valuable plants. Use drought-tolerant plants and grasses for landscaping and reduce grass-covered areas. Cut your grass at least three inches high to shade the roots, making it more drought tolerant; keep your mower sharp for the healthiest grass. Try to water only in the evening or very early morning to minimize evaporation. If you use porous pavement (gravel is a good example) instead of asphalt for driveways and walkways, the rain can recharge groundwater supplies instead of running off and contributing to erosion. Use a broom instead of a hose to clean off your driveway or sidewalk. Wash your car less often or wash it at a car wash where they clean and recycle the water. If you do wash your car at home, use a bucket of soapy water rather than running the hose. Keep a spring-loaded nozzle on the hose.

Figure 28. How to prevent pollution at home.

Land Pollution

Land pollution is the deterioration of the Earth's land surfaces, often directly or indirectly as a result of human activities and their misuse of resources. We know what this looks like. In fact, this is probably one form of pollution that needs very little definition. Much of it comes from waste in some form or another. Waste from garbage, pesticides, fertilizers, household products, and so on. It comes from us at home, from energy producers, manufacturing plants, farms, and other forms of industry. We dispose of it improperly and it ends up in the environment. We dispose of it properly and it still ends up in the environment, hopefully in a safer way. But this form of pollution is often right in front of us.

Solid and Hazardous Waste

Proper waste management is an essential part of society's public and environmental health. The Resource Conservation and Recovery Act (RCRA), passed in 1976, created the framework for America's hazardous and non-hazardous waste management programs. Materials regulated by RCRA are known as "solid wastes" and can also receive an additional classification of "hazardous" depending on the material.

Municipal Solid Waste and Its Common Components

Municipal solid waste (MSW) — more commonly known as trash or garbage — consists of everyday items we use and then throw away, such as product packaging, grass clippings, furniture, clothing, bottles, food scraps, newspapers, appliances, paint, and batteries. This comes from our homes, schools, hospitals, and businesses. This is our excess everything (Figure 29).

Global solid waste generation, if left unchecked, is likely to increase 70 percent by 2025, rising from more than 3.5 million tons per day in 2010 to more than six million tons per day. The waste from cities alone is already enough to fill a line of trash trucks 3,000 miles long every day. The global cost of dealing with all that trash is also rising. We spent $205 billion in 2010 and are expected to reach $375 billion by 2025, with the sharpest cost increases in developing countries.

In 2013, Americans generated about 254 million tons of trash and recycled and composted about 87 million tons of this material, equivalent to a 34.3% recycling rate. On average, we recycled and composted 1.51 pounds of our individual waste generation of 4.40 pounds per person per day (Figure 30).

That means that the average person generates over 1600 pounds per year. If that same person lived to be 80 years old, he would generate over 64 tons of trash in his lifetime! Americans produce a lot of waste.

Have you ever seen a picture of a landfill? Been to the dump? Seen where you trash went? It isn't a pretty sight. Out of all of the trash we generate, more than half ends up in landfills.

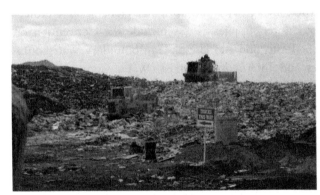

Figure 29. Managing waste is a major pollution issue.

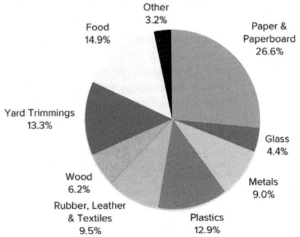

Figure 30. Most MSW can be recycled.

The Beauty of Landfills

As the industrial revolution revolved, we saw an increase in the amount of garbage produced. We tried letting pigs eat the trash, but that wasn't very practical. We tried piling it up outside of town, but the smell was awful and it was a breeding ground for disease. We tried burning it. That didn't work — we ended up with a lot of pollution and an inability to see the Los Angeles skyline. We went back to piling it up outside of town (or at least it used to be outside of town).

The landfills of today are different than the dumps of yesteryear. We go through a careful process of construction and maintenance in an attempt to keep the trash right where it is and as "sanitary" as possible. Essentially we bury it — dump it in a gigantic open area lined with several layers of protection and then carefully stack, level, and eventually cover the debris.

When MSW is first deposited in a landfill, it undergoes an aerobic (with oxygen) decomposition stage when little methane is generated. Then, typically within less than 1 year, anaerobic conditions are established and methane-producing bacteria begin to decompose the waste and generate methane.

Landfills are the third-largest source of human-related methane emissions in the United States, accounting for approximately 15.4 percent of these emissions in 2015. At the same time, methane emissions from landfills represent a lost opportunity to capture and use a significant energy resource.

Landfills have their merits, at least in the US where we seem to have space, but they also have their drawbacks. Despite careful engineering, they can leak liquids into the groundwater that can be toxic. Not all of the contents of the landfill completely degrade either. The process they undergo to engineer the waste often serves to preserve much of it rather than facilitate breakdown.

Are We Running Out of Space?

We use landfills because we don't have a better solution and, for now at least, we have the space. This will not always be the case. In many areas we have lots of room. In others, like New York City, we don't. Some cities are forced to haul their trash long distances, even to other states for disposal. This means more gas emission for transport and more opportunity for waste to end up everywhere but where it is supposed to (Figure 31).

Reusing and Donating Electronics	Preventing waste in the first place is preferable to any waste management option, including recycling. Donating used (but still operating) electronics for reuse extends the lives of valuable products and keeps them out of the waste stream for a longer period of time. Donating electronics allows schools, nonprofit organizations and lower-income families to obtain equipment that they otherwise could not afford. Businesses can also take advantage of tax incentives for donated computer equipment.
Recycling Electronics	If donation for reuse or repair is not a viable option, households and business can send their used electronics for recycling. Recycling electronics helps reduce pollution that would be generated while manufacturing a new product and the need to extract valuable and limited virgin resources. Electronic recycling also reduces the energy used in new product manufacturing.
Buying Green	Environmentally responsible electronics use involves not only proper end-of-life disposition of obsolete equipment, but also purchasing new equipment that has been designed with environmentally preferable attributes. Green electronics contain fewer toxic constituents. The use of recycled materials in new products promotes the following benefits: More energy efficient, more easily upgraded or disassembled, uses minimal packaging, offers leasing or take back options, meets performance criteria and shows they are more environmentally preferable.

Figure 31. E-waste is a serious pollution issue.

Hazardous Waste

Hazardous waste is a waste with properties that make it potentially dangerous or harmful to human health or the environment. The universe of hazardous wastes is large and diverse. Hazardous wastes can be liquids, solids, or contained gases. They can be the by-products of manufacturing processes, discarded used materials, or discarded unused commercial products, such as cleaning fluids (solvents) or pesticides. In regulatory terms, a hazardous waste is a waste that appears on one of the four RCRA hazardous wastes lists or that exhibits one of the four characteristics of a hazardous waste — ignitability, corrosivity, reactivity, or toxicity.

EPA developed a regulatory definition and process that identifies specific substances known to be hazardous and provides objective criteria for including other materials in the regulated hazardous waste universe. This identification process can be very complex, so EPA encourages generators of wastes to approach the issue using the series of questions described below:

Examples of Hazardous Waste include, but are not limited to:

Chemical wastes require special disposal methods because they present an immediate and long term threat to public health. Some sites in the US have experienced significant toxic threats and have had to be closed down for clean-up. These are called **Superfund** sites.

A Superfund site is any land in the United States that has been contaminated by hazardous waste and identified by the EPA as a candidate for cleanup because it poses a risk to human health and/or the environment. These sites are placed on the National Priorities List (NPL). EPA's Superfund program is responsible for cleaning up some of the nation's most contaminated land and responding to environmental emergencies, oil spills, and natural disasters. To protect public health and the environment, the Superfund program focuses on making a visible and lasting difference in communities, ensuring that these places are returned to livable, workable, areas.

Here are some examples of hazardous waste:

- Unused and surplus reagent grade chemicals

- Intermediates and byproducts generated from research & educational experiments

- Batteries

- Anything contaminated by chemicals

The Hazardous Waste Identification Process

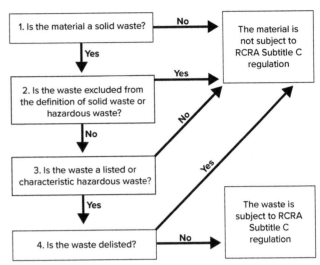

Figure 32. Flowchart used to identify hazardhous waste.

- Used oil of all types

- Spent solvents including water based

- Mercury containing items

- Photographic film processing solutions and chemicals

- Pesticides

- Non-returnable gas cylinders

- Non-empty aerosol cans

- Chemically contaminated sharps

- Finely divided powders

- Contaminated syringes, needles, GC syringes, razor blades, pasteur pipettes, pipette tips

- Equipment and apparatus containing hazardous waste

- Computer/electronic equipment

- Toner cartridges

- Ethylene glycol

- Paints - both oil and latex

- Fluorescent light bulbs

- Light ballasts

- Light ballasts

- Preserved specimens

- Custodial and industrial cleaners
- Uncured Resins(Phenolic, Epoxy, Styrene, etc.)
- Dye and glazes

- Degreasing solvents
- Brake/Transmission/Power Steering Fluids

Electronic Waste

So, you want a new phone? Again? Of course you do. We all do. There's a new one out each year and amazingly our old one just won't work as well as it used to. The problem is similar with computers, televisions, printers, and every other type of electronic gadget we own — planned obsolescence. They don't make them to last, partly because of money, and partly because technology is advancing at such a rapid pace that people *want* the new and improved items — your phone doesn't *need* to last because you will replace it anyway. But what happens to these electronics at the end of their lifecycle?

E-waste is a popular, informal name for electronic products nearing the end of their "useful life." Many of these products can be reused, refurbished, or recycled. Certain components of some electronic products contain materials that render them hazardous, depending on their condition and density (Figure 33).

E-waste is an emerging problem given the volumes of e-waste being generated and the content of both toxic and valuable materials in them. This fast growing waste stream is accelerating because the global market for personal computers (PC) is far from saturation and the average life span of a PC is decreasing rapidly. The life span of central processing units (CPU) had reduced from 4–6 years in

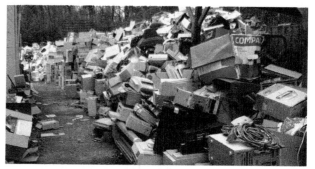

Figure 33. E-waste is common as new tech is created.

1997 to 2 years in 2005. Over the past two decades, the global market of electrical and electronic equipment (EEE) continues to grow exponentially, while the life span of those products becomes shorter and shorter. Predictably, the number of electrical devices will continue to increase on the global scale, and microprocessors will be used in ever increasing numbers in daily objects.

We cannot dispose of our e-waste in the same way as our MSW. If we do, not only are we throwing away precious metals — such as silver, gold, and palladium — that are used in the product, but we are also throwing toxic chemicals into the environment.

Resource Conservation

If you went to an elementary school in Oregon, you probably learned some version of the "Reduce, Reuse, Recycle" song. We on the west coast are fairly well educated in comparison to many parts of the nation. We are born and But we can always do more. Recycling and composting prevented 87.2 million tons of material away from being disposed in 2013, up from 15 million tons in 1980. This prevented the release of approximate-

ly 186 million metric tons of carbon dioxide equivalent into the air in 2013 — equivalent to taking over 39 million cars off the road for a year.

There are a lot of ways to minimize waste and a good first step is to avoid creating trash in the first place. This is what we call source reduction — starting at the very beginning of the chain of waste — and stopping it before it starts.

Reduce

We are all at a link in the chain. Making a new product requires a lot of materials and energy — raw materials must be extracted from the earth, and the product must be fabricated then transported to wherever it will be sold. This is one of the first links. You, the consumer,

can only do so much to control that step. Products need to be made and sold.

So, how do we reduce? For manufacturers, there are ways that reduction can take place. When was the last time you ordered something online and it came in a box

Environmental Protection Hierarchy

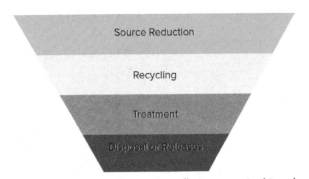

Figure 34. Environmental protection pollution prevention hierarchy.

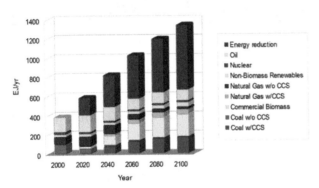

Figure 35. Environmental goals into the future.

6 times too big? Or, even worse, a box inside a box filled with non-recyclable packaging materials (Styrofoam, for example)? The companies that make your products do have the ability to reduce, significantly (Figure 36).

Practicing the three R's helps keep items out of landfills, can save you money, and keep harmful chemicals and pollutants out of the environment. So how do we reduce at home? This is the main link in the chain that we can break.

Buy what you need — Check your pantry and make a shopping list before you buy

Refuse — This could be the fourth "R" in the song. Say no to silly freebies, single-use plastics, and things you know you won't use or that will pose a disposal problem.

Be thrifty — If you have six scarves that you never wear, do you need another?

Speak up — Tell manufacturers what you think about their wasteful packaging. If they don't get the point, use a different vendor.

Reuse

This is a broad term with no one distinct definition. There are many ways that an item can be reused depending on the context. At home, there are some common items that frequently pose a problem and some easy ways to handle them:

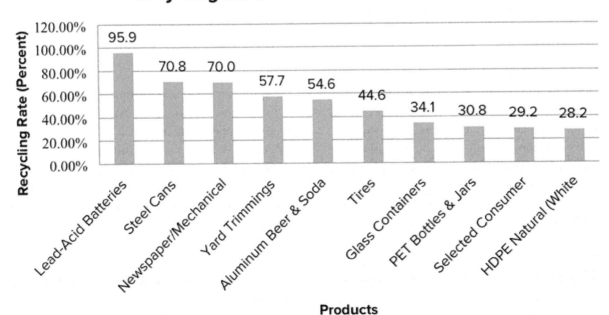

Figure 36. Some products are recycled more frequently than others.

- Buy reused or recycled products when you can. This keeps the 3R chain intact.

- Donate your old items to local churches, community centers, thrift stores, schools and nonprofit organizations. Many may accept a variety of donated items, including used books, working electronics and unneeded furniture.

- Repurpose your unwanted items. Consider how you might utilize an item as something else. Empty coffee cans, for example, make good storage containers.

- Carry your own reusable shopping bags to the store to eliminate the need for paper or plastic.

Recycle

Recycling is the process of collecting and processing materials that would otherwise be thrown away as trash and turning them into new products. Recycling can benefit your community and the environment by reducing the amount of waste in landfills, conserving natural resources, and reducing emissions involved in the manufacturing and transportation of new products. Familiar items that can be recycled include paper, cardboard, aluminum, tin, glass, and most plastic.

Recycling includes the three steps, which create a continuous loop, represented by the familiar recycling symbol.

Step 1: Collection and Processing — There are several methods for collecting recyclables, including curbside collection, drop-off centers, and deposit or refund programs. After collection, recyclables are sent to a recovery facility to be sorted, cleaned and processed into materials that can be used in manufacturing. Recyclables are bought and sold just like raw materials would be, and prices go up and down depending on supply and demand in the United States and the world.

Step 2: Manufacturing — More and more of today's products are being manufactured with recycled content. Common household items that contain recycled materials include paper, plastic, aluminum, and glass (many of the things we turn in curbside). Recycled materials are also used in new ways such as recovered glass in asphalt to pave roads or recovered plastic in carpeting and park benches.

Step 3: Purchasing New Products Made from Recycled Materials — You help close the recycling loop by buying new products made from recycled materials. As mentioned above, there are thousands of products that contain recycled content. When you go shopping, look for products that can be easily recycled, or are made from recycled content.

Reducing Food Waste

Most people don't realize how much food they throw away every day — from uneaten leftovers to spoiled produce. About 95 percent of the food we throw away ends up in landfills or combustion facilities. In 2014, we disposed of more than 38 million tons of food waste. By managing food sustainably and reducing waste, we can help businesses and consumers save money, provide a bridge in our communities for those who do not have enough to eat, and conserve resources for future generations.

As mentioned earlier, one easy way is to plan ahead. Plan a menu for the week, check your pantry, and make a list. Plan your menu to use the leftovers from each meal for another meal, perhaps one you can freeze. Avoid buying items in bulk that you've never tried before or that you know you can't consume, even if it's cheaper. The goal is to buy only what you need.

Make use of your leftovers and food that's about to go bad. If your bananas are about to rot, make banana bread or put them in the freezer for smoothies. Have leftover pot roast? Make soup! Think before you put something in the trash.

Composting

Compost is organic material that can be added to soil to help plants grow. Food scraps and yard waste currently make up 20 to 30 percent of what we throw away, and should be composted instead. Making compost keeps these materials out of landfills where they take up space and release methane, a potent greenhouse gas (Figure 37).

All composting requires three basic ingredients:

Browns — This includes materials such as dead leaves, branches, and twigs.

Greens — This includes materials such as grass clippings, vegetable waste, fruit scraps, and coffee grounds.

Water — Having the right amount of water, greens, and browns is important for compost development.

Your compost pile should have an equal amount of browns to greens. You should also alternate layers of organic materials of different-sized particles. The brown materials provide carbon for your compost, the green materials provide nitrogen, and the water provides moisture to help break down the organic matter.

If you don't have the discipline to compost on your own, many waste companies offer composting services.

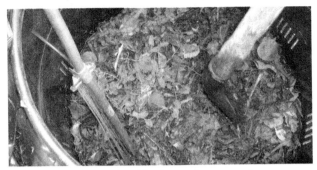

Figure 37. Manage yard and food waste by composting.

All you need to do is save the waste and put it in the proper bin at the curb. They'll do the rest.

Energy Recovery

We can also use garbage to create energy. **Energy recovery** from the combustion of municipal solid waste is a key part of the non-hazardous waste management hierarchy, which ranks various management strategies from most to least environmentally preferred. Energy recovery ranks below source reduction and recycling/reuse but above treatment and disposal.

Confined and controlled burning, known as combustion, can not only decrease the volume of solid waste destined for landfills, but can also recover energy from the waste burning process. This generates a renewable energy source and reduces carbon emissions by offsetting the need for energy from fossil sources and reduces methane generation from landfills.

The Mass Burn Process

At an MSW combustion facility, the waste is placed into a combustion chamber to be burned. The heat released from burning converts water to steam, which is then sent to a turbine generator to produce electricity.

The remaining ash is collected and taken to a landfill where a high-efficiency baghouse filtering system captures particulates. As the gas stream travels through these filters, more than 99 percent of particulate matter is removed. The facility transports the ash residue to an enclosed building where it is loaded into covered, leak-proof trucks and taken to a landfill designed to protect against groundwater contamination. Ash residue from the furnace can be processed for removal of recyclable scrap metals.

Other Environmental Health Concerns

Since we have learned the environmentally damaging effects of our 19th and 20th century industrial practices and started seeking solutions, we do so with a sense of caution. What technology that saves us from toxic air today is the problem we need to solve tomorrow? This question is most often raised when we talk about nuclear power.

Nuclear Power

Many power plants, including **nuclear power** plants, heat water to produce electricity. These power plants use steam from heated water to spin large turbines that generate electricity. Nuclear power plants use heat produced during nuclear fission to heat water (Figure 38).

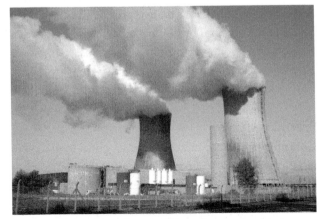

Figure 38. Steam rising from cooling nuclear power plants.

In **nuclear fission**, atoms are split apart to form smaller atoms, releasing energy. Fission takes place inside the reactor of a nuclear power plant. At the center of the reactor is the core, which contains uranium fuel. The uranium fuel is formed into ceramic pellets. Each ceramic pellet produces roughly the same amount of energy as 150 gallons of oil. These energy-rich pellets are stacked end to end in 12-foot metal fuel rods. A bundle of fuel rods, sometimes hundreds, is called a fuel assembly. A reactor core contains many fuel assemblies.

The heat produced during nuclear fission in the reactor core is used to boil water into steam, which turns the turbine blades. As the turbine blades turn, they drive generators that make electricity. Afterward, the steam is cooled back into water in a separate structure at the power plant called a cooling tower. The water can then be reused.

Nuclear power plants generate about 20% of US electricity. The United States has 99 nuclear reactors at 61 operating nuclear power plants located in 30 states. Thirty-five of the plants have 2 or more reactors. Nuclear power has supplied about one-fifth of annual US electricity since 1990.

The United States generates more nuclear power than any other country. Of the 31 countries in the world that have commercial nuclear power plants, the United States has the most nuclear capacity and generation. France has the second-highest nuclear electricity generation and obtains about 75% of its total electricity from nuclear energy. Fifteen other countries generate more than 20% of their electricity from nuclear power.

Nuclear power reactors do not produce direct carbon dioxide emissions. Unlike fossil fuel-fired power plants, nuclear reactors do not produce air pollution or carbon dioxide while operating. However, the processes for mining and refining uranium ore and making reactor fuel all require large amounts of energy. Nuclear power plants also have large amounts of metal and concrete, which require large amounts of energy to manufacture. If fossil fuels are used for mining and refining uranium ore, or if fossil fuels are used when constructing the nuclear power plant, then the emissions from burning those fuels could be associated with the electricity that nuclear power plants generate.

Nuclear energy produces radioactive waste. The primary environmental concern related to nuclear power is the creation of radioactive wastes such as uranium mill tailings, and spent (used) reactor fuel, among others. These materials can remain radioactive and dangerous to human health for thousands of years. Radioactive wastes are subject to special regulations that govern their handling, transportation, storage, and disposal to protect human health and the environment.

The radioactivity of nuclear waste decreases over time through a process called radioactive decay. The amount of time it takes for the radioactivity of material to decrease to half its original level is called the radioactive half-life. Radioactive waste with a short half-life is often stored temporarily before disposal to reduce potential radiation doses to workers who handle and transport the waste. This storage system also reduces the radiation levels at disposal sites.

By volume, most of the waste related to the nuclear power industry has a relatively low level of radioactivity. High-level radioactive waste consists of irradiated or spent nuclear reactor fuel (i.e., fuel that is no longer useful for producing electricity). The spent reactor fuel is in a solid form, consisting of small fuel pellets in long metal tubes called rods.

Spent Reactor Fuel Storage and Reactor Decommissioning

Spent reactor fuel assemblies are highly radioactive, and initially, must be stored in specially designed pools of water. The water cools the fuel and acts as a radiation shield. Spent reactor fuel assemblies can also be stored in specially designed dry storage containers. An increasing number of reactor operators now store their older spent fuel in dry storage facilities using special outdoor concrete or steel containers with air cooling. The United States does not currently have a permanent disposal facility for high-level nuclear waste.

When a nuclear reactor stops operating, it must be decommissioned. Decommissioning involves safely removing from service the reactor and all equipment that has become radioactive and reducing radioactivity to a level that permits other uses of the property. This is largely where controversy arises. Once a reactor is decommissioned, what do we do with it? Are there harmful effects to the neighborhoods near these radioactive plants?

Nuclear Reactor Safety and Security Features

An uncontrolled nuclear reaction in a reactor could result in widespread contamination of air and water. The risk of this happening at nuclear power plants in the United States is considerably small because of the diverse and redundant barriers and numerous safety systems in place at nuclear power plants, the training and skills of the reactor operators, testing and maintenance activities, and the regulatory requirements and oversight of the US Nuclear Regulatory Commission. A large area surrounding nuclear power plants is restricted and guarded by armed security teams. US reactors also have containment vessels that are designed to withstand extreme weather events and earthquakes.

Despite this, we have seen other countries sustain large loss due to problems with their reactors. This combined with controversy over whether or not people living near the reactors are exposed to any level of radioactivity makes them a hot topic of debate (you need only drive down the Pacific Coast Highway toward San Diego to see San Onofre sitting empty, quietly situated on the beach between cozy little cities). When decommissioned reactors sit idly, people get nervous. The future of nuclear energy will likely depend on how the nation decides to store and protect waste long-term and how comfortable they can make the community.

Radiation

We are exposed to a variety of naturally-occurring radiation in the environment that has an effect on our health. Energy emitted from a source is generally referred to as radiation. Examples include heat or light from the sun, microwaves from an oven, X rays, and gamma rays from radioactive elements. The World Health Organization defines **ionizing radiation** as radiation with enough energy so that during an interaction with an atom, it can remove tightly bound electrons from the orbit of an atom, causing the atom to become charged or ionized.

Ionizing radiation has sufficient energy to cause chemical changes in cells and damage them. Some cells may die or become abnormal, either temporarily or permanently. By damaging the genetic material (DNA) contained in the body's cells, radiation can cause cancer. Fortunately, our bodies are extremely efficient at repairing cell damage.

A very large amount of radiation exposure (acute exposure) can cause sickness or even death within hours or days. Such acute exposures are extremely rare.

Chronic and Acute Exposure

In general, the amount and duration of radiation exposure affects the severity or type of health effect. There are two broad categories of health effects: chronic (long-term) and acute (short-term).

Chronic exposure is continuous or intermittent exposure to radiation over a long period of time. With chronic exposure, there is a delay between the exposure and the observed health effect. These effects can include cancer and other health outcomes such as benign tumors, cataracts, and potentially harmful genetic changes (see Chapter 9). Current studies are not yet clear as to whether doses of low-level radiation causes cancer. Experts disagree over the exact definition and effects of "low dose," US

radiation protection standards are based on the premise that any radiation dose carries some risk, and that risk increases directly with dose.

Background radiation is present on Earth at all times. The majority of background radiation occurs naturally from minerals and a small fraction comes from man-made elements, such as nuclear weapons testing and medical procedures. Naturally occurring radioactive minerals in the ground, soil, water, and your body produce background radiation, as does cosmic radiation from outer space (people at higher altitudes are exposed to more cosmic radiation).

Radioactive Material in the Earth and in Our Bodies

Uranium and thorium naturally found in the earth are called primordial (existing since the formation of the solar system, naturally occurring). Trace amounts of uranium, thorium and their decay products can be found everywhere. Traces of radioactive materials can be found in the body, mainly naturally occurring potassium-40. Potassium-40 is found in the food, soil, and water we ingest, allowing it to be absorbed into our bodies.

48% of the average American's dose of radiation, however, comes from medical procedures. This total does not include the dose from radiation therapy used in the treatment of cancer, which is typically many times larger.

UV Radiation

Ultraviolet radiation is ubiquitous in sunlight and comes in three main types: UV-A, UV-B, and UV-C. Our atmosphere protects us from UV-C, which quickly damages cells, and is used to decontaminate surfaces and kill germs on food. UV-A causes premature skin aging, damages cells at the genetic level, and causes melanin release, which is a relatively ineffective defense against sun exposure. UV-A damage is what causes a sun tan. People who purposefully expose themselves to UV-A via tanning beds are 75% more likely to develop melanoma, a cancer which metastasizes quickly. UV-B causes sunburn, which is a defense response to UV-B damage that is similar to what happens with an open wound. The body reacts to UV-B damage as if it is an infection, which is why the skin becomes inflamed and puffy — blood and white blood cells are rushing to the surface of the skin.

The best defense against UV-A and UV-B radiation damage is to minimize exposure to the sun by staying out of it, wearing sun-protective clothing, and by correctly applying broad spectrum sunscreen with a 30+ SPF rating. If the label on the sunscreen does not indicate it is broad spectrum, then it will only protect against UV-B radiation.

SPF

SPF is a measure of how much solar energy (**UV radiation**) is required to produce sunburn on protected skin (i.e., in the presence of sunscreen) relative to the amount of solar energy required to produce sunburn on unprotected skin. As the SPF value increases, sunburn protection increases (Figure 39).

Generally, it takes less time to be exposed to the same amount of solar energy at midday compared to early morning or late evening because the sun is more intense at midday relative to the other times. Solar intensity is also related to geographic location, with greater solar intensity occurring at lower latitudes. Because clouds absorb solar energy, solar intensity is generally greater on clear days than cloudy days.

In addition to solar intensity, there are a number of other factor that influence the amount of solar energy that a consumer is exposed to:

- Skin type

- Amount of sunscreen applied

- Reapplication frequency

Fair-skinned consumers are likely to absorb more solar energy than dark-skinned consumers under the same conditions. Because sunscreens wear off and become less effective with time, the frequency with which they are reapplied is critical to limiting absorption of solar radiation. The reapplication frequency is also impacted by the activities that consumers are involved in. For example, consumers who swim while wearing sunscreen need to reapply the sunscreen more frequently because water may wash the sunscreen from the body. In addition,

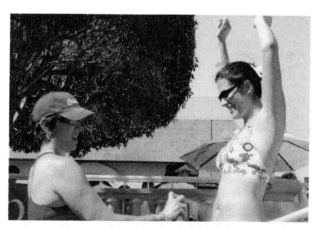

Figure 39. Always apply sunscreen to avoid UV radiation.

high levels of physical activity require more frequent reapplication because the activity may physically rub off the sunscreen and heavy sweating may wash off the sunscreen. In general, more frequent reapplication is associated with decreased absorption of solar radiation.

SPF does not inform consumers about the time that can be spent in the sun without getting sunburn. Rather,

SPF is a relative measure of the amount of sunburn protection provided by sunscreens. It allows consumers to compare the level of sunburn protection provided by different sunscreens. For example, consumers know that SPF 30 sunscreens provide more sunburn protection than SPF 8 sunscreens.

Noise Pollution

"Turn that noise down!" How many times have you heard someone from an older generation refer to your music as noise? Plenty. That's because to them it's pollution — an unwelcome, unwanted sound that disturbs their peace. The traditional definition of noise is "unwanted or disturbing sound." Sound becomes unwanted when it either interferes with normal activities such as sleeping, conversation, or disrupts or diminishes one's quality of life. The fact that you can't see, taste, or smell it may help explain why it has not received as much attention as other types of pollution, such as air pollution, or water pollution. The air around us is constantly filled with sounds, yet most of

us would probably not say we are surrounded by noise. Though for some, the persistent and escalating sources of sound can often be considered an annoyance. This "annoyance" can have major consequences, primarily to one's overall health (Figure 40).

Noise pollution adversely affects the lives of millions of people. Studies have shown that there are direct links between noise and health. Problems related to noise include stress related illnesses, high blood pressure, speech interference, hearing loss, sleep disruption, and lost productivity. Noise Induced Hearing Loss (NIHL) is the most common and often discussed health effect, but research has shown that exposure to constant or high levels of noise can cause countless adverse health effects.

NIHL can make it hard to understand speech in noisy environments, such as restaurants. NIHL can be caused by a one-time exposure to an intense "impulse" sound, such as an explosion, or by continuous exposure to loud sounds over an extended period of time, such as noise generated in a woodworking shop.

Recreational activities that can put you at risk for NIHL include target shooting and hunting, snowmobile riding, listening to MP3 players at high volume through earbuds or headphones, playing in a band, and attending loud concerts. Harmful noises at home may come from sources including lawnmowers, leaf blowers, and woodworking tools.

Sound is measured in units called decibels. Sounds of less than 75 decibels, even after long exposure, are unlikely to cause hearing loss. However, long or repeated exposure to sounds at or above 85 decibels can cause hearing loss. The louder the sound, the shorter the amount of time it takes for NIHL to happen. Here are the average decibel ratings of some familiar sounds (Figure 41).

NIHL is associated with increased aggression, decreased helpful behavior, reduced motivation and task performance, and even impaired cognitive development in children.

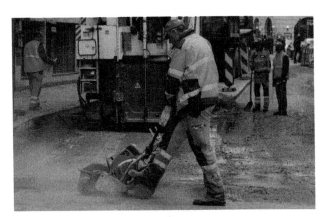

Figure 40. Noise pollution at work.

Noise Type	Decibels
A humming refrigerator	45
Normal conversation	60
Noise from heavy city traffic	85
A motorcycle	95
An MP3 player at maximum volume	105
Sirens	120
Firecrackers and firearms	150

Figure 41. Average decibel levels of common sounds.

Noise Pollution at Work

According to the CDC, noise pollution is especially prominent in the workplace. There are an estimated 16 million people working in the Manufacturing Sector, which accounts for approximately 13% of the US workforce. According to the Bureau of Labor Statistics, occupational hearing loss is the most commonly recorded occupational illness in manufacturing (17,700 cases out of 59,100 cases), accounting for one in every nine recordable illnesses. More than 72% of these occur among workers in Manufacturing. These numbers are particularly disturbing considering that a person's hearing loss must be determined to be work-related — and the hearing loss must be severe enough that the worker has become hearing impaired — in order to be considered recordable. Many more workers would have measurable occupational hearing loss but would not yet have become hearing impaired.

Protecting Your Hearing

If you know you are going to be in a high-decibel environment, use ear protection. Earplugs and sound-canceling earmuffs (Figure 42) are inexpensive and easy to keep on hand. In the context of work, adequate hearing protection is that which reduces noise exposure to below 85 decibels over the course of an average work shift of eight hours. Some people won't wear hearing protection because they think it makes them look silly. That's a silly reason to permanently damage your ears.

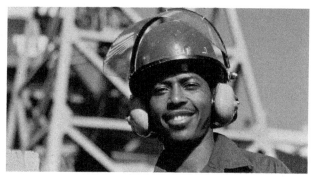

Figure 42. Always wear ear protection in loud environments.

Conclusion

This chapter discussed the different types of pollution, their effects on the health of the environment and the population, and ways that you can help reduce your exposure to pollution. Your next steps should be to assess the ways you can reduce your individual pollutants and encourage others around you — at work and in your community — to reduce overall pollution and improve environmental health for all people. Think about why it is important to you to be environmentally aware, and consider strategies that you could use to reduce, reuse and recycle to make a personal impact on the planet.

Text Acknowledgments

Chapter 1

This chapter reuses content from the following openly licensed sources:

Our World in Data (https://ourworldindata.org/life-expectancy/).

HE 250: Personal Health, Portland Community College (https://www.oercommons.org/authoring/14221-he-250-personal-health-portland-community-college/view).

This chapter reuses content in the Public Domain from the following US Government sources:

Centers for Disease Control and Prevention (https://www.cdc.gov).

Office of The Assistant Secretary for Planning and Evaluation (https://aspe.hhs.gov).

Healthy People 2020 (https://www.healthypeople.gov).

Eunice Kennedy Shriver National Institute of Child Health and Human Development (https://www.nichd.nih.gov).

US Department of Health and Human Services (https://www.hhs.gov).

This chapter reuses content under fair use from the following international non-profit organizations:

World Health Organization (http://www.who.int/about/mission/en/).

Chapter 2

This chapter reuses content in the Public Domain from the following US Government sources:

Centers for Disease Control and Prevention (https://www.cdc.gov).

National Center for Biotechnology Information (https://www.ncbi.nlm.nih.gov).

Office of Disease Prevention and Health Promotion (www.health.gov).

National Institute of Diabetes and Digestive and Kidney Diseases (https://www.niddk.nih.gov).

Oregon Department of Education (www.oregon.gov/ODE).

National Weather Service (http://www.nws.noaa.gov).

Environmental Protection Agency (www.epa.gov).

National Institutes of Health (http://www.nih.gov).

This chapter reuses content under fair use from the following national non-profit organizations and scholarly sources:

Medicine & Science in Sports and Exercise (http://journals.lww.com/acsm-msse/Abstract/2011/07000/Quantity_and_Quality_of_Exercise_for_Developing.26.aspx).

American College of Sports Medicine (http://www.acsm.org/public-information/articles/2016/10/07/basic-injury-prevention-concepts).

Asthma and Allergy Foundation of America (http://www.aafa.org/page/exercise-induced-asthma.aspx).

Chapter 3

This chapter reuses content in the Public Domain from the following US Government sources:

National Heart, Lung, and Blood Institute (https://www.nhlbi.nih.gov/health/health-topics/topics/phys/benefits).

Centers for Disease Control and Prevention (https://www.cdc.gov).

National Center for Biotechnology Information (https://www.ncbi.nlm.nih.gov).

Office of Disease Prevention and Health Promotion (www.health.gov).

National Cancer Institute (https://training.seer.cancer.gov/anatomy/cardiovascular/).

US National Library of Medicine (https://medlineplus.gov).

National Institutes of Health (http://www.nih.gov).

This chapter reuses content under fair use from the following national non-profit organizations and scholarly sources:

American Lung Association (http://www.lung.org/lung-health-and-diseases/lung-disease-lookup/copd/living-with-copd/physical-activity.html).

Harvard Health Publishing at Harvard Medical School (http://www.health.harvard.edu/blog/resting-heart-rate-can-reflect-current-future-health-201606179806).

National Academy of Sports Medicine (http://blog.nasm.org/weight-loss-specialist/myths-of-weight-management-you-have-to-exercise-at-a-low-intensity-to-burn-fat/).

American College of Sports Medicine (http://www.acsm.org/about-acsm/media-room/news-releases/2011/08/01/acsm-issues-new-recommendations-on-quantity-and-quality-of-exercise).

American College of Sports Medicine (https://www.acsm.org/docs/brochures/high-intensity-interval-training.pdf).

Chapter 4

This chapter reuses content in the Public Domain from the following US Government sources:

National Cancer Institute (https://training.seer.cancer.gov/anatomy/muscular/).

US Department of Health and Human Services (https://www.hhs.gov/fitness/).

Social Security Administration (https://www.ssa.gov/planners/retire/1943.html).

National Center for Biotechnology Information (https://www.ncbi.nlm.nih.gov).

National Institute on Alcohol Abuse and Alcoholism (https://pubs.niaaa.nih.gov/publications/arh27-4/317-324.htm).

National Human Genome Research Institute (https://www.genome.gov/dnaday/q.cfm?aid=5905&year=2006).

Centers for Disease Control and Prevention (https://www.cdc.gov).

Office of Disease Prevention and Health Promotion (www.health.gov).

National Institutes of Arthritis and Musculoskeletal and Skin Diseases (https://www.bones.nih.gov/health-info/bone/bone-health/exercise/exercise-your-bone-health).

National Institute on Aging (https://www.nia.nih.gov/research/intramural-research-program/dynamics-health-aging-and-body-composition-health-abc).

US National Library of Medicine (https://medlineplus.gov).

National Institute on Drug Abuse (https://www.drugabuse.gov).

Office on Women's Health (https://womenshealth.gov).

Office of Dietary Supplements (https://ods.od.nih.gov).

This chapter reuses content under fair use from the following national non-profit organizations and scholarly sources:

PubChem Open Chemistry Database (https://pubchem.ncbi.nlm.nih.gov/compound/creatine).

PT Direct Tools for Personal Training Success (http://www.ptdirect.com/training-design/anatomy-and-physiology/skeletal-muscle-roles-and-contraction-types).

Therapeutic Advances in Cardiovascular Disease (http://journals.sagepub.com/doi/pdf/10.1177/1753944708089701).

American College of Sports Medicine (http://acsm.org/about-acsm/media-room/news-releases/2011/08/01/acsm-issues-new-recommendations-on-quantity-and-quality-of-exercise).

American College of Sports Medicine (https://www.acsm.org/docs/brochures/resistance-training.pdf).

Chapter 5

This chapter reuses content in the Public Domain from the following US Government sources:

Centers for Disease Control (https://www.cdc.gov).

Office of Disease Prevention and Health Promotion (www.health.gov).

National Center for Biotechnology Information (https://www.ncbi.nlm.nih.gov).

National Institute of Neurological Disorders and Stroke (https://www.ninds.nih.gov/Disorders/Patient-Caregiver-Education/Fact-Sheets/Low-Back-Pain-Fact-Sheet).

National Institute on Aging (https://go4life.nia.nih.gov/exercises/flexibility).

US National Library of Medicine (https://medlineplus.gov).

National Institutes of Arthritis and Musculoskeletal and Skin Diseases (https://www.niams.nih.gov/health-topics/kids/healthy-joints).

National Institutes of Health (https://newsinhealth.nih.gov).

Genetic and Rare Diseases Information Center (https://rarediseases.info.nih.gov/diseases/2081/ehlers-danlos-syndrome-hypermobility-type).

US Department of Veterans Affairs (https://www.move.va.gov/docs/NewHandouts/PhysicalActivity/P33_SampleFlexibilityProgramForBeginners.pdf).

This chapter reuses content under fair use from the following national non-profit organizations and scholarly sources:

Harvard Health Publishing at Harvard Medical School (http://www.health.harvard.edu/staying-healthy/exercising-to-relax).

American College of Sports Medicine (http://www.acsm.org/about-acsm/media-room/news-releases/2011/08/01/acsm-issues-new-recommendations-on-quantity-and-quality-of-exercise).

Chapter 6

This chapter reuses content in the Public Domain from the following US Government sources:

National Institute of General Medical Sciences (https://publications.nigms.nih.gov/insidelifescience/fats_do.html).

National Heart, Lung, and Blood Institute (https://www.nhlbi.nih.gov/health/health-topics/topics/obe/causes).

National Center for Biotechnology Information (https://www.ncbi.nlm.nih.gov).

Centers for Disease Control (https://www.cdc.gov).

US National Library of Medicine (https://medlineplus.gov/ency/article/007199.htm).

Center for Clinical Interventions (http://www.cci.health.wa.gov.au/docs/set%20point%20theory.pdf).

National Institute on Aging (https://www.nia.nih.gov/health/what-menopause).

Surgeon General's Report (https://www.surgeongeneral.gov/library/reports/50-years-of-progress/sgr50-chap-10.pdf).

National Institute of Diabetes and Digestive and Kidney Diseases (https://www.niddk.nih.gov/health-information/weight-management/bariatric-surgery/types).

National Institute of Mental Health (https://www.nimh.nih.gov/health/statistics/prevalence/eating-disorders-among-children.shtml).

US National Library of Medicine (https://medlineplus.gov).

Office on Women's Health (https://womenshealth.gov).

Federal Trade Commission (https://www.consumer.ftc.gov/articles/0261-dietary-supplements).

This chapter reuses content under fair use from the following national non-profit organizations and scholarly sources:

University of Hawai'I Windward Community College (http://krupp.wcc.hawaii.edu/BIOL100L/nutrition/energy.pdf).

National Eating Disorders Collaboration (http://www.nedc.com.au/body-image).

Bradley University (https://www.bradley.edu/sites/bodyproject/male-body-image-m-vs-f/).

Academy of Nutrition and Dietetics (http://www.eatright.org/resource/health/weight-loss/fad-diets/staying-away-from-fad-diets).

Academy of Nutrition and Dietetics (http://www.eatright.org/resource/health/weight-loss/your-health-and-your-weight/healthy-weight-gain).

The Center for Eating Disorders (https://eatingdisorder.org/eating-disorder-information/osfed/).

Chapter 7

This chapter reuses content in the Public Domain from the following US Government sources:

US Department of Health and Human Services (https://www.hhs.gov/fitness/).

Office of Disease Prevention and Health Promotion (www.health.gov).

Choose MyPlate (https://www.choosemyplate.gov/nutrition-nutrient-density).

Centers for Disease Control (https://www.cdc.gov).

National Institute on Aging (https://www.nia.nih.gov/health/smart-food-choices-healthy-aging).

US Department of Agriculture (https://www.usda.gov/).

US National Library of Medicine (https://medlineplus.gov).

National Institute of Diabetes and Digestive and Kidney Diseases (https://www.niddk.nih.gov/health-information/digestive-diseases/celiac-disease/eating-diet-nutrition).

Food and Drug Administration (https://www.accessdata.fda.gov/scripts/InteractiveNutritionFactsLabel/factsheets/Dietary_Fiber.pdf).

National Institutes of Health (https://newsinhealth.nih.gov).

Australian Government Department of Health (https://www.eatforhealth.gov.au/food-essentials/fat-salt-sugars-and-alcohol/fat).

National Center for Complementary and Integrative Health (https://nccih.nih.gov/health/antioxidants/introduction.htm).

Office of Dietary Supplements (https://ods.od.nih.gov/factsheets/VitaminC-HealthProfessional/).

US Geological Survey (https://water.usgs.gov/edu/propertyyou.html).

National Heart, Lung, and Blood Institute (https://www.nhlbi.nih.gov/files/docs/public/heart/dash_brief.pdf).

This chapter reuses content under fair use from the following national non-profit organizations and scholarly sources:

Harvard Health Publishing at Harvard Medical School (https://www.health.harvard.edu/staying-healthy/the-truth-about-fats-bad-and-good).

Harvard School of Public Health (https://www.hsph.harvard.edu/nutritionsource/gluten/).

Harvard School of Public Health (https://www.hsph.harvard.edu/nutritionsource/carbohydrates/added-sugar-in-the-diet/).

Harvard School of Public Health (https://www.hsph.harvard.edu/nutrition-source/2017/04/24/removing-trans-fats-from-restaurant-menus-associated-with-drop-in-heart-attacks-and-strokes/).

Oregon State University Linus Pauling Institute Micronutrient Information Center (http://lpi.oregonstate.edu/mic/minerals).

Chapter 8

This chapter reuses content in the Public Domain from the following US Government sources:

National Institute of Mental Health (https://www.nimh.nih.gov/health/publications/stress/index.shtml).

Centers for Disease Control (https://www.cdc.gov).

National Center for Complementary and Integrative Health (https://nccih.nih.gov/health/stress).

National Center for Biotechnology Information (https://www.ncbi.nlm.nih.gov).

Substance Abuse and Mental Health Services Administration (https://www.samhsa.gov/samhsaNewsLetter/Volume_22_Number_3/working_with_anger/).

State of New Hampshire Employee Assistance Program (https://das.nh.gov/wellness/Docs/Percieved%20Stress%20Scale.pdf).

This chapter reuses content under fair use from the following national non-profit organizations and scholarly sources:

Harvard Health Publishing at Harvard Medical School (https://www.health.harvard.edu/staying-healthy/understanding-the-stress-response).

American Psychological Association (http://www.apa.org/monitor/2011/01/stressed-america.aspx).

American Psychological Association (http://www.apa.org/news/press/releases/stress/2015/snapshot.aspx).

American Psychological Association (http://www.apa.org/topics/anger/control.aspx).

American Psychological Association (http://www.apa.org/topics/personality/).

American Psychological Association (http://www.apa.org/news/press/releases/stress/2013/sleep.aspx).

Anxiety and Depression Association of America (https://adaa.org/living-with-anxiety/women/facts).

Anxiety and Depression Association of America (https://adaa.org/understanding-anxiety/related-illnesses/other-related-conditions/stress/physical-activity-reduces-st).

University of New Mexico Open Library College Success (http://open.lib.umn.edu/collegesuccess/chapter/10-5-stress/).

Chapter 9

This chapter reuses content in the Public Domain from the following US Government sources:

Centers for Disease Control (https://www.cdc.gov).

National Heart, Lung, and Blood Institute (https://www.nhlbi.nih.gov).

National Institute of Neurological Disorders and Stroke (https://www.ninds.nih.gov/Disorders/All-Disorders/Cerebral-Arteriosclerosis-Information-Page).

National Cancer Institute (www.cancer.gov).

National Institute of Diabetes and Digestive and Kidney Diseases (https://www.niddk.nih.gov/health-information/diabetes/overview/what-is-diabetes).

US National Library of Medicine (https://medlineplus.gov).

This chapter reuses content under fair use from the following national non-profit organizations and scholarly sources:

American Heart Association (http://www.heart.org/HEARTORG/Conditions/HeartAttack/WarningSignsofaHeartAttack/Angina-in-Women-Can-Be-Different-Than-Men_UCM_448902_Article.jsp#.WepxpBNSwlJ).

World Health Organization (http://www.who.int/tobacco/quitting/benefits/en/).

Harvard Health Publishing at Harvard Medical School (http://www.health.harvard.edu/blog/mild-high-blood-pressure-in-young-adults-linked-to-heart-problems-later-in-life-201506238100).

Harvard Health Publishing at Harvard Medical School (http://www.health.harvard.edu/heart-health/race-and-ethnicity-clues-to-your-heart-disease-risk).

Harvard Health Publishing at Harvard Medical School (https://www.health.harvard.edu/blog/should-kids-have-their-cholesterol-checked-201112224020).

Harvard Health Publishing at Harvard Medical School (https://www.health.harvard.edu/heart-health/11-foods-that-lower-cholesterol).

Chapter 10

This chapter reuses content in the Public Domain from the following US Government sources:

Centers for Disease Control (https://www.cdc.gov).

National Center for Biotechnology Information (https://www.ncbi.nlm.nih.gov).

US National Library of Medicine (https://medlineplus.gov).

National Institute of Allergy and Infectious Diseases (https://www.niaid.nih.gov).

Health and Human Services Secretary's Minority AIDS Initiative Fund (https://www.hiv.gov/hiv-basics/overview/about-hiv-and-aids/what-are-hiv-and-aids).

This chapter reuses content under fair use from the following national non-profit organizations and scholarly sources:

American Association of Retired Persons (https://www.aarp.org/home-family/sex-intimacy/info-03-2013/sexually-transmitted-infections-should-you-worry.html).

Kaiser Family Foundation (https://www.kff.org/global-health-policy/fact-sheet/the-global-hivaids-epidemic/).

Trust for America's Health (http://healthyamericans.org/assets/files/Final%202014%20Report.pdf).

American Academy of Pediatrics (https://www.healthychildren.org/English/health-issues/conditions/infections/Pages/Overview-of-Infectious-Diseases.aspx).

American Academy of Family Physicians (http://www.aafp.org/afp/2015/0501/p652.html).

Chapter 11

This chapter reuses content in the Public Domain from the following US Government sources:

Centers for Disease Control (https://www.cdc.gov).

National Institute on Drug Abuse (https://www.drugabuse.gov).

US National Library of Medicine (https://medlineplus.gov).

National Center for Biotechnology Information (https://www.ncbi.nlm.nih.gov).

National Institute on Alcohol Abuse and Alcoholism (https://pubs.niaaa.nih.gov/publications/aa35.htm).

Department of Health and Human Services (https://betobaccofree.hhs.gov/about-tobacco/Smoked-Tobacco-Products/index.html).

Food and Drug Administration (https://www.fda.gov/TobaccoProducts/Labeling/RulesRegulationsGuidance/ucm297786.htm).

United Kingdom Smokefree National Health Service (https://www.nhs.uk/smokefree/help-and-advice/e-cigarettes).

National Cancer Institute (www.cancer.gov).

National Institutes of Health Office of Disease Prevention (https://prevention.nih.gov/tobacco-regulatory-science-program/about-the-FSPTCA).

This chapter reuses content under fair use from the following national non-profit organizations and scholarly sources:

Substance Abuse and Mental Health Services Administration (https://www.samhsa.gov/prescription-drug-misuse-abuse).

American Lung Association (http://www.lung.org/stop-smoking/i-want-to-quit/five-secrets-for-quitting-smoking.html).

Rice University (http://www.rice.edu/~jenky/sports/caffeine.html).

Brown University (https://www.brown.edu/campus-life/health/services/promotion/alcohol-other-drugs-alcohol/alcohol-and-your-body).

Chapter 12

This chapter reuses content in the Public Domain from the following US Government sources:

European Environment Agency (https://www.eea.europa.eu/soer/synthesis/synthesis/chapter5.xhtml).

Office of Disease Prevention and Health Promotion (https://www.healthypeople.gov).

United Nations Department of Economic and Social Affairs (http://www.un.org/en/development/desa/news/population/2015-report.html).

National Institute on Deafness and Other Communication Disorders (https://www.nidcd.nih.gov/health/noise-induced-hearing-loss).

Central Intelligence Agency World Factbook (https://www.cia.gov/library/publications/the-world-factbook/rankorder/2127rank.html).

Environmental Protection Agency (https://www.epa.gov).

National Center for Biotechnology Information (https://www.ncbi.nlm.nih.gov).

National Resources Conservation Service (https://www.nrcs.usda.gov/wps/portal/nrcs/detail/soils/use/?cid=nrcs142p2_054028).

National Institute of Environmental Health Sciences (https://www.niehs.nih.gov/health/topics/agents/water-poll/index.cfm).

US Energy Information Administration (https://www.eia.gov).

US Global Change Research Program (http://www.globalchange.gov/climate-change).

National Aeronautics and Space Administration (https://climate.nasa.gov).

Food and Drug Administration (https://www.fda.gov/aboutfda/centersoffices/officeofmedicalproductsandtobacco/cder/ucm106351.htm).

US Geological Survey (https://water.usgs.gov/edu/wusw.html).

Portland Water Bureau (https://www.portlandoregon.gov/water/article/32978).

California Department of Toxic Substances Control (http://www.dtsc.ca.gov/HazardousWaste/upload/HWMP_DefiningHW111.pdf).

CalRecycle (http://www.calrecycle.ca.gov/electronics/whatisewaste/).

This chapter reuses content under fair use from the following national non-profit organizations and scholarly sources:

World Health Organization (http://www.who.int/ionizing_radiation/about/what_is_ir/en/).

World Health Organization (http://www.who.int/topics/climate/en/).

World Population History (http://worldpopulationhistory.org/carrying-capacity/).

Wheeling Jesuit University Center for Educational Technologies (http://ete.cet.edu/gcc/?/bio_loss_of_diversity_humact/).

United Nations (http://www.un.org/sustainabledevelopment/takeaction/).

University of Delaware Office of Campus and Public Safety (http://www1.udel.edu/ehs/waste/chemical-waste-management.html).

Image Acknowledgments

Chapter 1

Figure 1.0. "Push-ups" by skeeze is licensed under Public Domain (https://pixabay.com/en/push-ups-exercise-fitness-workout-888024/).

Figure 1.1. "Multnomah falls" by AirHaake is licensed under CC BY 2.0 (https://www.flickr.com/photos/80519348@N02/33861704144).

Figure 1.3. "Top Ten Reported Impediments to Academic Performance – Past 12 Months" by ACHA-NCHAII is licensed under Public Domain (http://www.acha-ncha.org/docs/NCHA-II_WEB_SPRING_2015_REFERENCE_GROUP_EXECUTIVE_SUMMARY.pdf).

Figure 1.4. "Football Children" by Sasint is licensed under Public Domain (https://pixabay.com/en/football-children-sports-action-1807520/).

Figure 1.7. "Mental Health Concerns of American College Students – Past 12 Months" by ACHA-NCHAII is licensed under Public Domain (http://www.acha-ncha.org/docs/NCHA-II_WEB_SPRING_2015_REFERENCE_GROUP_EXECUTIVE_SUMMARY.pdf).

Figure 1.8. "Family Jump" by Evil Erin is licensed under CC BY 2.0 (https://www.flickr.com/photos/evilerin/3565026821).

Figure 1.9. "Meditation" by Maxlkt is licensed under Public Domain (https://pixabay.com/en/meditate-theravada-buddhism-monk-2105143/).

Figure 1.10. "RES Students Plant Trees for Earth Day" by US Air Force is licensed under Public Domain (https://commons.wikimedia.org/wiki/File:RES_students_plant_trees_for_Earth_Day_150422-F-NH180-004.jpg).

Figure 1.11. "Leading Causes of Death in the US Overall and By Age" by CDC is licensed under Public Domain (https://www.cdc.gov/nchs/data/nvsr/nvsr65/nvsr65_04.pdf).

Figure 1.12. "Leading Causes of Death by Gender" by CDC is licensed under Public Domain (https://www.cdc.gov/nchs/data/hus/hus16.pdf).

Figure 1.13. "Life Expectancy by Gender/Country" by CDC is licensed under Public Domain (https://www.cdc.gov/nchs/data/hus/hus16.pdf).

Figure 1.14. "Life Expectancy by Race/Gender" by CDC is licensed under Public Domain (https://www.cdc.gov/nchs/data/hus/hus16.pdf).

Figure 1.15. "Improvements to Vaccines" by CDC Global is licensed under CC BY 2.0 (https://www.flickr.com/photos/cdcglobal/8190819133/).

Figure 1.16. "Health Care Provider" by travisdmchenry is licensed under Public Domain (https://pixabay.com/en/nurse-military-child-1796924/).

Figure 1.17. "Tokyo Infinity" and "Houses in a Woody Valley" by Jens Lelie and Pawel Nolbert are licensed under Public Domain (https://unsplash.com/photos/4u2U8EO9OzY and https://unsplash.com/photos/vIBkCjlYp3o).

Figure 1.18. "Mortality Rate" by CDC is licensed under Public Domain (https://www.cdc.gov/nchs/data/hus/hus15.pdf).

Figure 1.19. "Homicide Rate" by CDC is licensed under Public Domain (https://www.cdc.gov/nchs/data/hus/hus15.pdf).

Figure 1.20. "Suicide Rate" by CDC is licensed under Public Domain (https://www.cdc.gov/nchs/data/hus/hus15.pdf).

Figure 1.21. "Smoking Status by Race" by International Journal of Environmental Research and Public Health is licensed under (http://www.mdpi.com/1660-4601/13/10/1009/htm).

Figure 1.22. "Fighting Fires" by Jose L. Hernandez-Domitilo is licensed under Public Domain (https://media.defense.gov/2014/Aug/25/2000932712/-1/-1/0/140819-F-DT489-673.JPG).

Figure 1.23. "Healthy Food Retailer" by Kaleb Snay is licensed under Public Domain (https://media.defense.gov/2017/Mar/02/2001706379/670/394/0/170301-F-AE429-009.JPG).

Figure 1.25. "Brussels Marathon Runners" by Martins Zemlickis is licensed under CC BY 4.0 (https://unsplash.com/collections/420675/people-behavior-life-style?photo=NPFu4GfFZ7E).

Figure 1.26. "Fruits, Veggies, and Whole Grains " by dbreen is licensed under Public Domain (https://pixabay.com/en/carrot-kale-walnuts-tomatoes-1085063/).

Figure 1.27. "Meditation" by Marcos Moraes is licensed under CC BY 4.0 (https://unsplash.com/search/meditate?photo=LQ-n5xBg1rs).

Figure 1.28. "Stressor Examples" by APA is licensed under Public Domain.

Figure 1.29. "Second hand smoke effects" by US Army is licensed under Public Domain (https://www.army.mil/e2/c/images/2014/11/17/372309/original.jpg).

Figure 1.30. "Quitting Smoking Results" by NIH is licensed under Public Domain.

Figure 1.31. "Sleep" by claudioscott is licensed under Public Domain (https://pixabay.com/en/woman-girl-bella-read-sleep-2197947/).

Figure 1.32. "Critical Thinking About Health Care" by Ilmicrofono Oggiono is licensed under CC BY 2.0 (https://www.flickr.com/photos/115089924@N02/16256199615/).

Figure 1.33. "Friends" by Anna Vander Stel is licensed under CC BY 4.0 (https://unsplash.com/search/friends?photo=zimQNLdnKp0).

Figure 1.34. "How Spirituality Can Affect Important Clinical Issues" by Veteran's Affairs is licensed under Public Domain (https://www.ptsd.va.gov/professional/provider-type/community/fs-spirituality.asp).

Figure 1.35. "Calendar" by Dafne Cholet is licensed under CC BY 2.0 (https://www.flickr.com/photos/dafnecholet/5374200948).

Figure 1.38. "Pros and Cons of Smoking Cessation" by U.S. Department of Health & Human Services is licensed under Public Domain (https://www.cdc.gov/tobacco/campaign/tips/quit-smoking/guide/rewards-of-quitting.html).

Chapter 2

Figure 2.0. "Active" by Josh Marshall is licensed under Public Domain (https://unsplash.com/search/active?photo=BDI3NS0kZOM).

Figure 2.1. "BoysVarsity Soccer" by Selma Bears is licensed under CC BY 2.0 (https://www.flickr.com/photos/selmahighsoccer/8950173450/sizes/l).

Figure 2.2. "Freedom" by Dino Reichmuth is licensed under Public Domain (https://unsplash.com/search/freedom?photo=1tFd-Bb1pxk).

Figure 2.3. "Activity vs. exercise comparison" by Keit Trysh and Chris Hayashi are licensed under Public Domain (https://unsplash.com/search/exercise?photo=3cCe37VGDiQ and https://unsplash.com/collections/474021/active?photo=gbaeHydpgtE).

Figure 2.4. "Yoga" by Dave Rosenblum is licensed under CC BY 2.0 (https://www.flickr.com/photos/daverose215/9707554768/sizes/l).

Figure 2.8. "Moderate and Vigorous Intensity" by US Dept. of Health and Human Services is licensed under Public Domain.

Figure 2.9. "Strengthening Exercise" by N.W. Huertas is licensed under Public Domain (http://www.marines.mil/Photos/igphoto/2001610035/).

Figure 2.10. "Pilates" by UptownFitness is licensed under Public Domain (https://pixabay.com/en/weights-pilates-girls-1948837/).

Figure 2.11. "Kids Being Active" by sasint is licensed under Public Domain (https://pixabay.com/en/as-children-river-enjoy-water-1822704/).

Figure 2.12. "Skill-Related Fitness" by Skeeze is licensed under Public Domain (https://pixabay.com/en/high-jump-track-field-competition-695308/).

Figure 2.15. "Cyclist" and "Swimmer" by Dave Hosford are licensed under CC BY 2.0 and Public Domain (https://www.flickr.com/photos/baltimoredave/4715256656/sizes/l and https://pixabay.com/en/swimming-swimmer-female-race-78112/).

Figure 2.16. "Barriers to Physical Activity and How to Overcome Them" by CDC is licensed under Public Domain (https://www.cdc.gov/physicalactivity/basics/adding-pa/barriers.html).

Figure 2.17. "Hiking" and "Park Life" by Adam Bautz and Stan V Peterson are licensed under CC BY 2.0 and Public Domain (https://www.flickr.com/photos/130811041@N04/19824324090/sizes/l and https://pixabay.com/en/park-life-park-people-walking-life-2251981/).

Figure 2.18. "Running Shoes Display" by MarkBuckawicki is licensed under Public Domain (https://commons.wikimedia.org/wiki/File:Running_shoes_display.JPG).

Figure 2.19. "Wind chill index" by National Weather Service is licensed under Public Domain (http://www.nws.noaa.gov/om/cold/wind_chill.shtml).

Figure 2.23. "Smoggy day" by Alex Gindin is licensed under Public Domain (https://unsplash.com/photos/ifpBOcQlhoY).

Figure 2.24. "Air Quality Index Chart" by Air Now is licensed under Public Domain (https://airnow.gov/index.cfm?action=aqibasics.aqi).

Figure 2.25. "RPG wounded Iraq veteran exercising" by Virginia Reza is licensed under Public Domain (https://commons.wikimedia.org/wiki/File:RPG_wounded_Iraq_veteran_exercising_Army-dot-mil-2007-02-07-103140.jpg).

Figure 2.26. "Exercising During Pregnancy" by Ian Leones is licensed under Public Domain (http://www.marforres.marines.mil/Marine-Reserve-News-Photos/Marine-Reserve-Photos/igphoto/2001001198/).

Figure 2.28. "Compression Sleeve or Ace Bandage Wrap" by Martin R. Harris is licensed under Public Domain (https://commons.wikimedia.org/wiki/File:KICK-BOX008cropped.jpg).

Chapter 3

Figure 3.0. "Cardio Exercise" by hardloperhans is licensed under CC BY 2.0 (https://www.flickr.com/photos/hardloperhans/3648376652/).

Figure 3.1. "Diagram of Respiratory System" by Wikimedia is licensed under Public Domain (https://en.wikipedia.org/wiki/File:Respiratory_system_complete_en.svg).

Figure 3.2. "Exchange of Oxygen and CO2 in Alveoli" by Wikimedia is licensed under CC BY 3.0 (https://commons.wikimedia.org/wiki/File:2319_Fig_23.19.jpg).

Figure 3.3. "Circulation of Oxygen and Carbon Dioxide" by Wikipedia is licensed under CC BY 3.0 (https://commons.wikimedia.org/wiki/File:2101_Blood_Flow_Through_the_Heart.jpg).

Figure 3.4. "Heart with Blood Flow" by BurlesonMatthew is licensed under Public Domain (https://pixabay.com/en/heart-valve-circulatory-human-2222964/).

Figure 3.6. "Cardio Exercise" by ThomasWolter is licensed under Public Domain (https://pixabay.com/en/relay-race-competition-stadium-655353/).

Figure 3.7. "Asthma Before After" by Wikimedia is licensed under Public Domain (https://commons.wikimedia.org/wiki/File:Asthma_before-after-en.svg).

Figure 3.8. "Bronchitis" by Wikimedia is licensed under CC BY-SA 4.0 (https://commons.wikimedia.org/wiki/File:Bronchitis.png).

Figure 3.10. "Blood Pressure Cuff" by Morgan is licensed under CC BY 2.0 (https://www.flickr.com/photos/meddygarnet/3489151194/).

Figure 3.12. "Moderate and Vigorous Intensity Activity" by CDC is licensed under Public Domain (https://www.cdc.gov/nccdphp/dnpa/physical/pdf/PA_Intensity_table_2_1.pdf).

Figure 3.16. "Bicyclist" by Skeeze is licensed under Public Domain (https://pixabay.com/en/bicyclist-bicycling-biking-bike-569279/).

Figure 3.17. "Feel the Pain" by Ryan Labadens is licensed under Public Domain (http://www.403wg.afrc.af.mil/News/Photos/igphoto/2000862378/).

Chapter 4

Figure 4.0. "170713-N-JC445-028 Mediterranean Sea" by US Navy is licensed under Public Domain (https://www.flickr.com/photos/cne-cna-c6f/35135345094/).

Figure 4.1. "Paddle Boarding" by Don DeBold is licensed under CC BY 2.0 (https://www.flickr.com/photos/ddebold/19130073248/).

Figure 4.2. "Climbing" by Terry Robinson is licensed under CC BY-SA 2.0 (https://www.flickr.com/photos/suburbanadventure/4472605204/).

Figure 4.3. "Skeletal muscle" by Bruce Blaus is licensed under CC BY 3.0 (https://commons.wikimedia.org/wiki/File:Blausen_0801_SkeletalMuscle.png).

Figure 4.4. "Smooth muscle" by R. Bowen is licensed under Public Domain (https://ghr.nlm.nih.gov/art/large/muscle-fibers).

Figure 4.5. "Cardiac muscle" by Shutterstock is licensed under Public Domain (https://www.shutterstock.com/image-illustration/structure-skeletal-muscle-fiber-116410819?src=jmThxBNE0L1vXoKjxJoqMw-1-11).

Figure 4.6. "Muscle Anatomy" by Shutterstock is licensed under Public Domain (https://www.shutterstock.com/image-illustration/muscle-anatomy-199867766?src=hfdxHS6xrKZrCFeBL2n74Q-1-2).

Figure 4.7. "Sliding Filament Theory" by Gal Gavriel is licensed under CC BY-SA 4.0 (https://commons.wikimedia.org/wiki/File:%D7%9E%D7%91%D7%A0%D7%94_%D7%94%D7%9E%D7%95%D7%9C%D7%A7%D7%95%D7%9C%D7%94_-_Sliding_filament.gif).

Figure 4.8. "Endurance activity" by cellue communication is licensed under CC BY SA 2.0 (https://www.flickr.com/photos/131350192@N03/19270296086/).

Figure 4.9. "Marine Jumping " by U.S. Marine Corps is licensed under Public Domain (https://commons.wikimedia.org/wiki/File:USMC-05301.jpg).

Figure 4.10. "Might As Well Jump" by istolethetv is licensed under CC BY 2.0 (https://www.flickr.com/photos/istolethetv/3484450808/sizes/l).

Chapter 5

Chapter 6

Chapter 7

Figure 7.0. "Produce Market" by Patrick Feller is licensed under CC BY 2.0 (https://www.flickr.com/photos/nakrnsm/3815441846/).

Figure 7.2. "Estimated Calorie Needs" by US Office of Disease Prevention and Health Promotion is licensed under Public Domain (https://health.gov/dietaryguidelines/2015/).

Figure 7.4. "Breads" by FotoshopTofs is licensed under CC0 (https://pixabay.com/en/breads-cereals-oats-barley-wheat-1417868/).

Figure 7.5. "Danish Pancake with Raspberry" by Vegan Feast Catering is licensed under CC BY 2.0 (https://www.flickr.com/photos/veganfeast/5108221092/).

Figure 7.6. "Daily Carb Needs During Training" by Academy of Nutrition and Dietetics is licensed under Public Domain.

Figure 7.7. "Butter, Margarine, and Canola Oil" by Food and Drug Administration is licensed under Public Domain.

Figure 7.8. "Average Intake of Saturated Fats" by US Office of Disease Prevention and Health Promotion is licensed under Public Domain (https://health.gov/dietaryguidelines/2015/resources/2015-2020_Dietary_Guidelines.pdf).

Figure 7.9. "Comparison of Dietary Fats" by Vwalvekar is licensed under CC BY-SA 3.0 (https://commons.wikimedia.org/wiki/File:Comparison_of_dietary_fats.gif).

Figure 7.10. "Avocado" by Chad Miller is licensed under CC BY-SA 3.0 (https://www.flickr.com/photos/chadmiller/69170988/).

Figure 7.13. "Protein Functions and Types" by US National Library of Medicine-Genetics is licensed under Public Domain.

Figure 7.17. "Berries" by Tomasz Stasiuk is licensed under CC BY-SA 2.0 (https://www.flickr.com/photos/zstasiuk/5317397606/).

Figure 7.18. "Cooking" by congerdesign is licensed under Public Domain (https://pixabay.com/p-1013631/?no_redirect).

Figure 7.21. "Vitamin Supplements" by US Dept. of Defense is licensed under Public Domain (https://media.defense.gov/2017/Mar/31/2001725105/-1/-1/0/170322-F-OT558-0001.JPG).

Figure 7.22. "Spam Can Nutritional Label" by Lhe3460 is licensed under CC BY-SA 4.0 (https://commons.wikimedia.org/wiki/File:Spam_Can_Nutritional_Label.jpg).

Figure 7.23. "MyPlate" by US Dept. of Agriculture is licensed under Public Domain (https://commons.wikimedia.org/wiki/File:Myplate_blue.jpg).

Figure 7.31. "Nutrition Facts" by Food and Drug Administration is licensed under Public Domain (https://www.fda.gov/food/ingredientspackaginglabeling/labelingnutrition/ucm274593.htm#percent_daily_value).

Figure 7.32. "Plain and Fruit Yogurt Nutrition Facts Comparison" by Food and Drug Administration is licensed under Public Domain (https://www.fda.gov/food/ingredientspackaginglabeling/labelingnutrition/ucm274593.htm#percent_daily_value).

Figure 7.33. "Celery" and "Peaches" by 821292 and Celine Nadeau are licensed under CC0 and CC BY-SA 3.0 (https://pixabay.com/en/celery-vegetables-vegetable-green-692867/ and https://www.flickr.com/photos/celinet/4962398284/).

Figure 7.34. "Yellow and Red Onions" by Alexis Lamster is licensed under CC BY 2.0 (https://www.flickr.com/photos/amlamster/6608862125).

Chapter 8

Figure 8.0. "Relax" by Sole Treadmill is licensed under CC BY 2.0 (https://www.flickr.com/photos/149902454@N08/35507035266/sizes/l).

Figure 8.2. "Eustress" by AdinaVoicu is licensed under Public Domain (https://pixabay.com/en/study-girl-writing-notebook-1231393/).

Figure 8.6. "Learning" by CollegeDegrees360 is licensed under CC BY-SA 2.0 (https://www.flickr.com/photos/83633410@N07/7658284016/).

Figure 8.7. "Leading Stressors Among College Students" by National College Health Assessment is licensed under Public Domain (http://college.usatoday.com/2015/10/29/college-student-stress/).

Figure 8.13. "East Hollywood Art Cycle" by SupportPDX is licensed under CC BY 2.0 (https://www.flickr.com/photos/rocketboom/4432507224/sizes/l).

Figure 8.19. "Depression" by Ryan_M651 is licensed under CC BY 2.0 (https://www.flickr.com/photos/120632374@N07/13974181800/sizes/l).

Figure 8.21. "Cycle of Abuse" by Avanduyn is licensed under Public Domain (https://commons.wikimedia.org/wiki/File:Cycle_of_Abuse.png).

Figure 8.22. "Angst" by braerik is licensed under CC BY-SA 2.0 (https://www.flickr.com/photos/braerik/25022496121/sizes/l).

Figure 8.23. "Schedule" by fo.ol is licensed under CC BY-SA 2.0 (https://www.flickr.com/photos/forresto/488853222/sizes/l).

Figure 8.24. "Covey's Task Prioritizer" by Steven Covey is used by permission.

Figure 8.30. "Yoga Fitness Program" by Fort Meade is licensed under Public Domain (https://www.flickr.com/photos/ftmeade/7551022750/sizes/l).

Figure 8.31. "The Fall Salad" by organicboi is licensed under CC BY 2.0 (https://www.flickr.com/photos/141471286@N06/34854933566/).

Chapter 9

Figure 9.0. "Colon Biopsy" by Ed Uthmen is licensed under CC BY 2.0 (https://www.flickr.com/photos/euthman/4771852848/).

Figure 9.1. "Heart Attack Death Rate (adults 35+)" by CDC is licensed under Public Domain (https://www.cdc.gov/dhdsp/maps/national_maps/hd_all.htm).

Figure 9.4. "Atherosclerosis " by OpenStax College is licensed under CC BY 3.0 (https://commons.wikimedia.org/wiki/File:2113ab_Atherosclerosis.jpg).

Figure 9.5. "Atherosclerotic Artery" by National Institute of Health is licensed under Public Domain (https://www.nhlbi.nih.gov/health/educational/pad/about/what.html).

Figure 9.6. "Plaque Building Up" by CDC is licensed under Public Domain (https://www.cdc.gov/heartdisease/facts.htm).

Figure 9.7. "Heart with Muscle Damage and a Blocked Artery" by National Heart, Lung, and Blood Institute is licensed under Public Domain (https://www.nhlbi.nih.gov/health/health-topics/topics/heartattack/).

Figure 9.8. "Common Heart Attack Warning Signs" by American Heart Association is licensed under Public Domain (http://www.heart.org/HEARTORG/Conditions/HeartAttack/WarningSignsofaHeartAttack/Warning-Signs-of-a-Heart-Attack_UCM_002039_Article.jsp#.WXo19hMrKcY).

Figure 9.9. "Chest Pain" by Pexels is licensed under Public Domain (https://pixabay.com/en/adult-affection-chest-chest-pain-1846050/).

Figure 9.10. "Types of Stroke" by National Heart, Lung, and Blood Institute is licensed under Public Domain (https://www.nhlbi.nih.gov/health/health-topics/topics/stroke/types).

Figure 9.12. "Main Complications of Persistent High Blood Pressure" by FotoshopTofs is licensed under Public Domain (https://pixabay.com/en/anatomy-of-the-human-body-big-picture-1279987/).

Figure 9.13. "Blood Pressure Monitor" by geraldoswald62 is licensed under Public Domain (https://pixabay.com/en/blood-pressure-monitor-bless-you-1749577/).

Figure 9.14. "Blood Pressure Ranges" by American Heart Association is licensed under Public Domain.

Figure 9.17. "Top 10 Cancer Sites" by CDC is licensed under Public Domain (https://nccd.cdc.gov/uscs/toptencancers.aspx).

Figure 9.18. "Cancer development" by Webdicine is licensed under CC BY 2.0 (http://www.webdicine.com/3-stages-of-cancer-development.html).

Figure 9.19. "Sunbathing Newlyweds" by Mike Schinkel is licensed under CC BY 2.0 (https://www.flickr.com/photos/mikeschinkel/288584045/).

Figure 9.20. "Estimated Cancer Deaths in the US in 2016" by American Cancer Society is licensed under Public Domain (https://www.cancer.org/research/cancer-facts-statistics/all-cancer-facts-figures/cancer-facts-figures-2016.html).

Figure 9.21. "CAUTION Cancer Warning Signs" by National Cancer Institute is licensed under Public Domain (https://commons.wikimedia.org/wiki/File:Cancer_warning_signs.jpg).

Figure 9.23. "Insulin Screening Kit" by Alisha Vargas is licensed under CC BY 2.0 (https://www.flickr.com/photos/alishav/3534216143/).

Figure 9.24. "Family" by funkblast is licensed under CC BY 2.0 (https://www.flickr.com/photos/funkblast/103936734/).

Figure 9.25. "Risks from Smoking" by CDC is licensed under Public Domain (https://commons.wikimedia.org/wiki/File:Risks_form_smoking-smoking_can_damage_every_part_of_the_body.png).

Figure 9.26. "Runway Couple" by United States Army is licensed under CC BY 2.0 (https://www.flickr.com/photos/armymedicine/13452149373/).

Figure 9.27. "IMG_8510" by Oakridge Camp & Retreat Center is licensed under CC BY 2.0 (https://www.flickr.com/photos/oakridgecamp/13468501524/).

Figure 9.28. "Bowl of Granola" by Marco Verch is licensed under CC BY 2.0 (https://www.flickr.com/photos/30478819@N08/35094200403/).

Figure 9.29. "Depressed" by Sander van der Wel is licensed under CC BY-SA 2.0 (https://www.flickr.com/photos/jar0d/4649749639/).

Figure 9.30. "Apple and Pear" by Yves Geissbühler is licensed under Public Domain (https://commons.wikimedia.org/wiki/File:Apple_and_pear.jpg).

Figure 9.31. "Angry Woman" by LARA SCHNEIDER is licensed under CC BY 2.0 (https://commons.wikimedia.org/wiki/File:Angry_woman.jpg).

Figure 9.33. "A Multigenerational Slice of Life in Mumbai" by Dion Hinchcliffe is licensed under CC BY-SA 2.0 (https://www.flickr.com/photos/dionhinchcliffe/22090447908/).

Figure 9.34. "Cancer Prevention" by U.S. Air Force is licensed under Public Domain (https://media.defense.gov/2016/Jan/22/2001500554/-1/-1/0/AFG-160122-001.jpg).

Figure 9.35. "Vegetable Market" by Euro slice is licensed under CC BY 2.0 (https://www.flickr.com/photos/104021946@N05/23570543273/).

Chapter 10

Figure 10.0. "Handwashing" by U.S. Air Force photo/Staff Sgt. Corey Hook is licensed under Public Domain (https://media.defense.gov/2013/Feb/14/2000075261/-1/-1/0/121213-F-ZU607-001.JPG).

Figure 10.4. "Chain of Infection" by CDC is licensed under Public Domain (https://www.cdc.gov/ophss/csels/dsepd/ss1978/lesson1/section10.html).

Figure 10.5. "Epidemiologic Triad" by CDC is licensed under Public Domain (https://www.cdc.gov/ophss/csels/dsepd/ss1978/lesson1/section8.html).

Figure 10.8. "Clean Hands" by Arlington County is licensed under CC BY-SA 2.0 (https://www.flickr.com/photos/arlingtonva/4314530838).

Figure 10.9. "STI Estimates" by CDC is licensed under Public Domain (http://www.cdc.gov/std/stats/sti-estimates-fact-sheet-feb-2013.pdf).

Figure 10.1. "Chlamydia by Age" and "Gonorrhea by Age" by Delphi234 are licensed under Public Domain (https://commons.wikimedia.org/wiki/File:Chlamydia_in_the_US_by_age_and_sex.svg and https://commons.wikimedia.org/wiki/File:Gonorrhea_in_the_US_by_age_and_sex.svg).

Figure 10.11. "Healthy People 2020 and STIs" by U.S. Department of Health and Human Services is licensed under Public Domain (https://www.healthypeople.gov/2020/topics-objectives/topic/sexually-transmitted-diseases/national-snapshot).

Figure 10.12. "Throat Warts" and "Spinaliom" by GalliasM and Klaus M Peter are licensed under CC BY-SA 4.0 International (https://commons.wikimedia.org/wiki/File:Throat_Warts_-_HPV.jpg and https://commons.wikimedia.org/wiki/File:Spinaliom3.jpg).

Figure 10.13. "Female Sexual Anatomy" and "Male Sexual Anatomy" by CDC and Tsaitgaist are licensed under CC BY-SA 3.0 (https://commons.wikimedia.org/wiki/File:Scheme_female_reproductive_system-en.svg and https://commons.wikimedia.org/wiki/File:Male_anatomy_en.svg).

Figure 10.14. "Human Papillomavirus Testing" by BioMed Central is used by permission (https://bmcmedicine.biomedcentral.com/articles/10.1186/1741-7015-7-69).

Figure 10.15. "HPV Vaccine" by Benjamin W. Stratton is licensed under Public Domain (https://health.mil/News/Articles/2016/10/06/What-the-experts-want-you-to-know-about-the-HPV-vaccine).

Figure 10.16. "Chlamydia Screening Recommendations" by CDC is licensed under Public Domain (https://www.cdc.gov/std/tg2015/screening-recommendations.htm).

Figure 10.17. "Veteran Receiving Primary Care" by Veterans' Health is licensed under Public Domain (https://www.flickr.com/photos/veteranshealth/25347383620/).

Figure 10.18. "24 Weeks" by Sara Neff is licensed under CC BY 2.0 (https://www.flickr.com/photos/97725616@N06/14241752215/).

Figure 10.20. "Herpes Labialis" by Jojo is licensed under Public Domain (https://commons.wikimedia.org/wiki/File:Herpes_labialis_-_opryszczka_wargowa.jpg).

Figure 10.22. "Pregnant" by Jerry Lai is licensed under CC BY-SA 2.0 (https://www.flickr.com/photos/jerrylai0208/14281758292/).

Figure 10.23. "New HIV Diagnoses by Transmission Category" by CDC is licensed under Public Domain (https://www.cdc.gov/hiv/images/basics/statistics/statistics-basics-new-infections-by-category.png).

Figure 10.24. "AIDSVu Map of 2010 Rate of Adults and Adolescents Living with an HIV Diagnoses" by AIdsVU is licensed under CC BY-SA 4.0 (https://commons.wikimedia.org/wiki/File:AIDSVu_Map_of_2010_Rate_of_Adults_and_Adolescents_Living_With_an_HIV_Diagnoses.png).

Figure 10.25. "HIV-Timecourse" by Sigve is licensed under Public Domain (https://commons.wikimedia.org/wiki/File:Hiv-timecourse_copy.svg).

Figure 10.26. "HIV Screening Recommendations" by CDC is licensed under Public Domain (https://www.cdc.gov/std/tg2015/screening-recommendations.htm).

Figure 10.27. "Analisi Urina" by Federico Candoni is licensed under CC BY-SA 4.0 (https://commons.wikimedia.org/wiki/File:20150120_Analisi_Urina_1.jpg).

Figure 10.28. "HIV Testing" by Marcello Casal is licensed under CC BY 3.0 BR (https://commons.wikimedia.org/wiki/File:Oraquick.jpg).

Figure 10.29. "Diseased Livers" by Wellcome is licensed under CC BY 4.0 International (https://commons.wikimedia.org/wiki/File:Diseased_livers;_hepatitis,_syphilis,_angioma,_pylephlebitis_Wellcome_V0010282EL.jpg).

Figure 10.31. "Empty Rolled Condom" by Empcon54 is licensed under CC BY-SA 4.0 International (https://commons.wikimedia.org/wiki/File:Empty_rolled_condom.JPG).

Chapter 11

Figure 11.0. "Magic Pills" by Johnathan Silverberg is licensed under CC BY 2.0 (https://www.flickr.com/photos/jonathansilverberg/9194590737/).

Figure 11.1. "Past-Month Use of Selected Illicit Drugs" by National Institutes of Health is licensed under Public Domain (https://www.drugabuse.gov/publications/drugfacts/nationwide-trends).

Figure 11.2. "Health Care Costs of Substance Abuse" by National Institutes of Health is licensed under Public Domain (https://www.drugabuse.gov/publications/drugfacts/nationwide-trends).

Figure 11.3. "The Limbic System" by Bruce Blaus is licensed under CC BY 3.0 (https://commons.wikimedia.org/wiki/File:Blausen_0614_LimbicSystem.png).

Figure 11.4. "Drinking Status in the US" by CDC is licensed under Public Domain (https://www.cdc.gov/nchs/data/series/sr_10/sr10_260.pdf).

Figure 11.5. "Blood Alcohol Concentration " by CDC is licensed under Public Domain (https://www.cdc.gov/motorvehiclesafety/impaired_driving/impaired-drv_factsheet.html).

Figure 11.8. "Equivalent Servings of Different Drink Types" by National Institutes of Health is licensed under Public Domain (https://www.rethinkingdrinking.niaaa.nih.gov/How-much-is-too-much/What-counts-as-a-drink/How-Many-Drinks-Are-In-Common-Containers.aspx).

Figure 11.9. "Alcohol Poisoning PSA" by Stop Alcohol Deaths, Inc. is licensed under CC BY 2.0 (https://www.flickr.com/photos/stopalcoholdeaths/5525252988/).

Figure 11.10. "Library" by andrew_t8 is licensed under Public Domain (https://pixabay.com/en/library-la-trobe-study-students-1400312/).

Figure 11.11. "Drunk Man" by Mario Antonio Pena Zapatería is licensed under CC BY-SA 2.0 (https://commons.wikimedia.org/wiki/File:Drunk_man.jpg).

Figure 11.12. "Low-Risk Drinking Limits" by National Institutes of Health is licensed under Public Domain (https://www.rethinkingdrinking.niaaa.nih.gov/How-much-is-too-much/Is-Your-Drinking-Pattern-Risky/Whats-Low-Risk-Drinking.aspx).

Figure 11.13. "Women" by Susanne Nilsson is licensed under CC BY-SA 2.0 (https://www.flickr.com/photos/infomastern/34262951724/).

Figure 11.14. "31 Weeks Pregnant" by Jerry Lai is licensed under CC BY-SA 2.0 (https://www.flickr.com/photos/jerrylai0208/15514557255/).

Figure 11.15. "Cigarettes" by Klimkin is licensed under Public Domain (https://pixabay.com/en/cigarette-smoking-ash-habit-1642232/).

Figure 11.16. "E-Cigarette Starter Kit" by Ecig Click is licensed under CC BY-SA 2.0 (https://www.flickr.com/photos/ecigclick/16581902047/).

Figure 11.17. "How Tobacco Affects Your Body" by Office on Women's Health is licensed under Public Domain (https://www.girlshealth.gov/substance/smoking/index.html).

Figure 11.18. "What's Wrong with This Picture?" by alex yosifov is licensed under CC BY-SA 2.0 (https://www.flickr.com/photos/sashomasho/718292525/).

Figure 11.19. "Only the Last Time" by Morgan is licensed under CC BY 2.0 (https://www.flickr.com/photos/meddygarnet/4170136164/).

Figure 11.21. "Top of Mount Hood" by Tony Fischer is licensed under CC BY 2.0 (https://www.flickr.com/photos/tonythemisfit/3033524024/).

Figure 11.22. "No Smoking Sign" by smartSign is licensed under CC BY 2.0 (https://www.flickr.com/smartsignbrooklyn/10213459946/).

Figure 11.23. "Bodily Effects of Cannabis" by Mikael Häggström is licensed under Public Domain (https://commons.wikimedia.org/wiki/File:Bodily_effects_of_cannabis.png).

Figure 11.24. "DSC_0124" by USFS Region 5 is licensed under CC BY 2.0 (https://www.flickr.com/photos/usfsregion5/4888965362/).

Figure 11.25. "Marijuana Use After Medical Legalization" by PBS Newshour is used by permission (http://d3i6fh83elv35t.cloudfront.net/newshour/wp-content/uploads/2014/10/marijuana-use-afer-medical-legalization-NBER-1024x737.png).

Figure 11.26. "Drug Take-Back Day" by Barksdale Airforce Base is licensed under Public Domain (http://www.barksdale.af.mil/News/Article/635147/drug-take-back-day/).

Figure 11.27. "P1130349C" by Thirten of Clubs is licensed under CC BY-SA 2.0 (https://www.flickr.com/photos/thirteenofclubs/5520512981/).

Figure 11.28. "Overdose Deaths Involving Opioids" by CDC/NCHS is licensed under Public Domain (https://www.cdc.gov/drugoverdose/images/data/od_deaths_bytype.gif).

Figure 11.30. "Coffee Feathering" by Vivian Evans is licensed under CC BY-SA 2.0 (https://www.flickr.com/photos/vivevans/4106191761/).

Chapter 12

Figure 12.0. "US Navy" by Alesia Goosic is licensed under Public Domain (https://commons.wikimedia.org/wiki/File:US_Navy_110718-F-ET173-083_Cmdr._Mark_Riddle,_an_environmental_health_staff_member_from_the_Department_of_Sonsonate,_El_Salvador_Ministry_of_Health.jpg).

Figure 12.1. "Healthy People 2020 Environmental Health" by Offices of Disease Prevention and Health Promotion is licensed under Public Domain (https://www.healthypeople.gov/).

Figure 12.2. "Huge Crowds Gather in the Bogside" by Sinn Fein is licensed under CC BY 2.0 (https://www.flickr.com/photos/sinnfeinireland/33511256992/).

Figure 12.3. "Fertility Rate by Country" by CIA is licensed under Public Domain (https://www.cia.gov/library/publications/the-world-factbook/fields/2127.html).

Figure 12.4. "Fertility Rate by Region" by United Nations is licensed under Public Domain (http://www.un.org/en/development/desa/population/publications/pdf/fertility/world-fertility-patterns-2015.pdf).

Figure 12.5. "Fungi of Saskatchewan" by Sasata is licensed under CC BY-SA 3.0 (https://commons.wikimedia.org/wiki/File:Fungi_of_Saskatchewan.JPG).

Figure 12.6. "Anglers Using Electro Shock Fishing Techniques" by John Organ is licensed under Public Domain (https://commons.wikimedia.org/wiki/File:Anglers_using_electro_shock_fishing_techniques.jpg).

Figure 12.7. "World Energy Consumption by Fuel Source" by US Energy Information Administration is licensed under Public Domain (https://www.eia.gov/outlooks/ieo/pdf/0484(2016).pdf).

Figure 12.8. "Air Quality Index" by Environmental Protection Agency is licensed under Public Domain (https://airnow.gov/index.cfm?action=aqibasics.aqi).

Figure 12.9. "EPA Map of Radiation Zones " by Environmental Protection Agency is licensed under Public Domain (https://commons.wikimedia.org/wiki/File:EPA_Map_of_Radon_Zones.png).

Figure 12.1. "Origins of Acid Rain" by Environmental Protection Agency is licensed under Public Domain (https://commons.wikimedia.org/wiki/File:Origins_of_acid_rain.svg).

Figure 12.11. "Ozone Altitude UV graph" by NASA is licensed under Public Domain (https://commons.wikimedia.org/wiki/File:Ozone_altitude_UV_graph.svg).

Figure 12.12. "Total US Greenhouse Gas Emissions" by Environmental Protection Agency is licensed under Public Domain (https://www.epa.gov/ghgemissions/sources-greenhouse-gas-emissions).

Figure 12.13. "Ozone Hole 2015" by NASA is licensed under Public Domain (https://earthobservatory.nasa.gov/IOTD/view.php?id=86869).

Figure 12.14. "Total Emissions 2015 by Sector" by CDC is licensed under Public Domain.

Figure 12.15. "Global Carbon Dioxide Emissions by Region, 1990-2012" by Environmental Protection Agency is licensed under Public Domain (www.epa.gov/climate-indicators).

Figure 12.16. "US GHG Emissions Flow Chart" by World Resources Institute is licensed under Public Domain (http://www.wri.org/resources/charts-graphs/us-greenhouse-gas-emissions-flow-chart).

Figure 12.17. "Impact of Climate Change on Human Health" by CDC is licensed under Public Domain (https://www.cdc.gov/climateandhealth/effects/default.htm).

Figure 12.18. "Climate Change Threatens Your Health" by World Health Organization is licensed under Public Domain (http://www.who.int/globalchange/climate/infographics/en/).

Figure 12.20. "Stacken" by Janwikifoto is licensed under CC BY-SA 3.0 (https://commons.wikimedia.org/wiki/File:Stacken_0c149d_1755.jpg).

Figure 12.22. "Water Quality Testing Activity" by Shenandoah National Park is licensed under Public Domain (https://www.flickr.com/photos/snpphotos/36589911655/).

Figure 12.23. "Aquifers and Wells" by USGS is licensed under Public Domain (https://water.usgs.gov/edu/earthgwaquifer.html).

Figure 12.24. "An Oil Slick from the Oil Spill" by Martarano Steve is licensed under Public Domain (https://commons.wikimedia.org/wiki/File:An_oil_slick_from_the_oil_spill.jpg).

Figure 12.25. "Groundwater Pollution" by Foundation of Water Research is licensed under Public Domain (http://www.euwfd.com/assets/images/Groundwater-pollution02.jpg).

Figure 12.26. "Digging for Drinking Water in a Dry Riverbed" by DFID - UK Department for International Development is licensed under CC BY 2.0 (https://commons.wikimedia.org/wiki/File:Digging_for_drinking_water_in_a_dry_riverbed_(6220146368).jpg).

Figure 12.27. "Water Fountain 3" by joshme17 is licensed under CC BY 2.0 (https://www.flickr.com/photos/joshme17/1751994184/).

Figure 12.28. "Pollution Prevention Tips for Water Conservation" by Environmental Protection Agency is licensed under Public Domain (https://www.epa.gov/p2/pollution-prevention-tips-water-conservation).

Figure 12.29. "Landfill Face" by Ashley Felton is licensed under Public Domain (https://commons.wikimedia.org/wiki/File:Landfill_face.JPG).

Figure 12.30. "Total Municipal Solid Waste Generation 2014" by Environmental Protection Agency is licensed under Public Domain (https://www.epa.gov/sites/production/files/2016-11/panelizersidemswimage2014_0.jpg).

Figure 12.31. "Electronic Waste Tips" by Environmental Protection Agency is licensed under Public Domain (https://www.epa.gov/smm-electronics/basic-information-about-electronics-stewardship#03).

Figure 12.32. "Hazardous Waste Identification Process Flowchart" by Environmental Protection Agency is licensed under Public Domain (https://www.epa.gov/hw/learn-basics-hazardous-waste).

Figure 12.33. "Examples of Hazardous Waste" by Environmental Protection Agency is licensed under Public Domain.

Figure 12.33. "E-Waste" by Curtis Palmer is licensed under CC BY 2.0 (https://www.flickr.com/photos/techbirmingham/345897594/).

Figure 12.34. "Environmental Protection Hierarchy" by Environmental Protection Agency is licensed under Public Domain (https://www.epa.gov/p2).

Figure 12.35. "Projected Global Primary Electricity Consumption by Source" by Enescot is licensed under Public Domain (https://commons.wikimedia.org/wiki/File:Projected_global_primary_electricity_consumption_by_source,_over_the_21st_century,_for_a_climate_change_mitigation_scenario.png).

Figure 12.36. "Recycling Rates of Selected Products" by Environmental Protection Agency is licensed under Public Domain (https://www.epa.gov/sites/production/files/2015-09/documents/2012_msw_fs.pdf).

Figure 12.37. "Composting in the Escuela Barreales" by Diego Grez is licensed under Public Domain (https://commons.wikimedia.org/wiki/File:Composting_in_the_Escuela_Barreales.jpg).

Figure 12.38. "Eurodif Nuclear Power Plant, Tricastin, France" by IAEA is licensed under CC BY-SA 2.0 (https://www.flickr.com/photos/iaea_imagebank/8168889853/).

Figure 12.39. "Sunscreen" by Maggiejumps is licensed under CC BY 2.0 (https://www.flickr.com/photos/38494596@N00/443642299/sizes/l).

Figure 12.40. "Asphalt" by PxHere is licensed under Public Domain (https://pxhere.com/en/photo/1012613).

Figure 12.42. "Avondale Shipyard Worker" by John Messina is licensed under Public Domain (https://commons.wikimedia.org/wiki/File:AVONDALE_SHIPYARD_WORKER_WEARS_SPECIAL_EAR_MUFFS_FOR_PROTECTION_FROM_THE_HEAVY_LEVEL_OF_INDUSTRIAL_NOISE_POLLUTION_-_NARA_-_546041.jpg).

CPSIA information can be obtained
at www.ICGtesting.com
Printed in the USA
LVOW05s2215171117
556666LV00003B/6/P

9 781943 536344